Integrative Psychiatry

Weil Integrative Medicine Library

Published and Forthcoming Volumes

SERIES EDITOR

ANDREW T. WEIL, MD

Donald I. Abrams and Andrew Weil: *Integrative Oncology*
Timothy Culbert and Karen Olness: *Integrative Pediatrics*
Gerard Mullin: *Integrative Gastroenterology*
Victoria Maizes and Tieraona Low Dog: *Integrative Women's Health*
Randy Horwitz and Daniel Muller: *Integrative Rheumatology, Allergy, and Immunology*
Daniel A. Monti and Bernard D. Beitman: *Integrative Psychiatry*
Stephen DeVries and James Dalen: *Integrative Cardiology*

Integrative Psychiatry

EDITED BY

Daniel A. Monti, MD
Associate Professor of Psychiatry and Emergency Medicine
Director, Jefferson-Myrna Brind Center of Integrative Medicine
Jefferson Medical College of Thomas Jefferson University
Philadelphia, PA

Bernard D. Beitman, MD
Professor and Chair
Department of Psychiatry
University of Missouri School of Medicine

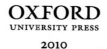

OXFORD
UNIVERSITY PRESS
2010

Published by Oxford University Press, Inc.
198 Madison Avenue, New York, New York 10016
www.oup.com

Library of Congress Cataloging-in-Publication Data
Integrative psychiatry / [edited by] Bernard Beitman, Daniel A. Monti.
p. ; cm.
Includes bibliographical references.
ISBN 978-0-19-538837-4
1. Mental illness—Alternative treatment.   2. Eclectic psychotherapy.   I. Beitman,
Bernard D.   II. Monti, Daniel A.
[DNLM: 1. Mental Disorders—therapy.   2. Complementary Therapies—
methods.   3. Psychotherapy—methods. WM 400 I605 2009]
RC480.5.I557 2009
616.89'14—dc22   2008042635

1 3 5 7 9 8 6 4 2
Printed in the United States of America
on acid-free paper

We dedicate this book to current psychiatrists willing to challenge current paradigms and to future psychiatrists for whom integrative psychiatry will become standard practice.

FOREWORD

ANDREW WEIL, MD

Series Editor

I ntegrative medicine and alternative medicine are not synonymous. Alternative medicine comprises all those therapies not taught in conventional (allopathic) medical schools, based on ideas of variable soundness, ranging from some that are sensible and worth including in mainstream medicine to others that are foolish and a few that are dangerous. The term "alternative medicine" has recently been incorporated into a broader term, "complementary and alternative medicine" or "CAM", used by the U.S. federal government and other institutions; the National Institutes of Health now has a national CAM center (NCCAM).

Neither "alternative" nor "complementary" captures the essence of integrative medicine. The former suggests replacement of conventional therapies by others; the latter adjunctive therapies, added as afterthoughts.

Integrative medicine does include ideas and approaches currently beyond the scope of conventional medicine as it is practiced today, but it neither rejects conventional therapies nor accepts alternative ones uncritically. Most importantly, it emphasizes principles that may or may not be associated with CAM, that is,

- *The natural healing power of the organism.* Integrative medicine assumes that the body has an innate capacity for healing, self-repair, regeneration, and adaptation to injury or loss. The primary goal of treatment should be to support, facilitate, and augment that innate capacity.
- *Whole person medicine.* Integrative medicine views patients as more than physical bodies. They are also mental/emotional beings, spiritual

entities, and members of particular communities and societies. These other dimensions of human life are relevant to health and to the accurate diagnosis and effective treatment of disease.

- *The importance of lifestyle.* Health and disease result from interactions between genes and all aspects of lifestyle, including diet, physical activity, rest and sleep, stress, the quality of relationships, work, and so forth. Lifestyle choices may influence disease risks more than genes and must be a focus of the medical history. Lifestyle medicine, which is one component of integrative medicine, gives physicians information and tools to enable them to prevent and treat disease more effectively.
- *The critical role of the doctor–patient relationship.* Throughout history, people have accorded the doctor–patient relationship special, even sacred, status. When a medically trained person sits with a patient and listens with full attention to his or her story, that alone can initiate healing before any treatment is offered. A great tragedy of contemporary medicine, especially in the United States, is that for-profit, corporate systems have virtually destroyed this core aspect of practice. If practitioners have only a few minutes with each patient—the time limit set by the managed care systems they work for—it is very unlikely they will be able to form the kind of therapeutic relationships that foster health and healing.

Furthermore, this special form of human interaction has been the source of greatest emotional reward for the physician, and its disappearance in our time is a main reason for rising practitioner discontent. Integrative medicine insists on the paramount importance of the therapeutic relationship and demands that health care systems support and honor it (e.g., by reimbursing physicians for time spent with patients rather than number of patients seen).

In essence, integrative medicine is conservative. It seeks to restore core values of the profession that have eroded in recent times. It honors such ancient precepts as Hippocrates' injunctions on physicians to "first do no harm" and "to value the healing power of nature." It is conservative in practice, favoring less invasive and drastic treatments over more invasive and drastic ones whenever possible, and it is fiscally conservative in relying less on expensive technology and more on simpler methods, *as appropriate to the circumstances of illness.*

I believe that applying the principles of integrative medicine to psychiatry can revitalize a field of medicine that is in trouble. It is ironic that psychiatry—the word comes from Greek roots meaning "soul doctoring"—has bought into the paradigm of scientific materialism more than almost any other specialty, a philosophical bias summed up in the motto that, "There can be no twisted thought without a twisted molecule." Working from that premise, conventional psychiatric treatment is now mostly synonymous with prescribing drugs.

If the currently popular psychiatric medications performed as their manufacturers claim in their advertising, mental health should be better than ever. We should be able to control anxiety and depression easily, manage psychosis, and even slow the progression of age-related dementia. Sadly, the clinical effectiveness of drug treatments for these common conditions is far from ideal. That is not to say that drugs are unnecessary; in fact, they often play an important role in the management of several major mental disorders. However, they should be viewed as a *component* of care when needed, and their usefulness should be re-evaluated regularly while other aspects of the patient are being addressed, such as diet, stress, activity level, relationships, and other factors. The issue is really one of judicious prescribing in the context of a comprehensive treatment approach versus overprescribing in the context of drugs as the solution to all of life's angst. I strongly question the wisdom of having so many people, children especially, on long-term treatment with antidepressants, antianxiety agents, stimulants, and neuroleptics. There is legitimate concern that these drugs may be much less benign than we once thought, which underscores the need to consider other options.

In the paradigm of integrative medicine, mind/body interactions are regarded as central to the healing process, with cause and effect not restricted to the unidirectional influence of physical reality on mental/emotional states. Twisted molecules may produce twisted thoughts, but disordered moods and emotions may also distort brain biochemistry. A great deal of research over the past 40 years demonstrates the power of emotions, moods, thoughts, and imagination to alter levels and functions of neurotransmitters, modify brain activity, even influence gene expression. Recent advances in brain imaging technology strongly support this new understanding by correlating states of consciousness with activity of specific brain areas.

Integrative psychiatrists have many more options to offer patients than their conventional counterparts. As alternatives to drugs, they can recommend dietary changes, dietary supplements, botanical remedies, exercise, relaxation training, a variety of mind/body therapies, and new forms of psychotherapy that can teach patients to be optimistic and to identify and restructure habitual patterns of thought that lead to negative moods and behaviors. Consumer demand for practitioners of this sort is high, but few are available.

Ever since I founded the Program in Integrative Medicine (now the Arizona Center for Integrative Medicine [AzCIM]) in 1994, I have worked to make training in integrative medicine available to psychiatrists and to stimulate research in integrative approaches to mental and emotional disorders. Several psychiatrists have completed our intensive integrative medicine fellowships (see www.integrativemedicine.arizona.edu). My colleagues and I at AzCIM are now developing a comprehensive curriculum in integrative medicine (in distributed learning format) that we intend to become a required, accredited part of all residency programs. We are also working to develop a more focused training program specifically for mental health professionals.

This series of volumes from Oxford University Press is intended to help practitioners in various medical specialties learn about strategies for managing common conditions not currently included in the medical school curriculum or in residency training. The editors of this volume, Drs. Daniel Monti and Bernard Beitman, have considerable expertise in both Psychiatry and Integrative Medicine, and they have contributed significantly to the literature in each. In this book they have done an excellent job of compiling a great deal of information to help practitioners understand and use integrative medical philosophy and methods to promote mental health and alleviate mental illness. I consider it a significant contribution to the emerging field of integrative psychiatry.

ACKNOWLEDGMENTS

W e would like to express our gratitude to Andrew Weil, MD, for the opportunity to contribute to this important Integrative Medicine textbook series. Andy has been a teacher and a friend, and we are humbled to have a small role in his mission to expand the horizons of health care and health preservation.

CONTENTS

IV   Mind

CONTRIBUTORS

John M. Balaicuis, MD, MS Ed
Fellow, Light Research Lab
Thomas Jefferson University
Philadelphia, PA

Bernard D. Beitman, MD
Professor
Department of Psychiatry
University of Missouri School of
    Medicine
Columbia, MO

George Brainard, PhD
Professor of Neurology
Professor of Biochemistry and
    Molecular Pharmacology
Thomas Jefferson University
Philadelphia, PA

James Caunt, BsE, MBA
Technical Director
Advanced Neurotherapy, PC
Wellesley, Massachusetts

Elif Celebi, PhD
Postdoctoral Fellow
Department of Psychiatry
University of Rochester Medical Center
Rochester, NY

Stephanie L. Coleman
Department of Educational, School,
    and Counseling Psychology
University of Missouri
Columbia, MO

Patricia A. Coughlin, PhD
Clinical Psychologist
Department of Psychiatry and Human
    Behavior
Thomas Jefferson University
Philadelphia, PA

Geraldine F. DePaula, MD
President, Aroma Medica
    Erdenheim, PA 19038
    www.AromaMedica.com

Karl Doghramji, MD
Professor of Psychiatry and Human
    Behavior
Director, Jefferson Sleep Disorders
    Center
Thomas Jefferson University
Philadelphia, PA

Joel S. Edman, DSc, FACN, CNS
Director of Integrative Nutrition
Jefferson-Myrna Brind Center of
    Integrative Medicine
Thomas Jefferson University
    Hospital
Philadelphia, PA

Howard L. Field, MD
Department of Psychiatry
Jefferson Medical College

Thomas Jefferson University
Philadelphia, PA

Bettina Herbert, MD
Instructor of Rehabilitation Medicine
  and Emergency Medicine
Jefferson-Myrna Brind Center of
  Integrative Medicine
Thomas Jefferson University Hospital
Philadelphia, PA

**Susan Kaye-Huntington, PsyD
ATR-BC**
Adjunct Associate Professor
University of Arts
Philadelphia, PA

**Doreen F. Lafferty, MAc, OTR/L,
NCTMB**
Licensed Occupational Therapist and
  Acupuncturist
Jefferson-Myrna Brind Center of
  Integrative Medicine
Thomas Jefferson University
  and Hospital
Philadelphia, PA

Bruce Y. Lee, MD
Departments of Medicine and
  Biomedical Informatics
University of Pittsburgh

Rajnish Mago, MD
Director, Mood Disorders
  Program
Thomas Jefferson University
Philadelphia, PA

Rajeev Mahajan, MBBS
Mood Disorders Program
Thomas Jefferson University Hospital
Philadelphia, PA

Denise E. Malkowicz, MD
Neurologist
Clinical Neurophysiologist and
  Epileptologist
Director of Clinical Research and
  Medical Education
Consultant in Neurology, Clinical
  Neurophysiology, Epileptology,
  Neurorehabilitation and
  Neurotherapy
The Institutes for the Achievement of
  Human Potential
Wyndmoor, PA
Medical Director
The Center for the Advancement
  of Neurorehabilitation and
  Neurotherapy
Bryn Mawr, PA

Donald McCown, MSW
Jefferson-Myrna Brind Center of
  Integrative Medicine
Thomas Jefferson University Hospital
Philadelphia, PA

Bernardo A. Merizalde, MD
Clinical Assistant Professor
  of Psychiatry and Emergency
  Medicine
Jefferson-Myrna Brind Center of
  Integrative Medicine
Thomas Jefferson University Hospital
Philadelphia, PA

Daniel A. Monti, MD
Associate Professor of Psychiatry
  and Emergency Medicine Director
Jefferson-Myrna Brind Center of
  Integrative Medicine
Thomas Jefferson University
  Hospital
Philadelphia, PA

Andrew B. Newberg, MD
Department of Radiology and
   Psychiatry
University of Pennsylvania Health
   System
Philadelphia, PA

**Caroline C. Peterson, MA,
ATR-BC, LPC**
Research Associate
Jefferson-Myrna Brind Center of
   Integrative Medicine
Thomas Jefferson University
   Hospital
Philadelphia, PA

Henry Pollard, PhD
Associate Professor
Department of Chiropractic
   Faculty of Science
Macquarie University
Sydney, Australia

Lynette Menefee Pujol, PhD
Assistant Professor of Psychiatry
   and Anesthesiology
Thomas Jefferson University
Philadelphia, PA

Diane Reibel, PhD
Research Associate Professor
Departments of Emergency Medicine
   and Physiology

Director of Professional Education
   and Development, Stress Reduction
   Program
Jefferson-Myrna Brind Center of
   Integrative Medicine
Thomas Jefferson University Hospital
Philadelphia, PA

Jolene Ross, PhD
Licensed Psychologist
Director and President
Advanced Neurotherapy, PC
Wellesley, MA

Linda Shrier, PhD
Assistant Professor of Psychiatry
Thomas Jefferson University
Philadelphia, PA

Marie Stoner, MEd, BCIAC
Jefferson-Myrna Brind Center of
   Integrative Medicine
Thomas Jefferson University Hospital
Philadelphia, PA

Jingduan Yang, MD Lic Ac
Psychiatry and Traditional Chinese
   Medicine
Jefferson-Myrna Brind Center of
   Integrative Medicine
Thomas Jefferson University and
   Hospital
Philadelphia, PA

PART I

Harnessing Daily Life

1

Dietary Guidelines for Psychiatric Patients

JOEL S. EDMAN

KEY CONCEPTS

- Diet can have an important role in the management of psychiatric disorders.
- One mechanism through which diet is helpful is that diet provides a range of vitamins and minerals that serve as cofactors for the synthesis of specific neurotransmitters.
- Dietary guidelines can also benefit specific psychiatric disorders and common comorbid symptoms through their influence on hypoglycemia/abnormal glucose tolerance, food intolerance, and possibly other effects.
- There is significant research to support the relationship between specific dietary factors and psychiatric disorders; however, many guidelines and recommendations come from years of clinical experience by many integrative medicine practitioners.
- Because there is a range of dietary and/or nutritional factors that may have an influence, and many individual factors that may provide a susceptibility to psychiatric symptoms or disorders, a comprehensive evaluation is needed in order to provide a unique and effective dietary and nutritional program.
- Since dietary changes and programs can be challenging, careful consideration should be given to what patients are willing and able to do.
- Significant future research is required to clarify the influence of dietary factors in specific psychiatric disorders, and to determine the most effective dietary and nutritional approaches to recommend.

Introduction

Healthy dietary guidelines are an important foundation approach to health and healing in integrative medicine, and are necessary to address in order to lessen patient symptoms and promote optimal wellness in people with psychiatric disorders. While dietary choices and practices can be closely linked to physical, emotional, and spiritual well-being, it can be challenging to evaluate how beneficial dietary modifications will be for psychiatric patients and to determine the best approach to take that will not add significantly to patient stresses. Even considering these issues, however, diet can have an important impact on well-being and produce specific psychiatric benefits. This is especially true when considering how unhealthy most people's diets are.

Dietary influences in nervous system function can occur in several ways. One primary characteristic of diet is that it provides essential vitamins and minerals that serve as cofactors for the synthesis of specific neurotransmitters. For example, the B complex vitamins (thiamine, riboflavin, pyridoxine, cobalamin, and folate) are cofactors for the synthesis of norepinephrine, dopamine, serotonin, GABA, and acetylcholine (Bell et al., 1992; Bradford, 1986). Dietary fatty acids also contribute to nerve cell membrane composition, fluidity, and resulting function. In addition, dietary antioxidants (e.g. vitamins C and E, selenium, and various phytonutrients) protect cell membranes from oxidative stress and aging, which could impair function over time. Also discussed are hypoglycemia/abnormal glucose tolerance, food intolerance, healthy fats or fatty acids, and other dietary factors.

How to approach patients with psychiatric symptoms and disorders to address dietary guidelines can be a challenge. However, integrative medical and nutritional approaches to these symptoms and disorders can provide an important framework from which dietary (and supplement) approaches can be presented. For example, an integrative medical practitioner could discuss the benefits of diet, supplements, exercise, relaxation techniques, and other modalities, and discuss approaches that the patient or client is open to consider. With nutrition, however, it should be remembered that supplements may have only limited benefit if the diet is very poor, so dietary improvements should be the basis for a good nutritional program.

A thorough clinical intake and physical examination is required, which should include questions about eating habits, foods preferred or avoided, typical meals and snacks, amounts eaten, and digestive function. Through this inquiry, suspected nutrient deficiencies or insufficiencies can be identified and later confirmed through specific diagnostic testing. These nutrient imbalances can usually be managed through a dietary and nutritional consultation, and then by providing appropriate information and recommendations. Consideration of nutritional supplementation will be addressed in Chapter 3.

While there is some research presented to support many of these dietary and nutritional factors, a significant amount of this information has been derived from many years of clinical experience, and when effectively applied can produce significant benefit. Because this field is evolving, references at the end will help readers understand where the current research is, but it will be important to monitor new information and research as it becomes available.

FACTORS LEADING TO NUTRITIONAL DEFICIENCY AND INSUFFICIENCY

There are many nutrition-related influences that can contribute to psychological distress and disorders. These factors will be different for each person, so the challenge is to carefully identify the unique combination of factors that are present, and to formulate an effective overall approach.

BIOCHEMICAL INDIVIDUALITY AND GENETIC POLYMORPHISMS

Roger Williams, an important early researcher of B complex vitamins (Williams & Saunders, 1934), proposed the role of nutrients to prevent diseases arising from above average demands for specific nutrients involved in cellular function due to genetic uniqueness; he called these conditions genetotrophic diseases. He popularized the term "biochemical individuality" and believed that major chronic degenerative diseases, such as heart disease, stroke, cancer, diabetes, and arthritis, as well as mental illness, behavior disorders, and alcoholism were "genetotrophic" diseases.

More recently, researchers led by Dr. Bruce Ames substantiated Dr. Williams's postulates of genetotrophic disease. They suggested that as many as one-third of mutations in a gene results in a lower level of enzyme activity, and that the administration of higher than dietary reference intake (DRI) levels of cofactors, in the form of specific vitamins and minerals, restores activity to near normal and even normal levels (Ames, Elson-Schwab, & Silver, 2002).

The most common gene mutations or polymorphisms are called "single nucleotide polymorphisms" or SNPs. SNPs will produce less functional translation of proteins and enzymes, and therefore can adversely affect biochemical and metabolic pathways.

The most common SNP may be found within the gene that codes for the methyl-tetra-hydrofolate reductase (MTHFR) enzyme. As a result of the

MTHFR SNP, extra dietary and supplemental folate (and other nutrients) may be required for neurotransmitter synthesis and methylation, and research suggests that this may be associated with depression, bipolar disorder, and schizophrenia (Gilbody, Lewis, & Lightfoot, 2007).

DIETARY AND METABOLIC INFLUENCES

From a dietary standpoint, we know that the standard American diet is not nutrient dense and can lead to nutritional deficiencies or insufficiencies for nutrients such as folate, magnesium, iron, and zinc, as well as inadequate phytonutrient intake (Biesalski, 2003; Vaquero, 2002). An example of this, which could easily occur, is that of an older patient who has never eaten very well, is taking a number of pharmaceuticals, and may have limited access to healthier food or lack the incentive to eat well. These factors could also be compounded by some degree of malabsorption from irritable bowel syndrome (IBS) or inflammatory bowel disease (IBD). In addition to inadequate nutrient intake and malabsorption, stresses or an acute incident, such as the loss of a family member or a motor vehicle accident, could contribute to physiological or metabolic stresses and/or loss of appetite, all of which could cause a vulnerability that could be the nexus of a psychiatric illness.

The increasing prevalence of overweight and obesity, and associated inflammation, can be a chronic metabolic stress that has nutritional consequences. The impact of this could be even broader, since research now suggests that aging is an inflammatory process (Napoli & Palinski, 2005). It would therefore be appropriate to address the effects of an anti-inflammatory diet and additional nutrient requirements when developing a dietary and nutritional program for either a new onset psychiatric disorder that occurs with aging, or other disorders in which inflammation may be present (e.g., IBD, CVD, RA, and others). Within the context of metabolic syndrome and inflammation, it is also important to note that the prevalence of depression in Type 2 Diabetes Mellitus (T2DM) is double the level of a normal population, and evidence suggests that the depression can worsen symptoms and/or glycemic control (Musselman, Betan, Larsen, & Phillips, 2003).

Finally, there is the question of environmental exposures to pollution, heavy metals, and chemicals from air, water, and food. These may contribute to nutritional imbalances by interfering with important nutrients, or by adding to nutritional requirements that may be involved with detoxification of these substances. This is an important challenge, however, since the current methods for assessing exposure or burden and treating it have not been effectively validated and remain controversial.

Because these factors can produce inadequate nutrient intake, poor digestion, decreased absorption, and utilization, as well as greater nutrient requirements, it is likely that there can be an "environmental" susceptibility to psychiatric disorders that could benefit from attention to healthy dietary guidelines and related interventions. The broad range of these influences suggests the importance of a comprehensive assessment process that will effectively identify the significant risks present for each patient.

Dietary Influences in Psychiatry

HYPOGLYCEMIA, ABNORMAL GLUCOSE TOLERANCE, AND INSULIN RESISTANCE

Hypoglycemia or abnormal glucose tolerance is an important consideration for neuropsychiatric disorders and symptoms. While this is controversial as a contributing factor to psychiatric disorders, abnormal glucose tolerance and insulin resistance for metabolic syndrome and associated characteristics are well accepted. It is possible, however, that these disorders represent two ends of a continuum, and both are representative of abnormal glucose tolerance. A primary factor is weight and its influence on insulin resistance, a central pathophysiological mechanism.

Although there has been little recent research, studies have suggested a significant relationship between affective disorders and abnormal glucose utilization and/or insulin resistance (Amsterdam, Schweizer, & Winokur, 1987). One study found significantly higher basal glucose levels, greater cumulative glucose responses during an oral glucose tolerance test (OGTT), larger cumulative insulin responses during the OGTT, and insulin resistance in depressives versus controls (Winokur, Maislin, Phillips, & Amsterdam, 1988). Some evidence suggests a greater prevalence in psychotic depression, melancholic depression, and bipolar disorder in comparison to neurotic depression or controls (Mueller, 1981). However, these findings have had some conflicting results, perhaps as a result of inconsistently examining factor effects from weight, age, activity level, diet, stress, and/or other potential influences.

In nine patients with panic disorder, OGTTs did produce typical hypoglycemia somatic complaints (palpitations and diaphoresis) as well as significant generalized anxiety symptoms according to the Zung Anxiety Scale (Uhde, Vittone, & Post, 1984). Also, those patients with the highest baseline anxiety levels tended to have the lowest glucose nadirs. However, no panic attacks were observed, so the authors concluded that "hypoglycemia is an unlikely cause." These results were supported by another study of insulin—induced hypoglycemia in which panic attacks were not elicited (Schweizer, Winokur, & Rickels, 1986). However, the authors of the latter study acknowledged the feasibility that the testing circumstances may have undercut the development of perceived panic. Finally, a study of cerebral glucose metabolism in women with panic disorders found significant abnormalities in PET scans, including increases in glucose metabolism in the left hippocampus and parahippocampal areas, as well as decreased metabolism in the right inferior parietal and right superior temporal regions (Bisaga et al., 1998).

There are also two other important studies of hypoglycemia in the medical and nutritional literature that need to be mentioned. In the first investigation (Chalew et al., 1984), the researchers actually called the condition "idiopathic post-prandial syndrome" (IPS). This research compared OGTTs in 19 patients with hypoglycemia or IPS versus 16 controls, and they also measured a full array of hormone levels, including epinephrine, norepinephrine, cortisol, glucagon, and growth hormone. What they found was significant differences between the two groups for all hormone levels at the OGTT nadir. In fact, there was no overlap between the two groups for epinephrine levels at the glucose nadir.

In the second excellent study (Blouin et al., 1993), the researchers compared subjects with bulimia and controls for their response to 25 g of injected glucose versus placebo. There were significant subject reports of fatigue, depression, and anxiety in bulimics injected with glucose in comparison to placebo and controls injected with glucose or placebo. Also, bulimics reported a significantly heightened urge to binge at 10 minutes and 60 minutes after the glucose injection.

Symptoms of hypoglycemia include fatigue, headaches, depression, anxiety, heart palpitations, irritability before meals, and possibly other symptoms. A review of hypoglycemia suggested that the symptoms could be categorized as adrenergic (e.g., anxiety, sweating, irritability) or neuroglycopenic (e.g., headache, fatigue, dizziness), although both are effects on the nervous system (Field, 1989). A prominent explanation is that epinephrine is a primary counter-regulatory hormone when blood glucose drops too low or too quickly. This notion is supported by Chalew's work (1984), although there are probably several other hormonal and/or cell receptor influences. For example, more recent research has found inadequate glucagon secretion (Leonetti et al., 1996) and decreased dehydroepiandrosterone sulfate (DHEA-S) levels (Altuntas, Bilir, Ucak, & Gundogdu, 2005). It is also likely that some individuals who are highly stressed and have higher circulating levels of epinephrine, will be more susceptible to hypoglycemic symptoms.

Causes of hypoglycemia include excessive sugar and refined carbohydrate intake, missing meals, excessive coffee or caffeine intake, inadequate dietary protein or fat (preferably healthy fat), significant stress and/or inadequate magnesium or chromium intake and/or status. While the most accurate test to identify hypoglycemia is an OGTT (insulin levels could also be measured), it can be a very unpleasant test, and there are several unresolved issues about the testing, such as optimal test length and diagnostic criteria. Common criteria for diagnosing hypoglycemia during a 5-hour OGTT include (a) plasma glucose < 55mg/dL; (b) glucose dropping > 100 mg/dL in 1 hour; (c) a flat OGTT curve; and/or (d) more than one peak during a 5-hour OGTT. It should be noted that early morning waking and some menopausal hot flashes may also be related to hypoglycemia. Early morning waking is particularly relevant to this text because of the importance of sleep and the significant adverse effect that insomnia can have on overall symptoms.

Although appropriate recommendations are indicated by addressing the list of causes or contributing factors listed above, assessing influences and applying dietary guidelines will be discussed later in this chapter. It is important to conclude this discussion of hypoglycemia by stating that consideration of abnormal glucose tolerance is important for all patients with neuropsychiatric disorders. This area remains controversial, however. Since there are many factors that influence this process, symptoms will vary in different people and are fairly broad, and there is not the significant and convincing evidence base of research that is required.

FOOD INTOLERANCE

The influence of food intolerance on nervous system functioning is also controversial. While there is a range of evidence to suggest that specific dietary components have neuromodulatory effects, the research is weak, and there are several important research gaps that need to be addressed. Food intolerance is a more useful and appropriate term than food allergy because the specific mechanisms of action go beyond immunologically based reactions, and they are not well understood. Research on exorphins and casomorphins provides a good example of other mechanisms of action.

The initial research on exorphins was reported in 1979, in which in vitro models of dairy (casein) and wheat (gluten) protein hydrolysates (using pepsin) showed opioid activation (Zioudrou, Streaty, & Klee, 1979). The proteins were four and five amino acid polypeptides that were exogenous in origin and had morphine-like activity, so they were called exorphins.

One research group has examined characteristics of five gluten exorphins (A4, A5, B4, B5, and C) and has shown in animal research that exorphin A5 can stimulate insulin secretion, suggesting pancreatic endocrine function modulation (Fukudome, Shimatsu, Suganuma, & Yoshikawa, 1995). Another group has examined milk-protein-derived opioid receptor ligands from alpha- and beta-casein, and alpha-lactalbumin and beta-lactoglobulin, and found that the beta casomorphin (derived from beta-casein) may have the most significant biological effects (Teschemacher, Koch, & Brantl, 1997). An example of this is an animal model study that found that beta-casomorphin modulated prolactin secretion (Nedvidkova, Kasafirek, Dlabac, & Felt, 1985).

A review by Reichelt and Knivsberg suggests that opioid peptides from foods have been found in significant levels in the urine of children with autistic disorders (Reichelt & Knivsberg, 2003). This research group and their colleagues have found similar results in attention deficit disorder (Hole et al., 1988), depression (Saelid, Haug, Heiberg, & Reichelt, 1985), schizophrenia (Reichelt et al., 1981), and celiac disease (Ek, Stensrud, & Reichelt, 1999).

While many integrative medicine practitioners recommend casein-free and gluten-free diets to children with autism, because they have observed significant clinical benefits and there is some research to support an association, these investigations have not been well controlled (Christison & Ivany, 2006). In addition, integrative medicine practitioners will usually also recommend supplements and behavioral or psychosocial approaches, as well as other modalities that can be beneficial. This makes it much more difficult to determine the degree to which the diet specifically has an effect.

Other pediatric research that illustrated this potential influence of food intolerance was done in children with epilepsy (Egger, Carter, Soothill, & Wilson, 1989). This study showed that a significant percentage of children with epilepsy and GI symptoms, headaches, and/or hyperactivity had some benefit from an elimination or oligoantigenic type of diet. Out of 24 children with generalized epilepsy, 18 had moderate improvement to complete control, as did 18 of 21 children with partial epilepsy; whereas none of the 16 children with epilepsy alone showed a response from the diet. In double-blind, placebo-controlled challenges, symptoms recurred in 15 of 16 subjects (8 had seizures).

In a subgroup of children with attention deficit hyperactivity disorder, this same research group was able to demonstrate that food not only affected clinical symptoms but also altered brain electrical activity (Uhlig, Merkenschlager, Brandmaier, & Egger, 1997). This study was done in 15 children following avoidance and ingestion of offending foods in a crossover design with blinded independent investigators reading topographic EEG mappings of brain electrical activity. Provoking foods were associated with an increase in beta 1 activity in the frontotemporal area of the brain.

It is important to note that there are a number of neurological syndromes that are associated with celiac disease (Wills, 2000). Also, one study of consecutive patients presenting to a neurology clinic (147 patients total—94 with a known diagnosis and 53 with no diagnosis), found that for those subjects with an idiopathic condition, 57% (30/53) had anti-gliadin antibodies (Hadjivassiliou et al., 1996). This is at least suggestive that wheat-derived peptides can significantly affect nervous system functioning.

While there is some evidence to support significant clinical influence, there are important unanswered questions that need to be addressed, including (a) what dietary components or peptides are most important; (b) whether there is scientific plausibility based on identifying circulating levels of exorphins, casomorphins, or other food components, and then whether they cross the blood brain barrier and promote adverse effects; (c) what the prevalence and degree of influence of these factors may be; (d) how susceptible individuals can be identified; and (e) what the impact is of eliminating these factors on circulating levels, and tissue and clinical responses.

Even without answers to these questions, the clinical influence can be assessed in patients. An effective way to try to test this is through the use of a rotation diet and/or elimination/challenge diet. While there are some tests that may identify food allergy or food intolerance, they have not been shown to have high specificity or reliability. Therefore, a clinical trial is appropriate, although there are differences of opinion regarding how exactly this should be done and for how long.

Rotation and elimination diets can also be useful for the significant numbers of psychiatric patients who present with comorbidities and psychosomatic disorders, such as stomach and intestinal disorders (IBS, IBD, and GERD), migraines, autoimmune disorders, chronic inflammatory or pain disorders, skin conditions, allergies, or others. These diets can be applied in three primary ways, including (a) a rotational diet (1–2 times per week of foods in Level 1 or Level 2)—this is a good way to begin, especially for those patients who may have difficulty with the diet and/or are resistant to it; and this diet can be followed for 2–4 weeks, or until they may be ready to proceed to the more restrictive protocol; (b) a "Level 1" elimination diet—avoid sugars, dairy, wheat, alcohol, and caffeine; and (c) a "Level 2" elimination diet—avoid foods from Level 1, plus other potentially offending foods such as peanuts, soy, other gluten grains (rye and barley), corn, oats, citrus, eggs, and any other foods that may be suspected. The patient's ability and willingness to comply even for a short time is important to consider.

HEALTHY DIETARY FAT AND ESSENTIAL FATTY ACIDS

The inclusion of significant amounts of healthy fatty acids in the diet is likely to be beneficial in several ways, including (a) its influence on nerve cell membrane fatty acid composition, membrane fluidity, and neuronal function;

(b) anti-inflammatory effects; (c) the adherence to a healthy dietary pattern, which would be similar to a Mediterranean-type diet or vegetarian-based diet; and (d) its help in balancing macronutrients and, therefore, in stabilizing glucose tolerance. Although dietary fats may be most important during infancy and childhood (for normal growth and development), and with aging, the effects can be important during any phase of life. These healthy fats include omega 3 fatty acids (primarily from specific types of fish, flax seeds, soy products, nuts/seeds, and dark green leafy vegetables) and monounsaturated fats (primarily from olive oil, olives, nuts/seeds, and avocado).

A recent review effectively addresses the importance of essential fatty acids in nerve cell membranes and their influence on cell membrane fluidity and physiological functions of the brain (Yehuda, Rabinovitz, & Mostofsky, 2005). Some of the specific functions thought to be affected include (a) membrane-bound enzyme activity; (b) number and affinity of membrane receptors; (c) ion channel function; (d) synthesis and activity of neurotransmitters; and (e) cellular signal transduction.

With regard to anti-inflammatory effects, a significant amount of the research and the best research is on omega 3 fatty acids and their influences on the eicosanoids (prostaglandins, leukotrienes, and thromboxanes), which mediate inflammation and related functions. While there are other dietary influences on inflammation that can promote inflammation (e.g., trans fats, saturated fats, and high glycemic index/load diets) or decrease inflammation (e.g., anti-oxidants, monounsaturated fat, and fiber/higher fiber dietary patterns), this research is getting a lot of attention and will continue to develop on a yearly basis (Kontogianni, Zampelas, & Tsigos, 2006). An example of the type of research that is needed is the effects of monounsaturated fat, since it probably has membrane and inflammatory influences, but this has not yet been carefully studied.

Research is accumulating that describes the inflammatory process associated with obesity, cardiovascular disease (Willerson & Ridker, 2004), cognitive dysfunction associated with aging, and aging in general (Napoli & Palinski, 2005). Since many patients will have one or more of these disorders, dietary guidelines that address anti-inflammatory effects could have benefits for these comorbid diseases but may also influence neuropsychiatric function and susceptibility to aging-related psychiatric disorders.

A recent meta-analysis suggested that omega 3 fatty acids did have anti-depressive effects, despite heterogeneity and publication bias in the included studies (Lin and Su, 2007). Although this research examined influences of supplemental EPA and DHA, there is research that has shown lower serum or red blood cell membrane levels of omega 3 fatty acids, or w3:w6 fatty acid ratios in patients with major depression (Kilkens, Honig, Maes, Lousberg, & Brummer, 2004; Maes et al., 1999). Still other research has found associations between chronic inflammatory disorders and affective disorders, such as the research of substance P, which has been tied to both the pathophysiology of inflammation, and to depression and anxiety (Rosenkranz, 2007).

Finally, it should be recognized that these influences are interrelated. For example, overweight or obesity can contribute to inflammation, and inflammation can contribute to oxidative stress of tissues, including neurological tissues. While healthy fats can contribute to more optimal cell-membrane fluidity and function, dietary and supplemental anti-oxidants will also help in protecting tissues from oxidative stress. At the same time, eicosanoid metabolism of fatty acids to less inflammatory or anti-inflammatory mediators is dependent on other factors, such as magnesium and zinc status, as well as cholesterol levels and aging, all of which can affect delta-6 desaturase enzyme activity. In addition, the inclusion of healthy dietary fat may promote the ingestion of a broader range of important nutrients and phytonutrients, as well as help in improving glucose tolerance. Therefore, future research will need to clarify the most important specific mechanisms involved, and the relative contributions that these factors have.

DIETARY FOLATE AND DEPRESSION

Investigations have documented a potential relationship between dietary folate and depression (Tolmunen et al., 2004). Other research suggests that this relationship may be more significant in men than women and for recurrent depression more than a single depressive episode (Astorg et al., 2008). Folate is important for methylation reactions and neurotransmitter synthesis. Since folate is found in healthy foods such as vegetables, whole grains, and beans, which are suggestive of healthier dietary patterns, it may be difficult to separate out the influence of folate specifically. However, other investigations have found that lower folate status was associated with poorer response to SSRIs and that folate supplementation may augment SSRI therapy in major depression (Alpert et al., 2002). The potential influence of folate and overall dietary guideline influences were supported by research that found that a Mediterranean dietary pattern was linked with depression prevention (Sanchez-Villegas, Henriquez, Bes-Rastrollo, & Doreste, 2006).

OTHER DIETARY FACTORS

To accurately and comprehensively describe the research and clinical practice that characterizes dietary influences in integrative psychiatry, it should be mentioned that there are other dietary factors that may have clinical influence and have been studied. Two examples of this are (a) the potential influence of dietary chemicals (e.g., pesticides, coloring agents, and preservatives) and their effects in children with ADHD and other disorders (Bateman et al., 2004); and (b) the area of diet and nutrition and behavior that includes associations with aggression, violence, and anti-social behavior (Benton, 2007).

Although these issues will arise periodically as research is published and/or advocacy groups are highlighted in media stories, it should be recognized that this research is very challenging to do and is always open to criticism. It is also likely that there are specific vulnerabilities in patient subpopulations from factors such as genetic polymorphisms or SNPs, and/or multifactorial influences that need to be in place for symptoms or a disorder that is affected by diet to manifest. Therefore, general studies that look at overall influences may miss some factors that are very important and have significant effects. Future research will hopefully be better designed and have more sensitive markers to evaluate these relationships, especially with regard to studying subpopulations.

Healthy Eating Behaviors and Relationship to Food

An important goal for integrative medicine and nutrition is to eat a natural, healthy diet that provides important nutrients for nervous system functioning, as well as one that may support other symptoms or disorders that may be present. As observed with the worsening problems of obesity and Type 2 Diabetes Mellitus (T2DM), however, this can be a very challenging objective.

Although it is beyond the scope of this chapter to discuss the range of evidence for the addictive potential of foods, it is important to note that there is increasing clinical and animal research that supports this relationship. Areas of research have included both sugar and carbohydrate addiction (Avena, Rada, & Hoebel, 2008; Spring et al., 2008), as well as the addictive qualities of high fat foods (Teegarden & Bale, 2007). A recent review paper discussed several aspects of this process, including the presence of chronic psychological stress, consequent influences on the HPA axis, a theoretical, reward-based stress eating model, and neuropeptide/endocrine dysregulation mediators that may be involved (Adam & Epel, 2007). A good illustration of some of these factors were observed in men recovering from substance abuse in which three main themes emerged, including excess weight gain, meaningful use of food, and a struggle to eat healthfully that varied by recovery stage (Cowan & Devine, 2008).

The emotional and physiological interrelationships that people have with food are complex. One recent study found that obesity was spread through the influences of social network (Christakis & Fowler, 2007). Other research suggests that many environmental factors increase food intake, including package size, plate, and glass sizes/shapes, lighting, socializing, variety, and others (Wansink, 2004). This same group found that people make as many as 200 decisions about food everyday.

As many integrative medicine practitioners may know, mindful eating is the focus of one of the eight sessions of the Mindfulness Based Stress Reduction (MBSR) program, the nationally recognized and well-researched approach developed by Jon Kabat-Zinn, PhD. In this practice, the full measure of attention and experience is brought to the process of eating—thoughts, feelings, smells, textures, etc.—which may provide an opportunity to be fully present to the healthy or unhealthy feelings that occur. Several other similar programs are in the process of being developed and researched.

One important consideration, which may or may not be specific to psychiatric practice, is that behavior change is difficult enough without the additional burden that depression, anxiety, and other psychiatric symptoms can add. Therefore, these guidelines may be more appropriate for patients with relatively stable or moderate conditions, or for those with significant knowledge, motivation, support, and/or resources. The process could also be started slowly by adding foods or making dietary changes that promote the inclusion of healthy foods (e.g., vegetables, fruits, bean products, healthy snacks such as nuts, and others), or by limiting potentially problematic foods (e.g., sugars, alcohol, caffeine, sodas, fast foods, and others).

The general approach and discussion of dietary change with patients can also be used to address a range of emotional, psychological, and spiritual issues—from addressing conflicted feelings, making choices, and employing restraint—to issues of self-care and personal responsibility. At the same time, comfort eating and food addiction can also present opportunities for talk therapies or other approaches to uncover or explore areas of trauma or conflict that have contributed to unproductive or unhealthy dietary patterns.

CONSIDERATIONS FOR PRACTICAL APPLICATION

Some practical issues have been addressed above. In general, the primary considerations are (a) knowledge of diet, dietary components, and health influence or impact; (b) shopping, cooking, and preparation time, as well as cost in some cases; and (c) what adjustments to make, and at what point in a treatment program; and (d) for how long should therapeutic guidelines be followed.

Knowledge, practices, and beliefs can be identified through a diet/food questionnaire, which could just be a description of one day's typical food intake, as well as through patient discussions. Another method to more clearly assess dietary patterns is to have patients fill out a 3- to 7-day food record, which may include daily symptoms, moods, and/or feelings. Individuals who have followed specific dietary guidelines or specific diets may be better able to make the recommended changes. An additional concern, for both patients and practitioners, is that there is often significant conflict or controversy regarding specific dietary guidelines or recommendations, which can result in considerable confusion. However, by taking a larger view of diet, it can be recognized that there is reasonably good agreement on basic healthy dietary (and lifestyle) recommendations that would be a good place to start. Then other, more controversial approaches could be considered for a period of time if desired.

Given some considerable controversies in nutrition and diet, another important option could be to refer to a knowledgeable and effective nutritionist or dietician who can support patient efforts more broadly, as well as be a good professional resource to the practitioner and patient regarding dietary and nutritional issues.

With respect to shopping, cooking, and preparation time, it may be helpful and important that a patient take time for this, and hopefully develop an ability to manage these tasks. While the degree to which this may be necessary will vary from person to person, it is a central feature of health and healing, especially in an integrative medical environment. Depending on how poor a patient's diet is and how much dietary change is made, some symptoms could improve within two weeks. In fact, some patients may have already made dietary changes in the past and observed that they feel better when they eat less sugar and refined flour products, dairy and/or wheat products, and/or made other dietary changes.

One empirical guideline to consider is that diet may need to change 25%–50% before it can have a significant enough influence on health and well-being (assuming that there is not a specific food or issue that is having an overriding effect). This is, in most cases, however, in addition to some changes in other integrative modalities, such as targeted nutritional supplementation, some regular exercise, movement and/or stretching, and some regular relaxation practice. It could also be important to have patients eat smaller but more frequent meals and snacks (e.g., four to six times per day, including three meals and one to three snacks, with the mid-afternoon snack being the most important), and to bring one to three healthy snacks to work or school so that they are readily available, and/or to set limits on specific, potentially problematic foods or beverages, such as sugar, caffeine, dairy, wheat, and alcohol.

Future Research

Because of the complexity of dietary research and the fact that it is not a funding priority, there has not been the range and depth of effective and meaningful research that is necessary to identify more effectively dietary influences on psychiatric-related illnesses and specific mechanisms that are involved. However, this deficiency is very slowly beginning to change for several reasons, including (a) significant interest in integrative medicine by the public, which has led the NIH to establish the National Center for Complementary and Alternative Medicine (NCCAM), where nutrition and lifestyle approaches, as well as other modalities, are being studied more carefully; (b) organizations, such as the Consortium for Academic Health Centers for Integrative Medicine and the Bravewell Collaborative, are actively promoting nutrition and lifestyle approaches for the prevention and treatment of disorders, and will soon begin practice-based research networks; (c) the public health problems of obesity and diabetes will necessitate a more effective approach to lifestyle factors, such as diet and exercise; and (d) the cost of medical care and the insurance system that supports it is almost at a breaking point, which will necessitate a move toward prevention and better care systems for chronic diseases.

Research priorities include more effective dietary research designs, reliable markers of nutritional status and dietary compliance, and research designs that can examine multifactorial influences on multifactorial disorders. This will, however, require significant time and resources.

Another important factor to investigate is dietary compliance and an examination of the various factors that promote this type of behavioral change. This will also need to be combined with more effective infrastructure to support these changes, as well as some insurance reimbursement to encourage a larger scale impact.

Summary and Conclusions

As this chapter describes, dietary guidelines that are part of an integrative medicine approach to care can have an important effect on physical and emotional symptoms that are important in psychiatric disorders. It is also evident that, while there is not as much effective research to support such approaches as may be desired, the research that has been done, combined with substantial clinical experience and logic, suggests the importance of addressing underlying contributing factors, such as dietary guidelines. This also provides a valuable opportunity to work with a patient in a comprehensive way, which allows him or her to be involved in the process of finding effective and helpful approaches, as well as taking responsibility for aspects of his or her care and well-being.

As described, key dietary factors include dietary nutritional composition, hypoglycemia, food intolerance, healthy dietary fat, and/or other possible effects. These guidelines could be addressed by (a) eating more whole foods (e.g., vegetables, beans, whole grains, fruit, and lean protein), and less refined flour products and processed foods; (b) eating smaller, more frequent meals (e.g., four to six times per day); (c) bringing two to three healthy snacks to work; (d) balancing meals for healthy protein, low carbohydrate vegetables, and complex carbohydrates; (e) rotating allergenic foods (e.g., dairy and wheat, only one to two times per week); and (f) setting limits on sugar (e.g., dessert, other than fruit, one to two times per week); caffeine (e.g., one cup of coffee per day at breakfast); and alcohol (e.g., one to two drinks per week). What can be a challenge is determining the exact approach to use, the appropriate point in time to apply it, and the time frame when a program should be used. Diet will also most likely be beneficial when it is linked directly to the use of targeted nutritional supplements, so that it can initiate biochemical influences more quickly, and promote more short-term benefits that will encourage longer term compliance. Ongoing research and clinical experience should help in determining the most important dietary influences in psychiatric disorders and the most effective clinical protocols to recommend.

REFERENCES

Adam, T. C., & Epel, E. S. (2007). Stress, eating and the reward system. *Physiology & Behavior, 91*, 449–458.

Alpert, J. E., Mischoulon, D., Rubenstein, G. E., Bottonari, K., Nierenberg, A. A., & Fava, M. (2002). Folinic acid (Leucovorin) as an adjunctive treatment for SSRI-refractory depression. *Annual Clinical Psychiatry, 14*, 33–38.

Altuntas, Y., Bilir, M., Ucak, S., & Gundogdu, S. (2005). Reactive hypoglycemia in lean young women with PCOS and correlations with insulin sensitivity and with beta cell function. *European Journal of Obstetrics, Gynecology, and Reproductive Biology, 119*, 198–205.

Ames, B. N., Elson-Schwab, I., & Silver, E. A. (2002). High-dose vitamin therapy stimulates variant enzymes with decreased coenzyme binding affinity (increased K(m)): Relevance to genetic disease and polymorphisms. *American Journal of Clinical Nutrition, 75*, 616–658.

Amsterdam, J. D., Schweizer, E., & Winokur, A. (1987). Multiple hormonal responses to insulin-induced hypoglycemia in depressed patients and normal volunteers. *American Journal of Psychiatry, 144*, 170–175.

Astorg, P., Couthouis, A., de Courcy, G. P., Bertrais, S., Arnault, N., Meneton, P., et al. (2008). Association of folate intake with the occurrence of depressive episodes in middle-aged French men and women. *British Journal of Nutrition, 100,* 183–187.

Avena, N. M., Rada, P., & Hoebel, B. G. (2008). Evidence for sugar addiction: behavioral and neurochemical effects of intermittent, excessive sugar intake. *Neuroscience and Biobehavioral Reviews, 32,* 20–39.

Bateman, B., Warner, J. O., Hutchinson, E., Dean, T., Rowlandson, P., Gant, C., et al. (2004). The effects of a double-blind, placebo-controlled, artificial food colorings and benzoate preservative challenge on hyperactivity in a general population sample of preschool children. *Archives of Disease in Childhood, 89,* 506–511.

Bell, I. R., Edman, J. S., Morrow, F. D., Marby, D. W., Perrone, G., Kayne, H. L., et al. (1992). Brief communication. Vitamin B1, B2, and B6 augmentation of tricyclic antidepressant treatment in geriatric depression with cognitive dysfunction. *Journal of the American College of Nutrition, 11,* 159–163.

Benton, D. (2007). The impact of diet on anti-social, violent and criminal behaviour. *Neuroscience and Biobehavioral Reviews, 31,* 752–774.

Biesalski, H.K., Brummer, R.J., Konig, J., O'Connell, M.A., Rechkemmer, G., Stos, K., et al. (2003). Micronutrient deficiencies. Hohenheim Concensus Conference. *European Journal of Nutrition, 42,* 353–363.

Bisaga, A., Katz, J. L., Antonini, A., Wright, C. E., Margouleff, C., Gorman, J. M., et al. (1998). Cerebral glucose metabolism in women with panic disorder. *American Journal of Psychiatry, 155,* 1178–1183.

Blouin, A. G., Blouin, J., Bushnik, T., Braaten, J., Goldstein, C., & Sarwar, G. (1993). A double-blind placebo-controlled glucose challenge in bulimia nervosa: psychological effects. *Biological Psychiatry, 33,* 160–168.

Bradford, H. (1986). *Chemical neurobiology. An introduction to neurochemistry.* New York: W.H. Freeman and Co.

Chalew, S. A., McLaughlin, J. V., Mersey, J. H., Adams, A. J., Cornblath, M., & Kowarski, A. A. (1984). The use of the plasma epinephrine response in the diagnosis of idiopathic postprandial syndrome. *JAMA, 251,* 612–615.

Christakis, N. A., & Fowler, J. H. (2007). The spread of obesity in a large social network over 32 years. *New England Journal of Medicine, 357,* 370–9.

Christison, G. W., & Ivany, K. (2006). Elimination diets in autism spectrum disorders: any wheat amidst the chaff? *Journal of Developmental and Behavioral Pediatrics, 27,* S162–S171.

Cowan, J., & Devine, C. (2008). Food, eating, and weight concerns of men in recovery from substance addiction. *Appetite, 50,* 33–42.

Egger, J., Carter, C. M., Soothill, J. F., & Wilson, J. (1989). Oligoantigenic diet treatment of children with epilepsy and migraine. *Journal of Pediatrics, 114,* 51–58.

Ek, J., Stensrud, M., & Reichelt, K. L. (1999). Gluten-free diet decreases urinary peptide levels in children with celiac disease. *Journal of Pediatric Gastroenterology and Nutrition, 29,* 282–285.

Field, J. B. (1989). Hypoglycemia. Definition, clinical presentations, classification, and laboratory tests. *Endocrinology and Metabolism Clinics of North America, 18,* 27–43.

Fukudome, S., Shimatsu, A., Suganuma, H., & Yoshikawa, M. (1995). Effect of gluten exorphins A5 and B5 on the postprandial plasma insulin level in conscious rats. *Life Sciences, 57,* 729–734.

Gibson, E. L. (2006). Emotional influences on food choice: sensory, physiological and psychological pathways. *Physiology & Behavior, 89,* 53–61.

Gilbody, S., Lewis, S., & Lightfoot, T. (2007). Methylenetetrahydrofolate reductase (MTHFR) genetic polymorphisms and psychiatric disorders: A HuGE review. *American Journal of Epidemiology, 165,* 1–13.

Hadjivassiliou, M., Gibson, A., Davies-Jones, G. A., Lobo, A. J., Stephenson, T. J., & Milford-Ward, A. (1996). Does cryptic gluten sensitivity play a part in neurological illness? *Lancet, 347,* 369–371.

Hole, K., Lingjaerde, O., Morkrid, L., Boler, J. B., Saelid, G., Diderichsen, J., et al. (1988). Attention deficit disorders: A study of peptide-containing urinary complexes. *Journal of Developmetnal and Behavioral Pediatrics, 9,* 205–212.

Kilkens, T. O., Honig, A., Maes, M., Lousberg, R., & Brummer, R. J. (2004). Fatty acid profile & affective dysregulation in irritable bowel syndrome. *Lipids, 39,* 425–431.

Kontogianni, M. D., Zampelas, A., & Tsigos, C. (2006). Nutrition and inflammatory load. *Annals of the New York Academy of Sciences, 1083,* 214–238.

Leonetti, F., Foniciello, M., Iozzo, P., Riggio, O., Merli, M., Giovannetti, P., et al. (1996). Increased nonoxidative glucose metabolism in idiopathic reactive hypoglycemia. *Metabolism, 45,* 606–610.

Lin, P. Y., & Su, K. P. (2007). A meta-analytic review of double-blind, placebo-controlled trials of antidepressant efficacy of omega-3 fatty acids. *Journal of Clinical Psychiatry, 68,* 1056–1061.

Maes, M., Christophe, A., Delanghe, J., Altamura, C., Neels, H., & Meltzer, H. Y. (1999). Lowered omega3 polyunsaturated fatty acids in serum phospholipids and cholesteryl esters of depressed patients. *Psychiatry Research, 85,* 275–291.

Mueller, D. P. (1981). The current status of urban-rural differences in psychiatric disorder. An emerging trend for depression. *Journal of Nervous and Mental Disease, 169,* 18–27.

Musselman, D. L., Betan, E., Larsen, H., & Phillips, L. S. (2003). Relationship of depression to diabetes types 1 and 2: epidemiology, biology, and treatment. *Biological Psychiatry, 54,* 317–329.

Napoli, C., & Palinski, W. (2005). Neurodegenerative diseases: insights into pathogenic mechanisms from atherosclerosis. *Neurobiology of Aging, 26,* 293–302.

Nedvidkova, J., Kasafirek, E., Dlabac, A., & Felt, V. (1985). Effect of beta-casomorphin and its analogue on serum prolactin in the rat. *Experimental and Clinical Endocrinology, 85,* 249–252.

Reichelt, K. L., Hole, K., Hamberger, A., Saelid, G., Edminson, P. D., Braestrup, C. B., et al. (1981). Biologically active peptide-containing fractions in schizophrenia and childhood autism. *Advances in Biochemical Psychopharmacology, 28,* 627–643.

Reichelt, K. L., & Knivsberg, A. M. (2003). Can the pathophysiology of autism be explained by the nature of the discovered urine peptides? *Nutritional Neuroscience, 6,* 19–28.

Rosenkranz, M. A. (2007). Substance P at the nexus of mind and body in chronic inflammation and affective disorders. *Psychological Bulletin, 133,* 1007–1037.

Saelid, G., Haug, J. O., Heiberg, T., & Reichelt, K. L. (1985). Peptide-containing fractions in depression. *Biological Psychiatry, 20,* 245–256.

Sanchez-Villegas, A., Henriquez, P., Bes-Rastrollo, M., & Doreste, J. (2006). Mediterranean diet and depression. *Public Health Nutrition, 9,* 1104–1109.

Schweizer, E., Winokur, A., & Rickels, K. (1986). Insulin-induced hypoglycemia and panic attacks. *American Journal of Psychiatry, 143,* 654–655.

Spring, B., Schneider, K., Smith, M., Kendzor, D., Appelhans, B., Hedeker, D., et al. (2008). Abuse potential of carbohydrates for overweight carbohydrate cravers. *Psychopharmacology* (Berl), *197,* 637–647.

Teegarden, S. L., & Bale, T. L. (2007). Decreases in dietary preference produce increased emotionality and risk for dietary relapse. *Biological Psychiatry, 61,* 1021–1029.

Teschemacher, H., Koch, G., & Brantl, V. (1997). Milk protein-derived opioid receptor ligands. *Biopolymers, 43,* 99–117.

Tolmunen, T., Hintikka, J., Ruusunen, A., Voutilainen, S., Tanskanen, A., Valkonen, V. P., et al. (2004). Dietary folate and the risk of depression in Finnish middle-aged men. A prospective follow-up study. *Psychotherapy and Psychosomatics, 73,* 334–339.

Uhde, T. W., Vittone, B. J., & Post, R. M. (1984). Glucose tolerance testing in panic disorder. *American Journal of Psychiatry, 141,* 1461–1463.

Uhlig, T., Merkenschlager, A., Brandmaier, R., & Egger, J. (1997). Topographic mapping of brain electrical activity in children with food-induced attention deficit hyperkinetic disorder. *European Journal of Pediatrics, 156,* 557–561.

Vaquero, M. P. (2002). Magnesium and trace elements in the elderly: Intake, status and recommendations. *Journal of Nutrition, Health & Aging, 6,* 147–153.

Wansink, B. (2004). Environmental factors that increase the food intake and consumption volume of unknowing consumers. *Annual Review of Nutrition, 24,* 455–479.

Willerson, J. T., & Ridker, P. M. (2004). Inflammation as a cardiovascular risk factor. *Circulation, 109,* II2–10.

Williams, R. J., & Saunders, D. H. (1934). The effects of inositol, crystalline vitamin B(1) and "pantothenic acid" on the growth of different strains of yeast. *Biochemistry Journal, 28,* 1887–1893.

Wills, A. J. (2000). The neurology and neuropathology of coeliac disease. *Neuropathology and Applied Neurobiology, 26,* 493–496.

Winokur, A., Maislin, G., Phillips, J. L., & Amsterdam, J. D. (1988). Insulin resistance after oral glucose tolerance testing in patients with major depression. *American Journal of Psychiatry, 145,* 325–330.

Wright, J. H., Jacisin, J. J., Radin, N. S., & Bell, R. A. (1978). Glucose metabolism in unipolar depression. *British Journal of Psychiatry, 132,* 386–393.

Yehuda, S., Rabinovitz, S., & Mostofsky, D. I. (2005). Essential fatty acids and the brain: from infancy to aging. *Neurobiology of Aging, 26* (Suppl 1), 98–102.

Zioudrou, C., Streaty, R. A., & Klee, W. A. (1979). Opioid peptides derived from food proteins. The exorphins. *Journal of Biological Chemistry, 254,* 2446–2449.

2

Exercise in the Treatment of Depressive Disorders

RAJNISH MAGO AND RAJEEV MAHAJAN

KEY CONCEPTS

- Treatment strategies that can supplement or be alternatives to antidepressant medications are needed because many patients decline or cannot tolerate antidepressant medications, or have a partial or no response to them.
- While the methodology of most studies on exercise has been less than rigorous, aerobic exercise may be considered as a potential sole treatment for mild depressive disorder, or as an adjunct to antidepressant medications.
- Potential advantages for exercise as a treatment for depressive disorders include an early onset of effect, a general lack of adverse effects, and improved physical functioning as an additional benefit.
- Overall, exercise as a treatment option is underutilized in clinical practice.
- Further research is needed to assess the efficacy of exercise using larger and well-designed studies. In addition, future research needs to further clarify the type, intensity, and frequency of exercise that is optimal.

Introduction

Depressive disorders, or "clinical depression," are highly prevalent, with a lifetime prevalence of 16.2% in the general population (Kessler et al., 2003). Antidepressant medications, which can treat some types of depressive disorders, have become the most frequently prescribed medications in the United States (Cohen, 2007). However, there are multiple potential problems with the use of antidepressant medications in the treatment of depressive disorders. First, antidepressant medications are not effective for all forms of clinical depression (e.g., adjustment disorder with depressed mood, and the all-too-frequently diagnosed "Depressive disorder not otherwise specified"). Second, antidepressant medications are efficacious in only a limited subgroup of even patients with major depressive disorder. A meta-analysis of clinical trials of antidepressant medications found that trials which did not find the medication to be more effective than placebo were more likely to remain unpublished, leading to a 32% overestimate of the size of the effect (Turner, Matthews, Linardatos, Tell, & Rosenthal, 2008). Another meta-analysis even found that, when unpublished data was included, antidepressant medications were more effective than placebo only for the most severely depressed patients (Kirsch et al., 2008).

Third, even including a placebo effect of the antidepressant, the Sequenced Treatment Alternatives to Relieve Depression (STAR*D) study found that in "real world" patients with major depressive disorder, treatment with citalopram led to "response" in only 47% of patients, and "remission " in only 33% (Trivedi, Rush, et al., 2006). In fact, a substantial proportion of patients failed to obtain remission of the depressive disorder even after trials of multiple medications or combinations of medications (Gaynes et al., 2008). Fourth, nonadherence to antidepressant medications is widespread, with 49% patients in "real-world" settings discontinuing the medication before completion of the continuation phase (Melartin et al., 2005), with side effects being a leading cause of this nonadherence. While the reasons for this nonadherence need to be carefully assessed and addressed in individual patients, realistically there is a need for other treatment options in patients who are unwilling to take antidepressant medications for any reason. Lastly, even among patients who are able and willing to take the antidepressant medication and do show a response to the treatment, a substantial proportion continue to have residual symptoms, which are associated with functional impairment and increased risk of relapse.

Thus, there is a pressing need for a variety of primary and adjunctive treatment options, including both biological and nonbiological interventions, that can be used alone or in combinations in patients whose depression is of mild or moderate severity, who are not able to tolerate antidepressant medications, or who have had limited response to antidepressant medications or psychotherapy.

In recent years, there has been increasing formal recognition of the potential role of exercise as a treatment for depressive disorders. Though it has long been known that exercise has positive effects on mental health, its potential utility is underrecognized, and it is not commonly utilized in mental health care (Callaghan, 2004). In addition, systematic research on the effectiveness of exercise as a treatment has been lacking until recently.

Methodological Problems in Research on Exercise

While the methodology of clinical trials of antidepressant medications has been well worked out, clinical trials assessing the efficacy of exercise as a treatment pose certain special challenges, and the appropriate designs of these trials are still evolving.

Two problems pertain to the issue of external validity or generalizability of the studies. First, such trials are subject to substantial enrollment bias. Subjects who have an aversion to more conventional treatments and a positive attitude toward exercise as an intervention for their problem are much more likely to participate in clinical trials of exercise. Even if exercise is found to be very effective, similar results may not be obtained when it is used in unselected patient populations. Second, depressive disorders are undoubtedly very heterogeneous and studies that find exercise to be effective for a certain subgroup of depressive disorders may not generalize to other patients with depressive disorders.

The other methodological challenges pertain to internal validity of these studies. First, placebo effects due to patients' expectations are quite pronounced in depressive disorders, and without an appropriate control group to take these into account, it is impossible to conclude that the specific nature of the intervention was the reason for patients' improvement. Placebo responses are probably even more likely in studies of exercise where patients tend to be self-selected for positive attitudes toward exercise. However, while it is relatively easy in studies of antidepressant medications to use a placebo pill that resembles the active antidepressant pill, the question arises as to what would constitute an adequate placebo for an exercise intervention. It is hard to conceal the nature of the intervention. Patients must believe that they are "exercising," yet not be exercising in the manner and to the degree that constitutes the treatment intervention being evaluated. For example, patients in the control group may be asked to do stretching exercises instead of a threshold level of aerobic exercise. Second, when the exercise intervention is provided in social settings, the benefits may be partly or entirely due to the social interaction and support and the behavioral activation that are inadvertently being provided. This effect may be reduced by including a treatment group where participants start to exercise but without increasing social interaction—for example, by exercising at home.

Examples of these methodological problems and of attempts to minimize them will be found in the studies discussed below, and should be kept in mind in critically evaluating the results of these studies.

Efficacy of Exercise in Depressive Disorders

Here we will describe the current level of evidence for the efficacy of exercise as a treatment for depressive disorders, including immediate effects, short-term effects, and long-term effects. Then, we will separately describe the potential efficacy of exercise as a treatment for patients with a depressive disorder and an inadequate response to antidepressant medications.

IMMEDIATE EFFECTS

While both antidepressant medications and psychotherapy usually require several weeks in order to produce meaningful benefits, exercise may produce immediate improvement in mood. It has been suggested that even a single bout of exercise can have a favorable impact on symptoms in patients who are feeling depressed (Bartholomew, Morrison, & Ciccolo, 2005; Pierce & Pate, 1994). In order to test this, 80 volunteers completed the Profile of Mood States-A questionnaire, and were divided into "depressed" and "nondepressed" groups based on depression scores on this questionnaire (Lane & Lovejoy, 2001). These subjects then participated in a 60-minute aerobic dance session and were reassessed at the end of the session. Subjects in both the "depressed" and "nondepressed" groups had a reduction in anger, confusion, tension, and fatigue. However, the improvement was significantly greater in participants who were classified as "depressed" before the exercise.

ACUTE PHASE

While there are tantalizing indications of the potential for improvement in patients when exercise is used as a treatment, the studies have small sample sizes and usually lack rigorous methodologies. A review and meta-analysis of 14 randomized controlled trials in adults suffering from depressive disorders of any severity did not find convincing evidence of the efficacy of exercise as a treatment for depressive disorders, in large part due to lack of good quality evidence on this topic (Lawlor & Hopker, 2001). On the other hand, subsequent reviews of exercise as a treatment for depression and other psychiatric disorders concluded that, while there is a relative lack of well-designed studies on this topic, existing data does support a role for exercise as an effective treatment for clinical depression (Barbour, Edenfield, & Blumenthal, 2007; Brosse, Sheets, Lett, & Blumenthal, 2002). The most recent meta-analysis of studies of exercise as a treatment for depression (Mead et al., 2008) noted that most studies did not conceal randomization adequately, use intent-to-treat analyses, or use clinician-rated scales as primary outcome measures. In this meta-analysis, exercise has a relatively large and statistically significant effect when 23 trials involving 907 patients were included. However, when only the three trials with more robust methodology (adequate concealment of treatment allocation, intent-to-treat analysis, and blinded assessment of the outcome measures) were combined, the effect was more moderate and statistically nonsignificant.

Recently a large and well-designed controlled clinical trial randomized 202 adults with major depressive disorder into four groups: supervised exercise, home-based exercise, sertraline (50–200 mg daily), and pill placebo (Blumenthal et al., 2007). The exercise schedule consisted of warm-up by 10 minutes of walking, followed by walking or jogging on a treadmill at 70%–85% of the patient's maximal heart rate for 30 minutes. After 16 weeks of treatment , 40% and 45% respectively of patients assigned to the home-based and supervised exercise groups achieved remission (according to the widely accepted criteria of not meeting criteria for major depressive disorder and having a score of less than 8 on the Hamilton Depression Rating Scale). These proportions were similar to that of the 47% of patients assigned to sertraline who achieved remission of the depression, and higher than the 31% remission rate with placebo, though the difference was not statistically significant ($p = 0.057$). However, when the 14 patients who showed 50% of greater improvement within 1 week (presumably placebo responders) were excluded, all active treatments were statistically significantly superior to placebo. This study addressed a number of the methodological concerns that have plagued previous studies—it had a moderately large sample size, included medication and pill placebo control groups, and included a group receiving home-based exercise to control for the effects of social interaction.

EXERCISE AS AN ADJUNCT TO ANTIDEPRESSANT MEDICATIONS

Exercise has also been evaluated as a potential adjunct to antidepressant medications (Pilu et al., 2007; Trivedi et al., 2006). In a small pilot study, 17 patients with unipolar, nonpsychotic depression, a Hamilton Depression Rating Scale score of 14 or greater after treatment with an antidepressant for at least 6 weeks, and physical inactivity (exercising $\leq$ 20 minutes, $<$3 days/week) were enrolled (Trivedi et al., 2006). While continuing their antidepressant medications, these patients participated in a 12-week exercise program, which consisted of both supervised and home-based exercise. On intent-to-treat analyses, a clinically and statistically significant decrease in clinician-rated (Hamilton Depression Rating Scale) and patient-rated (Inventory of Depressive Symptomatology-Self Report) depression scales was found. The findings of this study are tentative due to the small sample size and lack of a control group. In another small study of 30 female patients with major depressive disorder, randomization and a control group were used to study the potential utility of exercise as an adjunctive treatment (Pilu et al., 2007). Ten patients were randomly allocated to antidepressant medication plus exercise, while 20 controls received antidepressant medication alone in naturalistic treatment. Exercise treatment consisted of two 60-minute sessions per week involving strengthening exercises on cardio-fitness machines. After 8 months of treatment, the treatment group showed statistically significant improvement in Hamilton Depression Rating Scale and Clinical Global Impression scores, and in overall functioning compared to baseline, while the control group showed a smaller improvement that was not statistically significantly different from baseline. In addition to other limitations, the exercise group also received social interaction that was deliberately maximized by having the subjects stand in a circle while exercising.

Results are awaited from much larger, randomized, single-blind, dose comparison Treatment with Exercise Augmentation for Depression (TREAD) study which aims to overcome some of the limitations of prior studies (Trivedi et al., 2006).

LONGER-TERM EFFICACY

In addition to its potential efficacy in the acute treatment of depressive disorders, exercise may also reduce relapse rates during the continuation phase of treatment (Babyak et al., 2000; Blumenthal et al., 1999). In these studies, 156 adults aged 50 years or older were randomized into three groups—exercise, sertraline, and combination of exercise and sertraline—for 4 months (Blumenthal, 1999) and then over a further 6-month follow-up (Babyak, 2000). After 4 months of treatment, all three groups showed similar and statistically significant reduction in depression. After an additional 6-month follow-up, the exercise group showed higher remission and lower relapse rates compared to the sertraline or combination groups in the subgroup of patients who were in remission after the initial 4 months of treatment ($n = 83$). This data suggests that in patients who respond acutely to exercise as a treatment for depressive disorder, it may be efficacious as a continuation treatment as well.

Potential Advantages of Exercise as a Treatment

Depressive disorders are multidimensional syndromes with emotional symptoms, impaired physical and social functioning, and impaired quality of life. The increased physical activity may have greater positive effects on some of these aspects of depressive disorders than conventional treatments (Carta et al., 2008). The greater benefit of exercise in improving physical functioning may be especially helpful for elderly patients with depressive disorders (Brenes et al., 2007).

One of the most vexing limitations of treatment with antidepressant medications is that they usually require several weeks to produce significant improvement in depression. In those patients who can be thus engaged, initiation of an appropriate exercise regimen at the same time as the antidepressant medication may help to reduce the symptoms of depression during this lag period before antidepressant medications take effect (Knubben et al., 2007). These authors assessed this potential in a randomized controlled clinical trial of a 10-day exercise training program in 38 inpatients with major depressive disorder who were receiving antidepressant medications (Knubben et al., 2007). Twenty patients were randomized to aerobic exercise by brisk walking on a treadmill daily for 30 minutes and 18 patients to the control group of 30 minutes of stretching daily. Patients in the aerobic exercise group had statistically and clinically significantly greater improvement in clinician-rated and patient-rated severity of depression. Three times as many patients in the aerobic exercise group had a clinical response, as compared to those in the control group (65% versus 22%) within 10 days. Thus, exercise may have a useful role in producing early improvement in depression, though an optimum level of exercise with relatively high energy expenditure is probably required to produce benefits within a short period of time.

Patients with depressive disorder often suffer from comorbid physical and mental disorders, and exercise may be of particular value as a treatment for these patients due to its beneficial effects on these comorbid disorders. For example, exercise may reduce the morbidity and mortality due to cardiovascular diseases (Bjarnason-Wehrens et al., 2004; Lett, Davidson, & Blumenthal, 2005; Umpierre & Stein, 2007), and diabetes mellitus (Colberg, 2007; Wallberg-Henriksson, Rincon, & Zierath, 1998). Similarly, exercise may have beneficial effects in some anxiety disorders, like post-traumatic stress disorders (Manger,

2005; Newman & Motta, 2007), that may be comorbid with the depressive disorder.

Mechanism of Action of Exercise as a Treatment

Various potential mechanisms have been hypothesized to explain the efficacy of exercise in depressive disorders. Exercise may exert its antidepressant effect by increasing monoaminergic neurotransmission, similar to the effects of anti-depressant medications and electroconvulsive therapy (Ransford, 1982). It has also been proposed that the benefits of exercise in depression may be related to reduced endocrinologic stress, because reduced excretion of stress hormones like cortisol and epinephrine in the urine has been found after exercise in patients with depressive disorders (Nabkasorn et al., 2006). Lastly, increased release of endorphins from central opioid systems due to activation by contracting skeletal muscles during exercise has been considered as a potential mechanism (Thorén, Floras, Hoffmann, & Seals, 1990).

What Kind of Exercise, How Much, How Often, and For How Long

The two most common methods of exercise are aerobic or endurance training and strength or resistance training. Endurance training results in high aerobic capacity while resistance training increases muscle strength (Glowacki et al., 2004).

Most clinical trials in depressive disorders have focused on aerobic exercise. One study tested the efficacy of resistance training in 32 older patients (mean age 71 years) with various depressive disorders (major, minor, and dysthymia) who were randomized to 10 weeks of supervised resistance training or to an attention-control group (Singh, Clements, & Fiatarone, 1997). Statistically significantly greater reduction in clinician- and patient-rated depression was observed in patients in the resistance training group. Similarly, other studies have also supported aerobic and anaerobic exercise as being equally effective in the treatment of mild-to-moderate unipolar depressive disorders (Martinsen, 1994; Martinsen, Hoffart, & Solberg, 1989). Pending more specific guidance from further research, it is probably appropriate to collaborate with patients to recommend an individualized exercise plan consisting of either aerobic exercise or resistance training, and perhaps a combination of both.

Another aspect of exercise as a treatment is its intensity. In the 12-week randomized controlled Depression Outcomes Study of Exercise (DOSE) study

(Dunn, Trivedi, Kampert, Clark, & Chambliss, 2002, 2005), 80 young adults with mild-to-moderate major depressive disorder were randomized to exercise groups based on energy expenditure (17.5 kcal/kg/week or the "public health dose" versus 7.5 kcal/kg/week or the "low dose") and frequency (3 or 5 days). In addition, a placebo group engaged in 3 days/week of flexibility training. Patients in the higher energy expenditure exercise groups of either frequency had statistically significantly greater reduction in depression than those in the low dose or placebo groups, the latter two being essentially similarly improved. Given a certain level of energy expenditure, the frequency of exercise (3 versus 5 days) did not appear to affect the improvement in depression, though the number of patients in these subgroups was too small to draw this conclusion with confidence. At this time, it appears appropriate to recommend exercising for 30 minutes at 70%–85% of the patients' calculated maximal heart rate at least 3 and preferably 5 days a week.

While patients with mild-to-moderate depression can be motivated to exercise as a treatment for their depression, motivating patients with more severe depression to exercise can be very challenging, since lack of energy and interest are part of the syndrome of clinical depression. Providing supervised exercise with considerable support and encouragement, and exercising in groups, may assist in engaging patients in exercise. More severe patients may need to be treated with antidepressant medications before they are improved enough to participate in exercise. However, whenever possible, exercise should be started early in treatment due to its relatively rapid onset of action as discussed above.

In longer term treatment, assessment of patients' motivation to exercise is very important. As with other lifestyle changes, patients go through distinct stages of precontemplation, contemplation, preparation, action, and maintenance (see Prochaska & Diclemente, 1982; Zimmerman, Olsen, & Bosworth, 2000), before (hopefully) incorporating a change. Physicians should assess and assist patients' progress through these stages by making an individualized plan to motivate them to exercise on a regular basis (Heath & Stuart, 2002; Zimmerman et al., 2000).

Conclusions

1. While the research on exercise as a potential treatment of depressive disorders is certainly preliminary—even given the current data—due to the additional benefits of exercise and the usually innocuous nature of the intervention, exercise should probably be used as an adjunctive treatment in many or most patients with depressive disorders.

2. Exercise alone may be efficacious in some patients with mild depressive disorder, but at present, in most patients it is probably best used as an adjunct to antidepressant medications and/or psychotherapy.
3. Patients should be started on a regimen of systematic exercise as early as possible, because exercise may be especially helpful during the period when antidepressant medications and psychotherapy usually have a delayed onset of effect.
4. At this time, aerobic exercise of moderate intensity for at least 30 minutes, at least 3 days a week, appears to be the most reasonable recommendation. Perhaps this is no different than the public health recommendation for the general population.
5. Middle-aged or elderly patients, those with comorbid medical illnesses, and those at higher risk due to any reason should have a medical evaluation from their primary care physicians prior to starting an exercise regimen.

Future Research

A survey of physicians found that the most important barrier to integration of complementary and alternative treatments into routine clinical practice is the relative lack of scientific evidence supporting these treatments (Maha & Shaw, 2007). Appropriate and widespread utilization of exercise as a treatment for depressive disorders requires additional studies with (a) larger sample sizes; (b) narrowly defined subtypes of depressive disorders; (c) inclusion of representative samples of patients; and (d) use of a convincing placebo group. Besides further establishing the efficacy of exercise in the acute treatment of depressive disorders, further research should address (a) the role of exercise in continuation and maintenance treatment; (b) the type, intensity, and frequency of exercise that is optimal for these patients; and (c) the mechanism of action of exercise as a treatment for depressive disorders.

REFERENCES

Babyak M., Blumenthal, J. A., Herman S., Khatri P., Doraiswamy, M., Moore, K., et al. (2000). Exercise treatment for major depression: Maintenance of therapeutic benefit at 10 months. *Psychosomatic Medicine, 62,* 633–638.
Barbour, K. A., Edenfield, T. M., & Blumenthal, J. A. (2007). Exercise as a treatment for depression and other psychiatric disorders: A review. *Journal of Cardiopulmonary Rehabilitaion and Prevention, 27,* 359–367.

Bartholomew, J. B., Morrison, D., & Ciccolo, J. T. (2005). Effects of acute exercise on mood and well-being in patients with major depressive disorder. *Medicine and Science in Sports and Exercise, 37*, 2032–2037.

Bjarnason-Wehrens, B., Mayer-Berger, W., Meister, E. R., Baum, K., Hambrecht, R., & Gielen, S., Recommendations for resistance exercise in cardiac rehabilitation (2004). Recommendations of the German Federation for Cardiovascular Prevention and Rehabilitation. *European Journal of Cardiovascular Prevention and Rehabilitation, 11*, 352–361.

Blumenthal, J. A., Babyak, M. A., Doraiswamy, P. M., Watkins, L., Hoffman, B. M., Barbour, K. A., et al. (2007). Exercise and pharmacotherapy in the treatment of major depressive disorder. *Psychosomatic Medicine, 69*, 587–596.

Blumenthal, J. A., Babyak, M. A., Moore, K. A., Craighead, W. E., Herman, S., Khatri, P., et al. (1999). Effects of exercise training on older patients with major depression. *Archives of Internal Medicine, 25, 159*(19), 2349–2356.

Brenes, G. A., Williamson, J. D., Messier, S. P., Rejeski, W. J., Pahor, M., Ip, E., et al. (2007). Treatment of minor depression in older adults: A pilot study comparing sertraline and exercise. *Aging & Mental Health, 11*, 61–68.

Brosse, A. L., Sheets, E. S., Lett, H. S., & Blumenthal, J. A. (2002). Exercise and the treatment of clinical depression in adults: Recent findings and future directions. *Sports Medicine, 32*, 741–760.

Callaghan, P. (2004). Exercise: A neglected intervention in mental health care? *Journal of Psychiatric Mental Health and Nursing, 11*, 476–483.

Carta, M. G., Hardoy, M.C., Pilu, A., Sorba, M., Floris, A.L., Mannu, F.A., et al. (2008). Improving physical quality of life with group physical activity in the adjunctive treatment of major depressive disorder. *Clinical Practice and Epidemiology in Mental Health, 4*, 1.

Cohen, E. (July 9, 2007). CDC. Antidepressants most prescribed drugs in U.S. CNN. Retrieved Jan 1, 2008, from http://www.cnn.com/2007/HEALTH/07/09/antidepressants/index.html

Colberg, S. R. (2007). Physical activity, insulin action, and diabetes prevention and control. *Current Diabetes Reviews, 3*, 3176–3184.

Compton, W. M., Conway, K. P., Stinson, F. S., & Grant, B. F. (2006). Changes in the prevalence of major depression and co-morbid substance use disorders in the United States between 1991–1992 and 2001–2002. *American Journal of Psychiatry, 163*, 2141–2147.

Dunn, A. L., Trivedi, M. H., Kampert, J. B., Clark, C. G., & Chambliss, H. O. (2002). The DOSE study: A clinical trial to examine efficacy and dose response of exercise as treatment for depression. *Controlled Clinical Trials, 23*, 584–603.

Dunn, A. L., Trivedi, M.H., Kampert, J. B., Clark, C. G., & Chambliss, H. O. (2005). Exercise treatment for depression: Efficacy and dose response. *American Journal of Preventive Medicine, 28*, 1–8.

Gaynes, B. N., Rush, A. J., Trivedi, M. H., Wisniewski, S. R., Spencer, D., & Fava, M. (2008). The STAR*D study: Treating depression in the real world. *Cleveland Clinic Journal of Medicine, 75*, 57–66.

Glowacki, S. P., Martin, S. E., Maurer, A., Baek, W., Green, J. S., & Crouse, S. F. (2004). Effects of resistance, endurance, and concurrent exercise on training outcomes in men. *Medicine and Science in Sports and Exercise, 36*, 2119–2127.

Heath, J. M., & Stuart, M. R. (2002). Prescribing exercise for frail elders. *The Journal of American Board of Family Practice, 15*, 218–228.

Kessler, R. C., Berglund, P., Demler, O., Jin, R., Koretz, D., Merikangas, K. R., et al. (2003). National Comorbidity Survey Replication. The epidemiology of major depressive disorder: Results from the National Comorbidity Survey Replication (NCS-R). *JAMA, 289*(23), 3095–3105.

Kirsch, I., Deacon, B. J., Huedo-Medina, T. B., Scoboria, A., Moore, T. J., & Johnson, B. T. (2008). Initial severity and antidepressant benefits: A metaanalysis of data submitted to the Food and Drug Administration. *PLoS Medicine, 5*(2): e45. doi:10.1371/journal.pmed.0050045

Knubben, K., Reischies, F. M., Adli, M., Schlattmann, P., Bauer, M., & Dimeo, F. (2007). A randomised, controlled study on the effects of a short-term endurance training programme in patients with major depression. *British Journal of Sports Medicine, 41*, 29–33.

Lane, A. M., & Lovejoy, D. J. (2001). The effects of exercise on mood changes: The moderating effect of depressed mood. *The Journal of Sports Medicine and Physical Fitness, 41*, 539–545.

Lawlor, D. A., & Hopker, S. W. (2001). The effectiveness of exercise as an intervention in the management of depression: Systematic review and meta-regression analysis of randomised controlled trials. *British Medical Journal, 322*, 763–767.

Lett, H. S., Davidson, J., & Blumenthal, J. A. (2005). Nonpharmacologic treatments for depression in patients with coronary heart disease. *Psychosomatic Medicine, 67*(Suppl. 1), S58–S62.

Manger, T. A., & Motta, R. W. (2005). The impact of an exercise program on posttraumatic stress disorder, anxiety, and depression. *International Journal of Emergency Mental Health, 7*, 49–57.

Maha, N., & Shaw, A. (2007). Academic doctors' views of complementary and alternative medicine (CAM) and its role within the NHS: An exploratory qualitative study. *BMC Complementary and Alternative Medicine, 7*, 17.

Martinsen, E. W., Hoffart, A., & Solberg, O. (1989). Comparing aerobic with nonaerobic forms of exercise in the treatment of clinical depression: A randomized trial. *Comprehensive Psychiatry, 30*, 324–331.

Martinsen, E. W. (1994). Physical activity and depression: Clinical experience. *Acta Psychiatrica Scandinavica Supplementum, 377*, 23–27.

Mead, G. E., Morley, W., Campbell, P., Greig, C. A., McMurdo, M., & Lawlor, D. A. (2008). Exercise for depression. *Cochrane Database of Systematic Reviews, 4*, CD004366.

Melartin, T. K., Rytsala, H. J., Leskela, U. S., Lestela-Mielonen, P. S., Sokero, T. P., & Isometsa, E. T. (2005). Continuity is the main challenge in treating major depressive disorder in psychiatric care. *Journal of Clinical Psychiatry, 66*(2), 220–227.

Nabkasorn, C., Miyai, N., Sootmongkol, A., Junprasert, S., Yamamoto, H., Arita, M., et al. (2006). Effects of physical exercise on depression, neuroendocrine stress hormones and physiological fitness in adolescent females with depressive symptoms. *European Journal of Public Health, 16,* 179–184.

Newman, C. L., & Motta, R. W. (2007). The effects of aerobic exercise on childhood PTSD, anxiety, and depression. *International Journal of Emergency Mental Health, 9,* 133–158.

Pierce, E. F., & Pate, D. W. (1994). Mood alterations in older adults following acute exercise. *Perceptual and Motor Skills, 79*(1 Pt 1), 191–194.

Pilu, A., Sorba, M., Hardoy, M. C., Floris, A. L., Mannu, F., Seruis, M. L., et al. (2007). Efficacy of physical activity in the adjunctive treatment of major depressive disorders: Preliminary results. *Clinical Practice and Epidemiology in Mental Health, 3,* 8.

Prochaska, J. O., & Diclemente, C. C. (1982). Transtheoretical therapy. Toward a more integrative model of change. *Psychoterapy: Theory, Research and Practice, 19,* 276–288.

Ransford, C. P. (1982). A role for amines in the antidepressant effect of exercise: A review. *Medicine and Science in Sports and Exercise, 14,* 1–10.

Singh, N. A., Clements, K. M., & Fiatarone, M. A. (1997). A randomized controlled trial of progressive resistance training in depressed elders. *The Journals of Gerontology. Series A, Biological and Medical Sciences, 52,* M27–M35.

Thorén, P., Floras, J. S., Hoffmann, P., & Seals, D. R. (1990). Endorphins and exercise: Physiological mechanisms and clinical implications. *Medicine and Science in Sports and Exercise, 22,* 417–428.

Trivedi, M. H., Greer, T. L., Grannemann, B. D., Chambliss, H. O., & Jordan, A. N. (2006). Exercise as an augmentation strategy for treatment of major depression. *Journal of Psychiatric Practice, 12,* 205–213.

Trivedi, M. H., Greer, T. L., Grannemann, B. D., Church, T. S., Galper, D. I., Sunderajan, P., et al. (2006). TREAD: Treatment with Exercise Augmentation for Depression: Study rationale and design. *Clinical Trials, 3,* 291–305.

Trivedi, M. H., Rush, A. J., Wisniewski, S. R., Nierenberg, A. A., Warden, D., Ritz, L., et al. STAR*D Study Team. (2006). Evaluation of outcomes with citalopram for depression using measurement-based care in STAR*D: implications for clinical practice. *American Journal of Psychiatry,63,* 28–40.

Turner, E. H., Matthews, A. M., Linardatos, E., Tell, R. A., & Rosenthal, R. (2008). Selective publication of antidepressant trials and its influence on apparent efficacy. *New England Journal of Medicine, 358*(3), 252–260.

Umpierre, D., & Stein, R. (2007). Hemodynamic and vascular effects of resistance training: Implications for cardiovascular disease. *Arquivos Brasileiros de Cardiologia, 89,* 256–262.

Wallberg-Henriksson, H., Rincon, J., & Zierath, J. R. (1998). Exercise in the management of non-insulin-dependent diabetes mellitus. *Sports Medicine, 25,* 25–35.

Zimmerman, G. L., Olsen, C. G., & Bosworth, M. F. (2000). A 'stages of change' approach to helping patients change behavior. *American Family Physician, 61,* 1409–1416.

3

The Use of Nutritional Supplements in Psychiatric Practice

JOEL S. EDMAN AND DANIEL A. MONTI

KEY CONCEPTS

- Nutritional supplementation may have a role in psychiatric practice.
- Nutritional supplements may influence nervous system functioning through a variety of mechanisms, including neurotransmitter synthesis and activity; nerve cell membrane structure, fluidity, and function; cellular and mitochondrial energy production and support; cellular second messenger synthesis and activity; effects on HPA axis function; and others.
- A nutritional supplement program that includes multiple functionally interrelated nutrients will likely be more effective than individual nutrients.
- There is some research to support the relationship between specific nutritional supplements and psychiatric disorders, however, many recommendations are anecdotal and come from clinical experience.
- A comprehensive evaluation is needed in order to provide a thoughtfully tailored nutritional program.
- The potential benefits of nutritional supplementation will more likely be seen when combined with a foundational healthy diet, as well as other integrative medicine modalities, such as exercise/physical fitness, and relaxation and stress management techniques.
- More research is needed to clarify the influence of nutritional supplements in specific psychiatric disorders, and to determine the most effective nutritional supplement (and dietary) approaches to recommend.

■

Introduction

Nutritional supplementation may be a potentially useful adjunct to the management of the psychiatric patient. This chapter will build on the principles presented in the dietary chapter, with the goal of optimizing nutritional status and related physiological function, which relies on a foundation of a healthy, nutrient dense diet that is combined with targeted nutritional supplementation. A broad perspective that incorporates a range of different types of data is taken, particularly given the significant limitations of nutritional supplement research, much of which has major methodological weaknesses.

An estimated 50–55 percent of Americans take supplements (Radimer et al., 2004) and a recent estimate has suggested that supplement sales have increased to more than $23 billion per year (NIH, 2006). It is important for physicians to know what their patients are taking, the potential interactions with medications, and contraindications that should be considered and discussed. It is equally important to know what, if any, supplements may be making a positive contribution to the health status of patients.

Given the gaps between available data and clinical therapy, the use of nutritional supplements in clinical care relies to some degree on practice philosophy and orientation. For complementary and alternative medicine (CAM) practitioners as well as many integrative medicine physicians, supplements are a part of the framework of natural approaches that include diet, exercise, stress management, and other modalities.

There are several reasons supplements may be a beneficial adjunct for particular patients, including those with poor diet or gastrointestinal issues that may limit absorption of nutrients from food. Other issues include variations in soil nutritional content, micronutrient losses from food processing and cooking, and genetic polymorphisms or variations in individual nutrient requirements (Oakley, 1998).

The primary legislation that regulates all aspects of supplements, including manufacturing, quality control, labeling, and marketing, is The Dietary Supplement Health and Education Act (DSHEA) passed by Congress in 1994. The most important aspect of the legislation is that "dietary supplements" are regulated as food and are therefore not subject to the same FDA scrutiny as pharmaceuticals. Under DSHEA, manufacturers may distribute supplements without demonstrating safety and efficacy, as long as they do not make any health claims regarding specific diseases. The result is that there is a large range of supplements that practitioners may recommend or that patients may try on their own. We focus this discussion on those supplements that have some basis in data and are commonly used.

Patients and practitioners largely have the burden of identifying good products with adequate quality assurance procedures to insure that the contents listed on the supplement are accurate and that there is not environmental or processing contamination. Although most manufacturers make this information available and the NIH Office of Dietary Supplements (also established by DSHEA) can be helpful with this issue and other dietary supplement related information, it can be challenging to identify products that are manufactured with consistent quality standards.

ORTHOMOLECULAR PSYCHIATRY

There is a long history of nutritional supplement use in the treatment of psychiatric disorders from the Orthomolecular Psychiatry and Medicine movement. "Orthomolecular Medicine," as conceptualized by double-Nobel Laureate Linus Pauling, "aims to restore the optimum environment of the body by correcting imbalances or deficiencies based on individual biochemistry using substances natural to the body such as vitamins, minerals, amino acids, trace elements, and essential fatty acids." This was first presented by Dr. Pauling in the peer-reviewed journal, *Science,* in 1968 (Pauling, 1968).

Controversy and antagonism evolved regarding orthomolecular psychiatry and medicine, perhaps due to the conflicting model of healthcare and associated treatment modalities utilized at the time. For example, a 1973 APA taskforce issued a report, "Megavitamins and Orthomolecular Therapy in Psychiatry" (Lipton et al., 1973), rejecting the concept. Although there has been more research conducted and a better understanding of potential benefits of nutritional supplementation, there are important gaps in the data that make clear recommendations for supplements in psychiatric practice a challenge.

APPROACH TO RESEARCH AND EVIDENCE-BASE
FOR NUTRITIONAL SUPPLEMENTATION

There are a few models to explain how supplements can benefit a patient population, including (a) nutritional deficiency, (b) subclinical nutritional deficiency, (c) biological response modifiers, and (d) mass action effects (Ames, Elson-Schwab, & Silver, 2002).

Overt nutritional deficiency is well defined and most often utilized in medical and nutritional practice and research. Classic examples are iron and vitamin

B12 deficiencies that produce clinical symptoms, can be identified through laboratory analyses, and supplemented to monitor for symptom and assay changes.

More challenging is the evaluation of the other three research models in which there may be varying levels of supportive evidence from in vitro, animal, and clinical research. For example, a "subclinical magnesium deficiency" is the reason why many integrative medicine practitioners recommend magnesium despite normal serum or red blood cell magnesium levels (Olerich & Rude, 1994). Magnesium is a cofactor for over three hundred enzymes and is a calcium channel blocker. Research supports the influence of magnesium in glucose tolerance and diabetes, migraine headaches, hypertension, hormonal balance, allergies, muscle cramps, constipation, neurocognitive function, and possibly other disorders (Swain & Kaplan-Machlis, 1999; Ueshima, 2005). Because magnesium is often inadequate in the diet and can be depleted by chronic disease, it is often prescribed by integrative healthcare providers to help address a range of symptoms.

Omega-3 fatty acids, or fish oil supplements, are a good example of supplements that have biological response modifier effects. These supplements can enhance dietary influences and can effectively alter the synthesis of pro-inflammatory versus anti-inflammatory eicosansoids. Omega-3 fatty acids are potentially beneficial in a number of disorders due to their anti-inflammatory effects, and their impact on cellular membrane fluidity and function because of its effect on membrane fatty acid composition (Yehuda, Rabinovitz, & Mostofsky, 2005). There is no established nutritional status measure, although some studies have quantified blood levels and RBC membrane levels of specific omega-3 fatty acids or omega-3 to omega-6 fatty acid ratios (Tiemeier, Van Tuijl, Hofman, Kiliaan, & Breteler, 2003). Magnesium and omega-3 fatty acids are two good examples (among many) of important nutritional factors in which there are not accurate nutritional status measures available. This lack of effective assessment measures makes it much more difficult to conduct research that can quantify the effects of supplement recommendations.

With regard to "mass action" effects, a review by Ames and colleagues outlines the reported biochemical influences of high-dose vitamins on enzyme binding and activity in as many as 50 genetic diseases and many genetic polymorphisms (Ames et al., 2002). Further research is needed to elucidate the potential role of identifying SNPs and utilizing specific nutrients to influence how they are expressed.

Despite the challenges presented, the wealth of overall basic science and clinical data suggests a potential role for dietary supplementation, assuming a reliable source of products is identified. Table 3.1 describes an effective framework from which supplements can be recommended.

Table 3.1. Framework for Recommending Supplements.

Healthy diet as a foundation

Evidence base that includes a sound rationale and mechanism

Positive benefit-to-risk ratio

Defined dose and time frame to assess effects

Targeted populations to treat, such as: (a) patients with adverse or inadequate responses to medication; (b) patients or families who would like to try nutrition and/or natural therapies as part of their health care approach; or (c) vulnerable populations who may have inadequate dietary nutrient intake

Nutritional Supplements in Psychiatry

This section will present an overview of the most evidence-based nutrients and supplements that are recommended in clinical practice, as well as aspects of the rationale and evidence that supports their use. For most nutrients, definitive data is lacking, particularly in regard to treating a specific disorder. The focus is nutrient supplementation for a psychiatric practice.

VITAMINS

It is well accepted that vitamins, especially B complex vitamins, have an important influence on nervous system functioning. Although classic deficiencies of the B vitamins lead to disorders such as beriberi and Wernicke-Korsakoff Syndrome (thiamine), and pellagra (niacin), that affect brain function, this discussion is more about (a) the concepts of mild clinical and subclinical nutrient deficiency; (b) an evaluation of reasonable nutrient supplementation for functional effects (e.g., through biological response modification and mass action effects); and (c) thoughtful discussion about the rationale of combinations of nutritional supplements, as well as nutrient-augmented psychopharmacology.

Table 3.2, adapted from a recent review of important vitamin effects, lists known brain functions of selected vitamins (Kaplan, Crawford, Field, & Simpson, 2007). Of the vitamins included, vitamin B12 and folate have the most well-documented influences in psychiatry, but it is also important to note that they have interrelated biochemical and functional effects.

Vitamin B12 or cobalamin deficiency can produce a range of psychiatric symptoms including depression, irritability, mania, confusion, delusions, psychosis, and others (Hector & Burton, 1988). The two primary mechanisms

Table 3.2. Known Brain Functions of Selected Vitamins.

• Folate	• Can heighten serotonin function by slowing destruction of brain tryptophan (Cousens, 2000) • Functions as a cofactor for enzymes that convert tryptophan into serotonin, and for enzymes that convert tyrosine into norepinephrine/noradrenalin (Cousens, 2000) • Contributes to the formation of compounds involved in brain energy metabolism (Selhub, Bagley, Miller, & Rosenberg, 2000) • Involved in the synthesis of the monoamine neurotranmitters (Hutto, 1997) and in serotonin, dopamine, and noradrenergic systems (Bottiglieri et al., 2000)
• Cobalamin (Vitamin B12)	• Involved in synthesis of monoamine neurotransmitters (Hutto, 1997) • Involved in maintaining myelin sheaths on nerves for normal nerve conductance • Functions in folate metabolism; hence, deficiency can result in a secondary folate deficiency
• Thiamine (Vitamin B1)	• Functions as a coenzyme involved in the synthesis of acetylcholine, GABA, and glutamate (Bell et al., 1992) • Can mimic action of acetylcholine in the brain (Meador et al., 1993)
• Pyridoxine (Vitamin B6)	• Plays a basic role in synthesis of many neurotransmitters (dopamine, serotonin, norepinephrine, epinephrine, histamine, GABA); for example, serves as a cofactor for an enzyme involved in the last step in the synthesis of serotonin (Baldewicz et al., 2000) • Deficiency tends to selectively reduce brain production of serotonin and GABA (McCarty, 2000)
• Vitamin E	• Protects cell membranes from damage by free radicals (Berdanier, 1998) • May play a role in reducing brain amyloid beta peptide accumulation, known to be relevant in Alzheimer's disease (Muñoz, Solé, & Coma, 2005)
• Choline	• Plays essential roles in structural integrity of cell membranes, cell signaling (precursor to acetylcholine), and nerve impulse transmission; also is a major source of methyl groups for methylation reactions (Zeisel, 2000)

Adapted from Kaplan, B. J., Field, C. J., Crawford, S. G., & Simpson, J. S. A. (2007). Vitamins, minerals, and mood. *Psychological Bulletin, 133*(5), 747–760.

thought to be involved are methylation pathways that lead to neurotransmitter synthesis and function, and effects on neuronal myelinization. Susceptibility to clinical deficiency is increased with malabsorption or Inflammatory Bowel Disease (especially Crohn's Disease), vegan and vegetarian diets, and age-related factors, such as poor dietary choices, poor appetite, and hypochlorhydria. Deficiency effects may also occur in the absence of classical biomarker abnormalities, such as overtly low serum B12 and macrocytic anemia (Lindenbaum et al., 1988).

Since vitamin B12 deficiency can contribute to a wide variety of psychiatric symptoms and disorders, such as depression, mania, confusion, and psychosis, vitamin B12 could be tested in all psychiatric patients. Another approach would be to test B12 in patients if there is any question that it may be low, or if there is no apparent cause for the onset of the symptoms.

The most common form of vitamin B12 supplement is cyanocobalamin. Many integrative medicine practitioners believe that the methylcobalamin or hydroxycobalamin forms are better utilized, but there is no substantive evidence at this point to support that notion. Although there is some evidence that methylcobalamin can have beneficial effects for pain and parasthesia in diabetic neuropathy (Sun, Lai, & Lu, 2005), there does not appear to be any data comparing cyanocobalamin to methylcobalamin, especially in neuropsychiatric disorders. Some integrative medicine practitioners also recommend injectable or intravenous methyl-B12 as an alternative to oral supplementation.

Metabolically related to vitamin B12, folate is also an essential nutrient for nervous system function, with several research models implicating its significant influence in depression. Evidence suggests that (a) lower levels of folate are associated with depressive symptoms (Alpert, Mischoulon, Nierenberg, & Fava, 2000); (b) folate deficiency may be associated with worse treatment response (Fava et al., 1997); (c) folate supplementation may augment antidepressant pharmacotherapy (Alpert et al., 2002); and (d) elevated levels of homocysteine, which may be considered a functional deficiency of folate, may be related to depression (Folstein et al., 2007).

A particularly important folate-dependent reaction involves methyl-tetra-hydro-folate (MTHF) for the methylation and metabolism of homocysteine to form methionine; vitamin B12 is a cofactor for this enzymatic reaction. Methionine is, in turn, converted to S-adenosyl-methionine (SAMe), which is described below for its antidepressive effects and is involved in a range of important methylation reactions.

Folate is significantly inversely correlated with homocysteine levels, which may be a marker of inadequate methylation capacity for neurotransmitter synthesis. A recent review article also discusses the homocysteine hypothesis of depression (Folstein et al., 2007), again suggesting the association of elevated homocysteine with neurotransmitter deficiency, cerebral vascular disease, and depressed mood. Research is also increasingly finding elevated levels of homocysteine in a range of chronic, inflammatory, and/or aging-related disorders such as Parkinson's disease, RA, SLE, and IBD, which raises an interesting question about the interrelationship between homocysteine metabolism and inflammation.

Other B complex vitamins such as thiamine (B1), riboflavin (B2), niacin (B3), pantothenic acid (B5), and pyridoxine (B6) have important roles in nervous system functioning. For example, thiamine is important for acetylcholine production and cognitive function. A recent review documents a range of thiamine-dependent processes associated with neurological function and cognition, including oxidative stress, protein metabolism, peroxisomal functions, and genetic expression (Gibson & Blass, 2007).

Pyridoxine has most often been associated with depression, although the evidence is conflicting (Williams et al., 2005). A meta-analysis in premenstrual syndrome (PMS), however, found that B6 was beneficial for symptoms which included depression (Wyatt, Dimmock, Jones, & O'Brien, 1999). Riboflavin is a cofactor for converting vitamin B6 to its active form, pyridoxal 5 phospate, and is involved with flavoenzymes in the oxidative phosphorylation chain that produces mitochondrial energy in the form of ATP (Depeint, Bruce, Shangari, Mehta, & O'Brien, 2006). Pantothenic acid or pantethine is also important in energy production, since it is central to coenzyme A synthesis and the energy yielding processes of the mitochondrial Krebs cycle.

Nicotinic acid or niacin (vitamin B3) has been recommended as a treatment for schizophrenia (Hoffer & Osmond, 1964), although the concept has not been formally tested. Niacin and all of the B complex vitamins are reviewed in detail in a recent paper that outlines the important role of B complex vitamins on mitochondrial energy metabolism, function, and toxicity (Depeint et al., 2006). This could be an interesting direction for future research because there have been numerous studies evaluating the relationship between mitochondrial abnormalities in neurological disorders, and this is now a topic of investigation in psychiatry (Shao et al., 2008).

Vitamin D is another recent research topic in psychiatry, and there is significant prevalence of vitamin D deficiency in North America and worldwide (Hollick & Chen, 2008). Studies have shown significant improvement in mood from supplementing vitamin D in patients with seasonal affective disorder (SAD), which is logical since there is a seasonal variability in sun exposure and intensity which correlates with vitamin D levels (Lansdowne & Provost, 1998) (Dumville et al., 2006). Research also suggests that vitamin D is important for insulin sensitivity that may be associated with carbohydrate craving (Tai, Need, Horowitz, & Chapman, 2008), in addition to its well-known influence on calcium metabolism (an important cellular signaling mechanism) and immune function (Hollick & Chen, 2008).

Vitamin E effects on nervous system functioning are largely through protective influences on nerve cell membranes from oxidative stress. In tardive dyskinesia, supplementation with 1200 IU of vitamin E for 12 weeks was found to significantly reduce involuntary movement (Zhang et al., 2004). The recent controversy regarding the safety of tocopherols has led many practitioners to decrease doses recommended and to reinforce the importance of using mixed tocopherols and tocotrienols (Bjelakovic, Nikolova, Gluud, Simonetti, & Gluud, 2007). There have not been significant influences seen in other neuropsychiatric disorders (Berman & Brodaty, 2004).

Choline appears to influence several important nervous system functions including cell membrane structure, methylation, and cell signaling/neuronal impulse transmission. A Cochrane review of one form of choline, cytidine diphosphocholine (CDP-choline), concluded that there was a significant effect on short-to-medium term memory and behavior (Fioravanti & Yanagi, 2005). A well-designed study of lithium-treated bipolar patients (rapid cycling type) supplemented with choline found that there was a significant decrease in brain purine levels, suggesting that the choline may increase cell membrane phospholipid/phosphotidyl choline synthesis, which could improve energy status associated with ATP demand and mitochondrial dysfunction (Lyoo, Demopulos, Hirashima, Ahn, & Renshaw, 2003).

MINERALS

Some important mineral influences on brain function are listed in Table 3.3.

Magnesium may be one of the most important minerals that can influence nervous system functioning; however, the specific mechanisms involved are not well understood. It is a cofactor for over 300 enzymes in the body, including ATP synthesis. It is also one of the most common nutrients that can be overtly or subclinically deficient (due to poor diet, chronic disease, and other factors), eventhough there is not convincing data to support that assertion.

There is a range of research that has tied magnesium to nervous system disorders such as headaches/migraines (Mazzotta, Sarchielli, Alberti, & Gallai, 1999), seizures, and brain injury (Wong, Chan, Poon, Boet, & Gin, 2006). In migraine research, there is evidence of low levels of magnesium in migraine patients (Trauninger, Pfund, Koszegi, & Czopf, 2002), as well as supplementation research suggesting that magnesium can prevent migraines (Piekert, Wilimzig, & Kohne-Volland, 1996). Also, magnesium has been suggested

Table 3.3. Known Brain Functions of Selected Minerals.

• Magnesium	• Functions as a coenzyme; plays important role in the metabolism of carbohydrates and fats to produce ATP, and in the synthesis of nucleic acids (DNA and RNA) and proteins • Important for the active transport of ions (such as potassium and calcium) across cell membranes, and for cell signaling • Essential for more than 300 biochemical reactions in the body, including maintenance of normal nerve function (Wester, 1987)
• Zinc	• The most abundant intracellular trace element, with roles extending into protein synthesis, as well as structure and regulation of gene expression (Kuby, 1994) (Milne, 2000) • Cofactor for over 200 different enzymes; present in over 300 metalloenzymes involved in virtually all aspects of metabolism (Milne, 2000) • In the brain, serves in neurons and glial cells. Certain zinc-enriched regions (e.g., the hippocampus) are especially responsive to dietary zinc deprivation, which causes brain dysfunctions, such as learning impairment and olfactory dysfunction (Takeda, 2001)
• Iron	• Essential cofactor for the production of ATP energy in the brain • Plays an essential role in hemoglobin, ensuring there is sufficient oxygen in the brain for oxidative metabolism • Functions in the enzyme system involved in the production of serotonin, norepinephrine, epinephrine, and dopamine; for example, it is a cofactor in the metabolism of tyrosine to dopamine (Cousens, 2000) • Increases the binding of dopamine and serotonin to serotonin binding proteins in frontal cortex (Velez-Pardo, Jimenez Del Rio, Ebinger, & Vauquelin, 1995)

Adapted from Kaplan, B. J., Field, C. J., Crawford, S. G., & Simpson, J. S. A. (2007). Vitamins, minerals and mood. *Psychological Bulletin, 133*(5), 747–760.

as a mediator of vascular tone and neuronal excitability (Mazzotta et al., 1999).

Although there has been some research that has looked at magnesium in depression, for example, the results have been mixed. Some research suggests that magnesium would enhance limbic-hypothalamus-pituitary-adrenocortical function because it can suppress hippocampal kindling and reduce ACTH release (Murck, 2002). Research of magnesium status in major depression, however, has either found no differences between patients and controls, or higher blood magnesium levels (Widmer, Henrotte, et al., 1995). One explanation could be an enhanced sodium–magnesium exchange in erythrocytes of depressed patients (Widmer, Feray, et al., 1995). Significant challenges in this research are the poor magnesium status measures and the inadequate understanding of specific mechanisms involved. Other research suggests that magnesium is an N-methyl D-aspartate receptor agonist (Felsby, Nielsen, Arendt-Nielsen, & Jensen, 1996) and is inversely associated with inflammation (Mazur et al., 2007). Hence, it seems reasonable for the practicing psychiatrist to consider adequate magnesium in the diet and even moderate supplementation, though no data currently supports megadoses.

Zinc is similar to magnesium in that it is a cofactor for over 200 enzymes in the body, and there is not a great marker of zinc nutritional status. A recent review of zinc influences in depression suggests that the trace mineral is an antagonist of glutamate/N-methyl D-aspartate (NMDA) receptors and has antidepressant-like effects in animal models of depression (Nowak, Szewczyk, & Pilc, 2005). There have been no confirmatory human studies. In addition to being found in high levels in the hippocampus, zinc also modulates brain-derived neurotrophic factor gene expression.

While there is some clinical data to support an association between zinc and depression, there is not data to support the use of zinc as an antidepressant. In addition, since data is lacking regarding optimal zinc levels for depressed patients, the practicing psychiatrist might consider suggesting that patients have adequate zinc intake as part of the overall dietary and nutritional recommendations given.

There are other minerals in which there is some research supporting a significant influence in nervous system function and psychiatry including: (a) iron—see Table 3.3; (b) chromium—can mediate glucose tolerance and may be helpful for dysthymic disorder (McLeod, Gaynes, & Golden, 1999); and (c) selenium—has important antioxidant effects and thyroid function influences, including conversion of T4 to T3 (Papp, Lu, Holmgren, & Khanna, 2007). This may be important for energy level and metabolism associated with thyroid function, as well as antioxidant effects that could be protective of oxidative damage to nerve cells associated with aging and other factors. There are still other minerals and vitamins not mentioned in the previous section in which there may be influences in nervous system function, such as calcium, manganese, and vitamin C, but significant clinical data is lacking for supplementation beyond US DRI guidelines.

A final important point to make regarding minerals is that mineral status may have an important influence on heavy metal exposure and toxicity. Both animal and human research has found that iron deficiency is associated with increased blood lead levels (Wright, Tsaih, Schwartz, Wright, & Hu, 2003). Although zinc has received less attention, evidence supports zinc's role in blocking lead absorption and possibly impairing lead-mediated effects (Brewer, Hill, & Dick,

1985). Other investigators have questioned whether magnesium deficiency or sub-clinical deficiency could also contribute to susceptibility to heavy metal toxicity (Soldatovic et al., 2002). Although not well identified or understood, this is potentially important because of the influence that lead and other heavy metals may have on development and neurotoxicity in children and adults (Wasserman, Liu, Factor-Litvak, Gardner, Graziano, 2008).

MULTIPLE VITAMIN/MINERAL INFLUENCES AND NUTRIENT AUGMENTED PSYCHOPHARMACOLOGY

There is an increasing amount of investigation around the notion that supplementing multiple interrelated nutrients at one time and/or nutrient augmented psychotropic medication will more likely produce more benefits. The current available data is limited, and has been taken from correlational research and from nutritional or formula supplementation studies (Kaplan et al., 2007).

One investigation (Bell et al., 1990) showed that a group of consecutive psychiatric admissions with below median (but normal) blood levels of vitamin B12 and folate had significantly lower mini-mental state scores than subjects higher in one or both nutrients. A subsequent double-blind placebo-controlled study of geriatric inpatients with depression by the same research group found that 10 mg of vitamins B1, B2, and B6 (modest amounts) seemed to augment tricyclic antidepressant treatment effects (Bell et al., 1992).

In research on major depression, it was suggested that lower baseline blood folate levels were associated with a poorer response to fluoxetine (Fava et al., 1997) and, as previously presented, folate appeared to augment SSRI refractory depression (Alpert et al., 2002). In another study, unstable mood in children was shown to benefit from a 36-ingredient formula of relative high amounts of vitamins and minerals (Kaplan, Fisher, Crawford, Field, & Kolb, 2004).

OMEGA-3 FATTY ACIDS

The use of omega-3 fatty acids, particularly eicosapentenoic acid (EPA) and docosahexenoic acid (DHA), is likely beneficial for a range of neuropsychiatric disorders. In mood and depressive disorders, where much of the research has been done, the evidence for significant influences comes from a range of different study models, including dietary intake studies (Tanskanen et al., 2001), nutritional status (e.g., RBC omega-3 fatty acids and/or membrane omega-3:omega-6 fatty acid levels) correlational research (Kilkens, Honig, Maes, Lousberg, & Brummer, 2004), and supplementation investigations (Lin & Su, 2007). The common source of EPA and DHA is fish oil. Some plants such as flax and hemp are sources of alpha linolenic acid, a fatty acid that can convert into EPA and DHA. Most currently available data is on EPA and DHA from cold water fish.

A recent meta-analysis suggested that omega-3 fatty acids had significant antidepressant effects (Lin & Su, 2007). Studies included in this analysis used either EPA alone or EPA and DHA. The authors found that high-dose EPA (> 4 g/day) was significantly more effective than placebo, but not significantly more than the middle-dose (2 g/day) or low-dose (1 g/day) EPA.

Research also supports the use of omega-3 fatty acids as adjuvant therapy. In one study of 20 recurrent unipolar depressed patients on maintenance medication, four weeks of EPA at 2 g/day produced significant improvements in Hamilton depression scores (Nemets, Stahl, & Belmaker, 2002). In another randomized, double-blind, placebo-controlled study of adjuvant treatment in bipolar depression, EPA supplementation (1 or 2 g/day) for 12 weeks produced significant improvement in Hamilton depressions scores and global clinical measures (Frangou, Lewis, & McCrone, 2006).

There is also some further anecdotal support for using fish oils in the treatment of resistant depression (Puri, Counsell, Richardson, & Horrobin, 2002), bipolar depression (Chiu, Huang, Chen, & Su, 2005), major depression during pregnancy (Chiu, Huang, Shen, & Su, 2003), and postpartum depression (Freeman et al., 2006). It is noted that much of this literature is small pilot studies or case reports that require further research. Another recent double-blind, placebo-controlled trial of major depression found that low-to-moderate supplementation with DHA alone produced significant improvement (Mischoulon et al., 2008).

Although not well studied, the likely mechanism involved is the influence that these fatty acids have on cell membrane composition, fluidity, and function. Another possibility is effects on eicosanoid metabolism (prostaglandins, leukotrienes, and thromboxanes) and inflammation. As described previously, magnesium and zinc are important metabolic cofactors in fatty acid pathways.

AMINO ACIDS

S-adenosyl-methionine (SAMe) is an amino acid that is the major donor of methyl groups needed in the synthesis of monoamine neurotransmitters (dopamine, norepinephrine, and serotonin) and membranes, and is equally distributed throughout the brain (Baldassarini, 1998). It is made from a yeast fermentation process. A review of SAMe in major depressive disorder (MDD) suggests that there is extensive research spanning three decades to support its use (Papakostas, Alpert, & Fava, 2003). Although the exact mechanism is unknown, research suggests that SAMe can transfer a methyl group to membrane-bound phosphotidylethanolamine to produce phosphotidylcholine promoting membrane fluidity and function.

Although the data set on SAM-e is small and inconclusive, some interesting findings have been reported. In one study of partial or nonresponse to SSRIs or venlafaxine, SAMe supplementation produced a 50% response rate and 43% remission rate (Alpert et al., 2004). An interesting metabolic study of SAMe infusions administered by IV in healthy elderly patients showed that there were significant changes in EEG mapping and psychometry typical of antidepressants (Saletu et al., 2002). Controlled clinical trials of SAMe have generally given 800–1600 mg/day in divided doses.

Tryptophan and 5-hydroxytrophan (5-HTP) are amino acid precursors of the neurotransmitter serotonin. A Cochrane review of tryptophan and 5-HTP supplementation for depression concluded that available evidence suggested that it is beneficial for depression, eventhough further studies are required (Shaw, Turner, & Del Mar, 2002). It is notable that of the 108 trials identified in their search, only two were of sufficient quality to be considered reliable and therefore included in the analysis. Evidence suggests that tryptophan is converted to 5HTP in the body, which in turn is metabolized to serotonin, both peripherally and centrally, which may produce antidepressant effects (Lader & Herrington, 1981).

The use of tryptophan was discontinued for a time with the outbreak of eosinophil-myalgia syndrome (EMS) in 1989 and 1990 (Blackburn, 1997). A subsequent investigation found that this resulted from a contaminant in the microorganism-synthesized amino acid produced by a Japanese manufacturer, although there does still appear to be some controversy about this (Klarskov, Johnson, & Benson, 1999). The result of this situation is that there is a greater use of 5-HTP than tryptophan, although both are serotonin precursors, and more research and/or information is clearly needed.

Another important amino acid that has been examined in neuropsychiatric research is acetyl-L-carnitine, a form of "L-carnitine." A review of acetyl-L-carnitine (ALC) suggests that there are multiple potential benefits, including: (a) nervous system energy production (ATP) and phospholipid metabolism; (b) neuronal macromolecule effects for neurotrophic factors and neurohormones; and (c) synapse morphology and signal transduction (Pettegrew, Levine, & McClure, 2000). A subsequent pilot study by the same research group found that ALC was beneficial in geriatric depression (Pettegrew et al., 2002). In another study, a double-blind, randomized, controlled trial of ALC (500 mg bid) versus amisulpride (50 mg qid) in 204 patients with dysthymia, researchers found that both treatment groups improved significantly, with the ALC group having greater tolerability (Zanardi & Smeraldi, 2006).

Research has also found that ALC may be helpful for a range of other disorders, such as fatigue, ADHD, and pain. One recent study of elderly patients with fatigue showed that ALC supplementation had significant benefit (Malaguarnera et al., 2008), while another pilot study comparing ALC with amantadine for fatigue of MS, suggested that the ALC was more effective and better tolerated (Tomassini et al., 2004). With regard to ADHD, one recent DBPC multicenter study showed that ALC supplementation was associated with improvement in ADHD in Fragile X Syndrome boys (Torrioli et al., 2008), whereas another pilot study of just ADHD did not find a significant effect (Arnold et al., 2007). Finally, investigations of fibromyalgia (Rossini et al., 2007) and neuropathic pain from diabetes and HIV (Chiechio, Copani, Gereau, & Nicoletti, 2007) have shown that ALC may be of benefit.

OTHER SUPPLEMENTS

A recent review of inositol in psychiatric disorders suggests that there is support for its use as an adjunct to treating bipolar disorder, but the data is limited overall, and even more so for other psychiatric disorders (Kim, McGrath, & Silverstone, 2005). This is the case despite reports associating myo-inositol and the phosphotidyl-inositol second messenger signaling pathway with the pathophysiology and/or treatment of major depression, panic, obsessive compulsive disorder (OCD), eating disorders, and schizophrenia.

A brief report of inositol augmentation of lithium or valproate for bipolar depression (Evins et al., 2006), illustrates many of the issues that need to be considered in the use of inositol. Although four of the nine subjects on inositol (6–20 g/day based on tolerability) in this small study had >50% improvement in study citeria versus zero of eight on placebo ($p=0.053$), there was significant variability in the response. Two subjects on inositol had >50% worsening of criteria, three had no change, and four had >50% improvement.

Another nutritional supplement that targets cell membrane composition and function is phosphatidylserine. Although there is some animal and human research suggesting potential benefit for stress physiology (Hellhammer et al., 2004) and memory impairment (Jorissen et al., 2001), other research is negative, and there is not enough data to effectively evaluate whether it is clinically helpful or not, or in what circumstances (Amenta, Parnetti, Gallai, & Wallin, 2001).

The adrenal androgen, dihydroepiandosterone (DHEA), which has been recommended for depression, has been found to decrease with aging in both men and women. Research has also shown that depression is associated with alterations in DHEA secretion (both increased and decreased), so this supplement may influence HPA axis function (Yaffe et al., 1998).

In one study using DHEA as monotherapy, it was found that supplementation was beneficial for mid-life major and minor depression (Schmidt et al., 2005). This research was a 6 week DBPC crossover trial of 23 men and 23 women given 90 mg/day for 3 weeks and 450 mg/day for 3 weeks (and 6 weeks of placebo). The authors noted that they examined several markers of response (e.g., pre-treatment DHEA levels), but no measures predicted response. Other research has suggested that DHEA is beneficial for nonmajor depression associated with HIV/AIDS (Rabkin, McElhiney, Rabkin, McGrath, & Ferrando, 2006).

There may be many other nutrients or nutritional supplements that may be of benefit to psychiatric symptoms or disorders, but the research is not currently available. The challenge to conducting this type of research includes obtaining the kind of information clinicians need, such as (a) optimal nutrient form, dose, and duration of supplementation; (b) rationale and mechanism(s) of action; (c) reliable nutritional status measures and neuropsychiatric markers; and (d) clinical benefit assessment. These issues must be addressed with well-controlled trials and sufficient power to detect significant effects.

Practical Considerations

A solid nutritional foundation is an important aspect of Integrative Medicine philosophy, as are individualized assessment and care plans. A challenge with supplementation is that it often makes sense to do it, but the clinician is left to fill in the gaps where testing and research is lacking. Some rely on nutritional and functional testing, which is an interesting and controversial issue. Validated common testing would include serum vitamin B12, folate, and homocysteine, as well as other nutrient measures such as other B complex vitamin levels, 25 hydroxy vitamin D, and red blood cell (RBC) magnesium and zinc. Some tests commonly used by integrative medicine practitioners, but not well validated, are urinary panels for neurotransmitter metabolites, cellular metabolic profiles, fatty acid profiles, detoxification profiles, and others. While many practitioners may find these useful, their validity as clinical tools are yet to be determined.

With regard to nutritional supplementation, one approach is to recommend a foundational program that has reasonably good supportive data. Such a program might include a comprehensive multivitamin and mineral complex, omega-3 fatty acids/fish oil and a calcium/magnesium/zinc mineral supplement. Additional targeted supplements could be focused on antidepressive effects, anxiety, sleep, cellular energetics, and/or other aspects of a patient's circumstances. For example, if depression were the diagnosis, SAMe could be added on a trial basis to the foundation program, which would already include good quantities of B complex vitamins and folate in the multivitamin and mineral, and fish oil/omega-3s.

A final point to note is that there are potential nutrient–drug interactions to be aware of and monitor, although these interactions can be difficult to identify and quantify. For example, it is known that fish oil influences blood clotting ability, and patients are recommended to stop all fish oil one week prior to surgery. Other examples include high doses of folate possibly having adverse influences on sleep, seizure activity, and/ or gastrointestinal symptoms, as well as the potential for SAMe to produce nausea, flatulence, and diarrhea in some patients (Shneider & Lovett, 2007). Questions have also been raised about the potential use of tryptophan or 5-HTP in conjunction with antidepressant medication, which may increase the susceptibility to serotonin syndrome.

Future Research

Further research is needed to validate all aspects of nutritional supplement use in psychiatric practice, as well as to develop clinically effective treatment protocols. Some important methodological challenges include determining adequate levels of all nutrients, identifying biochemical, functional, and/or clinical markers that could assess significant influences, and controlling for a range of potentially confounding factors.

Probably one of the most important issues is how to best translate what is known in the basic sciences to the clinical setting, especially in regard to multiple interrelated influences from (a) nerve cell membrane composition and function from fatty acids, second messengers, and protective antioxidants; (b) neurotransmitter synthesis from precursor amino acids, vitamin/mineral cofactors and methylation pathways; (c) cellular metabolism and energetics; (d) stress physiology and HPA axis function; and (e) genetic polymorphism influences.

Summary and Conclusions

As this chapter describes, nutritional supplement recommendations that are part of an integrative medicine approach may play a role in psychiatric care. Nutrient and nutritional supplement influences on nervous system function and psychiatry is clearly an evolving area of research and understanding. An important first step in the use of nutritional supplements is a thorough history and physical evaluation that includes some laboratory testing. A variety of vitamins, minerals, fatty acids, amino acids, and other nutrients or nutritional supplements can influence nervous system functioning and some may possibly affect mood, anxiety, cognition, and a range of other psychological and/or comorbid symptoms or disorders. With regard to implementing a nutritional supplement program, it would be important to effectively develop a regimen and integrative medicine approach that could be evaluated periodically. Ongoing research and clinical experience should focus on understanding the influences of supplements on metabolic and functional biochemical variables that impact specific psychiatric disorders, as well as the most effective clinical protocols to recommend.

REFERENCES

Alpert, J. E., Mischoulon, D., Nierenberg, A. A., & Fava, M. (2000). Nutrition and depression: Focus on folate. *Nutrition, 16,* 544–546.

Alpert, J. E., Mischoulon, D., Rubenstein, G. E. F., Bottonari, K., Nierenberg, A. A., & Fava, M. (2002). Folinic acid (leucovorin) as an adjunctive treatment for SSRI-refractory depression. *Annals of Clinical Psychiatry, 14*(1); 33–38.

Alpert, J. E., Papakostas G., Mischoulon, D., Worthington, J. J., Peterson, T., Mahal, Y., et al. (2004). S-adenosyl-L-methionine (SAMe) as an adjunct for resistant major depressive disorder: An open trial following partial or nonresponse to selective serotonin reuptake inhibitors or venlafaxine. *Journal of Clinical Psychopharmacology, 24*(6), 661–664.

Amenta, F., Parnetti, L., Gallai, V., & Wallin, A. (2001). Treatment of cognitive dysfunction associated with Alzheimer's disease with cholinergic precursors. Ineffective treatments or inappropriate approaches? *Mechanical Ageing Development, 122*(16), 2025–2040.

Ames, B. N., Elson-Schwab, I., & Silver, E. A. (2002). High-dose vitamin therapy stimulates variant enzymes with decreased coenzyme binding affinity (increased km): Relevance to genetic disease and polymorphisms. *American Journal of Clinical Nutrition, 75*(4), 616–658.

Arnold, L.E., Amato, A., Bozzolo, H., Hollway, J., Cook, A., Ramadan, Y., et al. (2007). Acetyl-L-carnitine (ALC) in attention-deficit/hyperactivity disorder: A multi-site, placebo-controlled pilot trial. *Journal of Child Adolescent Psychopharmacology, 17*(6), 791–802.

Baldessarini, R. J. (1987). The neuropharmacology of S-adenosyl-methionine (SAMe). *American Journal of Medicine, 83,* 95–103.

Baldewicz, T. T., Goodkin, K., Blaney, N. T., Shor-Posner, G., Kumar, M., Wilkie, F. L., et al. (2000). Cobalamin level is related to self-reported and clinically rated mood and to syndromal depression in bereaved HIV-1+ and HIV-1- homosexual men. *Journal of Psychosomatic Research, 48*(2), 177–185.

Bell, I. R., Edman, J. S., Marby, D. W., Satlin, A., Dreier, T., Liptzin, B., et al. (1990). Vitamin B12 and folate status in acute geropsychiatric inpatients: Affective and cognitive characteristics of a vitamin nondeficient population. *Biological Psychiatry*, 27(2), 125–137.

Bell, I. R., Edman, J. S., Morrow, F. D., Marby, D. W., Perrone, G., Kayne, H. L., et al. (1992). Brief communication: Vitamin B1, B2, and B6 augmentation of tricyclic antidepressant treatment in geriatric depression with cognitive dysfunction. *Journal of the American College of Nutrition*, 11(2), 159–163.

Berdanier, C. D. (1998). Advanced nutrition micronutrients. *CRC Press*, 100.

Berman, K., & Brodaty, H. (2004). Tocopherol (vitamin E) in Alzheimer's disease and other neurodegenerative disorders. *CNS Drugs*, 18(12), 807–825.

Bjelakovic, G., Nikolova, D., Gluud, L. L., Simonetti, R. G., & Gluud, C. (2007). Mortality in randomized trials of antioxidant supplements for primary and secondary prevention: Systematic review and meta-analysis. *JAMA*, 297(8), 842–857.

Blackburn, W. (1997). Eosinophilia myalgia syndrome. *Seminars in Arthritis and Rheumatism*, 26(6), 781–784.

Bottiglieri, T., Laundy, M., Crellin, R., Toone, B. K., Carney, M. W. P., & Reynolds, E. H. (2000). Homocysteine, folate, methylation, and monoamine metabolism in depression. *Journal of Neurology Neurosurgery and Psychiatry*, 69(2), 228–232.

Brewer, G. J., Hill, G., & Dick, R. D. (1985). Interactions of trace elements: Clinical significance. *Journal of the American College of Nutrition*, 4(1), 33–38.

Bryan, J. (2008). Psychological effects of dietary components of tea: Caffeine and L-theanine. *Nutrition Reviews*, 66(2), 82–90.

Chiechio, S., Copani, A., Gereau, R. W., & Nicoletti, F. (2007). Acetyl-L-carnitine in neuropathic pain: Experimental data. *CNS Drugs*, 21(S1), 31–38.

Chiu, C., Huang, S., Chen, C., & Su, K. (2005). Omega-3 fatty acids are more beneficial in the depressive phase than in the manic phase in patients with bipolar I disorder [2]. *Journal of Clinical Psychiatry*, 66(12), 1613–1614.

Chiu, C. C., Huang, S. Y., Shen, W. W., & Su, K. P. (2003). Omega-3 fatty acids for depression in pregnancy. *American Journal of Psychiatry*, 160(2), 385.

Cousens, G. (2000). *Depression-free for life*. New York: William Morrow.

Depeint, F., Bruce, W. R., Shangari, N., Mehta, R., & O'Brien, P. J. (2006). Mitochondrial function and toxicity: Role of the B vitamin family on mitochondrial energy metabolism. *Chemico-Biological Interactions*, 163(1–2), 94–112.

Dumville, J. C., Miles, J. N. V., Porthouse, J., Cockayne, S., Saxon, L., & King, C. (2006). Can vitamin D supplementation prevent winter-time blues? A randomised trial among older women. *Journal of Nutrition, Health and Aging*, 10(2), 151–153.

Evins, A. E., Demopulos, C., Yovel, I., Culhane, M., Ogutha, J., Grandin, L. D., et al. (2006). Inositol augmentation of lithium or valproate for bipolar depression. *Bipolar Disorders*, 8, 168–174.

Fava, M., Borus, J. S., Alpert, J. E., Nierenberg, A. A., Rosenbaum, J. F., & Bottiglieri, T. (1997). Folate, vitamin B12, and homocysteine in major depressive disorder. *American Journal of Psychiatry*, 154(3), 426–428.

Felsby, S., Nielsen, J., Arendt-Nielsen, L., & Jensen, T. S. (1996). NMDA receptor blockade in chronic neuropathic pain: A comparison of ketamine and magnesium chloride. *Pain*, 64(2), 283–291.

Fioravanti, M., & Yanagi, M. (2005). Cytidinediphosphocholine (CDP-choline) for cognitive and behavioural disturbances associated with chronic cerebral disorders in the elderly. *Cochrane Database of Systematic Reviews (Online)*, (2).

Folstein, M., Liu, T., Peter, I., Buel, J., Arsenault, L., Scott, T., et al. (2007). The homocysteine hypothesis of depression. *American Journal of Psychiatry*, *164*(6), 861–867.

Frangou, S., Lewis, M., & McCrone, P. (2006). Efficacy of ethyl-eicosopentaenoic acid in bipolar depression: Randomised double-blind placebo-controlled study. *British Journal of Psychiatry*, *188*, 46–50.

Freeman, M. P., Hibbeln, J. R., Wisner, K. L., Brumbach, B. H., Watchman, M., & Gelenberg, A. J. (2006). Randomized dose-ranging pilot trial of omega-3 fatty acids for postpartum depression. *Acta Psychiatrica Scandinavica*, *113*(1), 31–35.

Gibson, G. E., & Blass, J. P. (2007). Thiamine-dependent processes and treatment strategies in neurodegeneration. *Antioxidants & Redox Signaling*, *9*(10), 1605–1619.

Hector, M., & Burton, J. R. (1988). What are the psychiatric manifestations of vitamin B12 deficiency? *Journal of the American Geriatrics Society*, *36*(12), 1105–1112.

Hellhammer, J., Fries, E., Buss, C., Engert, V., Tuch, A., Rutenberg, D., et al. (2004). Effects of soy lecithin phosphatidic acid and phosphatidylserine complex (PAS) on the endocrine and psychological responses to mental stress. *Stress*, *7*(2), 119–126.

Hoffer, A., & Osmond, H. (1964). Treatment of schizophrenia with nicotinic acid—A ten year follow-up. *Acta Psychiatrica Scandinavica*, *40*, 171–189.

Holick M. F., & Chen, T. C. (2008). Vitamin D deficiency: A worldwide problem with health consequences. *American Journal of Clinical Nutrition*, *87*(4), 1080S–1086S.

Hutto, B. R. (1997). Folate and cobalamin in psychiatric illness. *Comprehensive Psychiatry*, *38*(6), 305–314.

Jorissen, B. L., Brouns, F., Van Boxtel, M. P., Ponds, R. W., Verhey, F. R., Jolles, J., et al. (2001). The influence of soy-derived phosphatidylserine on cognition in age-associated memory impairment. *Nutritional Neuroscience*, *4*(2), 121–134.

Kaplan, B. J., Crawford, S. G., Field, C. J., & Simpson, J. S. A. (2007). Vitamins, minerals, and mood. *Psychological Bulletin*, *133*(5), 747–760.

Kaplan, B. J., Fisher, J. E., Crawford, S. G., Field, C. J., & Kolb, B. (2004). Improved mood and behavior during treatment with a mineral-vitamin supplement: An open-label case series. *Journal of Child and Adolescent Psychopharmacology*, *14*, 115–122.

Kilkens, T. O. C., Honig, A., Maes, M., Lousberg, R., & Brummer, R. M. (2004). Fatty acid profile and affective dysregulation in irritable bowel syndrome. *Lipids*, *39*(5), 425–431.

Kim, H., McGrath, B. M., & Silverstone, P. H. (2005). A review of the possible relevance of inositol and the phosphatidylinositol second messenger system (PI-cycle) to psychiatric disorders—focus on magnetic resonance spectroscopy (MRS) studies. *Human Psychopharmacology*, *20*(5), 309–326.

Kimura, K., Ozeki, M., Juneja, L. R., & Ohira, H. (2007). L-theanine reduces psychological and physiological stress responses. *Biological Psychology*, *74*(1), 39–45.

Klarskov, K., Johnson, K. L., & Benson, L. M., (1999). Eosinophilia myalgia syndrome case-associated contaminants in commercially available 5-hydroxytryptophan. *Advances in Experimental Medical Biology*, *467*, 461–468.

Kuby, J. (1994). *Immunology*. New York: W.H. Freeman and Company.

Lader, M., & Herrington, R. (1981). Drug treatment in psychiatry-psychotropic drugs. In H. Praag, H. Lader, O. Rafaelsen, & E. Sachar (Eds.), *Handbook of biological psychiatry.* Vol. 5, New York: Marcel Dekker.

Lansdowne, A. T. G., & Provost, S. C. (1998). Vitamin D3 enhances mood in healthy subjects during winter. *Psychopharmacology, 135*(4), 319–323.

Lin, P., & Su, K. (2007). A meta-analytic review of double-blind, placebo-controlled trials of antidepressant efficacy of omega-3 fatty acids. *Journal of Clinical Psychiatry, 68*(7), 1056–1061.

Lindenbaum, J., Healton, J.B., Savage, D.G., Brust, J.C., Garrett, T.J., Podell, E.R., et al. (1988). Neuropsychiatric disorders caused by cobalamin deficiency in the absence of anemia or macrocytosis. *New England Journal Medicine, 318*(26), 1720–1728.

Lipton, M., Ban T. A., Kane F. J., et al. (1973). *Taskforce report on megavitamin and orthomolecular therapy in psychiatry.* Washington DC: American Psychiatric Association.

Lyoo, I. K., Demopulos, C. M., Hirashima, F., Ahn, K. H., & Renshaw, P. F. (2003). Oral choline decreases brain purine levels in lithium-treated subjects with rapid-cycling bipolar disorder: A double-blind trial using proton and lithium magnetic resonance spectroscopy. *Bipolar Disorders, 5*(4), 300–306.

Malaguarnera, M. Gargante, M.P., Cristaldi, E., Colonna, V., Messano, M., Koverech, A., et al. (2008). Acetyl L-carnitine (ALC) treatment in elderly patients with fatigue. *Archives of Gerontology and Geriatrics, 46*(2), 181–190.

Mazur, A., Maier, J. A. M., Rock, E., Gueux, E., Nowacki, W., & Rayssiguier, Y. (2007). Magnesium and the inflammatory response: Potential physiopathological implications. *Archives of Biochemistry and Biophysics, 458*(1), 48–56.

Mazzotta, G., Sarchielli, P., Alberti, A., & Gallai, V. (1999). Intracellular Mg++ concentration and electromyographical ischemic test in juvenile headache. *Cephalalgia, 19*(9), 802–809.

McCarty, M. F. (2000). High dose pyridoxine as an "anti-stress" strategy. *Medical Hypotheses, 54*(5), 803–807.

McLeod, M. N., Gaynes, B. N., & Golden, R. N. (1999). Chromium potentiation of antidepressant pharmacotherapy for dysthymic disorder in 5 patients. *Journal of Clinical Psychiatry, 60*(4), 237–240.

Meador, K. J., Nichols, M. E., Franke, P., Durkin, M. W., Oberzan, R. L., Moore, E. E., et al. (1993). Evidence for a central cholinergic effect of high-dose thiamine. *Annals of Neurology, 34*(5), 724–726.

Milne, D. B. (2000). Laboratory assessment of trace element and mineral status. *Clinical Nutrition of the Essential Trace Elements and Minerals: The Guide for Health Professionals,* 69–90.

Mischoulon, D., Best-Popescu, C., Laposata, M., Merens, W., Murakami, J. L., Wu, S.L., et al. (2008). A double-blind dose-finding pilot study of docosahexaenoic acid (DHA) for major depressive disorder. *European Neuropsychopharmacology,* Epub, June 5.

Muñoz, F. J., Solé, M., & Coma, M. (2005). The protective role of vitamin E in vascular amyloid beta-mediated damage. *Sub-Cellular Biochemistry, 38,* 147–165.

Murck, H. (2002). Magnesium and affective disorders. *Nutritional Neuroscience, 5*(6); 375–389.

National Institutes of Health State-of-the-science conference statement: Multivitamin/mineral supplements and chronic disease prevention. (2006). *Annual Internal Medicine, 145,* 364–371.

Nathan, P. J., Lu, K., Gray, M., & Oliver, C. (2006). The neuropharmacology of L-theanine (N-ethyl-L-glutamine): A possible neuroprotective and cognitive enhancing agent. *Journal of Herbal Pharmacotherapy, 6*(2), 21–30.

Nemets, B., Stahl, Z., & Belmaker, R. H. (2002). Addition of omega-3 fatty acid to maintenance medication treatment for recurrent unipolar depressive disorder. *American Journal of Psychiatry, 159,* 477–479.

Nowak, G., Szewczyk, B., & Pilc, A. (2005). Zinc and depression. an update. *Pharmacological Reports, 57*(6), 713–718.

Oakley, G. P., Jr. (1998). Eat right and take a multivitamin. *New England Journal of Medicine, 338*(15), 1060.

Olerich, M. A., & Rude, R. K. (1994). Should we supplement magnesium in critically ill patients? *New Horizons* (Baltimore, Md.), *2*(2), 186–192.

Papakostas, G. I., Alpert, J. E., & Fava, M. (2003). S-adenosyl-methionine in depression: A comprehensive review of the literature. *Current Psychiatry Reports, 5*(6), 460–466.

Papp, L. V., Lu, J., Holmgren, A., & Khanna, K. K. (2007). From selenium to selenoproteins: Synthesis, identity, and their role in human health. *Antioxidants and Redox Signaling, 9*(7), 775–806.

Pauling, L. (1968). Orthomolecular psychiatry. Varying the concentrations of substances normally present in the human body may control mental disease. *Science, 160*(825), 265–271.

Piekert, A., Wilimzig, C., & Kohne-Volland, R. (1996). Prophylaxis of migraine with oral magnesium: Results from a prospective, multi-center, placebo-controlled and double-blind randomized study. *Cephalalgia, 16,* 257–263.

Pettegrew, J. W., Levine, J., Gershon, S., Stanley, J. A., Servan-Schreiber, D., Panchalingam, K., et al. (2002). 31P-MRS study of acetyl-L-carnitine treatment in geriatric depression: Preliminary results. *Bipolar Disorders, 4*(1), 61–66.

Pettegrew, J. W., Levine, J., & McClure, R. J. (2000). Acetyl-L-carnitine physical-chemical, metabolic, and therapeutic properties: Relevance for its mode of action in alzheimer's disease and geriatric depression. *Molecular Psychiatry, 5*(6), 616–632.

Puri, B. K., Counsell, S. J., Richardson, A. J., & Horrobin D. F. (2002). Eicosapentaenoic acid in treatment-resistant depression. *Archives of General Psychiatry, 59*(1), 91–92.

Rabkin, J. G., McElhiney, M. C., Rabkin, R., McGrath, P. J., & Ferrando, S. J. (2006). Placebo-controlled trial of dehydroepiandrosterone (DHEA) for treatment of non-major depression in patients with HIV/AIDS. *American Journal of Psychiatry, 163*(1), 59–66.

Radimer, K., Bindewald B., Hughes, J., Ervin, B., Swanson, C., & Picciano, M. F. (2004). Dietary supplement use by US adults: Data fromm the National Health and Nutrition Examination Survey, 1999–2000. *American Journal of Epidemiology*, *160*(4), 339–349.

Rossini, M., Di Munno, O., Valentini, G., Bianchi, G., Biasi, G., Cacace, E., et al. (2007). Double-blind, multicenter trial comparing acetyl L-carnitine with placebo in the treatment of fibromyalgia patients. *Clinical and Experimental Rheumatology*, *25*(2), 182–188.

Saletu, B., Anderer, P., Linzmayer, L., Semlitsch, H. V., Lindeck-Pozza, E., Assandri, A., et al. (2002). Pharmacodynamic studies on the central mode of action of S-adenosyl-L-methionine (SaMe) infusions in elderly subjects, utilizing EEG mapping and psychometry. *Journal of Neural Transmission*, *109*(12), 1505–1526.

Schmidt, P. J., Daly, R. C., Bloch, M., Smith, M. J., Danaceau, M. A., Simpson St. Clair, L., et al. (2005). Dehydroepiandrosterone monotherapy in midlife-onset major and minor depression. *Archives of General Psychiatry*, *62*(2), 154–162.

Selhub, J., Bagley, L. C., Miller, J., & Rosenberg, I. H. (2000). B vitamins, homocysteine, and neurocognitive function in the elderly. *American Journal of Clinical Nutrition*, *71*(2).

Shao, L., Martin, M. V., Watson, S. J., Schatzberg, A., Akil, H., Myers, R. M., et al. (2008). Mitochondrial involvement in psychiatric disorders. *Annals of Medicine*, *40*(4), 281–295.

Shaw, K., Turner, J., & Del Mar, C. (2002). Tryptophan and 5-hydroxytryptophan for depression. *Cochrane Database of Systematic Reviews (Online)*, (1).

Soldatovic, D., Matovic, V., Vujanovic, D., Guiet-Bara, A., Bara, M., & Durlach, J. (2002). Metal pollutants and bioelements: Retrospective of interactions between magnesium and toxic metals. *Magnesium Research : Official Organ of the International Society for the Development of Research on Magnesium*, *15*(1–2), 67–72.

Sun, Y., Lai, M., & Lu, C. (2005). Effectiveness of vitamin B12 on diabetic neuropathy: Systematic review of clinical controlled trials. *Acta Neurologica Taiwanica*, *14*(2), 48–54.

Swain, R., & Kaplan-Machlis, B. (1999). Magnesium for the next millennium. *Southern Medical Journal*, *92*(11), 1040–1047.

Tai, K., Need, A. G., Horowitz, M., & Chapman, I. M. (2008). Vitamin D, glucose, insulin, and insulin sensitivity. *Nutrition*, *24*(3), 279–285.

Takeda, A. (2001). Zinc homeostasis and functions of zinc in the brain. *BioMetals*, *14*(3–4), 343–351.

Tanskanen, A., Hibbeln, J.R., Hintikka, J., Haatainen, K., Honkalampi, K., & Niinamaki, H. (2001). Fish consumption, depression and suicidality in a general population. *Archives of General Psychiatry*, *58*, 512–513.

Tiemeier, H., Van Tuijl, H. R., Hofman, A., Kiliaan, A. J., & Breteler, M. M. B. (2003). Plasma fatty acid composition and depression are associated in the elderly: The Rotterdam study. *American Journal of Clinical Nutrition*, *78*(1), 40–46.

Tomassini, V., Pozzilli, C., Onesti, E., Pasqualetti, P., Marinelli, F., Pisani, A., et al. (2004). Comparison of the effects of acetyl L-carnitine and amantadine for the treatment of fatigue in multiple sclerosis: Results of a pilot, randomised, double-blind, crossover trial. *Journal of Neurological Science*, *218*, 103–108.

Torrioli, M.G., Vernacotola, S., Peruzzi, L., Tabolacci, E., Mila, M., Militerni, R., et al. (2008). A double-blind, parallel, multicenter comparison of L-acetylcarnitine with placebo on the attention deficit hyperactivity disorder in Fragile X Syndrome boys. *American Journal of Medical Genetics*-Part A, *146ª*, 803–812.

Trauninger, A., Pfund, Z., Koszegi, T., & Czopf, J. (2002). Oral magnesium load test in patinets with migraine. *Headache, 42*, 114–119.

Ueshima, K. (2005). Magnesium and ischemic heart disease: A review of epidemiological, experimental, and clinical evidences. *Magnesium Research, 18*(4), 275–284.

Velez-Pardo, C., Jimenez Del Rio, M., Ebinger, G., & Vauquelin, G. (1995). Manganese and copper promote the binding of dopamine to 'serotonin binding proteins' in bovine frontal cortex. *Neurochemistry International, 26*(6), 615–622.

Wasserman, G. A., Liu, X., Factor-Litvak, P., Gardner, J. M., & Graziano, J. H. (2008). Developmental impacts of heavy metals and undernutrition. *Basic and Clinical Pharmacology and Toxicology, 102*(2), 212–217.

Wester, P. O. (1987). Magnesium. *American Journal of Clinical Nutrition, 45*(5 Suppl.), 1305–1312.

Widmer, J., Feray, J. C., Bovier, P., Hilleret, H., Raffin, Y., Chollet, D., et al. (1995). Sodium-magnesium exchange in erythrocyte membranes from patients with affective disorders. *Neuropsychobiology, 32*(1), 13–18.

Widmer, J., Henrotte, J. G., Raffin, Y., Bovier, P., Hilleret, H., & Gaillard, G. M. (1995). Relationship between erythrocyte magnesium, plasma electrolytes and cortisol, and intensity of symptoms in major depressed patients. *Journal of Affective Disorders, 34*(3), 201–209.

Williams, A., Cotter, A., Sabina, A., Girard, C., Goodman, J., & Katz, D. L. (2005). The role for vitamin B-6 as treatment for depression: A systematic review. *Family Practice, 22*(5), 532–537.

Wong, G. K. C., Chan, M. T. V., Poon, W. S., Boet, R., & Gin, T. (2006). Magnesium therapy within 48 hours of an aneurysmal subarachnoid hemorrhage: Neuro-panacea. *Neurological Research, 28*(4), 431–435.

Wright, R. O., Tsaih, S., Schwartz, J., Wright, R. J., & Hu, H. (2003). Association between iron deficiency and blood lead level in a longitudinal analysis of children followed in an urban primary care clinic. *Journal of Pediatrics, 142*(1), 9–14.

Wyatt, K. M., Dimmock, P. W., Jones, P. W., & O'Brien, P. M. S. (1999). Efficacy of vitamin B-6 in the treatment of premenstrual syndrome: Systematic review. *British Medical Journal, 318*(7195), 1375–1381.

Yaffe, K., Ettinger, B., Pressman, A., Seeley, D., Whooley, M., Schaefer, C., et al. (1998). Neuropsychiatric function and dehydroepiandrosterone sulfate in elderly women: A prospective study. *Biological Psychiatry, 43*, 694–700.

Yehuda, S., Rabinovitz, S., & Mostofsky, D. I. (2005). Essential fatty acids and the brain: From infancy to aging. *Neurobiology of Aging, 26*(Suppl.)

Zanardi, R., & Smeraldi, E. (2006). A double-blind, randomised, controlled clinical trial of acetyl-L-carnitine vs. amisulpride in the treatment of dysthymia. *European Neuropsychopharmacology, 16*(4), 281–287.

Zeisel, S. H. (2000). Choline: An essential nutrient for humans. *Nutrition, 16*(7–8), 669–671.

Zhang, X. Y., Zhou, D. F., Cao, L. Y., Xu, C. Q., Chen, D. C., & Wu, G. Y. (2004). The effect of vitamin E treatment on tardive dyskinesia and blood superoxide dismutase: A double-blind placebo-controlled trial. *Journal of Clinical Psychopharmacology, 24*(1), 83–86.

4

Botanicals of Interest to Psychiatrists

HOWARD L. FIELD

KEY CONCEPTS

- Nature provides a rich menu of herbal medicines for the treatment of psychiatric disorders. Because each medicine derives from a different source, contains different active principles, and has a different application, each must be studied thoroughly and used carefully.
- The use of herbal medicines differs from that of chemical pharmaceuticals, which are usually tested, packaged, and administered as single agents in defined dosages.
- Clinical evidence of effectiveness and toxicity of natural agents varies greatly as do methods for assessing their efficacy. Systems of evaluation have developed in a rather unsystematic fashion in the United States. The regulation, legality, standards, and control of their use also vary greatly throughout the world.
- An account of the most frequently used phytopsychopharmaceuticals with their biologic effects, indications, side effects, and interactions can be useful to the clinician.

■

Introduction

Psychoactive plant substances are so ubiquitous in nature that it is impossible to walk through an ordinary back yard garden without encountering plants with central nervous system effects. Our knowledge of these plants have come from serendipitous discovery by traditional healers, as well as from practitioners with sophisticated theories of disease: the imbalance of vital forces in Chinese and Ayurvedic medicine; or humeral imbalance theories originating in Greco-Roman medicine that formed the basis of medical practice until recent times.

In psychiatry, as in all areas of medicine, botanicals were the chief sources of treatment until the first third of the twentieth century when they began to be supplanted by synthetic chemicals. Even now, a quarter of all prescription medications are derived from herbal sources. By the second third of the past century, disappointment with the failures and toxicity of synthetic drugs, together with a wish for more authentic natural treatments, led to an upsurge in the use of herbal medicines in the West. In developing countries, herbal remedies administered by traditional practitioners never lost favor.

Regulations and Control

There are significant differences between the regulation and use of herbal preparations in the United States and in other parts of the world. In the United States regulation of herbal preparations is unsatisfactory as no governmental agency has undertaken to evaluate their effectiveness. A succession of federal laws endeavored to correct the problems of the previous legislation. The Federal Food and Drugs Act of 1906 and Federal Food, Drug, and Cosmetic Act of 1938 were enacted to remedy egregious abuse of drugs. The Federal Food and Drug Administration, authorized to oversee pharmaceuticals, hewed to increasingly rigid evaluation procedures, refusing to modify the strict criteria used for new synthetic chemical drugs in evaluating natural products (Davis, 1999). This approach meant that herbal medicines were marketed as foodstuffs without need for evaluation of effectiveness. The Dietary Supplement and Health Education Act of 1994 was enacted to remedy these failures of regulation. The FDA was empowered not only to protect against dangerous, toxic, and unsanitary products, but also to monitor safety, evaluate the truthfulness of advertising claims, and set standards in processing of botanicals. Product labels were required to contain lists of ingredients, potential side effects and contraindications, and special warnings. Manufacturers were not permitted to claim effectiveness of their products for specific diseases or symptoms. A tiny fraction of the many available products were evaluated and approved for sale as over-the-counter medications. Drug evaluation in the United States has stalled because the evaluating agencies have not felt able to undertake testing. The methods designed to evaluate new chemical drugs from the pharmaceutical industry do not transfer well to natural products (Weill, 1999). It seems unfortunate that, while older chemical drugs are used without proof of efficacy because of their long history of use, natural products have not been granted this latitude. Most botanicals continue to be sold in the United States as food rather than medicine. Supplements are found in retail stores in such perfusion as to overwhelm the ability of agencies to inspect them.

In Europe and Asia, the regulation and evaluation of herbal medicines took a less rigid, more practical course (DeSmet, 2005). France and Germany acted to accept bibliographic and anecdotal evidence in preparations with a long history of use and with demonstrated plausible pharmacologic effects. Agencies have simplified the registration process, and specified dose and potency. In 1978, Commission E of the German Institute for Drugs and Medical Products began to evaluate botanicals, publishing monographs covering description of the plants involved, methods of preparation, chemical content and action of the principle components, standards of purity and content of active principles, allowable adulterants (Blumenthal, 1998). The resulting formulary is accepted by herbal practitioners in many places including the United States. An English translation and a more recent revision have been published (Blumenthal, 2000). Although there were considerable differences between European countries, the European community has begun to harmonize the disparate standards. The European Scientific Cooperative on Phytotherapy has published monographs on 50 botanicals. The World Health Organization (WHO) has also issued drug monographs covering botanicals from many areas of the world. The character of the herb, methods of preparation, purity, and uses are specified comprehensively by the WHO. Six of the WHO monographs cover herbals useful in psychiatry.

Problems in Evaluation of Botanicals

Evaluation of the efficacy of natural products has not been easy. National differences in diagnosis and evaluation procedures often lead to different outcomes. For example, the first procedures used for evaluation of Hypericum in Germany were emphatically rejected by American researchers. Even now, there are many criticisms of the scientific purity of clinical trials (Gagnier, 2006). Herbal medicines contain many constituents. Growing conditions, harvesting procedures, and methods of preparation may account for considerable variation in the products. Confronting these difficulties, the Commission E created three categories based on proven effectiveness and safety: safe and effective, neutral, unsafe. The neutral category described drugs whose therapeutic effectiveness had not been evaluated by scientific methods, but posed no significant risk to the user.

Botanicals in Current Practice

Botanical medicines have been used in many nervous and mental disorders including insomnia, anxiety, depression, psychosis, dementia, and fatigue/ exhaustion syndromes. In addition to single botanical agents, the practitioner will encounter many combinations of herbal medicines designed to achieve a desired result. Because of the lack of coherent regulation, the phrase *caveat emptor* applies in this country. The purchaser must be aware of the source of the product, its stated composition and strength, along with various side effects and warnings on the label. Inappropriate combinations of various elements, and the interaction of botanicals with other phytochemicals and synthetic prescription medicines, may be important. This is particularly so in the many remedies that combine different herbs to achieve the desired response. Even after careful reading, the consumer may be at risk from wide discrepancy in strength of preparations from those that are listed on the label (Bauberg, 2000; Straus, 2002). Toxic adulterants have dogged the herbal medicine industry (Marcus & Grollman, 2002). As a further caveat, some writers have pointed out potential dangers of consumer self-diagnosis (Ernst, 2007).

With increased clinical trials and basic scientific exploration, the field of herbal medicine is changing rapidly. Sources of current information can be invaluable. These include the PDR for Herbal Medicine (PDR, 2004) and the Natural Medicines Comprehensive Database (NMCD, 2003). Even more timely information can be obtained on internet sites: www.naturaldatabase. com, which is said to be updated on a daily basis, and the National Institute of Health Center for Comprehensive and Alternative Medicine's web site, www. nccam.nih.gov.

Although some of these remedies are both powerful and specific, many have milder, more diffuse actions. Unlike pharmaceutical drugs, natural remedies tend not to bulldoze the patient into desired states of alertness, sleep, or calmness and should be combined with other alternative methods. The following accounts are intended to be descriptive rather than prescriptive. The practioner and user should evaluate the package label for strength, dose, side effects, and possible interactions. Because of the diversity of phytopharmaceuticals, it may be helpful to classify the two dozen herbal medicines described below into three groups: those with at least some evidence of clinical effectiveness, those which have been found ineffective or have not been tested, and a final group that the psychiatrist may encounter as a result of their addictive or neurotoxic properties or legal status. This classification is somewhat arbitrary; members may belong in more than one category. In addition, assignment to either effective or ineffective, safe or unsafe categories will change with further investigation. It should be noted that even many of those listed as unproven, contain substances with central nervous system activity. Three of the botanicals listed are refined by pharmaceutical manufacturers and sold as prescription medications.

1. Botanicals with some evidence of clinical effectiveness

Coffea arabica, Coffea robusta

Botany

A small tree of the tropics with handsome glossy leaves. The red berries are fermented or dried, then roasted. Production of coffee forms the basis of the economy in many tropical areas. The principle active component, caffeine, a methylxanthene, acts as a central stimulant, increasing monoamines through antagonism of adenosine. At the usual doses (90–140 mg in a cup of coffee), the effect is of heightened alertness, increased reaction speed, and a mild euphoria. Caffeine stimulates gastric acid and is diuretic. Other methylxanthene compounds including theophylline and theobromine have similar effects. Caffeine is found in a number of botanicals, including *Cola acumenata* (cola soft drinks), *Ilex paraguariensis* (mate), *Camellia sinensis* (tea), and *Theobroma cacao* (chocolate). Each of these stimulants have different proportions of various methylxanthenes.

Use

Coffee and other caffeine containing substances are a common antidote to fatigue. They have been used universally as social beverages in Europe and the Americas since the fifteenth century. Tea has been accepted in Asia for many centuries. There is suggestion that coffee has a beneficial effect in Parkinson's disease. Commission E has approved coffee charcoal for use in intestinal disorders, but not the roasted berry, for reasons that seem obscure.

Cautions

These substances may cause anxiety, insomnia, cardiac arrhythmias, and gastric irritation. Increased amounts of caffeine result in increasing anxiety. Tolerance develops and there may be withdrawal symptoms (fatigue, headache). When combined with other stimulants, an additive effect may cause complications. Caffeine crosses the placenta and is secreted in breast milk where it may cause restlessness and poor sleep in nursing infants

Ginko biloba

Pharmacology

A deciduous tree of China, planted as a shade tree throughout the world. It is dioecious, the fruits having a strong odor that offends some people, but the nuts are highly prized as both foodstuff and medicine in Asia. The active principles are found in the leaves, which contain a complex mixture of phytochemicals, including flavenoids, biflavenoids, sesquiterpenes, diterpenes. Ginkolides are believed to account for much of the biologic activities. Ginkolide B inhibits platelet activating factor, which is responsible for many inflammatory processes. Flavenoids are antioxidants and protect against ischemic damage. Ginko acts to relax vascular smooth muscle.

Use

Standardized extracts of dried Ginko leaves are available for administration; 120–240 mg of dry extract or 1.5 ml of fluid extract daily. The WHO and Commission E approve Ginko for the symptomatic relief of organic brain dysfunction, intermittent claudication, vertigo, and tinnitus of vascular origin. Ginko extract may slow the cognitive and social deterioration in mild cognitive impairment, Alzheimer's and multi-infarct dementia. However, its ability to slow progression to dementia has been questioned in recent studies (DeKosly, 2008). It increases exercise tolerance in vascular conditions of the lower extremity. It is possibly effective when used in premenstrual syndrome, altitude sickness, and age-related macular degeneration.

Cautions

The inhibition of platelet aggregation suggests caution in patients with bleeding disorders. Interaction with anticoagulant and platelet inhibiting drugs may occur. Interactions with anticonvulsants and antidepressants have been reported. Its safety in pregnancy and nursing has not been documented.

Humulus lupulus (HOPS)

Biology

A tall dieocious perennial vine cultivated for commercial use of the inflorescence and fruit cones, which contain the aromatic, bitter tasting elements used in brewing. Hops contains a complex mixture of acylphoroglucinols, humulones, lupulones humulene, myrcene, flavenoids, and others. The volatile oil has been noted to induce excitement followed by sleep in experimental animals. The active agents induce sleep and reduce anxiety. The extract of hops has antimicrobial activity and binds to estrogen receptors.

Uses

Hops is approved by Commission E for nervousness and insomnia. The use of hops in flavoring beer has a long tradition. It is difficult to separate the effect of hops from that of ethanol in producing the disinhibiting and sedating effects of beer. Nevertheless, hops is an effective sedative and calming agent. A tea is prepared by infusion of 1 g of cone with 0.3 L of boiling water for 15 minutes. Capsules, standardized liquid, and alcoholic extracts are available.

Cautions

Excessive dose of hops, in combination with ethanol or other sedative agents, may reduce alertness to dangerous levels. Its safety in pregnancy has not been established.

Hypericum perforatum (ST. JOHN'S WORT)

Biology

A perennial plant with attractive yellow flower, blooming in late June at about the time of St. John's day. Indigenous to Europe, it has been planted throughout the world. It is a prolific plant. Ranchers in America have attempted to eradicate it because it is felt to sensitize cattle to sunburn. The flowers and leaves are collected for drying. Hypericum is produced by many sources, sold in large quantities, and has been extensively studied. Hypericum contains the naph-thodianthones hypericin and pseudohypericin, the flavenoids hyperocide, quercitrin, isoquecitrin, the acylphoroglucinol hyperforin, numerous other compounds. The antidepressant effect was at first attributed to hypericin, but now hyperforin is felt to be the active agent. Actually a combination of several compounds may better explain its activity. The herb has been shown to inhibit monoamine reuptake, and down-regulate monoamine receptors in the brain. St John's wort has some antiviral and antibacterial properties.

Uses

St. John's wort is approved by Commission E for anxiety and depressive moods. Studies have demonstrated antidepressant activity in mild to moderated depression. A large controlled study demonstrated its lack of effectiveness in major depression (Hypericum Depression Trial Study Group, 2002). Effectiveness in other conditions is controversial. It has been shown to reduce anxiety. The herb has a long history of use for skin conditions and wounds and is still recommended for that purpose. It is available in many forms including capsules, pellets, tablets, tincture, fluidextract, injection, transdermal patches, and dried herb in doses ranging from 125 to 1000 mg. The most common dose is 300 mg capsule or tablet TID. The growing conditions, preparation, and storage can have marked effect on potency of the product. St. John's wort capsules have been standardized to contain 0.3 % hyperforin.

Cautions

Photosensitization is observed in large doses. Hypericum induces cytochrome P450 enzymes. Thus one can expect reduction in blood levels of drugs metabolized by this enzyme system. These include cyclosporine, indinavir, barbiturates, estrogens, and theophylline. There may be a tendency to toxic interactions with a number of antidepressants. Its safety in pregnancy has not been documented.

Panax ginseng, Panax cinquifolium

Biology

A perennial plant native to northern Asia. *Panax cinquifolium* is a North American native with similar properties. The roots of both varieties are harvested in the wild and cultivated and dried as part of a brisk commercial trade. *Panax* should not be confused with Siberian Ginseng, which is an entirely different plant, although with some similar qualities. The principal active components are the ginsenosides, a group of several dozen triterpene saponins with different biologic activities. In addition, the root contains many other compounds with biologic activity. Different components both bind to and block nicotinic acetylcholine receptors. There are antineoplastic, antioxidant, anticoagulant, and antiviral effects. Ginseng induces the alcohol oxidizing system, activates lipoprotein lipase lowering blood lipids, and stimulates insulin to hypoglycemic effect. Many of the components of Ginseng have a steroidal nucleus and mimic endogenous steroid hormones.

Use

Controlled studies of the effect of Ginseng on cognitive function have yielded mixed results. Studies confirm hypoglycemic and antiviral properties. The WHO monograph lists Ginseng as restorative agent for enhancement of mental and physical capacities in cases of weakness, exhaustion, tiredness, loss of concentration, and during convalescence. Commission E approves Ginseng for lack of stamina. Accounts of Ginseng's enhancement of sexual virility may account for its enormous popularity in Asia and the West. It may be beneficial for exhaustion and debility. The dried root may be made into tea. More common are the many types of fluidextract and capsules containing dried root supplied in numerous sizes.

Cautions

Side effects include Mastalgia, vaginal bleeding, and arterial hypertension. Side effects are dose related. Combination with caffeine containing drugs may raise blood pressure. Interactions with antidiabetic drugs, warfarin, NSAIDs, MAOIs, and loop diuretics have been reported. Ginseng is not recommended in pregnancy.

Piper methysticum (KAVA)

Botany

A deciduous bush of the South Pacific. It has been long used in Polynesian rituals aimed at dissipating hostility. The rhizome contains lactones and chalcones. The pyrones—including kavain, dihydrokavain, methysticin, yangonine, and desmethylyangonine—have central muscle relaxant, anticonvulsant, sedative, and analgesic properties through inhibition at neuronal ion channels. They potentiate GABA-a, inhibit norepinephrine uptake, and increase serotonin and dopamine.

Use

The rhizomes are prepared by maceration, in native culture by mastication. The drug is prepared by several manufacturers as a powder or extract. Controlled studies have demonstrated a reduction of anxiety symptoms equal to that obtained with the standard benzodiazepines.

Cautions

Kava increases the risk of suicide in depressed patients. Dose-related side effects include weight loss, liver conditions, depressed alertness, impaired reflexes, skin rash, and discoloration. Kava potentiates the effects of alcohol, benzodiazepines, and barbiturates. It should be discontinued after 3 months use. The NIH discontinued research on kava because of a number of cases of liver damage resulting from use of the herb. Kava is contraindicated in pregnancy.

Rauwolfia serpentina

Botany

A small shrub native to South Asia. The root is collected and dried commercially. Its use in medicine has so depleted the supply that the pharmaceutical industry has been forced to turn to a related species, *Rauwolfia vomitoria*, or else synthesis to obtain the active alkaloid. The active alkaloids include reserpine, reserpinine, serpentine, serpetenine, ajmaline, and others. The effect of reserpine is to deplete both peripheral and the central nervous system of all catacholamines by limiting their reabsorption. Rauwolfia is dispensed as the alkaloid, reserpine, or preparations containing the powdered whole root.

Use

Rauwolfia is currently used to treat essential hypertension, but was one of the first agents shown to be effective in treatment of acute schizophrenia. It has a sedative effect and gradually ameliorates agitation, delusions, hallucinations, and other psychotic symptoms. Rauwolfia was gradually replaced in psychiatry by synthetic drugs on account of its side effects. It is obtainable through prescription. Dose of the refined alkaloid varies from 0.1 mg to 1 mg.

Cautions

Snakeroot (another name for Rauwolfia) causes severe nasal congestion, somnolence, erectile dysfunction, and depression. In depressed patients it increases the severity of symptoms. It increases the depressant effects of alcohol, barbiturates, and benzodiazepines, and antagonizes the effects of levodopa and other anti-Parkinson medicines. Administration with digitalis glycosides results in marked bradycardia. Long-term use may lead to breast tumors, some of which become malignant.

Valeriana officinalis

Biology

A European native shrub of moderate height. It is cultivated for its medicinal uses. The roots are dried in preparation of the medicine. The active principles include iridoids, sesqueterpines, pyridine alkaloids, and caffeic acid derivatives. The combination of compounds is central depressant, sedative, anxiolytic. The herb effects an increase of central GABA. Controlled trials indicate decreased sleep latency and improved quality of sleep.

Use

The botanical is supported as a mild sedative by the WHO Monograph. Commission E approves this herb for nervousness and insomnia. Recent publications have reported Valerian to be ineffective when compared to placebo in double-blind studies on anxiety. These remain to be replicated.

Cautions

Valerian may potentiate other CNS depressants. Long-term use may cause headaches, restlessness, insomnia, and cardiac dysfunction.

2. Botanicals That Have Not Demonstrated Clinical Effectiveness or Have Not Been Adequately Tested

Artemesia absinthium (WORMWOOD)

Biology

A small shrub with deeply incised silvery grey leaves, an aromatic odor, and bitter taste, it is found through the world. Its leaves and stems are the source of medicinal elements, the volatile oils include thujone, cis-epoxy ocimeme, and chrysanthenyl acetate. The flavoring elements include absinthine, anabsinthine, and matricine. The leaf is said to have a cholegogic effect and to inhibit the growth of some bacteria and protozoa. A related species has found to be active against malaria.

Use

The leaf and extracts are approved by Commission E for use in loss of appetite, dyspepsia, and liver and gallbladder complaints. The folk use of wormwood as a vermifuge, appetite stimulant, and digestive has never been demonstrated. The liqueur beverage, absinthe, was banned for most of the twentieth century because it was felt to cause seizures, brain damage, and addiction. While it is true that thujone precipitates seizures, it is difficult to determine what proportion of the notorious effects were the result of ethanol. Wormwood continues to be used as a flavoring agent in various bitter wines such as Vermouth. The dried leaf may be used in tea at 1 g per cup.

Cautions

A distilled oil preparation is dangerous because of the high levels of active substances. Wormwood may cause gastrointestinal symptoms. Chronic, excessive use leads to central nervous system disorders. Its use in pregnancy is contraindicated.

Artemisia vulgaris (MUGWORT)

Biology

A weedy plant of moderate height, native to North America and now found throughout the world. The roots and aerial parts of the plant are used in medicine. The herb contains cineol, camphor, linalool, thujone, sesquiterpene lactones, flavenoids, and hydroxycoumarins.

Use

The drug is used as a tonic, sedative, and digestive. Psychophysiologic activity has never been evaluated in scientific studies. It is reputed to be a vermifuge, but this use has not been evaluated. In Chinese medicine, mugwort is used in moxibustion. It is sold as a tincture and dried herb used for tea.

Cautions

Mugwort is not safe for use in pregnancy on account of its arborfacient actions.

Eleutherococcus senticosus (SIBERIAN GINSENG)

Biology

Siberian Ginseng is often confused with, and sold as, *Panax ginseng*. Despite some common effects, the plants are different and have different components. It is a shrub native to Northeast Asia. The roots are dried and used as tea extracted. The herb contains a complex mixture of lignans, sterols, steroid glycosides, coumarins, saponins, phenypropanols, and several provitamins. Various components have been noted to stimulate the immune system, inhibit platelet aggregation, stimulate the pituitary adrenal axis. There may also be anti-inflamatory, sedative, anabolic, gonadotropic, and antiviral properties, however these have not been demonstrated by careful clinical trials.

Use

Commission E recommends Siberian Ginseng for lack of stamina and tendency to infection. It has been used to increase resistance to stress and infections, to improve memory and concentration. Siberian Ginseng has not been as well studied as Panax.

Cautions

The drug is contraindicated in hypertension. Possible drug interactions include digoxin, antidiabetic agents, and anticoagulants. Its safety in pregnancy has not been documented.

Lavender agustifolia (ENGLISH LAVENDER)

Biology

A fine-leafed, aromatic shrub indigenous to the Mediterranean, but cultivated in all temperate regions. The fresh and dried flowers are processed to extract the aromatic oil. Lavender is used in cosmetics and food as well as medicine. The herb contains the volatile oils linalool, linalyl acetate, acimene, cineole, and other elements. Central nervous system depressant effects have been demonstrated in animals. An effect on the limbic system of the brain can be demonstrated in humans upon inhalation. The active ingredients shorten sleep latency and increase duration of sleep.

Uses

Lavender is approved by Commission E for loss of appetite, nervousness and insomnia, circulatory disorders, and dyspeptic complaints. Lavender may be taken as tea prepared by infusing 3 g of dried flowers in 300 mL of boiling water for 15 minutes. In addition, inhalation of the essential oil may give a therapeutic effect. Lavender is also been used in baths.

Cautions

No ill effects have noted at ordinary quantities.

Leonurus cardiaca (MOTHERWORT)

Biology

A shrub with bright red flowers and an unpleasant odor. It is native to northern Europe, but now established in the wild in North America. The aerial portions of the plant are dried and prepared as tinctures and fluid extracts. Compounds include stachydrine, leocardin, leonuride, flavenoids, leonurinine, bufenolide, betonicine, ursolic acid, and others. The herb has a mild sedative effect. Its glycocodes act to inhibit cardiac activity, stimulate uterine smooth muscle, and inhibit coagulation. Motherwort stimulates the release of oxytocin. Ursolic acid inhibits tumor growth.

Use

Motherwort is available in extracts and tinctures. Tea made by infusion of 3 g of dried herb in 250 mL of boiling water. In folk medicine, motherwort was used to decrease the anxiety often experienced by mothers. It is approved by Commission E for nervous heart complaints. It has a chronotropic effect, slowing the heart rate.

Cautions

No serious side effects have been noted at ordinary doses. Excess of 3 g per day has been known to cause diarrhea and uterine bleeding. Motherwort may increase the effect of sedatives and herbs containing cardiac glycosides. It is not recommended in pregnancy.

Lycopus virginicus (BUGLEWEED)

It is a perennial herb of North America. Lycopus europraus (gypsywort) is a close European relative with similar pharmaceutical effects. The dried stems and leaves are used. The plant contains several active ingredients: including caffeic acid derivatives rosmaric and lithospermic acids, lefteolin glycosides, flavenoids acacetine and apigenein, and others. The herb has pituitary effects including inhibition of prolactin and gonadal and thryroid hormones.

Use

Approved for nervousness, insomnia, and premenstrual syndrome by Commission E.

Cautions

Because of its effects on the thyroid, bugleweed should not be given to patients with hypothyroidism. It may interfere with tests of thyroid function. Prolonged use may result in thyroid enlargement. Sudden discontinuation may result in rebound release of pituitary trophic hormones. It is contraindicated in pregnancy.

Matricaria recutita (GERMAN CHAMOMILE)

Botany

A European plant about 1 foot tall, bearing daisy-like flowers with white petals and yellow centers. The aromatic, bitter-tasting flowers are dried. Matricaria should not be confused with Anthemis nobilis, a low-growing ground cover, or Anthemis cotula. Although both of these have some active elements, the more potent German chamomile is used in most preparations. Diverse components account for the variety of effects of this herb. Chamazulene and apigenen have anti-inflamatory effects. Chamazulene is an antioxidant. Flavenoids such as apigenen exert anxiolytic effects. On the body surface, the herb inhibits bacteria, tumor formation, and inflammation.

Use

Although the Commission E approval is limited to oral, dermatologic, and infectious problems, the WHO monograph mentions its usefulness in the restlessness and insomnia associated with nervous disorders. Chamomile has a long history of use as an anxiolytic and sedative. There have been no comprehensive, controlled evaluations. Teas prepared from this herb are often offered as bedtime beverages. Tea may be prepared from 3 g of dried flowers infused in 250 mL of boiling water for 10 minutes. Capsules, tincture, and liquid extract are also available.

Cautions

Matricaria may potentiate the effects of sedative and anticoagulant herbs. It may precipitate violent allergic reactions in persons sensitive to other members of the composite family.

Melissa officinalis (LEMON BALM)

Biology

Lemon balm is a small perennial plant of the mint family native to the Mediterranean but cultivated throughout the world. The leaves are dried and used as tea. Distillation provides an essential oil. The herb contains a complex mixture of volatile substances including geranial (citral a), neral (citral b), citronellal, linalool, geraniol, rosmaric acid, eugenol glycoside, and many other compounds. These act as sedative and calming agents. The herb is most effective when used within a few months of harvest. The source of the sedative effects have not been determined.

Use

Commission E approves for nervous and insomnia. The herb is used as a culinary flavoring agent. It may be taken as a tea made by infusion of 3 g of leaves in 250 mL of water. It is also sold in capsule form.

Cautions

The herb is relatively benign. It may potentiate sedatives and interfere with thyroid replacement therapy.

Papaver species: Papaver rhoeas (CORN POPPY), *Eschscholzia californica* (CALIFORNIA POPPY)

Biology

Papaver somniferum, the opium poppy, has been thoroughly treated in standard textbooks of pharmacology. Its two cousins—one a native of Europe, the other of North America—may be considered together. Both are annual plants with bright attractive yellow-to-red flowers. Flower heads and aerial parts are dried. Both herbs have a variety of alkaloids, but relatively sparse content of the alkaloid, opium. The alkaloids of corn poppy include rhoeadine, isorhoeadine, rheoagenine, and others. The California poppy contains the alkaloids californidine, eschscholzine, protopine, cyptopine, and others. Alkaloids of the California poppy have been shown to bind to benzodiazepine receptors. Californidine has been shown to promote sleep and decrease anxiety in animals; however, there have been no controlled human trials with either herb to confirm sedative and calming effects, and Commission E withholds support for the use of these poppy products.

Use

The dried flowers and petals are used in teas prepared by steeping 1–3 g of dried herb in 250 mL of water for 15 minutes. Infusions and extracts may be found. The indications are for insomnia and anxiety.

Cautions

Poppy may potentiate the effects of sedatives. These herbs have not been evaluated for safety in pregnancy

Passiflora incarnata (PASSIONFLOWER)

Biology

A tall perennial vine native to the Americas. It is grown as an ornamental. The fruits are edible. Medicine is made of the dried leaves and shoots. Biologically active ingredients include many flavenoids and the glycoside, gynocardine. Studies have been unable to prove sedative efficacy.

Use

Commission E approves this botanical for nervousness and insomnia. Passionflower has been given for insomnia, hysterical agitation, and anxiousness. It is prepared as capsules and fluid extract. A tea may be prepared by infusion of the dried leaves. Clinical studies to confirm its effectiveness are lacking.

Cautions

No side effects are reported at the ordinary doses.

Scutellaria (SCULLCAP)

Botany

An attractive native American wildflower with bitter taste. It is cultivated in other areas for its medicinal properties and as a ornamental. The aerial portions of the plant are dried and powdered. The plant contains a complex mixture of flavenoids and volatile oils, which have not been thoroughly explored. No studies have been performed to confirm its physiologic effects.

Use

Scullcap has been prescribed for hysteria, anxiety, and other nervous disorders. The herb has not been subjected to controlled evaluation of therapeutic efficacy. It is prepared as powder and as a fluid extract.

Cautions

No known adverse side effects reported with moderate use of this medicine. Large amounts may cause vertigo, somnolence, and confusion. Scullcap may potentiate other sedative substances. Its safety in pregnancy has not been established.

3. Botanicals That Are Illegal, or Have toxic or Addictive Characteristics

Atropa belladonna (BELLADONNA)

Biology

A European wildflower now cultivated throughout the world for the pharmacologic properties of its leaves and roots. It is a plant with three interesting features: it is poisonous; it has a fascinating history having been used to dilate the pupils of women in order to enhance their attractiveness, and drug manufacturers extract the active alkaloids for use as single agents. The active compounds include atropine, hyoscyamine, and scopolamine. These are powerful anticholinergic agents acting as antagonists at the peripheral muscarinic parasympathetic autonomic receptors and in the brain, where they produce a characteristic delirium with agitation, confusion, and hallucinations.

Use

Belladonna may be obtained as powder and liquid extract for gastrointestinal conditions. Commission E lists the leaf for liver and gall bladder complaints in dose of 50 to 100 mg of leaf. Commercially, atropine and scopolamine are extracted from the plant and prepared as an injection for use in anesthesia and other purposes. Capsules containing atropine, hyoscyamine, scopolamine, and phenobarbital are available in most pharmacies with a prescription. Due to the variable amounts of alkaloid in the plants and their extreme toxicity, manufacturers carefully control the strength of alkaloids in the products. The direct use of the plant materials is dangerous.

The significance of belladonna for psychiatrists involves its recreational use to induce hallucinations. It should be noted that a number of other anticholinergic substances, such as *Hyoscyamus niger* (Henbane), *Mandragora* species (Mandrake), *Datura* species (Thorn Apple and Jimson Weed), *Solanum dulcamara* (Bittersweet nightshade) all contain tropane alkaloids and have similar effects. Even more ubiquitous deliriants are the leaves of solanaceous garden vegetables such as tomatoes, potatoes, and peppers. Recently, the recreational use of tropane alkaloids has declined with the increased illegal use of other psychotomimetic substances.

Cautions

Anticholinergic drugs increase heart rate, impair bodily temperature through inhibition of perspiration, and slow gastrointestinal motility. Hyperthermia and cardiac arrhythmias may be fatal. Toxic effects are increased in the elderly. Atropa and similar botanicals are contraindicated in fever, acute narrow angle glaucoma, and gastro esophageal reflux disorder. The frenzy of delirium may threaten life. These agents should not be used for recreational purposes. Their use in pregnancy is limited.

Cannabis sativa (MARIJUANA)

Biology

The hemp plant is a large shrub reaching considerable height in warm climates. Pictures of the characteristic leaf pattern have been so widely circulated that by now it must be one of our more familiar plants. The plant is dioecious, the inflorescence of the female plant being the richest source of resin-containing active ingredients. The plant is now bred for maximum cannabinol production. Cannabinoids characterize the plant. 9-tetrahydrocannabinol is the most thoroughly studied of these; however, there are many other cannabinoids as well as flavinoids and other elements in this plant. Cannabinoid receptors have been demonstrated in several areas of the brain. Naturally occurring neuromodulators of these receptors, such as anandamide, stimulate release of dopamine in the mesolimbic reward system, as does cannabinol. The usual dose produces a reduction of drive, concentration, thinking, memory, and perception of time. Sensory impressions are heightened or altered. The usual mood is euphoric, but can be anxious. In larger amounts, cannabis may be hallucinogenic. The drug stimulates appetite and reduces nausea. It reduces intraocular pressure.

Use

Cannabis yielded a useful fiber; the seeds were a prized food for canaries. However, these uses are now halted. The recreational use of cannabis is the basis of an enormous underground agriculture. The plant has been bred for enhanced content of alkaloids. Marijuana may be taken by mouth as tea or extract but the most common route is inhalation of smoke. In the past, the drug was frequently prescribed for nervous conditions and listed in the USP; it is now subject to criminal prosecution. Cannabis has been used for symptoms of AIDS and certain malignancies on account of its antiemetic and appetite-stimulating properties. A preparation of one of its components, delta-9-tetrahydrocannabinol (Marinol) is manufactured for that purpose. The use of cannabis has been the ground for bitter political debate.

Cautions

Side effects include dry mouth and a pathognomonic conjunctival injection. Long-term use of smoked cannabis may cause bronchial and pulmonary inflammation and neoplasm. Reports have suggested the occurrence of an amotivational syndrome consequent to heavy long-term use. A number of studies report permanent changes in the structure of the brain. The reports of permanent changes with occasional use are less convincing than those with chronic or excessive use. Cannabinols cross the placental barrier and are secreted in breast milk. They may impair fetal development and, hence, are contraindicated in pregnancy and breast-feeding.

Catha edulis (KHAT)

Biology

An evergreen tree native to East Africa, it is a prime recreational substance in Islamic countries, where the religion proscribes alcohol. The phenethylamine compounds, cathine, and cathinone are chief active agents. Norpseudoephedrine, norephedrine, and related compounds contribute to stimulating effects. The more volatile cathinone dissipates rapidly. The ingredients have a sympathomimetic and central stimulating action, which result in alertness, euphoria, suppression of hunger.

Use

The fresh leaves may be chewed, made into paste, or taken as tea. The drug is said to increase self-regard, alertness, and act as an aphrodisiac. Many countries attempt to restrict its recreational use. The World Health Organization has declared it a drug of abuse. It is banned in many countries and is a schedule 1 controlled substance in the United States.

Cautions

Excitement, hypertension, and appetite suppression result from Khat use. Long-term use leads to apathy and anorexia. The drug may be habituating, and a withdrawal syndrome of depression and fatigue result from sudden cessation. The effects in pregnancy have not been documented.

Ephedra sinica AND OTHER SPECIES

Biology

Ephedra sinica is a commonly used botanical used in Chinese medicine as Ma Huang; however, *Ephedra* species are widely distributed throughout temperate regions. The aerial portions of the plant are dried and used as tea. More commonly, a fluid extract is used as tincture or capsules. The active principles are the alkaloids ephedrine, pseudophedrine, norephedrine, and norpseudoephedrine. These are powerful peripheral sympathomimetic and central nervous system stimulants.

Use

Ephedrine and pseudoephedrine are extracted from the plant and used as decongestants in commercial cold medicine and nose drops. Ephedra root may be used as tea at 0.5 to 3 g per cup, but more commonly as extracts. It is approved for treatment of cough and bronchitis by Commission E and the WHO. There is no evidence that it increases stamina in athletes. Ephedrine has been abused for its stimulant properties and, furthermore, is a raw material for illegal stimulants in the underground drug economy.

Cautions

Ephedrine products have been popular in pharmacies and health food stores, they are sold over the counter to control appetite and increase energy. It is well to note that ephedrine is never used alone in Asian medicine, but rather combined with other botanicals that modify its effects. Its use in nose drops results in rebound nasal turgor. It can be habituating with chronic use. Ephedrine increases blood pressure and is contraindicated in hypertension. Other contraindications include thyrotoxicosis, pheochromocytoma, and lower urinary tract obstruction. It is contraindicated in pregnancy. Drug interactions, some potentially fatal, include MAOI, stimulants, and other sympathomimetic drugs.

Erythroxylum coca (COCAINE)

Botany

A shrubby tree native to the Andes mountains of South America, but cultivated elsewhere in mountainous regions. The fibrous leaves are dried or chewed in their native environment. The chemical processing of coca leaves is the basis of a large illegal enterprise. The plant contains a number of active substances, but chief agent is the tropane alkaloid, cocaine. Cocaine is a local anesthetic agent. It stimulates release of monoamine neurotransmitters and blocks their reuptake. Its strongest effect is on dopamine, which accounts for the prominent euphoria. Other effects,—such as hypertension, irritability, restlessness, anxiety, paranoia—may result from excess of other monoamines.

Use

It has been used as a local anesthetic. Leaves are chewed by Andean workers to increase stamina on long journies. Cocaine's use is illegal in most countries.

Cautions

Use in pregnancy causes fetal abnormalities. Coca may be habituating. Adrenergic effects may lead to acute vascular events of cardiac and cerebral arteries, although such untoward effects are more common with the refined alkaloid, cocaine.

Summary

This chapter has attempted to summarize the current state of herbal pharmacopoeia in psychiatry. Table 4.1, which contains the most common herbal psychotropic medicines, may be helpful in prescribing. Doses are difficult to quantitate because of the variation of potency. Also, many of these medicines, particularly those used for insomnia and anxiety, are sold in combination. The growth of interest in this area has produced two contrasting effects. On a positive note, interest has insured increased funding for scientific exploration of botanicals and of the differences between herbal and ordinary medical practice. More disturbing developments are the uncontrolled proliferation of products, lack of standardization, wide disparity in outlets selling herbal products. The enthusiasm of the consumer, who often feels that these products are healthy and one can never have too much health, may lead to injudicious and excessive use of these products. Taking a complete history is important as the practitioner may uncover bizarre mixtures, contaminated, or unsanitary medicines, as well as ones that are carefully produced and used.

Table 4.1. Some Common Phytopsychopharmaceuticals.

Herbal	Indications	Dose	Side Effects
Coffea	Somnolence, fatigue	90–100 mg	Anxiety, cardiac arrhythmia, gastric irritation
Ginko	Organic cognitive disfunction, memory impairment	120–240 mg	Potentiates anticoagulants
Hops	Insomnia, anxiety	1 g of strobile as tea, 1–2 mL tincture	Somnolence, potentiates depressants
Hypericum	Depressive disorder	900 mg daily	Photosensitivity, induces CYP450 enzymes, lowers levels of several medicines
Ginseng	Stress, fatigue, cognitive impairment	100–400 mg daily	Hypertension, mastalgia, interactions with a number of drugs
Rauwolfia	Schizophrenia, anxiety, insomnia	0.05–1 mg	Hypotension, nasal congestion, potentiates depressants, increased incidence of breast tumors with chronic use
Valerian	Insomnia, anxiety	300–900 mg at bedtime. 300–450 TID	Potentiates depressants

REFERENCES

Beaubrun, G., & Gray, G. E. (2000). A review of herbal medicines for psychiatric disorders. *Psychiatric Services, 51*(9), 1130–1134.

Blumenthal, M., & Busse, W. R. (1998). Complete German Commission E monographs; therapeutic guide to herbal medicines/developed by a special expert committee of the German Federal Institute for Drugs and Medical Devices. Integrative Medicine Communications, Boston, MA.

Blumenthal, M., Goldberg, A., & Brinkmann, J. eds. (2000). *Herbal medicine: expanded commission E monographs*. Integrative Medicine Communications, Newton, MA.

Davis, D. L. (1999). Opening comments from the Department of Health and Human Services, 7. In D. Eskinazi (Ed.), *Botanical Medicine*. Larchmont, NY: Mary Ann Liebert, Inc.

DeKosky, S. T., Williamson, J. D., Fitzpatrick, A. L., et al. (2008). *Ginko biloba* for prevention of dementia: A randomized controlled trial. *Journal of the American Medical Association, 300*(19), 2253–2262.

DeSmet PAGM (2002). Herbal remedies. *New England Journal of Medicine, 347*(25), 2046–2056.

DeSmet PAGM (2005). Herbal medicine in Europe—relaxing regulatory standards. *New England Journal of Medicine, 352*(12), 1176–1178.

Ernst, E. (2007). Herbal medicine: Buy one get two free. *Postgraduate Medical Journal, 83*, 615–616.

Gagnier, J. J., DeMelo, J., Boon, H., Rochon, P., Bombardier, C. (2006). Quality of reporting of randomized controlled trials of herbal medicine interventions. *American Journal of Medicine, 119*, 800.e1–800.e11.

Hypericum Depression Trial Study Group The effect of Hypricum perforatum (St. John's wort) in major depressive disorder: A randomized controlled trial (2002). *JAMA, 287*(10), 1807–1814.

Marcus, D. M., & Grollman, A. P. (2002). Botanical medicines—the need for new regulations. *New England Journal of Medicine, 347*(25), 2073–2076.

Sarris, J. (2007). Herbal medicine in the treatment of psychiatric disorders: A systematic review. *Phytotherapy Research, 21*, 703–716.

Straus, S. E. (2002). Herbal Medicines—what's in the bottle? *New England Journal of Medicine, 347*(25), 1997–1998.

Thompson Health Care (FIRM) *Physicians Desk Reference for Herbal Medicines*, 3rd edn (2004). Montvale, NJ

Thomson, P. D. R. (2003). *Natural medicines comprehensive database* (5th edn). Stockton, CA: Therapeutic Research Faculty.

Weill, A. T. (1999). Botanical efficiency in the clinical setting. In D. Eskinazi (Ed.), *Botanical medicine.* Larchmont, NY: Mary Ann Liebert Inc., pp. 43–44.

World Health Organization (WHO) Monographs on selected medicinal plants, v. 1 (1999). Geneva: World Health Organization.

5

Art Therapy in the Context of Creative Expressive Therapies

SUSAN KAYE-HUNTINGTON AND CAROLINE C. PETERSON

KEY CONCEPTS

- Creative arts and expressive therapies have grown since their introduction in the field of mental health since the mid-twentieth century.
- Developmental, psychodynamic, learning, and self-regulatory theories have contributed to the rationale for the use of creative expressive modalities.
- Creativity and play, with their body-centered sensing in activities, are posited to be significant contributors to overall well-being.
- Combining the nonverbal and verbal, creative expressive therapists employ multi-modal approaches to support skills reparation in both receptive and expressive domains.
- Evidence-based outcomes in art, music, dance, and narrative expressive therapies have moved beyond case studies to clinical outcomes research.
- A neurodevelopmental approach in the art therapy field has increasingly focused on the role of the use of imagery in bilateral coordination and integration and in self-regulation.
- The 50-year development of arts-based assessments to gain insight into cognitive and emotional functioning has advanced towards factor correlations with differential diagnosis.
- Evidence points to the use of art therapy in clinical populations diagnosed with PTSD, behavioral disorders, in medical problems and somatic symptoms, and in the treatment of self-esteem and mood.

Introduction

In the domain of Complementary and Alternative Medicine (CAM), creative arts therapies utilizing art, music, movement, and drama as well as other expressive therapies incorporating poetry and narrative writing have been increasingly utilized as beneficial therapeutic interventions in the treatment of a range of psychosocial issues for both children and adults.

The theoretical underpinnings for the use of the arts as clinical modalities include ego psychology, object relations theory, existential and phenomenological perspectives, developmental psychology, learning theory, and, most currently, self-regulation theory and neurodevelopmental models. Those who pioneered the development of the creative arts and expressive therapies referenced the contributions of Freud (1908, 1989) and Jung (1956), for their theories related to the symbolic unconscious and active imagination, respectively. However, Winnicott (1953, 1971) is the most cited theorist, given his clarity about the importance of play as the freedom to be creative and the therapeutic utility of the objects of play.

This chapter offers an overview of the dominant modes of theory and practice in the creative arts and expressive therapies, briefly highlighting outcomes research in music and dance/movement, and in the drama and expressive writing domains. In the latter segment of the chapter, a more comprehensive treatment of art therapy as a therapeutic modality is given.

Organizing Inner and Outer Experience: Fine Tuning Expressive and Receptive Domains in the Creative Arts and Expressive Therapies

Freud (1908, 1989) compared the process of creativity to children's play, whereby the natural movement of play reflects an inherent metaphor in reality that in the arts therapies, represents the doorway to insight, reconciliation, and growth. This capacity to discern internal reality as an emergent function of creativity was described by Maslow (1968) as "self-actualizing creativeness," which he described as a capacity for persons to perceive:

> [t]he fresh, the raw, the concrete, the idiographic, as well as the generic, the abstract, the rubricized, the categorized and the classified. Consequently, (those who see in this way) live far more in the real world of nature than in

the verbalized world of concepts, abstractions, expectations, beliefs and stereotypes that most people confuse with the real world. (p.137)

Maslow suggested that this quality of attending "is well expressed in Rogers' phase: *openness to experience*" (p. 138). In his influential article "*Towards a Theory of Creativity*," Maslow's colleague Carl Rogers (1954) proposed a constructionist view of creativity, describing possible conditions within the individual for creativity including: "*Openness to experience, an internal locus of evaluation*, and *the ability to toy with elements and concepts* (an ability to play spontaneously)" (p. 353–355). "It is from this spontaneous toying and exploration that there arises…(from) the creative seeing of life in a new and significant way…there emerges one or two evolutionary forms with the qualities which give them a more permanent value" (p. 355). These *evolutionary forms* of *permanent value that emerge from creativity* are at the heart of clinically successful outcomes in creative expressive therapies.

Within the therapeutic milieu of creative arts, "inner states are externalized or projected into the arts media, transformed in health promoting ways and then re-internalized by the client" (Johnson, 1998, p. 85). Following on Winnicott's (1953) concept of the holding environment between the mother and child in early development as a "transitional phenomenon," the creatively expressed products (image, poem, dance song) serve as symbolic *transitional objects* and provide a means to distinguish between fantasy-related inner objects and the fact-based outer reality/objects. From a clinical perspective, the ability to think in symbols is related to object permanence and constancy, and to self-other differentiation and awareness, and represents a cognitive (Piaget, 1962) and affective (Mahler, 1975) achievement that supports the capacity for self-regulation.

In this way, creative expressive tasks related to life experiences can potentially alter threat and other schemas, and positively affect self-regulatory coping skills, as both objective and subjective representations are present within the emergent expressed forms. This outcome is derived both organically and as a result of the participant's active expression as creator (subjective role) and as observer of what is created (objective role). It is felt that this dual role supports the cultivation of autonomous functioning so important in the resolution of mental health challenges, and offers participants the opportunity to perceive themselves and the world more clearly as well as to play an active role in their own well-being (Peterson, 2006; Monti et al., 2006).

In summary, negotiating the emergent expressed representations in free and structured creative tasks may be understood as a parallel process to the integration and appraisal of coping outcomes in self-regulation (Levanthal, 1984). When done in the context of a therapeutic process, the completed sculpture, picture, dance, song, or poem expressed is perceived externally and held as an internalized personal reference that is posited to mediate coping procedures.

Creative Arts and Expressive Therapy Utilization

Over the last half century, the use of creative expressive modalities as primary and adjunctive treatments has been incorporated into the care of persons with psychiatric diagnosis, as well as for those with medical illness experiencing anxiety, depression, and stress-related disorders. As a result, creative arts and expressive therapies outcomes research has been increasingly reported in peer-reviewed journals.

CREATIVE EXPRESSIVE THERAPIES REVIEW

Music Therapy: "Within a therapeutic relationship with a music therapist, persons receiving music therapy explore both their expressive and receptive capacities, playing or listening to music, creating song lyrics, and improvising using standards of treatment developed under the aegis of the licensing body for credentialed music therapists" (American Music Therapy Association, 2007). Music therapy has been reported to be of benefit in the treatment of children, adolescents with at-risk behaviors, depression, and in geriatric populations with a range of mental health issues.

Music therapy is often used as an adjunctive treatment for children with autism, and a meta-analysis of reported outcomes suggests the potential for improved communication and behavioral skills (Gold & Wigram, 2006). To assess the efficacy of music therapy with adolescents with a range of psychiatric diagnoses, 11 studies ($n = 188$) of limited sample size were analyzed and revealed that music therapy has a medium-to-large positive effect (ES =. 61). Although this review had several limitations, the largest effects were seen in the treatment of behavioral and developmental disorders using psychodynamic and humanistic rather than behavioral models of treatment (Gold, Voracek, & Wigram, 2004). In a review of studies of persons diagnosed with schizophrenia, global state improvements, including a reduction in negative symptoms and an increase in social functioning, were reported, particularly when 20 or more sessions of music therapy were used (Gold, Heldal, Dahle, & Wigram, 2005).

The use of music therapy in the treatment of addictions appeared to be particularly useful in group work with music therapy as a means to reduce isolation in the newly sober (Winkleman, 2003). In addition, music therapy supported the cultivation of new modes for stress reduction and relaxation as a coping mechanism to prevent relapse (James, 1988). In an analysis of 22 music therapy interventions that provided quantitative outcomes, stress-based arousal decreased (Pelletier, 2004).

Dance Therapy: "Given that many criteria for differential diagnosis in psychiatry relate to both symptoms experienced in the body or the functional capacity for activities of daily living, dance movement therapy has particular clinical relevance to integrated approaches to well being." (American Dance Therapy Association, 2007). Standards for practice and professionalism have been established in the field for over 40 years.

Though the literature suggests a depth of work in geriatrics, physical rehabilitation, and children, overall there are few randomized clinical trials on the use of dance movement therapy. However, as with the other creative arts therapies, there is a current trend to assess the impact of these often nonverbal, body-centered modalities.

In a Korean study of middle-school seniors with mild depression—mean age of 16—40 students were randomized to a 12-week dance movement therapy (DMT) group or a control group. Those participating in the DMT group had significant reductions in psychological distress on a valid and reliable measure; their plasma serotonin concentration increased and dopamine concentration decreased, as well, indicative of neurophysiological change underlying improvements on self-report measures (Jeong, 2005).

While patients with dementia and Alzheimer's disease experience severe cognitive losses and suffer emotional change, they still manifest their lives through their bodies. Numerous reports of work with social dancing or dance learning in geriatric settings suggest that dance/movement therapy can be a significant resource for connection, expression, clinical assessment, and learning (Hokkanen, 2003; Paolo-Bengtsson, 1998; Rosler, 2002).

Drama and Narrative Expressive Therapies: Drama therapy accommodates using nonverbal and verbal approaches, including theatrical enactments, pantomime, and puppetry (National Association for Drama Therapy, 2007). Significant to the use of these dramatic forms for advancing clinical goals are clients' abilities to tell their stories and the exploration of role play that this modality affords (Landy, 1990). A recent meta-analysis of five clinical trials with a total of 210 subjects of the use of drama therapy, with persons with schizophrenia or schizophrenia-like diagnoses, failed to produce significant findings due to variations in approach that included drama therapy, social drama group, psychodrama, and role playing. This outcome underscores research challenges facing creative arts and expressive therapists (Ruddy & Dent Brown, 2007).

Another expressive therapy that uses the exploration of story, role, and relationship is expressive writing. Research on the process of expressive writing was initiated by Pennebaker and colleagues (1984). The process includes numerous prescribed elements, including disclosure of both emotions and cognitions around the traumatic event (Pennebaker & Beall, 1986; Ullrich & Lutgendorf, 2002). The *languaging* process itself is posited as being of particular importance because it provides a structure to support integrating, reframing, and resolving traumatic experiences. Reductions in psychological distress resulting from the use of expressive writing have been correlated with a number of positive physiological outcomes (Esterling, 1994; Pennebaker, Kiecoult-Glaser, & Glaser, 1988; Rude, Gortner, & Pennebaker, 2004). In the medical arena, persons with rheumatoid arthritis and asthma in a randomized clinical trial of expressive writing had significant decreases in disease severity (Smyth, 1999).

Art Therapy

The focus on art therapy for the remainder of this chapter allows for further elaboration on possible mechanisms of actions in at least one expressive therapy, which potentially could be applied to others. Data increasingly supports the use of art therapy in clinical populations diagnosed with PTSD, behavioral disorders, in medical problems and somatic symptoms, and in the treatment of self-esteem and mood.

Art therapy is based on the belief that "the creative process involved in the making of art is healing and life-enhancing (American Art Therapy Association, 2007)." Art therapists have a board certification procedure and are licensed for practice dependent on the state in which they practice. The establishment of art therapy as a profession was influenced by the evolving field of psychoanalysis, developmental theories such as Jean Piaget's, and the ideas of the late-nineteenth-century progressive education movement (Junge, 1994). Margaret Naumberg (1966), one of the founders of the art therapy profession developed what she called "dynamically oriented art therapy," which advanced the view that spontaneous art making provided the ground for the psychotherapeutic process to unfold and for the development of insight. Edith Kramer (1971), another influential American theorist in the development of art therapy, theorized that the value of the process of art making, and the problem solving around producing an aesthetically satisfying picture or sculpture, supported the development of a healthy ego.

Art therapy is reported to have developed along a somewhat parallel course in Great Britain, with the use of art therapy expanding in psychiatric settings in both countries during and after World War II, most notably in the United States at the Menninger Clinic (Junge, 1994). In Germany and other parts of Europe, art therapy developed as part of the anthroposophical medicine tradition based on the theories of Rudolph Steiner (Howard, 1998).

Kwiatkowska (1978) was a critical influence in the development of family art therapy and assessment. Her work at St. Elizabeth's Hospital in Washington, D.C. served as a model for art therapists including Landgarten (1981), whose use of family systems theory supported "here and now family interchange approach through art task orientation." Art therapist Judy Rubin (1978) proposed a studio-based orientation to art therapy, which she described as supportive of a "framework for freedom." Myra Levick (1983) proposed an intensive art psychotherapeutic model in which the client's verbal associations to artwork supported the cultivation of insight and working through. Working from object relations theory, Arthur Robbins (1987) used Mahler's phases of development in working from the provision of structure and mirroring within the sensory domains of the art experience, through working with boundaries towards rapprochement.

Harriet Wadeson (1980), author of what is considered a classic art therapy text, *Art Psychotherapy*, synthesized the advantages of art therapy to include six factors: imagery, decreased defenses, objectification (distancing from the completed art production), permanence, spatial matrix, and creative and physical energy (pp. 8–12). Wadeson (1987) worked at the National Institute of Mental Health in the 1960s and, based on her work there, she expanded the approach espoused by Naumberg (1966) related to transference and projection, integrating elements from Jung (shadow side), Gestalt (disowned parts), and the existential tradition.

Laurie Wilson's (1987) work has focused on symbolic expression in art therapy following principles of ego psychology advanced by Beres (1965), who suggested that symbols "stand for" rather than "stand in" for what they represent, and thus are equal and not substitutes (Wilson, 1987, p. 45). Attributing dysfunctions in symbolic processing as the underlying problem in schizophrenia, aphasic disorders, and mental retardation, her work has focused on how picture-image making as symbolic language by her clients is indicative of both cognitive functioning and energy directed towards stimulus, both of which are amenable to mediation and moderation through the art therapy process towards supporting enhanced self-regulation (pp. 44–62) (Figure 5.1).

Other approaches reflect historic influences in psychotherapy and psychology, including Rhyne's *Gestalt Art Therapy* (1973), psycho-educational approaches to art therapy in the treatment of populations of emotionally and mentally disturbed children (Silver, 1987), and behavioral approaches (Ach-Feldman & Kunkel-Miller, 1987; Roth, 1987). McNiff (1992) sees the art

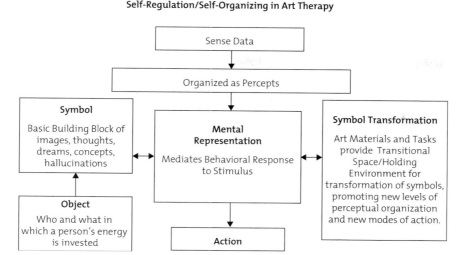

FIGURE 5.1. Proposed mechanism of action in art therapy derived from L. Wilson (1987).

therapist as shaman or healer and has integrated other expressive therapies in his work.

The perspective that the process orientation in working with images in art therapy supports self-organizing from what is felt, to what may be described and understood in a meaningful way, has been well described as encouraging a dynamic exchange in the mind–body by Achterberg (1985) and Lusebrink (1990). Others have described art therapy in terms of potentiating the therapeutic alliance (Luzzatto & Gabriel, 1998).

This dynamic exchange described by Achterberg (1985) is operationalized in terms of images in the prefrontal cortex linking conscious levels of information processing with physiological shifts in the body. This is facilitated by the right hemisphere as an image bank, with its strong link both to affect (emotion) and to the autonomic nervous system that regulates our internal environment, including our fight/flight response and capacity to evoke calm. Achterberg describes the role of stored images in the prefrontal cortex in self-regulatory processes operating as a gateway between emotion and direct experience in our physical bodies (pp. 113–126).

The utilization of this essential role of images and image expression in ordering our experience in art therapy is described by Lusebrink (1990) within a neuro-developmental model. This unfolds from the kinesthetic (the physical engagement in art making), through sensory gateways, to the perception of the sense experience (creation of form and structure in relation to the plasticity of the art media), towards affective (form evokes feeling evokes form), supported by cognitive domains (organizing the whole), toward the symbolic (conscious and unconscious mind senses into form conceptually) (pp. 91–110).

In their integrated theory of art psychotherapy, Luzzatto and Gabriel (1998) suggest that the introduction of visual imagery shifts and enhances the nature of the therapeutic setting "from a bipolar field of verbal psychotherapies to a tripolar field where the three poles are the patient, the therapist, and the image (within which) there are three dimensions: expressive-creative, cognitive-symbolic, and interactive-analytic" (p.743).

Assessment: General Issues and Problems in Utilizing Art-Based Assessment

Art therapists have long utilized visual images as a method of gaining insight into cognitive and emotional functioning. Measures of human figure drawings have been used to assess cognitive development, personality, and psychopathology (Buck, 1948; Goodenough, 1926; Hammer, 1958; Harris, 1963; Koppitz, 1968; Machover, 1949; Naglieri, 1988). Human figure drawings have also been successfully utilized to differentiate among individuals with specific problems, such as depression and anxiety (Tharinger & Stark, 1990), thought impairment (White, Wallace, & Huffman, 2004), quality of relationship attachment (Milne, Greenway, & Best, 2005), and schizophrenia (Lev-Wiesel & Shvero, 2003). In addition to figure drawings, children demonstrate changes in all aspects of their drawing development—the use of color, composition, and line, etc.—that are age and stage related; and these, too, have been studied in some detail as a means of understanding normal visual/ perceptual development (Golomb, 1992; Levick, 1983, 1989; Lowenfeld & Brittain, 1987; Malchiodi, 2003; Rubin, 2005).

Art therapists have used a variety of assessment measures, but as Vick (2003) points out, "The key difference is the art therapy perspective that the making and viewing of the art have inherent therapeutic potential for the client" (p. 8). In consequence, art therapists have tended to use materials and directives in a less formal and more expressive manner, preferring to emphasize the client's role in interpreting their own artwork (2003). Art therapists have struggled with developing formalized assessments in the context of a discipline that has often preferred to use informal clinical assessment processes. Pioneers of art therapy, such as Kwiatkowska (1978), Rubin (1978/1984, 2005), Ullman and Dachinger (1975/1996), and Landgarten (1993) created evaluation procedures that included the use of multiple drawings with varying levels of structure in which the client's art process and verbal association were central to the evaluative process.

The need for appropriate quantitative assessment measures has been recognized, and art therapy literature has recently been enriched by these (Gantt, 2001; Kaplan, 2003). A number of art therapists have developed standardized assessments (Cohen, Mills, & Kijak, 1994; Gantt & Tabone, 1998, 2001; Silver, 1996), and there are on-going efforts to evaluate art content formally (Kaplan, 2003; Gantt & Tabone, 1998, 2001; Hacking, 2000; Hacking, Foreman, & Belcher, 1996). Nonetheless, some argue that combinations of qualitative and quantitative methods need to be balanced in order to maintain the values that are central to the practice of art therapy as distinct from other disciplines (McNiff, 1987).

Assessment: Commonly Utilized Assessment Procedures

HUMAN FIGURE DRAWING

There are a number of specific assessments that are frequently used by art therapists. These form the basis on which art therapists begin to understand the clients with whom they work. In general, the rationale for using these techniques is that they are less threatening and more revealing of personal information than direct questioning, and especially effective in working with children who may have difficulty putting their thoughts into words (Groth-Marnet, 1997).

The Goodenough Draw-A-Man Test (1926) was probably the earliest assessment of intelligence in children to use drawings, and was used exclusively to determine a child's cognitive abilities. Naglieri (1988) updated Harris' work (1963) creating the "Draw a Person: A Quantitative Scoring System," including standard scores, percentiles, age equivalents, clear scoring criteria, and modern representative norms. Subsequently, he has added additional scoring and validity criteria for detecting emotional disturbance (Groth-Marnat, 1997). A correlational study (Hagood, 2002) comparing the DAPs of 34 primary school subjects with two other measures of cognition—the Colored Progressive Matrices (CPM) and the British Picture Vocabulary Scale (BPVS)—found, overall, statistically significant correlations among measures.

Two interesting recent studies have examined the use of self-figure drawings (Lev-Wiesel, Aharaoni, & Bar-David, 2002; Lev-Wiesel & Shvero, 2003). In the first, the authors attempted to identify indices that might reflect schizophrenia. Sixty adults (30 diagnosed with schizophrenia and 30 controls, were compared with regard to visual elements that indicated symptoms associated with schizophrenia. Indices were drawn from the literature (e.g., Hammer, 1997; Koppitz,

1968) and results suggested that self-figure drawings of adults with schizophrenia differed significantly from controls. In the second, the authors (Lev-Wiesel et al., 2002) utilized self-figure drawings to study the effect of blindness on self-representations and self-concept in relation to artistic development, and the use of sensory, as opposed to visual cues, to complete the drawing task. In a study of 15 born-blind adults 18–25 years old, they found the stage of artistic development was consistent with the subjects' biological ages, despite their lack of vision, and that body representation of the senses was accurately drawn without distortion.

Machover (1949) was the first to formally utilize drawings as projective tools to assess personality with her Draw-a-Person (DAP). The projective rationale assumed that the individual's image represented attitudes and feelings about the self and others. Subjects were asked to "draw a picture of a person," and "draw a person of the opposite sex." Subjects were encouraged to respond to specific questions about the images. At the same time, Buck (1948) developed the House-Tree-Person (HTP) assuming that, in addition to a person, an image of a tree and a house could also carry symbolic meaning for individuals (Groth-Marnet, 1997). Koppitz (1968) examined developmental maturity in children, as well as interpreting the drawings for self-attitudes and self-image. She examined images for "emotional indicators," which were partially based on Machover's work. Koppitz developed easy-to-score scales, which were normed on 1,856 public school children from a wide range of socioeconomic strata, ethnicities, and cultural backgrounds, but it is noted that the validity and reliability of the projective aspects of this drawing protocol have not been established.

KINETIC FAMILY DRAWING

The Kinetic Family Drawing (KFD) (Burns & Kauffman, 1987) was developed in response to an increased interest in clinical work with families. In this assessment, the subject is asked to "Draw your family doing something." The person is then asked to describe the image or to tell a story about it. It is anticipated that the request to present the family in a shared activity will reveal aspects of the individual's experience in the family system and the nature of family relationships.

A study of 52 children by Tharinger and Stark (1990) found that, while Burns and Kauffman's quantitative scoring system utilizing individual emotional indicators did not effectively distinguish between children with mood disorders and normal children, a more global qualitative appraisal did. The goal of their DAP Integrative System, was to score a figure drawing on the rater's impressionistic sense of the severity of overall psychological functioning of the individual. In a similar manner, the authors constructed the KFD Integrative System, which measured relative accessibility of family members, degree to which family members seemed engaged with one another, appropriateness of the underlying structure, and relative "humanness" of family figures. These measures were successful in differentiating depressed and normal children (1990). The Integrative DAP was also successful in differentiating children with depression/anxiety from normal controls. The success of this more global assessment procedure suggests that this may be an effective way to evaluate emotional functioning in children.

Milne, Greenway, and Best (2005) used the Kinetic Family Drawing to assess the quality of attachment relationships. They hypothesized that similarities and differences between children's representations of themselves and of their parents would relate to correlates in their behavior. Results were correlated with the Behavioral Assessment System for Children (BASC, Reynolds & Kamphaus, 1992) and the Child Behavior Checklist (CBCL, Achenbach, 1991). Their study of 56 Australian children between 5 and 13 years (mean age 10.22) found that hypotheses were partially supported. The number of similarities in boys' drawings of themselves and each of their parents was inversely related to "negative" behavioral characteristics and to a lesser extent positively related to adaptive behaviors.

The Kinetic School Drawing (KSD; Prout & Celmer, 1984), a variation of the KFD in which subjects are asked to draw people at school doing something, has been developed to assess attitudes towards experiences at school. In their study of the drawings of 100 fifth grade students, significant correlations were found among a number of dimensions thought to measure negative affect and academic achievement.

THE FORMAL ELEMENTS OF ART THERAPY SCALE

Gantt and Tabone (1998, 2003) developed a rating system using a single picture (Person Picking an Apple From a Tree, PPAT, Lowenfeld, 1947). The system utilizes a set of 14 scales based on global and formal attributes of drawings (prominence of color, color fit, implied energy, space, integration, logic, realism, problem-solving, developmental level, details of objects and environment, line quality, person, rotation, perseveration). Scoring on specific scales is based on the overall impression the images make on raters. Excellent interrater reliability (.88 and up) has been established on the various scales. At the time of their development, the authors keyed these formal graphic equivalents to symptoms as described in the *Diagnostic and Statistical Manual of Mental*

Disorders (DSM III, American Psychiatric Association, 1980), which allowed them to distinguish between diagnostic groups of depression, bipolar disorder, and schizophrenia (Gantt, 1990).

There are a number of interesting studies utilizing the FEATS. White, Wallace, and Huffman (2004) used the measure to identify thought impairment in a population of children with emotional and behavior disorders. This study of 53 children between the ages of 8–16 in treatment at a therapeutic day school examined FEATS rated drawings and compared them to scores on the Child and Adolescent Functional Assessment Scale (CAFAS, Hodges, 2000). The CAFAS was designed to rate functional impairment in children and adolescents, ages 7–17. Scores on the "thinking" scale were used as the dependent variable in this study. Students with moderate or severe impairment in their thinking (as rated on the CAFAS) were distinguished on the FEATS from others without thought impairment. Of note, this study did not result in a clear differentiation of diagnostic categories; thought impairment was measured in a number of diagnoses—aspergers disorder, ADHD, bipolar disorder and depresssion. Rockwell and Dunham (2006) assessed the FEATS to distinguish substance use disorders from normal controls ($N = 40$). They found that the aggregate score from twelve scales was able to correctly categorize 85% of the group members—80% for the experimental group and 90% for the controls—suggesting that the FEATS may be a useful instrument in predicting a diagnosis of substance related disorders.

A scoring scale, the descriptive Assessment for Psychiatric Art (DAPA), based on formal properties of artwork has been developed by Hacking and Foreman (Hacking, Foreman, & Belcher, 1996; Hacking & Foreman, 2000). They argue that formal characteristics may be better in distinguishing diagnostic groups and are easier to operationalize and rate. Subjects (86 patients and 23 controls) representing a variety of diagnoses in mixed sex inpatient psychiatric units were included. No specific visual theme was requested of participants. In the rating guide (the DAPA rating guide V.3, available from its authors), the authors (Hacking & Foreman, 2000) defined 15 scales that referenced a variety of formal visual elements (i.e., color intensity, line quality, etc.) and found that two general effects significantly differentiated subjects: the controls used a range of colors and produced more complete pictures; the controls' pictures were more positive in emotional tone than those of all the patient groups. They also report that "diagnostic differences between patient groups were fewer, but showed up on different and more consistent scales within diagnoses, than those differentiating between patients and controls." The authors found the DAPA to be a "sufficiently robust instrument to deal with a variety of less controlled circumstances common in everyday clinical practice" (2000, p.8).

DIAGNOSTIC DRAWING SERIES

The Diagnostic Drawing Series (DDS) (Cohen, Hammer, & Singer, 1988) has been well researched, and its norming, validity, and reliability as an instrument to assist with the establishment of formal diagnosis, keyed to the *Diagnostic and Statistical Manual of Mental Disorders*, fourth edition (1994), has been documented (Cohen, Hammer, & Singer, 1988; Cohen & Mills, 2000; Cohen, Mills, & Kijak, 1994; Couch, 1994; Fowler & Ardon, 2002; Mills, 1989). As with the FEATS, the emphasis in this assessment procedure is on scoring the formal elements of an image and developing a profile of responses (an alternative form of the DDS has been developed for children—The Diagnostic Drawing Series for Children, DDS-C: Sobel & Cox, 1992). In a Dutch study, Fowler and Ardon (2002) administered the DDS to patients diagnosed with Dissociative Disorder or Dissociative Disorder NOS, with the goal of examining the reliability and validity of the DDS in the assessment of Dissociative Disorders. They compared raters' assessments utilizing the DDS with results of the Structured Clinic Interview for DSM-IV Dissociative Disorders; they also considered whether the results of the DDS profile for DID could be utilized to develop an actuarial decision making process for the DDS. The DDS has also been used with a number of other diagnostic groupings (Couch, 1994; Kessler, 1994; Mills & Cohen, 1993).

Intervention and Treatment

Consistent with the theoretical underpinnings reviewed, art therapy may be effective as an adjunctive treatment for disorders with a strong sensory/affective component, problems with self-regulation and body image, and difficulties negotiating unresolved experiences. Evidence-based treatment outcome studies are most frequent in the areas of post-traumatic stress disorder (Chapman, Morabito, Ladakakos, Schreier, & Knudson, 2001; Collie et al., 2006; Gantt & Tinnin, 2007; Talwar, 2007), stress associated with medical problems (Council, 1999; Delue, 1999; Monti et al., 2006; Nainis et al., 2006; Theorell et al., 1998), behavioral disorders (Rosal, 1993; Saunders & Saunders, 2000; Tibbets & Stone, 1990), problems with self-esteem and mood (DiPetrillo & Winner, 2005; Gussak, 2006; Hartz & Thick, 2005; Rosal, McCulloch-Vislisel, & Neece, 1997), anxiety (Curry & Kasser, 2005), and sexual abuse (Pifalo, 2006). Art therapy can, of course, be utilized throughout the lifespan to treat a wide variety of problems.

Art therapy treatment interventions range from supportive to intensive, which also is reflected in the literature (Peterson, 2006).

Art Therapy Intervention with Specific Populations

MEDICAL ART THERAPY

Utilizing a grounded theory method (interview and observation) in an international study of British and American children, Rollins (2005) explored and compared the everyday nature of stressors experienced by children with cancer, their coping mechanisms, and the use of drawing to enhance communication. Participants (N = 22) were children 7–18 years of age and of both sexes, receiving treatment for cancer, of mixed ethnicity (primarily in the United States; in the United Kingdom almost exclusively Caucasian). The author used unstructured interviews, which included a question guide, focused (semistructured) interviews, observation, Person Picking an Apple from a Tree (PPAT) drawing evaluated utilizing the Formal Elements of Art Therapy Scale (FEATS), Scariest Image Drawing, and a closure drawing in which children were asked to "draw a picture of wherever you would like to be right now if you could be anywhere in the world. This can be a real place or a make believe place." The author found that the drawing process did enhance the children's ability to discuss issues beyond the content of the image drawn. The results of the FEATS assessment suggested that, in spite of indications of fatigue or depression, children were able to perceive themselves as resourceful and somewhat in control. Of note, the author points out that, regardless of ethnicity and culture, based on the similarity of their FEATS assessments, children in the study experienced childhood cancer in a similar manner.

Another study with children (N = 33, ages 5–10 years old) (DeLue, 1999), utilizing a pre–post test, control group design, measured whether "mandala" drawings could reduce stress and induce relaxation. Mandala drawings were used based on Jung's assertion that they may have a calming and centering effect on the maker. Peripheral skin temperatures and heart rates were monitored during a 15-minute drawing task in which experimental subjects were asked to color in a pre-drawn circle. In contrast, controls were provided with problem solving puzzles and activities. Findings on measures of heart rate for the experimental group suggested a significant reduction in autonomic arousal. The author suggests that the task's ability to reduce stress might be particularly appropriate for children who are hospitalized, traumatized, or physically ill.

Mindfulness Based Art Therapy (MBAT) (Monti et al., 2006) combines art making with mindfulness meditation, verbalization, and a mindful art activity in a supportive group therapy milieu. MBAT groups were formulated to help participants develop specific self-regulation skills through utilizing mindfulness-based stress reduction and using arts media in response to specific arts tasks (Figure 5.2). In a randomized, controlled trial, women ($N = 111$) with a variety of cancer diagnoses were paired by age and randomized into experimental and wait- list control groups. Subjects who completed the 8-week group protocol ($N = 93$), showed significant reduction in symptoms of distress (as measured by the Symptoms Checklist-90 Revised (SCLR-90-R), and improvements in quality of life as measured by the Medical Outcomes Study Short-Form Health Survey (SF-36).

Utilizing a quasi-experimental, pre- and post-test design, Nainis et al. (2006) examined the effect of a 1-hour art therapy session on pain, anxiety, and other symptoms common to adult cancer. Patients with a variety of cancer diagnoses ($N = 50$) completed the study. When the artwork was completed, the art therapist, with open-ended questions, encouraged the participants to discuss their productions. There were significant reductions in eight of nine symptoms measured by the Edmonton Symptom Assessment Scale (ESAS), with one surprising finding—a reduction in report of "tiredness," despite their using energy during the therapy session. There were also significant differences in most of the domains measured by the Spielberger State-Trait Anxiety Index (STAI-S). Many subjects stated that the art therapy session distracted them and focused

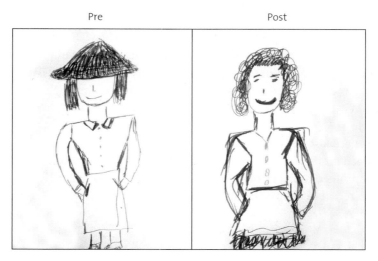

Pre   Post

FIGURE 5.2. MBAT pre–post self-picture assessment (SPA). By completing a complete self-picture before and after an 8-week multimodal program—including meditation, creative expression, and group support—a participant accounts nonverbally for her own experience of state change (used with permission).

their attention on something positive, that therapy was calming and relaxing, that they felt productive and worthwhile in the process, and so on (2006).

POST-TRAUMATIC STRESS DISORDER AND TRAUMA

As described by Chapman et al. (2001), although Post-Traumatic Stress Disorder (PTSD) in children has been extensively studied, the literature on treatment research has been sparse. The emotional sequelae of traumatic physical injury can be significant and can include grief reactions, psychological retreat, and other defensive behavioral patterns. Some children develop PTSD symptoms, including flashbacks, avoidance of thoughts and feelings about the event, hyperarousal in response to trigger stimuli. In an effort to address this problem, Chapman conducted a prospective, randomized, controlled, cohort design study of children 7–17 years old who had been admitted to a Level I Trauma Center for traumatic injuries. Measures were administered at intervals of 1 week, 1 month, and 6 months, post hospital discharge. Pre- and posttest measures included the University of California at Los Angeles Children's Post-Traumatic Stress Disorder Index, Child or Adolescent version (PTSD-I), University of California at Los Angeles Children's Post-Traumatic Stress Disorder Index, Parent Version, Post-Traumatic Stress Disorder Diagnostic Scale, Family Environment Scale, and Nursing Checklist. The authors also utilized the Chapman Art Therapy Treatment Intervention (CATTI), which includes a graphic kinesthetic activity and a series of directives designed to elicit drawings to complete a narrative about the event. Each drawing narrative is followed by the opportunity for verbalization related to each image. While no significant differences in intervention and standard hospital treatment was seen in PTSD-I scores, there were significant differences in all PTSD (Cluster C) avoidance symptoms after 1 week, and the decrease sustained after 1 month.

There are also reports of art therapy interventions for PTSD with adults (Gantt & Tinnin, 2007). In addition, Talwar (2007) developed an art therapy trauma protocol (ATTP) designed to address nonverbal, somatic memory of traumatized individuals. This protocol has not yet been formally tested.

MOOD AND SELF-CONCEPT

A number of studies of art treatment interventions have addressed problems with mood and self-esteem in both adults and children. Rosal et al. (1997)

integrated the use of monthly art therapy tasks into ninth-grade English classes in an urban high school, with the goals of reducing dropout rates and improving attitudes toward school, family, and self. The authors reported that, while it was difficult to separate the interactive effect of the curriculum from art therapy, they found that at post-test, 25.4% more students reported that they "made friends easily," a strong indicator of perceived power to affect people around them. In addition to these changes in attitude, none of the 50 students had dropped out of school or failed the academic year. Petrillo and Winner (2005) investigated whether art making improved mood, utilizing two experiments with college undergraduates between the ages of 18 and 22 ($N = 62$ for both experiments). Their findings, similar to those of DeLue (1999) with regard to anxiety, were that mood valence increases significantly more in making a drawing than after solving a puzzle. They suggested that improved mood was related to the expression of meaning and feelings though the construction of free drawings. In a controlled study by Gussak (2006) with adult male prison inmates ($N = 44$), the Formal Elements of Art Therapy Scale (FEATS) and the Beck Depression Inventory-Short Form (BDI II) were used to measure the effects of group art therapy on decreasing depression and increasing socialization skills. The author found that overall changes in mood in the experimental group were supported by the BDI II; however, results from the post treatment FEATS scores did not suggest that there were any changes in socialization and problem-solving abilities. Thus, the results were mixed.

Conclusion

Given the early and ongoing use in human society of image expression, sound/rhythm, and dance/movement to support both narrative creation and supplication in personal and collective rituals, creative arts and expressive therapists view their work as grounded across cultures and time. Today, expressive therapists work with individuals and groups of all ages to provide services in every domain of healthcare and in education settings. Advances and theoretical developments in general medicine, psychology, and psychiatry have influenced these therapies over time.

The methods used in these therapies to integrate and expand beyond the verbal, towards sensing inwardly through body engagement and perceptual organizing, are being met by advances in neuroscience, physiological, and psychological outcomes assessment and intervention, lending credence to their utilization in the field of integrative psychiatry.

REFERENCES

Aach-Feldman, S., & Kunkel-Miller, C. (1987). A developmental approach to art therapy. In Rubin, J.A. (Ed.), *Approaches to Art Therapy: Theory and Technique.* Bristol, PA: Brunner/Mazel, pp. 251–274.

Achterberg, J. (1985). *Imagery in healing: Shamanism and modern medicine.* Boston, MA: New Sciences Library.

Alton, T. A., & Krout, R. E. (2005). Development of the Grief Process Scale through music therapy songwriting with bereaved adolescents. *The Arts in Psychotherapy, 32,* 131–143.

American Art Therapy Association. (2007). Information and Membership Brochure, Mudelein, IL, http://www.arttherapy.org/./about.html

American Dance Therapy Association, 2007, Columbia, Maryland, http://www.adta.org/about.html

American Music Therapy Association (2007). Silver Spring, Maryland, http://www.musictherapy.org/quotes.html

American Psychiatric Association (1980).*Diagnostic and statistical manual of mental disorders* (3rd edn.). Washington, D C: author.

American Psychiatric Association (1994).*Diagnostic and statistical manual of mental disorders* (4th edn.). Washington, D C: author.

Arieti, S. (1976). *Creativity. The magic sysnthesis.* New York: Basic Books.

Beres, D. (1965). Symbol and object. *Bulletin of the Menninger Clinic, 29,* 3–23.

Bojner-Horwitz, E. Theorell, T., & Anderberg, U. M. (2003). Dance/movement therapy and changes in stress-related hormones: a study of fibromyalgia patients with video interpretation. *The Arts in Psychotherapy, 30:* 255–264.

Buck, J. N. (1948). The house-tree-person technique: A qualitative and quantitative scoring manual. *Journal of Clinical Psychology, 4,* 317–396.

Burns, R. C., & Kauffman, S. H. (1970). *Kinetic family drawings (K-F-D): An introduction to understanding children through kinetic drawings.* New York: Brunner/Mazel.

Burns, R. C., & Kauffman, S. H. (1972). *Actions, styles, and symbols in Kinetic Family Drawings (K-F-D).* New York: Brunner/Mazel.

Chapman, L., Morabito, D., Ladakakos, C. Schreier, H., & Knudson, M. M. (2001). The effectiveness of art therapy interventions in reducing post traumatic stress disorder (PTSD) symptoms in pediatric trauma patients. *Art Therapy: Journal of the American Art Therapy Association, 18*(2): 100–104.

Cohen, B. M., Mills, A., & Kijak, A. K. (1994). An introduction to the Diagnostic Drawing Series: A standardized tool for diagnostic and clinical use. *Art Therapy: Journal of the American Art Therapy Association, 11*(2): 105–110.

Cohen, B. M., Hammer, J. S., & Singer, S. (1988). The Diagnostic Drawing Series: A systematic approach to art therapy evaluation and research. *The Arts in Psychotherapy, 15*(1): 11–21.

Collie, K., Backos,A., Malchiodi, C., & Spiegel, D.(2006). Art therapy for combat-related PTSD: Recommendations for research and practice. *Art Therapy: Journal of the American Art Therapy Association, 23*(4), 157–164.

Couch, J. B. (1994). Diagnostic Drawing Series: Research with older people diagnosed with organic mental syndrome and disorders. *Art Therapy: Journal of the American Art Therapy Association, 11*(2): 111–115.

Council, T. (1999). Art therapy with pediatric cancer patients. In C. Malchiodi (Ed.), *Medical art therapy with children.* London: Jessica Kingsley Publishers.

De Petrillo, L., & Winner, E. (2005). Does art improve mood? A test of a key assumption underlying art therapy. *Art Therapy: Journal of the American Art Therapy Association, 22*(4): 205–212.

Delue, C. H. (1999). Physiological effects of creating mandalas. In C. Malchiodi (Ed.), *Medical Art Therapy with Children.* London: Jessica Kingsley Publishers, pp. 33–49.

Esterling, B. A., Antoni, M. H., Fletcher, M. A., Margulies, S., & Schneiderman, N. (1994). Emotional disclosure through writing or speaking modulates latent Epstein-Barr virus antibody titers. *Journal of Consulting and Clinical Psychology, 62*, 130–140.

Freud, S. (1908). Creative writers and daydreaming. In P. Gay (Ed.), (1989). *The freud reader.* New York: W.W. Norton & Co., pp. 436–444.

Gantt L., & Tinnin, L. (2007). Intensive trauma therapy of PTSD and dissociation: An outcome study. *The Arts in Psychotherapy, 34*, 69–80.

Gantt, L., & Tabone, C. (1998). *The Formal Elements Art Therapy Scale: The rating manual.* Morgantown, WV: Gargoyle Press.

Gantt, L. & Tabone, C.(2003). The formal elements art therapy scale and "draw a person picking and apple from a tree." In C. Malchiodi (Ed.), *Handbook of art therapy.* New York: Guilford Press, pp. 420–427.

Gantt, L. (2001) The formal elements art therapy scale: A measurement system for global variables in art. *Art Therapy: Journal of the American Art Therapy Association, 18*(1), 50–55.

Gold, C., & Wigman, T. (2006). Music therapy for autism spectrum disorders. *Cochrane Database of Systematic Review,* Issue I.

Gold, C., Heldal, T. O., Dahle, T., & Wigram, T. (2005). Music therapy for schizophrenia or schizophrenia-type illnesses. *The Cochrane Database of Systematic Reviews,* 3.

Gold, C., Voracek, M., & Wigram, T. (2004). Effects of music therapy for children and adolescents with psychopathology. A meta-analysis. *Journal of Child Psychology and Psychiatry, 45*(6), 1054–1063.

Golomb, C. (1992). *The child's creation of the pictorial world.* Berkeley, CA: University of California Press.

Goodenough, F. L. (1926). *Drawings as measures of intellectual maturity.* New York: Harcourt, Brace, and World.

Groth-Marnat, G. (1997). *Handbook of Psychological Assessment.* New York: John Wiley & Sons.

Gussak, D. (2006). Effects of art therapy with prison inmates: A follow-up study. *The Arts in Psychotherapy, 33*(3), 188–198.

Hacking, S., Foreman, D., & Belcher, J. (1996) The descriptive assessment for psychiatric art: A new way of quantifying paintings by psychiatric patients. *Journal of Nervous and Mental Disorders, 184*, 425–430.

Hacking, S., & Foreman, D. (2000). The descriptive assessment for psychiatric art (DAPA): Update and further research. *Journal of Nervous and Mental Disorders, 188*(8), 525–529.

Hagood, M. M. (2002). A correlational study of art-based measures of cognitive development: Clinical and research implications for art therapists working with children. *Art Therapy: Journal of the American Art Therapy Association, 19*(2), 63–68.

Harris, D. B. (1963). *Children's drawings as measures of intellectual maturity: A revision and extension of the goodenough draw-a-man test.* New York: Harcourt Brace Janovich.

Hendricks, C. B. (2001). A study of the use of music therapy techniques in a group for the treatment of adolescent depression. *Dissertation Abstracts International Section A. Humanities and Social Sciences, 62*(2-A), 472.

Hodges, K. (2000). *Child and adolescent functional assessment scale.* Ann Arbor, MI: Functional Assessment Systems.

Hokkanen, L., Rantala, L., Remes, A. M., Harkonen, B., Viramo, P., Winblad, I. (2003). Dance/movement therapeutic methods in management of dementia. *Journal of the American Geriatrics Society, 51*(4), 576–577.

Howard, M. (Ed.) (1998). New directions in art In *Art as a spiritual activity: Selected lectures on the visual arts.* Hudson, NY: Anthroposophic Press, pp. 93–107.

James, M. R. (1988). Self-monitoring inclination and adolescent clients with chemical dependency. *Journal of the American Association for Music Therapy, 2*(25), 94–102.

Jeong, Y. J., Hong, S. C., Lee, M. S., Park, M. C., Kim, Y. K., & Suh, C. M. (2005). Dance movement therapy improves emotional responses and modulates neurohormones in adolescents with mild depression. *International Journal of Neuroscience, 115*(12), 1711–20.

Johnson, D. R. (1998). On the therapeutic action of the creative arts therapies: The psychodynamic model. *Arts in Psychotherapy, 25*(2), 85–99.

Jung, C. (1956). *Symbols of transformation: Collected works*, Vol. 5. Princeton, NJ: Princeton University Press.

Junge, M. (1994). *A history of art therapy in the United States.* Mudelein, IL: American Art Therapy Association.

Koppitz, E. M. (1968). *Psychological evaluation of children's human figure drawings.* New York: Grune & Stratton.

Kramer, E. (1971). *Art as therapy with children.* New York: Schocken.

Kramer, E., & Wilson, L. (1979). *Childhood and art therapy: Notes on theory and application.* New York: Schocken.

Kwiatkowska, H. Y. (1978). *Family therapy and evaluation through art.* Springfield, IL: Charles C. Thomas.

Landgarten, H. (1981). *Clinical art therapy: A comprehensive guide.* New York: Brunner/Mazel.

Landgarten, H. (1993). *Magazine photocollage: A multicultural assessment and treatment technique*. New York: Brunner/Mazel.

Landy, J. R. (1990). The concept of role in drama therapy. *Arts in Psychotherapy*, *17*(3), 223–230.

Leventhal H., Zimmerman R., & Gutmann, M. (1984). Compliance: A self-regulation perspective. In W. D. Gentry (Ed.), *Handbook of behavioral medicine*. New York: Guilford Press, pp. 369–436.

Levick, M. F. (1983). *They could not talk and so they drew: Children's styles of coping and thinking*. Springfield, IL: Charles C. Thomas.

Levick, M. (1989). *The Levick Test of Cognitive and Emotional Development*. (Available from Myra F. Levick, 21710 Palm Circle, Boca Raton, FL 33433.)

Lev-Wiesel, R., & Shvero, T. (2003). An exploratory study of self-figure drawings of individuals diagnosed with schizophrenia. *The Arts in Psychotherapy*, *30*: 13–16.

Lev-Wiesel, R., Aharoni, S., & Bar-David, K. (2002). Self-figure drawings of born-blind adults: stages of artistic development and the expression of the senses. *The Arts in Psychotherapy*, *29*, 253–259.

Lowenfeld, V., & Brittain, W. L. (1987). *Creative and mental growth* (8th edn). Englewood Cliffs, NJ: Prentice Hall Career & Technology.

Lowenfeld, V. (1947). *Creative and mental growth*. New York: Macmillan

Lumley, M. A., Tojek, T. M., Maclem, D. J. (2002). The effects of written emotional disclosure among repressive and alexithymic people. In S. J. Lepore, & J. M. Smyth (Eds.), *The writing cure: How expressive writing promotes health and emotional well-being*. American Psychological Association, Washington, D. C.: 75–95.

Lusebrink, V. B. (1990). *Imagery and visual expression in therapy*. New York: Plenum Press.

Luzzatto, P., & Gabriel, B. (1998). Art psychotherapy. In J. Holland (Ed.), *Psycho-oncology*. New York: Oxford University Press, pp. 743–766.

Machover, K. (1949). *Personality projection in the human figure*. Springfield, IL: Charles C. Thomas.

Mahler, M., Pine, F., & Bergman, A. (1975) *The psychological birth of the human infant*. New York: Basic Books.

Margulies, S., & Schneiderman, N. (1994). Emotional disclosure through writing or speaking modulates latent Epstein-Barr virus antibody titers. *Journal of Consulting and Clinical Psychology*, *62*, 130–140.

Maslow, A. (1968). *Towards a psychology of being* (2nd edn). Toronto, ON: Van Nostrand.

McNiff, S. (1992). *Art as medicine*. Boston, MA: Shambala.

McNiff, S. A. (1987). Research and scholarship in the creative arts therapies. *The Arts in Psychotherapy*, *14*, 285–292.

Mills, A., & Cohen, B. A. (1993). Facilitating the identification of multiple personality disorder through art: The diagnostic drawing series. In E. Kluft (Ed.), *Expressive and functional therapies in the treatment of multiple personality disorder*. Springfield, IL, Charles C. Thomas, pp. 39–66.

Milne, L. C., Greenway, P., & Best, F. (2005). Children's behaviour and their graphic representation of parents and self. *The Arts in Psychotherapy, 32*, 107–119.

Monti, D., Peterson, C., Shakin-Kunkel, E., Hauck, W. W., Pequignot, E., Brainard, G. C., et al. (2006). A randomized, controlled trial of mindfulness-based art therapy (MBAT) for women with cancer. *Psycho-Oncology, 15*, 363–373.

Naglieri, J. A. (1988). *Draw-a-person: A quantitative scoring system*. San Antonio, TX: The Psychological Corporation.

Nainis, N., Paice, J. A., Ratner, J., Wirth, J., Lai, J., & Shott, S.(2006). Relieving symptoms in cancer: Innovative use of art therapy. *Journal of Pain and Symptom Management, 31*(2), 162–169.

National Association for Drama Therapy (2007). Pittsford, NY, http://www.nadt.org/about.html

Naumberg, M. (1966). *Dynamically oriented art therapy*. New York: Grune & Stratton.

Palo-Bengtsson, L., Winblad, B., & Ekman, S. L. (1998). Social dancing: A way to support intellectual, emotional and motor functions in persons with dementia. *Journal of Psychiatric & Mental Health Nursing, 5*(6), 545–554.

Pelletier, C. L. (2004). The effect of music on decreasing arousal due to stress: A meta-analysis. *Journal of Music Therapy, 41*(3): 192–214.

Pennebaker, J. W., & Beall, S. K. (1986). Confronting a traumatic event: Toward an understanding of inhibition and disease. *Journal of Abnormal Psychology, 93*, 473–476.

Pennebaker, J. W., Kiecoult-Glaser, J., & Glaser, R. (1988). Disclosure of traumas and immune function: Health implications for psychotherapy. *Journal of Consulting and Clinical Psychology, 56*, 239–245.

Pennebaker, J. W., & O'Heeron, R. C. (1984). Confiding in others and illness rate among spouses of suicide and accidental death victims. *Journal of Abnormal Psychology, 95*, 274–281.

Peterson, C. (2006). Art therapy. In B. Rakel, & E. MacKenzie (Eds.), *Holistic approaches to healthy aging: Complementary and alternative medicine for older adults*. New York: Springer Publishing, pp. 111–134.

Piaget, J. (1962). *Play, dreams and imitation in childhood*. New York: W.W. Norton & Sons.

Pifalo, T. (2006). Art therapy with sexually abused children and adolescents: Extended research study. *Art Therapy: Journal of the American Art Therapy Association, 23*(4), 181–185.

Prout, H. T., & Celmer, D. (1984). School drawings and academic achievement: A validity study of the Kinetic School Drawing technique. *Psychology in the Schools, 21*, 176–180.

Reynolds, C. R., & Kamphaus, R.W. (1992). *Behaviour assessment system for children: Manual*. Circle Pines, MN: American Guidance Service, Inc.

Rhyne, J. (1973). The gestalt art experience. Monterey, CA: Magnolia Street Publishers.

Robbins, A. (1987). An object relations approach to art therapy. In J. A. Rubin (Ed.), *Approaches to art therapy: Theory and technique*. Bristol, PA: Brunner/Mazel, pp. 63–74.

Rockwell, P. & Dunham, M. (2006). The utility of the Formal Elements Art Therapy Scale Assessment for substance use disorder. *Art Therapy: Journal of the American Art Therapy Association, 23*(3), 104–111.

Rogers, C. R. (1954). Towards a theory of creativity. *ETC: A Review of General Semantics, 11*(4), pp. 350–358.

Rollins, J. A. (2005). Tell me about it: Drawing as a communication tool for children with cancer. *Journal of Pediatric Oncology Nursing, 22*(4), 203–222.

Rosal, M., McCulloch-Vislisel, S., & Neece, S. (1997). Keeping students in school: An art therapy program to benefit ninth-grade students. *Art Therapy: Journal of the American Art Therapy Association, 14*(1), 30–36.

Rosal, M. (1993). Comparative group art therapy research to evaluate changes in locus of control in behavior disordered children. *The Arts in Psychotherapy, 20*(3), 231–241.

Rosler, A., Seifritz, E., Krauchi, K., Spoerl, D., Brokuslaus, I., Proserpi, S. M., et al. (2002). Skill learning in patients with moderate Alzheimer's disease: A prospective pilot-study of waltz-lessons. *International Journal of Geriatric Psychiatry, 17*(12), 1155–1156.

Roth, E. A. (1987). A behavioral approach to art therapy. In J. A. Rubin (Ed.), *Approaches to art therapy: Theory and technique.* Bristol, PA, Brunner/Mazel, pp. 213–233.

Rubin, J. A. (1978/1984). *Child art therapy: Understanding and helping children through art.* New York: Van Nostrand Reihold/Wiley, pp. 173–187.

Rude, S. S., Gortner, E. M., & Pennebaker, J. W. (2004). Language use of depressed and depression-vulnerable college students. *Cognition and Emotion, 18*, 1121–1133.

Ruddy, R. A., & Dent-Brown, K. (2007) Drama therapy for schizophrenic and schizophrenic like illnesses. *Cochrane Database of Systematic Reviews* (1).

Saunders, E., & Saunders, J. (2000). Evaluating the effectiveness of art therapy through a quantitative, outcomes-focused study. *The Arts in Psychotherapy, 27*(2), 99–106.

Silver, R. (1989). *Developing cognitive and creative skills through art: Programs for children with communications disorders and learning disabilities.* Mamaroneck, NY: Albin Press.

Silver, R. (1996). *Silver drawing test of cognition and emotion* (3rd edn). Sarasota, FL: Ablin Press.

Smyth, J. M., Stone, A. A., Hurewitz, A., & Kaell, A. (1999). Effects of writing about stressful experiences on symptom reduction in patients with asthma and rheumatoid arthritis. *Journal of the American Medical Association, 281*, 1304–1309.

Talwar, S. (2007). Accessing traumatic memory through art making: An art therapy trauma protocol (ATTP). *The Arts in Psychotherapy, 34*, 22–35.

Tharinger, D. J., & Stark, K. (1990). A qualitative versus quantitative approach to evaluating the Draw-A-Person and Kinetic Family Drawing: A study of mood and anxiety-disorder children. *Psychological Assessment, 2*(4), 365–375.

Theorell, T., Konarski, K., Westerlund, H., Burell, A., Engstrom, R., Lagercrantz, A., et al. (1998). Treatment of patients with chronic somatic symptoms by means of art psychotherapy: A process description. *Psychotherapy and Psychosomatics, 67*, 50–56.

Tibbetts, R., & Stone, B. (1990). Short-term art therapy with seriously emotionally disturbed adolescents. *The Arts in Psychotherapy, 17*(2), 139–146.

Ullrich, P. M., & Lutgendorf, S. K. (2202). Journaling about stress events: Effects of cognitive processing and emotional expression. *Annals of Behavioral Medicine, 24,* 244–250.

Ulman, E., & Dachinger, P. (1975/1996). *Art therapy in theory and practice.* New York: Schocken Books.

Vick, R. (2003). A brief history of art therapy. In C. Malchiodi (Ed.), *Handbook of art therapy,* New York: Guilford Press, pp. 5–15.

Wadeson, H. (1980). *Art psychotherapy.* New York: John Wiley.

Wadeson, H. (1987). An eclectic approach to art therapy. In J. A. Rubin (Ed.), *Approaches to art therapy: Theory and technique.* Bristol, PA, Brunner/Mazel, pp. 277–298.

White, C. R., Wallace, J. & Huffman, L. (2004). Use of drawings to identify thought impairment among students with emotional and behavioral disorders: An exploratory study. *Art Therapy: Journal of the American Art Therapy Association, 21*(4): 210–218.

Wilson, L. (1987). Symbolism in art therapy: Theory and critical practice. In J. A. Rubin (Ed.), *Approaches to art therapy: Theory and technique.* Bristol, PA: Brunner/Mazel, pp. 44–62.

Winkleman, M. (2003). Complementary therapy for addiction: "drumming out drugs." *American Journal of Public Health, 93*(4), 647–651.

Winnicott, D. W. (1953). Transitional objects and transitional phenomenon. *International Journal of Psychoanalysis, 34,* 89–97.

Winnicott, D. W. (1971). *Playing and reality.* New York: Basic Books.

6

Aromatherapy in Psychiatry

GERALDINE F. DEPAULA AND DOREEN F. LAFFERTY

KEY CONCEPTS

- Aromatherapy is a branch of herbal medicine using very concentrated plant extracts called essential oils (EOs).
- There are many conditions for which EOs are useful.
- There are safety considerations in using these potent EOs.
- There are many routes of administration of EOs.
- Research has indicated that inhalation of dilute grapefruit EO enhances the functioning of the sympathetic nervous system.
- Similarly, research has shown that inhalation of dilute lavender EO enhances the functioning of the parasympathetic nervous system.
- Olfaction of EOs can directly stimulate the five parts of the olfactory cortex. These five parts are connected to the hypothalamus, thalamus, hippocampus, and amygdala.
- EOs can affect GABA (the major down-regulating neurotransmitter in the central nervous system) receptors.
- EOs affecting GABA and GABAA receptors can improve sleep, and decrease the symptoms of depression and complex partial seizures.
- EO blends are selected on an individualized basis.
- Administration of EO blends led to improved sleep patterns and decreased unfavorable events in nursing home patients, often allowing a decrease in medications.
- EO blends are useful in smoking cessation programs.
- We have focused only on psychiatric uses of EOs; however, there are *many* other uses of EOs.
- Consult a trained aromatherapist for recommendations on EOs if you are interested in clinical use of EOs but do not have time for further study.

■ There is room for future research using EOs as we look for safe, effective, and less costly ways to approach common health issues.

■

Introduction

Aromatherapy is a branch of herbal medicine using very concentrated plant extracts called essential oils (EOs). This chapter is to inform you of the most basic information about EOs and some of the available research about EOs that is relevant to psychiatry. We hope this will encourage you to consider and use EOs with your patients to augment the strategies you already know and use. We will present some strategies for the safe and effective use of EOs with your patients.

What Is an Essential Oil?

Aromatherapy is the controlled use of EOs to promote balance and harmony in the body, mind, and spirit. An EO is a volatile, highly concentrated extract from plants, various parts of plants (flowers, leaves, roots, seeds, sap, or bark) depending on the EO. Each specific EO is composed of many individual molecular constituents; the particular constituents and their ratios are unique to a particular EO. Essential oils serve many functions in maintaining the life and health of a plant. They protect the plant by preventing attack from herbivores, insects, bacteria, viruses, and fungi. Essential oils also attract insects for pollination, help to heal wounds in the plant, prevent dehydration, and help the plant survive difficult growth conditions (Price, 1995, 1999).

How Essential Oils Are Obtained

True EOs are obtained through steam distillation and expression. Steam distillation is a process in which plant material and water are placed in a still and heated. The steam and volatile constituents rise and are put through a condenser. As the steam cools, the EO and water separate. The EO is lipophilic and usually rises to the top of the water. It is decanted off for use. (The water portion contains the water soluble constituents and is known as a hydrosol or "water," such as rose water.)

Expression is a process used to extract EO from citrus fruits. The rind of the citrus fruit is squeezed until the oil globules burst and the essential oil is collected. EOs are stored in amber-, cobalt-, or violet-colored glass bottles in a cool, dry place to prevent degradation and evaporation. Many EOs can dissolve plastic, and plastic is porous and will allow oxidation of the EOs. An orifice reducer is used to control easily the number of drops dispensed for treatment, and is a safety feature (Price, 1983, 1987).

Safety Considerations

Safe use of EOs is important. They should be stored out of reach of children as 10–20 mL could be lethal to a child if ingested. Good ventilation of the massage therapy room and mixing or rebottling areas is strongly recommended. There are a small number of essential oils that are hazardous and are not used in aromatherapy. For a complete list of essential oils that are restricted in *undiluted form* because of their potentially hazardous nature, please refer to *Essential oil safety: A guide for health care professionals* written by Robert Tisserand and Tony Balacs. Care is used with pregnant women, babies and children, as well as people with cancer and epilepsy. Generally, EOs are administered to these populations in greater dilution. EOs are diluted in a carrier before use to prevent overdose and side effects such as skin and mucus membrane irritation. If skin irritation or sensitization occurs, wash the skin with unperfumed soap to remove the oils, expose skin to the air, and apply mild corticosteroid cream. Cold-pressed vegetable oils, such as grapeseed, fractionated coconut, or jojoba can be used as carrier oils (Kusmirek, 2002). Some EOs cause dermal phototoxic reactions. These reactions are caused when certain constituents, such as psorolens or furanocumarins, are altered by ultraviolet light, making the skin more sensitive to burning and damage (Tisserand, 1995). This can be completely prevented if the EOs presented in Table 6.1 are not exposed to sunlight or UV lamps for at least 12 hours after application on the skin (Tisserand, 1995, 1996).

Routes of Administration

Routes of administration for treatment with EOs include olfactory through inhalation, topical, oral, rectal, and vaginal. Appropriate dilution to prevent irritation to mucous membranes is important. Olfactory and topical routes of administration are most common. EOs can be inhaled from a tissue, steam inhalation, through the air from a diffuser, or directly from the bottle. Topical administration methods include massage, baths, compresses, lotions, and oils.

Table 6.1. Essential Oils at Risk for Being Phototoxic.

Common Name	Latin Name
Taget	*Tagetes patula*
Bergamot	*Citrus bergamia*
Cumin	*Cumimum cyminum*
Lime	*Citrus aurantifolia*
Angelica root	*Angelica achangelica*
Rue	*Ruta graveolens,*
Opopanax	*Commiphora erythraea*
Orange (bitter)	*Citrus arantium*
Lemon	*Citrus limonum*
Grapefruit	*Citrus paradises*

When using EOs in a bath, avoid those that cause irritation to mucus membranes, such as peppermint (*Mentha piperita*), citrus oils, oregano (*Origanum vulgare*), and spicy oils, such as cinnamon (*Cinnamomum verum*), clove (*Syzygium aromaticum*), and nutmeg (*Myristica fragrans*) (Price, 1983, 1987).

Research Findings

We will now describe some of the more recent research on pharmacological effects of some EOs, and later combine that with some practical applications in psychiatry and general medicine.

There is very good evidence that some essential oils affect the autonomic nervous system through olfactory administration. Grapefruit EO (*Citrus paradisii*) and its major constituent limonene (95.26%) were studied in rats (Shen et al. 2005; Tanida, Niijima, Shen, Nakamura, & Nagai, 2005). These two studies showed increased blood pressure and heart rate; increased metabolism of both brown and white adipose tissue; increased production of glycerol, a by-product of fat metabolism; decreased appetite and weight loss over 6 weeks; increased adrenal and renal sympathetic nerve activity; and decreased parasympathetic gastric vagal nerve activity. The doses for these effects was tiny: 1:100 dilution of grapefruit EO or limonene in anesthetized rats and 1:10,000 dilution for grapefruit EO administered for 15 minutes a day, three times a week, for unanesthetized rats. The authors showed that these effects are a central action extended to the periphery, clearly the result of olfaction. They used many methods to block olfaction and others to block the pathways from olfaction to peripheral action, showing it was, indeed, olfaction that led to these peripheral effects.

The same authors (Shen et al., 2005; Tanida et al., 2005) did parallel studies with lavender EO (*Lavendula angustifolia*) and its major constituent linalool (48.15%), again, in rats. Here they found increased parasympathetic activity of the gastric vagal nerve and decreased activity of enervation to the adrenals, brown and white adipose tissue (with decreased glycerol levels), and decreased blood pressure. The longer-term studies showed an appetite increase and weight gain with a 1:100,000 dilution of lavender EO 15 minutes daily for 33 days. Again, these results were demonstrated effective via olfaction, using the same elimination studies as in those above.

Haze, Sakai, and Gozu (2002), studying humans, used six EOs (2% concentrations in triethyl citrate, which they used as their control) by inhalation and measured systolic blood pressure fluctuations [SPB-LF] (after inhalation for 3 minutes), and plasma catecholamine (adrenalin [A], noradrenalin [NA], and dopamine [DA] levels, after inhalation for 7 minutes). I simplified the results by creating a table listing the EOs, their measurement, and its level of significance or insignificance (ns) (used by permission, G. DePaula, M.D.). See Table 6.2.

Before we get into a discussion of GABA receptors, we will describe very briefly the pathways for olfaction. The olfactory nerves are found in the third and upper second turbinates in the nasal cavity. The nerve endings, sitting in a thin mucus layer, are the most exposed nerve endings in our bodies. The olfactory nerves go through the cribriform plate of the ethmoid bone of the skull directly to the olfactory bulb, an out-pouching of the central nervous system (CNS) known as the first cranial nerve. From the bulb, the olfactory tracts go directly to the five parts of the olfactory cortex: the anterior olfactory

Table 6.2. Essential Oils and Their Sympathetic Effects in Humans.

Essential Oil	SBP-LF	A	NA	DA
Pepper (*Piper nigrum L*), corns	up, $p<0.05$	up, $p<0.1$	ns	ns
Estragon (*Artemisia dracunculus*), entire plant	up, $p<0.05$			
Fennel (*Foeniculum vulgare*), seeds	up, $p<0.05$			
Patchouli (*Pogostemon patchouli*), leaves	dn, $p<0.01$			
Rose (*Rosa damascena*) flowers, steam distillate	dn, $p<0.01$	dn, $p<0.01$	ns	ns
Grapefruit (*Citrus paradises*), cold-pressed	up, $p<0.05$	ns	ns	ns

nucleus, the olfactory tubercle, the orbitofrontal cortex, the piriform cortex, and the enterorhinal cortex. The olfactory tubercle projects to the medial dorsal nucleus of the thalamus. The piriform cortex projects to several hypothalamic and thalamic nuclei, the hippocampus and amygdala. The enterorhinal cortex sends messages to the amygdala and hippocampus. (Lledo, Gheusi, & Vincent, 2004) You can see that the pathways described here connect to the autonomic pathways that were demonstrated in the above research. And now we will show that these pathways can affect GABA receptors and that they influence many physiological functions.

Essential oils can also affect GABA receptors. GABA is the predominant down-regulating neurotransmitter in the CNS. Disruptions in these receptors can contribute to familial seizures (Bowser, 2002) and drug-resistant mesial temporal lobe epilepsy (Ragozzino, 2005). Freichel, Potschka, Ebert, Brandt, and Loscher (2006) studied the role of GABA, the number of GABA neurons and GABA upregulation of the remaining neurons in the piriform cortex of the temporal lobe, the largest region of the olfactory cortex with direct connections to other limbic structures, including the amygdala, hippocampus, and enterorhinal cortex. This relates to the role of the limbic system in complex partial seizures. Too few GABAA receptors can contribute to panic attacks (Cameron, 2007). GABAA receptors are important in sleep induction (Harrison, 2007) and management of insomnia (Roth, 2007)

Hossain, Aoshima, Koda, & Kiso (2004) studied fragrances—*cis*-jasmone, jasmine lactone, linalool oxide and methyl jasminate—from oolong tea on GABAA receptors and, in a second study, on sleeping time in mice after pentobarbital administration. In the first study, they used GABAA receptors cultivated on frog eggs. They compared the response of GABA to responses of GABA plus one of the above components. All of the combinations elicited a stronger response ($p<0.05$) than GABA alone, with *cis*-jasmone and methyl jasminate potentiating the greatest response. Then, with these two substances, they studied the dose–potentiation relationship to the saturation level, beyond which there was no further potentiation. In addition, they studied the GABA dose–response curve. These studies showed that addition of *cis*-jasmone or methyl jasminate lowered the dose of GABA needed to trigger a response. This showed that these two substances enhanced GABA binding to GABAA receptors. They also used a diethyl ether extract of oolong tea with GABA on the frog eggs; this inhibited the GABAA receptors in a noncompetitive manner, because the extract contained the caffeine substances of the tea. In the second study, with pentobarbital treated mice, they compared sleep time of pentobarbital alone, or with either *cis*-jasmone or methyl jasminate. The combinations each prolonged sleep time in the mice compared to pentobarbital alone, supporting enhanced GABAA receptor activity.

Another study done using GABAA receptors on frog eggs showed that certain EOs and other fragrances (colognes with a lavender base, but also other nonplant-based ingredients) potentiated the GABAA receptor's response in the presence of GABA in low concentrations (Aoshima, 1999). This showed that *Lavandula officinalis*, *Lavandula hybrica*, and three lavender-based colognes all potentiated the response of GABAA receptors in a manner similar to benzodiazepines, barbiturates, steroids, and anesthetics.

Koo et al. (2003) did a study using the hexane extract of *Acorus gramineus* rhizomes in mice. They used brain homogenized after 7, 14, or 30 days of exposure to the extract to measure levels of GABA, NADPH, a GABA metabolite, and the GABA transaminase enzyme that converts GABA to NADPH. They also measured levels of glutamate, an excitatory neurotransmitter, in mice treated with pentylenetetrazole (PTZ) in a dose sufficient to cause convulsions, comparing mice exposed to EO to those not exposed. Other mice were given pentobarbital to induce sleeping. Sleeping time increases were then measured and compared to that induced by chlorpromazine or a control group.

They found concentrations of GABA increased, but concentrations of its metabolite NADPH decreased, while GABA transaminase remained the same. This indicates an inhibition of the enzyme, causing an increased concentration of GABA. In the mice treated with PTZ (to induce convulsions) alone, the levels of GABA were decreased, and levels of glutamate were increased. In the mice also exposed to EO for 30 days, and then to PTZ, the GABA and glutamate levels were nearly at control group levels. The convulsive activity in the mice was compared among controls, and mice breathing the extract for 7, 14, or 30 days. Onset of seizures took progressively longer, the duration and recovery time became progressively shorter, and the severity less, as the number of exposure days increased. And, significantly, the seizure lethality for the control group was 71.4%; for the 7- and 14-day EO exposure groups, 14.3%, and for the 30-day exposure group, none. For the sleep prolongation study, the mice were exposed to the EO for 2, 5, or 10 hours and given pentobarbital. The sleep time increased with each increase in exposure.

Betts (2003) reported on a series of 100 patients from his neurology clinic who had intractable epilepsy, mostly complex partial seizures with secondarily generalized tonic-clonic attacks. The patients were self-selected and each selected her or his EO, the EO was "highly diluted," and some patients changed the EO they first selected. The methods used were determined by the resources available to his clinic at the time: thus some patients received a full body massage twice, one month apart with their chosen EO; others received no massage. Most received training in hypnosis with their EO; some received both treatments. Across the population studied, 30% were seizure free for a year after treatment, 32% had a 50% reduction in seizure frequency, 33% had no or only transient positive effect, and 5% were worse.

Goel, Kim, & Lao (2005) used young healthy men (16) and women (15) in sleep laboratory studies with lavender EO versus water diffused 2 minutes out of 10, times three at the beginning of sleep. This small and intermittent exposure of 6 minutes total means the effects are due to olfactory administration, not absorption through the lungs. This protocol showed increases in the percentage of slow-wave sleep, enhancing the restorative property of sleep. All subjects reported "higher vigor" after sleep with lavender exposure. In the women subjects, the EO also contributed to an increase in stage 2 (light) sleep and a decrease in REM sleep.

Another sleep study, done by Lee and Lee (2006), used 42 female college students complaining of insomnia. Measurements of sleep parameters and depression were taken weekly. The first week was control, the second week a 60% lavender concentration was used, the third week was control, and the fourth week a 100% lavender concentration was used. Sleep variables (length of time to fall asleep, severity of insomnia, and self-satisfaction with sleep) were all improved with 60% and 100% concentrations ($p = 0.0001$ for all three, and both concentrations). Depression was improved for 100% concentration only ($p = 0.002$). Insomnia can be a problem associated with anxiety and/or depression. In this study, it is clear that improving sleep patterns can help mild depression.

There is a study by Komori, Fujiwara, Tanida, & Nomura (1995) in rats using the forced swimming test, a reliable means of screening antidepressant effects. Lemon EO and its major constituent, citral, both reduced immobility time and potentiated the effects of imipramine with olfactory stimulation. This was followed by a study with 12 depressed patients (Komori, Fujiwara, Tanida, Nomura, & Yokoyama, 1995). They found that the doses of antidepressants necessary to treat the depression could be reduced markedly with olfactory administration of lemon EO. In addition, they found neuroendocrine hormone levels and immune function normalized better than with antidepressants alone.

Treatment Options

So how can EOs be used by your patients to help with insomnia, anxiety, and/or depression? I have a selection process I use on an individualized basis after the problems have been identified in a thorough interview. The interview includes issues around the chief complaint(s), a review of systems, family context history, and work context history. I am looking for what bothers this person, the aggravations in his/her life, coping skills, what this person enjoys in his/her life, specific stressors, when and how he/she acts. This selection process enhances positive treatment outcomes. The process utilizes muscle testing as used by applied kinesiologists and other health professionals (Thie, 2005). It can be employed to assess quickly if the person is congruent with an EO. The author uses the following method to develop a blend of EOs:

- Select a number of EOs whose pharmacological effect is desired; keep bottle closed and label unknown to the patient to avoid preconceived notions from interfering with the result.
- The person holds upper extremity at a 90° angle of either forward or side extension. *Gentle* force is applied in the downward direction at the wrist to test muscle strength of the shoulder muscles. Demonstrate this to patient first and as your control. Then the patient holds the EO to his/her heart. If the muscle stays strong when tested, that particular essential oil is included in the group of EOs from which the blend will be chosen.
- Next, from that initial selection of EOs, the patient is asked to repeat muscle testing with deep, slow inhalation of each EO, with the patient's attention focused on how breathing in the EO vapors through the nose changes *in any way* how the patient *feels*. Listen carefully.
- From the second round of muscle testing, the patient will have selected some EOs that will assist with the presenting problem(s). From these, a blend is made for the patient for inhalation and/or topical application. A small amount of an additional EO may be added to make the blend more pleasing to the patient.

Once the blend is created and diluted, it can be used for inhalation, massage, or baths. The inhalation can be very important, because breathing in the scent can be associated with relaxation, hypnosis, meditation, visualization of success, and so on. When the association has been made, a state of classical conditioning is in effect; that means the state of relaxation, the object of visualizations, and such can be evoked by smelling the EO blend alone. This is augmented by the initial selection of EOs that have a pharmacological action desired/ needed by the patient's presenting problem(s). If the patient is on high doses of medication, and there is improvement in the clinical situation, one can try a very gradual decrease in medication. Over time, some people have decreased medication to levels without side effects. Some have been able to stop medication, especially hypnotics that may affect their function the following day.

In addition to this individualized approach, Jackie Farnell (personal communication, October 19 and 20, 2007) has done work with EOs in over 400 nursing homes. Her program won the "Best Practice Award" from South

Carolina Nursing Home Regulators in 2003. She created a blend of lavender and bergamot EOs to use at night. The nursing home staff reported a marked decrease in the "events" reported on the night shift and, by the second month, an 80% decrease in patient falls on the night shift. Another blend, frankincense and grapefruit EOs, was used during the daytime. There were fewer incidents of yelling, cursing, kicking, attempts to leave, wandering, sun downing, and crying. During the daytime, the patients wear little heart-shaped felt pins on their shirts, about 8 to 10 inches from their nose with a few drops of the diluted blend on the felt. In addition to the decrease in falls and other events, many of these patients have decreased doses, or been able to stop much, of the psychotropic medication they use, also improving their level of alertness. The Center for Medicare and Medicaid has expressed interest in her work and making it more available around the country.

Smoking cigarettes is a problem; many people find it very difficult to stop. Psychiatric patients have high rates of nicotine addiction, much higher than the general population. There are EOs that act on nicotinic acetylcholine receptors (DePaula, 2004). There are other EOs that provide some of the mental and adrenergic stimulation that nicotine does. Olfactory administration of Stop Smoking Aid by Aroma Medica® provides a very rapid change in mental state of the smoker craving a cigarette. After smelling the blend, if the smoker still craves a cigarette, I often use the question, "Can I wait 5 minutes?" That allows the EOs to work before the person smokes another cigarette, decreasing gradually the number smoked in a day without withdrawal symptoms. The EO blend also helps curb appetite, so that stopping smoking need not be associated with weight gain.

There are many additional uses for EOs, but we have restricted ourselves to psychiatric uses that are easy enough for you to incorporate into your practices. Should you not have enough time or experience, you could work along with a trained aromatherapist for the benefit of your patients.

Summary

We have presented to you essential oils, the most concentrated extracts from healing plants. We informed you of research using EOs that bears directly on their use for your patients. We explained some of the CNS connections for olfaction, showing how very central and powerful these connections are. We briefly reviewed the many roles of GABA and GABAA receptors and then showed several ways that EOs can influence them, giving you solid information for utilizing EOs with your patients.

We have not touched upon the many, many other uses for EOs. Among the many EOs available, there are some that are strongly antibacterial (effective for

MRSA), some strongly antiviral, and some strongly antifungal. We have not mentioned their use in relief of menstrual cramps, inflammation, and chronic pain or enhancement of wound healing. There are some EOs that act as muscle relaxants and mental stimulants simultaneously. We hope this chapter stimulates your curiosity to learn more about EOs. If you do not have enough time, please work along with a trained aromatherapist, for the benefit of you and your patients.

There is ample room for more research with EOs. Most of the current research is done in countries where herbal medicine never went out of style or use. We predict that pattern will continue, as major pharmaceutical companies do not invest in natural, nonpatentable products. As one author was told, "We wouldn't be able to protect our product (or investment) in the marketplace." There is still plenty of room for clinical research here, as we search for safer and less expensive methods to deal with many of these common issues.

REFERENCES

Astin, J. A., Shapiro, S., Eisenberg, D. M., & Forys, K. L. (2003). Mind–Body medicine: State of the science, implications for practice. *Journal American Board of Family Practice, 16*, 131–147.

Betts, T. (2003). Use of aromatherapy (with or without hypnosis) in the treatment of intractable epilepsy—a two year follow-up study. *Seizure, 12*, 534–538.

Bowser, D. N., Wagner, D. A., Czajkowski, C., Cromer, B. A., Parker, M. W., Wallace, R. H., et al. (2002). Altered kinetics and benzodiazepine sensitivity of a GABAA receptor subunit mutation [*gamma*2 (R43Q)] found in human epilepsy. *Proceedings of the National Academy of Sciences the United States of America, 99*(23), 15170–15175.

Cameron, O. G., Huang, G. C., Nichols, T., Koeppe, R. A., Minoshima, S., Rose, D., et al. (2007). Reduced *gamma*-aminobutyric acid A-benzodiazepine binding sites in insular cortex of individuals with panic disorder. *Archives of General Psychiatry, 64*(7), 793–800.

Davidson, R. J., Kabat-Zinn, J., Schumacher, J., Rosenkranz, M., Muller, D., Santorelli, S. F., et al. (2003). Alterations in brain and immune function produced by mindfulness meditation. *Psychosomatic Medicine 65*, 564–570.

DePaula, G., & Ranade, G. (2004). Ways to incorporate aromatherapy into a smoking cessation program. National Association for Holistic Aromatherapy, Conference Proceedings: *The World of Aromatherapy* V: 102–106.

Freichel, C., Potschka, H., Ebert, U., Brandt, C., & Loscher, W. (2006). Acute changes in the neuronal expression of GABA and glutamate decarboxylase isoforms in the rat piriform cortex following status epilepticus. *Neuroscience, 141*, 2177–2194.

Ghanta, V. K., Hiramoto, N. S., Solvason, H. B., Tyring, S. K., Spector, N. H., & Hiramoto, R. N. (1987). Conditioned enhancement of natural killer cell activity but not interferon, with camphor or saccarin–LiCl conditioned stimulus. *Journal of Neuroscience Research, 18*(1), 10–5.

Goel, N., Kim, H., & Lao, R. P. (2005). An olfactory stimulus modifies nighttime sleep in young men and women. *Cronobiology International, 22*, 889–904.

Harrison, N. L. (2007). Mechanisms of sleep induction by GABAA receptor agonists. *Journal of Clinical Psychiatry, 68* (Supplement 5), 6–12.

Haze, S., Sakai, K., & Gozu, Y. (2002). Effects of fragrance Inhalation on sympathetic activity in normal adults. *Japanese Journal of Pharmacology, 90*, 247–253.

Hossain, S. J., Aoshima, H, Koda, H., & Kiso, Y. (2004). Fragrances in oolong tea that enhance the response of GABAA receptors. *Bioscience, Biotechnology and Biochemistry, 68*(9), 1842–1848.

Komori, T., Fujiwara, R., Tanida, M., & Nomura, J. (1995). Potential antidepressant effects of lemon odor in rats. *European Neuropharmacology*, Dec 5(4), 477–480.

Komori, T., Fujiwara, R., Tanida, M., Nomura, J., & Yokoyama, M. M. (1995). Effects of citrus fragrance on immune function and depressive states. *Neuroimmunomodulation*, May-Jun 2(3), 174–180.

Koo, B.-S., Park, K.-S., Ha, J.-H., Park, J. H., Lim, J.-C., & Lee, D.-U. (2003). Inhibitory effects of the fragrance inhalation of essential oil from *Acorus gramineus* on central nervous system. *Biological & Pharmaceutical Bulletin, 26*(7), 978–982.

Kusmirek, J. (2002). *Liquid sunshine: Vegetable oils for aromatherapy.* England: Floramicus.

Lee, I. S., & Lee, G. J. (2006). Effects of lavender aromatherapy on insomnia and depression in women college students. *Taehan Kanho Hakhoe Chi, 36*(1), 136–143.

Lledo, P.-M., Gheusi, G., & Vincent, J.-D. (2004). Information processing in the Mammalian olfactory system. *Physiological Reviews, 85*, 281–317.

Price, S. (1983, 1987). *Practical aromatherapy: How to use essential oils to restore vitality* (2nd edn). Wellingborough, Northamptonshire, England: Thorsons Publishers Limited.

Ragozzino, D., Palma, E., Di Angelantonio, S., Amici, M., Mascia, A., Arcella, A., et al. (2005). Rundown of GABA type A receptors is a dysfunction associated with human drug-resistant mesial temporal lobe epilepsy. *Proceedings of the National Academy of Sciences of the United States of America, 102*(42),15219–15223.

Reibel, D. K., Greeson, J. M, Brainard, G. C., & Rosenzweig, S. (2001). Mindfulness-based stress reduction and health-related quality of life in a heterogeneous patient population. *General Hospital Psychiatry, 23*(4), July-August, 183–192.

Roth, T. (2007). A physiological basis for the evolution of pharmacotherapy for insomnia. *Journal of Clinical Psychiatry, 68*(Supplement 5), 13–17.

Shen, J., Niijima, A., Tanida, M., Horii, Y., Maeda, K., & Nagai, K. (2005). Olfactory stimulation with scent of grapefruit oil affects autonomic nerves, lipolysis and appetite in rats. *Neuroscience Letters, 380*, 289–294.

Shen, J., Niijima, A., Tanida, M., Horii, Y., Maeda, K., & Nagai, K. (2005). Olfactory stimulation with scent of lavender oil affects autonomic nerves, lipolysis and appetite in rats. *Neuroscience Letters, 383*, 188–193.

Tanida, M., Niijima, A., Shen, J., Nakamura, T., & Nagai, K. (2005). Olfactory stimulation with scent of grapefruit oil affects autonomic neurotransmission and blood pressure. *Brain Research, 1058*, 44–55.

Tanida, M., Niijima, A., Shen, J., Nakamura, T., & Nagai, K. (2006). Olfactory stimulation with scent of lavender oil affects autonomic neurotransmission and blood pressure in rats. *Neuroscience Letters, 398,* 155–160.

Teasdale, J. D., Segal, Z. V., Williams, M. G., Ridgeway, V. A., Soulsby, J. M., & Lau, M. A. (2000). Prevention of relapse in major depression by Mindfulness-Based Cognitive Therapy. *Journal of Consulting and Clinical Psychology, 68*(4), 615–623.

Tisserand, R., & Balacs, T. (1995). *Essential oil safety: A guide for health care professionals.* Edinburgh, Scotland: Churchill Livingstone.

PART II

Healing Systems

7

Acupuncture and Chinese Medicine

JINGDUAN YANG AND DANIEL A. MONTI

KEY CONCEPTS

- Chinese medicine is a complete system of healing that first appeared in written form around 100 BC. China, Japan, Korea, and Vietnam have since developed their own distinct versions of the original Chinese system.
- Chinese Medicine describes human physiology and psychology in term of *qi,* a vital energy that circulates through energetic channels called *meridians.* Chinese medicine uniquely relates specific mental and physical functioning to corresponding meridians.
- Qi balance is described in terms of yin and yang, which represent opposing energetic qualities.
- Human beings are considered healthy when the Qi circulating in each meridian is balanced in forces of yin and yang, sufficient in amount, and moving freely in the correct direction.
- As one of the major treatment modalities of Chinese medicine, acupuncture is the oldest and most commonly used medical procedure in the world.
- Acupuncture has been used alone or integrated with Western medicine to treat a variety of psychiatric conditions, such as depression, anxiety, insomnia, pain, and addiction.
- The literature to support the use of acupuncture is encouraging for some psychiatric problems, but too limited to draw definitive conclusions.

Introduction

Several practices that are considered part of complementary and alternative medicine (CAM) in the United States are derived from traditional health systems from other cultures (National Institute of Health, 1998). One that has become particularly popular over the past several decades is Chinese medicine, which is an ancient medical system that originated over 4,000 years ago in China (Jeon, 1998; Ong, Bodeker, Grundy, Burford, & Shein, 2005; Rister, 1999), forms of which are widely practiced today in the United States (Barnes, Powell-Griner, McFann, & Nahin, 2004). This chapter reviews some fundamental concepts of Chinese medicine with an emphasis on applications of acupuncture, particularly in regard to treatment of psychiatric problems.

Chinese medicine was a relatively complete body of knowledge at the time it was first documented in book form between 100 and 200 BC (Unschuld, 2003); however, over centuries, practitioners have amassed much additional information about the formulation and clinical indications of individual herbs and clinical applications of acupuncture (Hsu, 2007). Today, this ancient medical system is the major component of what is known as traditional Chinese medicine (TCM) in China (Scheid, 2002), Kempo in Japan (Rister, 1999; Tsumura, 1991), and traditional Korean medicine (Jeon, 1998).

The theoretic foundations of Chinese Medicine, such as theories of qi, meridians, yin and yang, organ function, five elements, and the relationship of human beings with nature, provide a unique system of understanding the internal and external factors that comprise human existence (Kaptchuck, 2000). In that context, Chinese medical interventions, such as acupuncture and herbal remedies, are considered to influence mind, body, and spirit at the same time (Hammer, 1991).

Clinical reports and reviews of the literature have suggested that Chinese medicine could potentially be useful in treating conditions that are similar to DSM-IV diagnoses, such as depressive disorders (Gallagher, Allen, & Hitt, 2001; Han, 2002; Luo, Meng, Jia, & Zhao, 1998; Manber, Schnyer, Allen, Rush, & Blasey, 2004; Yang, Liu, Luo, & Jia, 1994; Yu et al., 2007), anxiety disorders (Eich, Agelink, Lehmann, Lemmer, & Klieser, 2000; Gibson, Bruton, Lewith, & Mullee, 2007; Pilkington, Kirkwood, Rampes, Cummings, & Richardson, 2007), schizophrenia (Rathbone et al., 2007; Rathbone & Xia, 2005), pain disorders (Facco et al., 2007; Haake et al., 2007; Usichenko et al., 2007), insomnia (Kalavapalli & Singareddy, 2007), and addiction (He, Medbø, & Høstmark, 2001; Zhang, Gu, Wang, & Zahng, 2004). However, there are considerable limitations to this data set, which are discussed below, making definitive conclusions impossible at this time.

This chapter reviews theoretical constructs of classic Chinese medicine (as it is taught and practiced in China) and available evidence for its effectiveness, with an emphasis on acupuncture and mental health. The goal of this chapter is to provide a basic understanding of the system, how it is applied in daily practice, and to review available data regarding treatment of specific psychiatric problems.

Theoretical Framework of Chinese Medicine

Since Chinese medicine is inherited from an ancient civilization, our knowledge of the original system is incomplete. First, we do not know how Chinese medicine originated or how its creators came to conceptualize the energetic aspects of the human body, which is a significant component of the system (Li, 2006). Second, some valuable information may no longer be available due to the loss of ancient volumes (Chan & Lee, 2001). Third, texts were written in an ancient Chinese language, and interpreted by different scholars and practitioners at different times in different languages; therefore, these incarnations of translated texts may have resulted in lost information (Galambos, 1996). The best-known resource for the basic concepts of the original Chinese Medicine system are described in a Chinese version of the *Yellow Emperor's Internal Classics*, the first book to systematically describe Chinese medicine in 100 BCE (Huangdi Neijing Suwen, 1956).

CONCEPT OF *QI*

Qi (also spelled "Chi") is the essential concept in Chinese medicine. Much like the Chinese written characters, Qi has a variety of meanings and is used in different contexts. In the broadest sense, Qi means a form of energy that exists both inside and outside the human body. It can be further defined and classified according to the characteristics and constituents to which it is attached. For example, common terms describing human physiology—such as blood Qi (血气), defending Qi (卫气), organ Qi (脏腑之气), meridian Qi (经络之气), nutritional Qi (营气) (Chen & Deng, 2005)—and that describing pathogenic energy from outside—such as Qi for wind, dampness, heat, cold, and dryness—reflect that Qi is the energy behind every aspect or function of ourselves or the universe around us. In keeping with this concept, Qi also is part of the description of mental functions and emotions. In the Chinese language, emotions are followed by the word Qi; for example, anger is called "anger Qi (怒气)" and Joy is called "joyful Qi (喜气)" (Hangyu da zidian, 1995).

Qi is believed to come from two sources. The first is called "prenatal Qi," which is inherited from parents in a predetermined quantity; this kind of Qi does not increase and only decreases over time. Prenatal Qi resides in the kidney meridian and is distributed to other meridians in the course of development. It determines basic mental and physical constitution. Another kind of Qi is derived from environmental sources, such as air, food, and water. It is therefore called "postnatal Qi." The postnatal energies are mostly obtained through the lung and spleen meridians and then dispersed to every other meridian. Postnatal Qi is important to provide the energy for the body to function on a daily basis and also to replenish to a certain degree the prenatal Qi that decreases over time. Lack of postnatal Qi is the focus of most medicinal interventions, and its imbalance causes most of the difficulties with illnesses that people encounter (Holland, 2000).

Qi flows in networks of channels called "meridians." Direction of flow is important, and over time it has become described within the context of current anatomical knowledge. For example, Stomach Qi ideally moves downward to facilitate food to be digested; when it moves upward it will cause nausea and vomiting. Spleen Qi ideally moves upward and buoys internal organs in their places; when it moves downward it causes diarrhea, heavy menstruation, and prolapsed organs ensue. Lung Qi normally moves downward to disperse the Qi to the rest of the body; when it moves upward it causes wheezing and coughing. These energy pathways are intended to balance one another. For example, Heart Qi moves down to warm the entire body by circulating the blood; Kidney Qi moves up to balance the heat of the Heart Qi and to nourish the brain. Within this model, when the Heart Qi and Kidney Qi are disconnected, which often is due to deficiency of Kidney Qi, anxiety, panic attacks, and insomnia can occur. Liver Qi is dispersing in nature and facilitates directional free flow of Qi in the entire body; when it is stagnated, it causes pain in the entire body, particularly in the areas the liver meridians reach, such as neck and shoulder, and in deep connective tissues, and it causes depression (Chen & Deng, 2005).

YIN AND YANG

The quality of Qi is categorized into two major groups, Yin and Yang. Yin Qi manifests as the material foundation of the meridians, stillness, and the energies of dampness and coldness (Maciocia, 1989). Yang Qi is manifested as the

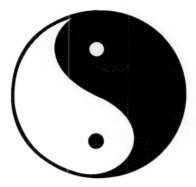

DIAGRAM 7.1. Ying-Yang symbol.

function of the meridians themselves, movements, and the energies of heat and wind, and dryness.

Yin and Yang are opposite energies but exist interdependently. Yang Qi needs Yin Qi's nourishment in order to function, and Yin Qi needs Yang Qi's function in order to be produced and utilized. The opposite nature of the two energies balances the other to have coordinated movement of all Qi and to regulate temperature and metabolism (Weyer, 1997). Similar regulatory mechanisms of opposite forces creating homeostasis are seen on the physical level in the human nervous, immune, and hormonal systems (Chan & Halpern, 2007).

As illustrated in the Tai Chi emblem, there is Yin Qi inside the Yang Qi and there is Yang Qi inside Yin Qi; the extreme of Yin energy is the beginning of Yang energy and vice versa. In a healthy state, the Yin Qi and Yang Qi have a circadian rhythm and are balanced by each other (Diagram 7.1).

When Yin Qi is deficient, Yang Qi will be relatively excessive. This can manifest in symptoms like hot flashes, night sweats, anxiety, restlessness, elevated blood pressure, and constipation. When Yang Qi is deficient, Yin Qi is relatively excessive, which can manifest in increasing feelings of coldness, fatigue, diarrhea, and slowed metabolism, with water retention, lower blood pressure, and psychomotor retardation.

When Yin Qi is excessive itself, Yang Qi is relatively deficient. Major depression is the extreme psychiatric manifestation of this imbalance; mania is the opposite, with extreme manifestation of excessive Yang Qi and deficiency of Yin Qi. The abnormal transition between extreme Yin and extreme Yang is similar to the pattern of cycling in bipolar disorders (Flaws & Lake, 2001).

A primary treatment goal of physicians of Chinese medicine is to balance Yin Qi and Yang Qi. When Yin is sufficient and Yang is balanced, both mental and physical health ensues.

MERIDIANS

Meridians are the main channels in which Qi circulates. Since meridians are nonphysical, energetic conduits, they are not observable with conventional scientific tools, though some feel they eventually may be visualized by new technology (Schlebusch, Maric-Oehler, & Popp, 2005). The 12 main meridians (Table 7.1) are named after the organ in which Qi is centered. For instance, the liver meridian includes the Qi centered in the liver and channels that connect the Qi at the liver to the parts of the body that are functionally dependent on the Qi at the liver, such as part of the brain, gallbladder, uterus, esophagus, spleen, stomach, eyes, genital area, breast, connective tissues, etc. (Figure 7.1).

Therefore, in Chinese medicine, the Liver really means the liver meridian, an energetic network rather than just an anatomic organ. In biomedicine, the body is connected by nerves, blood vessels, muscles, ligaments. In Chinese medicine, the body is connected by the meridians, and the pattern of connection does not correspond to the pathways of nerves and vessels (Li, 2006).

In addition to the 12 main meridians, there are some meridians that are connected to the main meridians but have a special area or functional focus, such as the "eight extraordinary meridians" at the same level as the main meridians (Table 7.2): Jing Bia for connecting Yin meridians and Yang meridians interiorly around the chest, abdomen, and head (Figure 7.2); Luo Mai for connecting Yin meridians with Yang meridians exteriorly in the extremities; Jin Jin for connecting muscular with skeletal functions; and Pi Bu, which connects to the surface of the skin and is the first defense of the body (Figures 7.3). Due to the complex web-like meridian connections, it can be difficult to find a point or technique for so-called sham acupuncture, because stimulation on any part of the body at any level could potentially affect a main meridian response. People tend to mistake the artificial lines that connect acupuncture points on the surface of the body as meridians (Figure 7.4).

FUNCTION OF THE MAIN MERIDIANS

Owing to the inclusive, interrelated, web-like nature of the meridian system model in Chinese medicine, specific connections between each meridian and physical and emotional functions are available, making it a rather complete paradigm for understanding physical and mental health (Chen & Deng, 2005). Cognitive and emotional expressions are viewed as components of Qi, and each meridian is responsible for specific mental functions and emotions (Flaws &

Table 7.1. Twelve Main Meridians.

Meridian	Points	Location	Partner
Lung	11	Begins in the upper chest below the clavicle and ends at the corner of the thumbnail	Large intestine
Large intenstine	20	Begins at the index fingernail and ends at the side of the nostril	Lung
Stomach	45	Begins at the face under the eye, moving down to the front side of body along center of foot, and ends outside the second toe nail	Spleen
Spleen	21	Begins at the big toe onto calf and thigh, groin, abdomen, medial chest and axilla, and ends at the fifth intercostal space of the chest	Stomach
Heart	9	Begins under armpit onto inner surface of arm and ends at the cornr of the fifth finger nail	Small intestine
Small intestine	19	Begins at the fifth finger, moving up to the side of hand, back of arm, shoulder, neck and face, and ends in the front of the ear	Heart
Urinary bladder	67	Begins at the inner corner of eye , moving over the head, down to the neck and back, and ends at the edge of the fifth toe nail	Kidney
Kidney	27	Begins at bottom of foot, moving up to the inside ankle, calf and thigh up center of body to chest along sternum, and ends beneath the clavicle	Urinary bladder
Pericardium	9	Begins at the lateral to the nipple, moving along the inside of the arm down to the middle of the forearm, and ends by the nail of the middle finger	Triple burner
Triple burner	23	Begins by the nail of fourth finger, moving up along the back of the hand and the arm, and ends at the point just lateral to the eyebrow	Pericardium
Gall bladder	44	Begins at outer corner of eye, moving around lateral side of the head, then down to the side of body and leg, and ends at the fourth toenail	Liver
Liver	14	Begins at the edge of big toenail, moving up inside the leg, groin area, and ends just under the rib cage at the tip of the ninth rib	Gall bladder
Ren (conception vessel	24	Begins below the navel on the midline, moving up along the chest, and ends at the lower lip	Du
Du (Governor vessel)	28	Begins at the tailbone, moving up to the back, then over the head, and ends at the upper lip	Ren

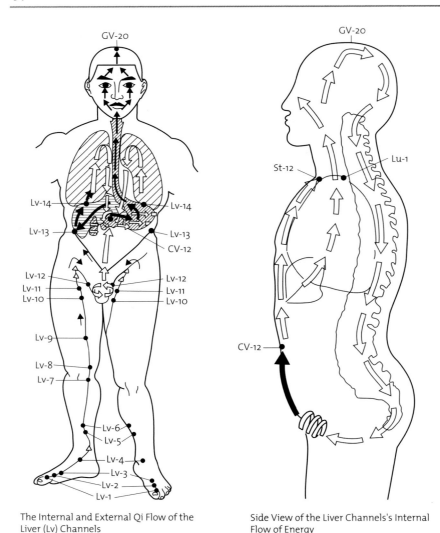

The Internal and External Qi Flow of the
Liver (Lv) Channels

Side View of the Liver Channels's Internal
Flow of Energy

FIGURE 7.1. Liver Meridian.

Lake, 2001). For example, grief is expressed through the lung meridian, and
people in a grieving process may be more susceptible to upper respiratory
infections. While the biomedical model might explain such an association in
terms of diminished immune responsiveness from the chronic stress of intense
grief, Chinese medicine would characterize the problem in terms of the emotional stressor causing imbalance in the lung meridian (that governs grief),
which becomes relatively Qi deficient.

Table 7.2. Eight Extraordinary Meridians.

Eight Extra Meridian	Area Supplies	Connecting Meridian	Function
Du Vessel	Posterior midline	Foot-Yangming and Ren	Governing channel of Yang meridians and reservoir of Yang qi of entire body
Ren Vessel	Anterior midline	Foot-Yangming and Du	Governing channel of Ying meridians and reservoir of Ying qi of entire body. In charge of reproductivity
Chong Vessel	First lateral line of the abdomen	Foot-Shaoyin	Reservoir of qi and blood in 12 main meridians, assiting Ren Mai in reproductivity
Dai Vessel	Lateral side of the lumbar region	Foot-Shaoyang	Regulate the function of all meridians, in particular, kidney meridian qi and essence
Yang Qiao Vessel	Lateral side of the lower extremities, shoulder, and head	Hand and Foot-Taiyang, Hand and Foot-Yangming, and Foot-Shaoyang	Regulate motions in lower extremities
Yin Qiao Vessel	Medial aspect of the lower extremities and eye	Foot-Shaoyin and Foot-Taiyang	Same as Yang Qiao
Yang Wei Vessel	Lateral aspect of the lower extremities, shoulder, and vertex	Hand and Foot-Taiyang, Du, Hand and Foot-Shaoyang, and Foot-Yangming	Regulate the flow of qi in the yin and yang meridians, and help maintain coordination and equilibrium between yin and yang meridians
Yin Wei Vessel	Medial aspect of the lower extremities, third lateral line of the abdomen and neck	Foot-Shaoyin, Foot-Taiyin, Foot-Jueyin, and Ren	Same as Yang Wei

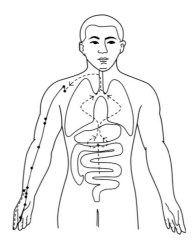

FIGURE 7.2. Jing Bia of the lung meridian.

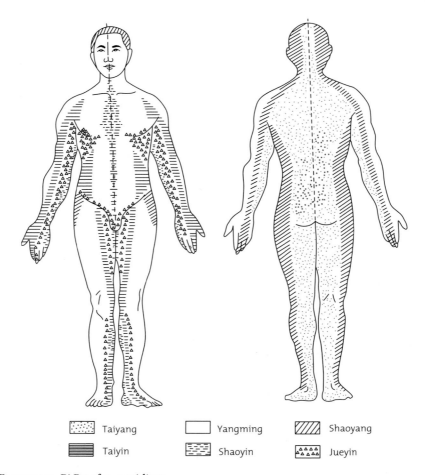

Taiyang	Yangming	Shaoyang
Taiyin	Shaoyin	Jueyin

FIGURE 7.3. Pi Bu of 12 meridians.

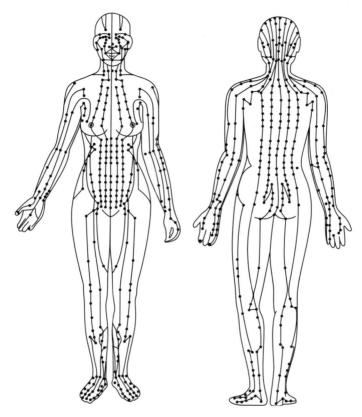

FIGURE 7.4. Artificial lines connecting acupuncture points.

In Chinese medicine, emotions and mental functions are not confined to the brain but viewed more as the interaction between the brain and each individual meridian. Another way of looking at it is that the brain is part of each individual meridian. Each meridian's health affects the brain, a so-called extraordinary organ in Chinese medicine (Sakatani, 2007).

Understanding the connections is important for identifying meridians that are related to clinical symptoms so that a treatment plan can be formulated. Integrative mental health professionals who utilize this system aim to identify the meridians involved in an overall presentation, which leads to specific connections with specific emotional states and mental functions. Having additional ways of categorizing signs and symptoms may potentially expand the range of treatment options.

FIVE ELEMENTS

In Chinese medicine, the human body is created as part of the natural universe and therefore shares the characteristics of nature. The five major pair of meridians share the nature of the five elements and energies and their relationship with each other (Table 7.3). The liver meridian shares the nature of wood and wind; the heart meridian, fire and heat; the spleen meridian, earth and dampness; the lung meridian, metal and dryness; and the kidney meridian, water and coldness.

There is also something called Shen and Ko cycles that explain the relationship of one element to another (Diagram 7.2). The Shen cycle describes the generative relationship of the five elements: wood can generate fire; fire can contribute to earth; earth can provide metal; metal can be melted into water; and water can help the growth of wood. Therefore, the emotions of those elements have the same generative (shen) relationship: fulfillment (liver) may generate joy (fire); the joy (heart) leads to self-confidence (earth); self-confidence to empowerment (metal), which leads to motivation (water); and the motivation may once again give the sense of fulfillment.

The Ko Cycle describes the degenerative relationship of the five elements: water extinguishes fire; fire melts metal; metal cuts wood; wood punctures earth; and earth blocks water (Connelly, 1994). Likewise, there is the same degeneration in the emotional aspect of these meridians: fear (kidney, water) can overshadow over-excitement (heart, fire); over-excitement can overshadow sadness (lung, metal); sadness can repress anger (liver, wood); anger can cover up worries (spleen, earth); and worry can overshadow fear (Huangdi Neijing Suwen, 1956). Sometimes correlations can be made between Chinese medicine and Western medicine. For example, a crying patient may be covering underlying anger; anger may manifest as being worried. Fear may be used to control impulses for excitement, and thrill-seeking behavior may be used to avoid grieving.

The homeostatic goal of a living system is for the five elements to be in balance. However, when one element is too excessive or deficient, it may affect that element's relationship among the other elements. An excessive wood energy, for example, may become rebellious for the control of the metal energy and overwhelm the earth energy. For example, when liver energy is stagnated with excessive anger and resentment, it can cause symptoms in the lung meridian, such as coughing, wheezing, and grief; as well as affect the Spleen meridian causing symptoms like indigestion, fatigue, and worrying. When one element is too deficient, it may fail to generate and control. For example, if Kidney Qi

Table 7.3. Five Elements.

Five Elements	Directions	Tastes	Colors	Environmental Factors	Seasons	Zang	Fu	Five Sensory Organs	Five Tissues	Emotions
Wood	East	Sour	Green	Wind	Spring	Liver	Gall-bladder	Eye	Tendon	Anger
Fire	South	Bitter	Red	Heat	Summer	Heart	Small Intestine	Tongue	Vessel	Joy
Earth	Middle	Sweet	Yellow	Dampness	Late summer	Spleen	Stomach	Mouth	Muscle	Worry
Metal	West	Pungent	White	Dryness	Autumn	Lung	Large intenstine	Nose	Skin and hair	Grief and melancholy
Water	North	Salty	Black	Cold	Winter	Kidney	Bladder	Ear	Bone	Fright and fear

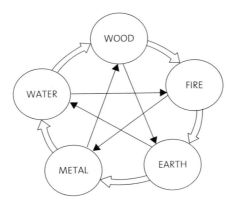

DIAGRAM 7.2. Shen/Ko relationship of five elements.

is very deficient, because of its relationships in the Shen and Ko cycle, it may cause deficiency in the liver meridian, such as poor sleep, dizziness and vertigo, and depression, as well as relative excess in the heart meridians, such as heart palpitations, anxiety, and insomnia (Chen & Deng, 2005). Therefore, clinical symptoms of a particular meridian/element imbalance may be a primary issue to that meridian/element or secondary to another meridian/element that is having a downstream effect. The experienced Chinese medicine practitioner has ways of assessing these issues and determining primary and secondary dysfunctions.

The theoretical frameworks of Chinese medicine provide a unique and holistic view of mind–body medicine. Whether or not this approach is viable and testable according to Western scientific standards, it is, nevertheless, a complete system for diagnosing and treating problems that are often challenging for the biomedical model to conceptualize, such as psychosomatic conditions, cognitive deficits, sleep disorders, mood disorders, anxiety disorders, sexual dysfunction, chemical dependence, and pain disorders. A more comprehensive description of the theories and clinical application of Chinese medicine can be found in a well written, recently compiled textbook (Flaws & Lake, 2001).

Acupuncture

According to Chinese medicine theory, meridians have points on the surface of the body that are constantly communicating with the outside environment. These surface points, also called acupoints, can be used to manipulate the status of qi via the meridians that reach far inside the body. This aspect of meridians is the foundation for acupuncture, moxabustion, Chinese herbal medicine, and Tui Na.

In the classic practice of Chinese medicine, the practitioner must evaluate a patient's qi status in the involved meridians and decide a treatment strategy accordingly, select and combine acupoints and manipulation techniques to restore the balance. This evaluation is done by well -trained practitioners who will make systematic inquiry to symptoms and examine signs, including use of a unique technique of tongue and pulse readings.

In modern times, Acupuncture is not always practiced in accordance with the theoretical framework of classic Chinese medicine, such as when acupuncture is used as a biochemical tool to stimulate nerves and muscles (Wong, 1999). Some add electric stimulation with the needles to enhance their efficacy, or replace them with hand manipulations (Dang, 1999). Others develop a fixed treatment protocol for every patient with a given condition, without making differentiation of qi status and meridians involved (Zhang & Lu, 2002). The inconsistency in how acupuncture is approached and utilized is reflected in the published research on acupuncture, and may be partially responsible for the differences among the studies reviewed here. When done in accordance to the principles of Chinese medicine, acupuncture, relies heavily on energetic evaluation that is dependent on the acupuncturist's clinical experience and training in conceptual and theoretical foundations of Chinese medicine (Liu, 2007). The individualized energy pattern differentiation and customized needling techniques make it difficult to create double-blinds and standardized experimental protocols (Paterson & Dieppe, 2005).

The efficacy of acupuncture and Chinese medicine in treating mental illness has been reported in studies of various types of design and quality. Although most of the studies from the People's Republic of China are case reports and non-RCT studies, they may have anecdotal value and, to some degree, inform future studies. Therefore, we focus our review of the literature on specific psychiatric diagnoses, to selected studies that appear to have reasonably good design, and a few compelling case series, with the understanding that no conclusive recommendations can be made from this overall data set.

ANXIETY DISORDERS

A systematic review of the literature on the efficacy of acupuncture in the treatment of anxiety revealed promising but insufficient evidence, due to the poor quality of the design of most studies and lack of reliable assessments (Pilkington et al., 2007). However, a better done RCT of auricular acupuncture on preoperative anxiety was more effective than acupuncture at a sham point.

In a placebo-controlled, randomized, modified double-blind study, 43 patients with minor depression, and 13 patients with generalized anxiety disorders, received body needle acupuncture (Du.20, Ex.6, He.7, Pe.6, Bl.62) versus sham acupuncture, and were assessed by the Clinical Global Impression Scale (CGI) before and after treatments. After completing a total of 10 acupuncture sessions, the experimental group (true acupuncture) group ($n = 28$) showed a significantly larger clinical improvement on the CGI, lower HAM-A scores as well as more responders (60.7% versus 21.4%; chi-square test, $p < 0.01$) as compared to the sham acupuncture group ($n = 28$) (Eich et al., 2000). The total sum of acupuncture sessions seemed important in this study, because no differences in the response rates were evident between the two groups at the point of five sessions.

A single-blind crossover trial was carried out comparing the effects of 4 weeks of either acupuncture or breath training on patients with hyperventilation syndrome (HVS). Ten (10) patients diagnosed with HVS were recruited to the trial and randomized into the two groups. Patients were crossed over from the treatment condition they were not assigned after a 1-week washout period. The results showed statistically significant treatment differences between acupuncture and breathing retraining, in favor of acupuncture. Reductions were found in the HAD A (anxiety) ($p = 0.02$) and Nijmegen (symptoms) ($p = 0.03$) scores (Gibson et al., 2007), suggesting that acupuncture may be beneficial in the management of HVS, although a large scale study is warranted.

In another study, 58 patients with generalized anxiety were randomly assigned to two groups, a medication group that used SSRI's and alprazolam, and the acupuncture group (Li, Zeng, & Zhuang, 2006) Both groups received treatment for six weeks. In addition to the Hamilton anxiety scale (HAM-A), clinical global impression (CGI), and treatment emergent symptom scale (TESS), the concentration of 5-hydroxytryptamine (5-HT) in platelets, and plasma levels of corticosterone (CS) and adrenocorticotropic hormone (ACTH) were measured before and after treatment. The results suggest that the clinical effects in the two groups were equivalent, while the adverse reaction found in the acupuncture group was less than that in the medication group ($p < 0.05$). The platelet concentration of 5-HT and plasma ACTH level decreased significantly in both groups after treatment with insignificant difference between the groups ($p < 0.05$) (Luo, Liu, & Mei, 2007).

Another pilot study showed that acupuncture may help people with post-traumatic stress disorder. The researchers analyzed depression, anxiety, and impairment in 73 people with a diagnosis of PTSD. The participants were assigned to receive either acupuncture or group cognitive-behavioral therapy over 12 weeks, or were assigned to a wait-list control group. The people in the control group were offered treatment or referral for treatment at the end of their participation. The researchers found that acupuncture provided treatment effects similar to group cognitive-behavioral therapy; both interventions were superior to the control condition. Additionally, treatment effects of both the acupuncture and the group therapy were maintained for 3 months after the end of treatment (Hollifield, Sinclair-Lian, Warner, & Hammerschlag, 2007). In a case series, cancer patients with traumatic stress symptoms were treated with Neuro-Emotional Technique, an intervention that links acupuncture points with psychological processing techniques. Pre- to post-outcome scores on psychological measures and autonomic reactivity to distressing cues showed marked improvement (Monti, Gomella, Peterson, & Kunkel, 2007).

A study examing immune variables in patients with anxiety indicated that acupuncture may positively impact immune functions such as chemotaxis, phagocytosis, lymphoproliferation and NK activity, and modulate superoxide anion levels and lymphoproliferation in women with anxiety. Effects appeared as early as 72 hours after a single session (Arranz, Guayerbas, Siboni, & De la Fuente, 2007).

An RCT of 100 elderly patients who received auricular acupressure at specific relaxation points while being transported to the hospital were reported to be less anxious and anticipated less pain than the sham treated group (Mora et al., 2007). Auricular acupuncture was also reported to help anxiety induced by dental work in a study of 67 patients who were randomized to three groups of auricular acupuncture, placebo acupuncture, and intranasal midazolam, and compared with a no-treatment group. The auricular acupuncture group and the midazolam group were significantly less anxious at 30 minutes as compared with patients in the placebo acupuncture group. In addition, patient compliance assessed by the dentist was significantly improved if auricular acupuncture or application of intranasal midazolam had been performed (Karst et al., 2007).

A combination of auricular acupuncture and body acupuncture is reported to be effective in reducing preoperative anxiety and intraprocedural analgesia in patients undergoing lithotripsy (Wang, Punjala, Weiss, Anderson, & Kain, 2007). The acupuncture group was less anxious prior to the procedure, and used a lesser amount of alfentanil and had lower pain scores on admission to the recovery room than those in the sham control group. Similar results were reported for patients who underwent cataract surgery in an RCT of 75 patients; the pre- and postprocedure anxiety were significantly less in the acupuncture group (Gioia et al., 2006). Another study suggested that acupuncture may also decrease the demand for sedative drugs and increase satisfactory sedation during colonoscopy (Fanti et al., 2004).

An animal study showed that acupuncture treatment reduced anxiety-like behavior in adult rats following maternal separation, and modulated the Neuropeptide Y immunohistochemistry in the basolateral amygdala (BLA).

It was noted that only acupuncture on the Heart 7 (seventh point on the heart meridians, known to help anxiety) acupoint produced the result, not the Stomach 36 (Park, Chae, et al., 2005).

Twenty-one patients meeting ICD-10 diagnosis of obsessive compulsive disorder who failed at least 2 years of adequate medication treatment were given, five times per week, electro-acupuncture at the point of GV20 (Bai Hui) and M-NH-1 (Yin Tang) for 6 weeks. The median Yale-Brown Obsessive Compulsive Scale (YBOCS) scores and HAM-A score improved after treatment. Among them, five were claimed cured (23.8%), four significantly improved, nine improved moderately, and three were nonresponsive (Zhang & Lu, 2002). These results should be considered within the context of the clear study limitations of a small sample size and a noncontrolled design. In addition, classic Chinese medicine pattern differentiation diagnosis was not used.

DEPRESSION

Depression is the most studied mental illness treated with acupuncture and herbal medicine. Results are promising, but again, there are clear methodological limitations in the majority of studies (Leo, 2007). Recent efforts have been made to improve the quality of research, such as using needle manipulation according to classic Chinese medicine theory (MacPherson, Thorpe, Thomas, & Geddes, 2004; Manber et al., 2004). We review a few that have particular interest and/or merit.

A randomized controlled pilot study of 61 women with major depression during pregnancy, with a 17-item Hamilton Rating Scale for Depression score above 14, suggested that the active acupuncture group showed a significantly higher response rate (69%) than both the sham acupuncture group (47%) and Massage group (32%) (Manber et al., 2004). However, the same group then investigated acupuncture as monotherapy in 152 patients with major depressive disorder and failed to demonstrate efficacy (Allen et al., 2006).

A study on 6-month depression relapse rates among women treated with acupuncture suggested that acupuncture designed in accordance with classic Chinese medicine produced results comparable to other validated treatments for depression, such as psychotherapies and medications (Gallagher et al., 2001). However, results for this group were less favorable in a small size RCT of 33 women who completed 8 weeks of acupuncture treatment; four (24%) of out of 17 women who achieved full remission at the conclusion of treatment experienced a relapse 6 months later (Gallagher et al., 2001).

In a nonrandomized comparison of electro-acupuncture (EA) and maprotyline (Han, Li, & Luo, 2002), 30 depressed patients were treated with EA and had comparable score reduction on the Hamilton Depression Rating Scale (HAM-D) and Self-Rating Scale for Depression (SDS) to the 31 patients treated with maprotyline. The same group (Han, Li, Luo, Zhao, & Li, 2004) replicated these findings and noted additionally that, after treatment, the plasma cortisol levels and the endothelin-1 (ET-1) levels of the two groups were decreased ($p < 0.01$), without significant between-group differences ($p > 0.05$). Two other small studies that compared acupuncture with amytrptyline reported similar positive efficacy between groups (Luo et al., 1998; Yang et al., 1994). A nonrandomized study comparing acupuncture with fluoxetine reported equal efficacy between two groups after 6 weeks of treatments (Lin, Li, Zhou, & Liu, 2005). A, RCT compared 22 patients with EA combined with paroxetine, to 20 patients treated with paroxetine alone for 6 weeks (Zhang et al., 2007). The significant improvement rate evaluated at the end of the 6-week treatment was notably higher in the group with combined therapies than that in the paroxetine alone (72.7% vs. 40.0%). All of these studies are methodologically limited by small samples, nonblinding, nonrandomized design, and short duration of treatment.

Using a special group of acupoints (GV 24, 20, 14, 11,9) and needling techniques called Governor Vessels Daoqi, a small RCT compared the efficacy of acupuncture combined with antidepressants or antidepressants alone in a small group of patients with depression and dyssomnia (Wang, Jiang, & Wang, 2006). HAM-D and Pittsburgh Sleep Quality Index (PSQI) scores were measured before and after 4 weeks of treatments for both groups. Combined therapy appeared superior to antidepressants alone. However, the short treatment duration and variety of antidepressants involved limit the value of the study.

Mechanisms of acupuncture effects on depression with or without antidepressants were explored in the following studies.

Scalp acupuncture (SA) used to treat depression was shown to positively affect regulation of cortex-limbic circuitry dysfunction and increase glucose metabolism in various brain regions (Huang et al., 2005). In this study, 12 depressive patients were treated by scalp acupuncture on middle line of vertex (MS5), middle line of forehead (MS1) and bilateral lateral line 1 of forehead (MS2), once a day for 6 days per week, and received PET before and after the 6-week acupuncture treatment protocol. SA increased glucose metabolism at bilateral frontal lobes, bilateral parietal lobes, right occipital lobe, right caudate nucleus, right cingulate gyrus, and left cerebellum and decreased metabolism at right temporal lobe and bilateral thalamus.

A study measuring GTP-binding-protein (G protein) in platelet membranes in patients with major depression revealed significantly increased G-alpha-i and G-alpha-q in depressed patients. Although electro-acupuncture and fluoxetine both produced similar clinical efficacy in patients with moderate depression, fluoxetine failed to reduce levels of G protein alpha subtypes in this small study (Song, Zhou, Fan, Luo, & Halbreich, 2007).

SCHIZOPHRENIA

There are very limited scientific data on the use of acupuncture for patients with schizophrenia. Cochrane Schizophrenia Group (Rathbone & Xia, 2005) has analyzed five randomized clinical trials comparing acupuncture, electro-acupuncture, and laser-acupuncture with antipsychotic alone, and antipsychotic combined with acupuncture. Owing to the problematic study designs and poor methodology, no conclusions could be drawn except for the possibility that acupuncture combined with antipsychotic medications may potentially produce fewer medication-related side effects.

INSOMNIA

A recent review of the effectiveness of auricular acupuncture (AA) on insomnia included six RCTs that cumulatively included 402 patients treated with AA among 673 participants. The improvement rates produced by AA were encouraging; however, given the overall poor quality of the studies, it was concluded that further clinical trials with higher design quality, longer duration of treatment, and longer follow-up were needed. (Chen et al., 2007).

Another review was recently published that considered RCTs on acupuncture and its variations such as acupressure, auricular acupuncture, seed therapy (herbal or metal seed placed on the relevant meridian) and transcutaneous electrical acupoint stimulation (TEAS). Based on the findings from individual trials, the review suggested that acupuncture and acupressure may help to improve sleep quality scores when compared to sham acupuncture (SMD = −1.08, 95% CI = −1.86 to −0.31, p=0.006) or no treatment (SMD −0.55, 95% CI = −0.89 to −0.21, p=0.002). TEAS also resulted in better sleep quality score in one trial (SMD = −0.74, 95% CI = −1.22 to −0.26, p=0.003). Again, due to the great variability in acupuncture techniques and evaluative measurements, definitive conclusions or recommendations from this review cannot be made (Cheuk, Yeung, Chung, & Wong, 2008).

PAIN DISORDERS

There is some suggestion that meridian and acupuncture points may have chemical and physiological configurations (Pearson, Colbert, McNames,

Baumgartner, & Hammerschlag, 2007; Schlebusch et al., 2005; Shen et al., 2006; Usichenko, Lysenyuk, Groth, & Pavlovic, 2003; Wick, Wick, & Wick, 2007), and biological markers associated with acupuncture treatment include release of endorphins (Ulett, Han, & Han, 1998), affects on neurotransmitters and hormone levels (Ma, 2004), increased blood circulation (Sandberg, Lundeberg, Lindberg, & Gerdle, 2003; Tsuchiya, Sato, Inoue, & Asada, 2007), and affects on immune variables (Cabyoglu, Ergne, Tan, 2006). Neuroimaging studies have shown that acupuncture affects brain regions involved with pain perception, emotions, and cognitive functioning(Dhond, Kettner, & Napadow, 2007; Lundeberg, Lund, & Näslund, 2007; Yoo, Teh, Blinder, & Jolesz, 2004).

RCTs examining efficacy of acupuncture on migraine and tension headaches have revealed promising, but mixed, results (Linde et al., 2005, 2007; Vincent, 1989). A recent prospective, randomized controlled study of 160 patients suffering from migraine without aura, suggested that acupuncture plus Rizatriptan was more effective than the drug alone, and acupuncture seemed to decrease the amount of Rizatriptan needed to manage symtoms (Facco et al., 2007). This study had several merits. First, it used traditional Chinese medicine diagnoses and selected acupuncture points and techniques accordingly; second, it used a needle with a blunt tip that did not penetrate the skin for the sham control; and third, it used an additional sham acupuncture group that did not follow TCM diagnoses and treatment.

A recent German acupuncture trial for chronic lower back pain showed both therapeutic and sham acupuncture as twice as effective as conventional therapies (a combination of drugs, physical therapy,and exercise; Haake et al., 2007). This was a randomized, multicenter, blinded, parallel-group trial with three groups totalling 1,162 patients aged 18–86 years. It is unclear why the sham acupuncture group did so well, but possible explanations include placebo effects and the fact that in classic Chinese medical theoryit is difficult to find a point on the body that will not affect meridians in some way because of the complexity of the meridian system. In 121 patients undergoing ambulatory arthroscopic knee surgery with standard general anesthesia, a RCT (Usichenko et al., 2007) with intention-to-treat analysis showed that patients from the control group ($n=59$) required significantly more ibuprofen than patients from the auricular acupuncture group ($n=61$).

A small RCT from China on elctro-acupuncture in relieving labor pain (Qu & Zhou, 2007) studied 36 primipariaras randomly divided into either the electro-acupuncture group or control group. The electro-acupuncture group exhibited a lower pain intensity and better degree of relaxation ($p = 0.018, p = 0.031$) as well as increased release of ß-endorphin and 5-HT in peripheral blood at the end of first stage($p = 0.037, p = 0.030$).

ADDICTIONS

The Acupuncture Consensus Panel of the United States National Institutes of Health (National Institute of Health, 1998) stated that acupuncture "may be useful as a supportive treatment, or acceptable alternative, or part of a comprehensive program" in drug-addiction therapy, including nicotine dependency. However, despite success in several small studies, an RTC and updated review of studies of auricular acupuncture on cocaine dependence could not confirm that auricular acupuncture was effective as a sole treatment(D'Alberto, 2004; Gates, Smith, & Foxcroft, 2006; Kim, Schiff, Waalen, & Hovell, 2005; Margolin et al., 2002). Likewise, a large RCT of auricular acupuncture for alcohol dependence failed to show efficacy of auricular across 503 patients (Bullock et al., 2002). There is some suggestion it may be useful as an adjunctive treatment for alcohol withdrawal symptoms (Karst et al., 2007) but, that too, has not been a consistent result (Kunz, Schulz, Lewitzky, Driessen, & Rau, 2007).

Smoking Cessation

Acupressure using beads on acupoints in the ears was used to treat patients on nicotine replacement therapies (NRT) for smoking cessation (White, Moody, & Campbell, 2007). This open-label, randomized pilot study was unable to detect any effects of acupressure on smoking withdrawal as an adjunct to the use of NRT. Of note, this study used only one or two points on the ear, instead of the standard five that normally are recommended.

Chinese investigators used a modified acupuncture technique called wrist ankle acupuncture (Zhang et al., 2004) in a RCT with a control group treated with traditional acupuncture points. Both groups used the "smoking cessation point"(an empirical point between L7 and LI5). In the experimental group, patients received additional needles implanted subcutaneously at points at the ankle and wrist for 24 hours every other day for 4 weeks of treatment. Out of 30 in each group, the experimental group had 28 subjects who were able to quit for more than 1 year in comparison with 14 in the other group.

Researchers in Taiwan combined auricular acupressure with an internet-assisted smoking cessation program (Chen, Yeh, & Chao, 2006) and found that it was more effective than using acupressure alone. An RCT examined the effectiveness of combining acupuncture and education for smoking cessation (Bier, Wilson, Studt, & Shakleton, 2002), showing acupuncture and education, alone and in combination, significantly reduce smoking; however, combined they show a significantly greater effect at 18-month follow-up, particularly in subjects with greater pack-year histories.

Korean investigators attempted to evaluate genetic determinants for responsiveness to acupuncture for smoking cessation (Park, Kim, et al., 2005). They found that people who responded favorably had a higher DRD2*A2 allele frequency than low responders, suggesting that DRD2 TaqI A polymorphism could be related to acupuncture responsiveness in smoking cessation treatment.

Conceptual Integration of Biomedicine and Chinese Medicine

Some investigators who are familiar with both modern Western medicine and Chinese medicine have noticed conceptual similarities between the biomedical model of allostasis/altostatic load and the emotional motor system (EMS), with the ancient paradigm of Chinese medicine (Tan, Tillisch, & Mayer, 2004). Both systems stress the fundamental importance of homeostasis in the body. In the process of allostasis, Western medical homeostatic mechanisms involve ascending monoaminergic systems (including the serotonergic, noradrenergic, and cholinergic pathways), the hypothalamic-pituitary-adrenal (HPA) axis, endogenous pain modulation networks, and autonomic pathways(McEwen, 2003), while Chinese medicine involves balancing yin and yang, qi, blood, and essence (which is the physical manifestation of qi). The functional somatic syndromes described in modern medicine are comparable to patterns of energetic imbalance in Chinese medicine. Both systems explore the complicated interaction of physical and emotional stressors in the genesis of symptoms and diseases. The EMS is a parallel set of outputs from limbic and paralimbic circuits, which generate distinct patterns of body functions("body map") associated with specific emotions (fear, anger, joy, etc.; Holstege, Bandler, & Saper, 1996). Similarly, Chinese medicine has long recognized that specific emotional stress produces imbalance of qi in specific meridians and results in specific physical and mental dysfunctions (Maciocia, 1989).

CLINICAL VIGNETTES

In clinical practice, Chinese medicine can play a complementary role to conventional therapies, particularly when there are chronic health issues that have limited options in conventional biomedicine, and in cases where complementary medicine might offer improved quality of life and symptomatic relief without side effects. Below is a case example of how Chinese medicine can be integrated in the biomedical treatment of psychiatric issues. This case was taken from our practice, with alterations in identifying information to assure confidentiality.

Kathleen was a 65-year-old physician in private practice. She was referred for a Chinese medicine evaluation by her psychoanalyst, who believed that her psychotropic medications were causing cognitive side effects. After many trials of different medications in the last 20 years, including virtually every category of psychotropic agents, Kathleen's current regimen included Wellbutrin and Nortriptyline. Although she felt these medications had helped to some degree, she continued to have a depressed mood, low interest in pleasurable activities , poor memory and concentration, and fatigue. Additional constitutional symptoms were elicited in the Chinese medicine assessment. She also complained of lower back and knee pain, urinary incontinence, lack of sexual desire, tinnitus, and decreased hearing. These symptoms suggested a severe kidney qi/essence deficiency. The Chinese medicine physical examination revealed a tongue that was dry with cracks and little coating, which also is a sign of kidney qi/essence/yin deficiency. Her liver pulse was thin, rapid, and wiry, which in Chinese Medicine is a sign of liver yin deficiency with qi stagnation. Hence, all of her physical and emotional symptoms were explained by yin/essence/qi deficiency in her kidney and liver meridians and also qi stagnation in the liver meridian, and these diagnoses were confirmed by the Chinese physical examination. The patient received twice weekly acupuncture treatment for 3 months and Chinese herbal remedies. Although this was a classic approach, a multimodal treatment makes it impossible to know what the relative contribution of each modality is to the treatment effect. After 2 weeks of treatement, patient reported improvement in mental clarity, sleep, and energy. She later reported reduced lower back and knee pain, decreased urinary incontinence. She had sex with her husband for the first time in 3 years. Over time, she discontinued two medications and was able to decrease the dosage of a third. This case illustrates how Chinese medicine is a mind–body–energy system of health that may be useful with functional disorders that are challenging to conceptualize and treat with conventional Western medicine alone.

CLINICAL CONSIDERATIONS

While the available evidence does not support the use of Chinese medicine/acupuncture as a sole therapy for psychiatric problems, there may be a role for this approach in an integrative model that is primarily guided by biomedicine with an integration of complementary therapy. It has been our clinical experience that Chinese medicine most often does not replace medication and conventional psychotherapies. Patients need to be screened for serious psychopathology and safety issues, and carefully evaluated for the need for medication or the continued use of medication. If the acupuncturist is not a psychiatrist, then decisions about medication changes need to be deferred to the clinical judgment of the psychiatrist who is working with the patient. Finally, due to financial and logistical reasons, patients can rarely receive acupuncture on a daily basis, which is the ideal approach in the classic Chinese model and the typical treatment in China, even when Western medicine is also part of the treatment plan. Therefore, the Westernized treatment schedule for acupuncture that is common in the United States makes it difficult to predict how long a course of acupuncture will be needed to see a clinical effect.

Conclusions

Chinese medicine in general, and acupuncture in particular, for the treatment of psychiatric problems has nonconclusive, but encouraging supportive data for some types of anxiety; mixed data with a positive lean for depression and pain; and extremely limited data for other issues. Overall, the majority of studies in the field suffer from problematic methodological design and lack of standardized treatment approaches among studies, making definitive conclusions and recommendations impossible. Nonetheless, this system of health has a several thousand year history that has been developed and documented with countless case descriptions that could potentially provide a unique perspective when considering possible complementary approaches to enhance the treatment plan of complicated mind–body problems.

REFERENCES

Abbott, R. B., Hui, K.-K., Hays, R. D., Li, M.-D., & Pan, T. (2007). A randomized controlled trial of Tai Chi for tension headaches. *Evidence-Based Complementary and Alternative Medicine, 4,* 107–113.

Allen, J. J, Schnyer, R. N., Chambers, A. S., Hitt, S. K., Moreno, F. A., & Manber, R. (2006). Acupuncture for depression: A randomized controlled trial. *Journal of Clinical Psychiatry, 67,* 1665–1673.

American Academy of Medical Acupuncture (2004). Doctor, what's this acupuncture all about? A brief explanation. December 14, available from www.medicalacupuncture.org/acu_info

Arranz, L., Guayerbas, N., Siboni, L., & De la Fuente, M. (2007). Effect of acupuncture treatment on the immune function impairment found in anxious women. *American Journal of Chinese Medicine*, *35*, 35–51.

Barnes, P. M., Powell-Griner, E., McFann, K., & Nahin, R. L. (2004). Complementary and alternative medicine use among adults: United States (2002), CDC Advance Data Report #343.

Bier, I. D., Wilson, J., Studt, P., Shakleton, M. (2002). Auricular acupuncture, education, and smoking cessation: A randomized, sham-controlled trial. *American Journal of Public Health*, *92*, 1642–1647.

Bosco, J., & Silva, G. (2007). Acupuncture for mild to moderate emotional complaints in pregnancy—a prospective, quasi-randomized, controlled study. *Acupuncture in Medicine*, *25*, 65–71.

Bullock, M.L., Kiresuk, T. J., Sherman, R. E., Lenz, S. K., Culliton, P. D., Boucher, T. A., et al. (2002). A large randomized placebo controlled study of auricular acupuncture for alcohol dependence. *Journal of Substance Abuse Treatment*, *22*, 71–77.

Cabyoglu, M., Ergne, N., & Tan, U. (2006). The Mechanism of acupuncture and clinical applications. *International Journal of Neuroscience*, *116*, 115–125.

Chan, B., & Halpern, G. M. (2007). *The Yin and Yang of cancer: Breakthroughs from the east and the west*. Square One Publishers.

Chan, K., & Lee, H. (2001). *The way forward for Chinese medicine*. CRC Press, Taylor & Francis Group.

Chen, H. H., Yeh, M. L., Chao, Y. H. (2006). Comparing effects of auricular acupressure with and without an internet-assisted program on smoking cessation and self-efficacy of adolescents. *Journal of Alternative Complementary Medicine*, *12*, 147–152.

Chen, H. Y., Shi, Y., Ng, C. S., Chan, S. M., Yung, K. K. L., & Zhang, Q. L. (2007). *Journal of Alternative and Complementary Medicine*, *13*(6), 669–676.

Chen, X., & Deng, L. (2005). *Chinese acupuncture and moxibustion* (2nd edn). Beijing, China: Foreign Languages Press.

Cheuk, D. K. L., Yeung, W. F., Chung, K. F., & Wong, V. (2008) *Acupuncture for insomnia*.

Cochrane Database of Systematic Reviews Issue 1.

Connelly, D. M. (1994). *Traditional acupuncture: The law of the five elements* (2 Sub edn). Traditional Acupuncture Institute.

D'Alberto, A. (2004). Auricular acupuncture in the treatment of cocaine/crack abuse: A review of the efficacy, the use of the National Acupuncture Detoxification Association protocol, and the selection of sham points. *Journal of Alternative Complementary Medicine*, *10*, 985–1000.

Dang, Y. (1999). *Acupuncture and moxibustion*. Beijing, China: Academy Press.

Dhond, R. P., Kettner, N. & Napadow, V. (2007). Do the neural correlates of acupuncture and placebo effects differ? *Pain*, *128*, 8–12.

Eich, H., Agelink, M. W., Lehmann, E., Lemmer, W., & Klieser, E. (2000). Acupuncture in patients with minor depressive episodes and generalized anxiety: Results of an experimental study. *Fortschritte der Neurologie-Psychiatrie*, *68*, 137–144.

Facco, E., Liguori, A., Petti, F., Zanette, G., Coluzzi, F., & Nardin, M. D. (2007). Traditional acupuncture in migraine: A controlled, randomized study. *Headache, 48,* 398–407

Fanti, L., Gemma, M., Passaretti, S., Guslandi, M., Testoni, P. A., Casati, A., et al. (2004).

Electroacupuncture analgesia for colonoscopy. A prospective, randomized, placebo-controlled study. *Gastroenterology, 126,* 355–356.

Flaws, B., & Lake, J. (2001). *Chinese medical psychiatry—a textbook and clinical manual.* Boulder, CO: Blue Poppy Press.

Galambos, I. (1996). The origins of Chinese medicine. The early development of medical literature in China. Available from www.logoi.com.

Gallagher, S. M., Allen., J. J. B., & Hitt, S. K. (2001). Six-month depression relapse rates among women treated with acupuncture. *Complement Therapies in Medicine, 9,* 216–218.

Gates, S., Smith, L. A., & Foxcroft, D. R. (2006) Auricular acupuncture for cocaine dependence. *Cochrane Database Systematic Reviews,* (1), CD005192.

Gibson, D., Bruton, A., Lewith, G. T., & Mullee, M. (2007). Effects of acupuncture as a treatment for hyperventilation syndrome: A pilot, randomized crossover trial. *Journal of Alternative and Complementary Medicine, 13,* 39–46.

Gioia, L., Cabrini, L., Gemma, M., Fiori, R., Fasce, F., Bolognesi, G., et al. (2006). Sedative effect of acupuncture during cataract surgery: Prospective randomized double-blind study. *Journal of Cataract & Refractive Surgery, 32,* 1951–1954.

Haake, M., Muller, H., Shade-Brittinger, C., Basler, H. D., Schafer, H., Maier, C., et al. (2007), German acupuncture trials for chronic lower back pain. *Archives of Internal Medicine, 167,* 1892–1898.

Hammer, L. (1991). *Dragon rises, red bird flies: Psychology, energy and Chinese medicine.* Station Hill Press.

Han, C., Li, X., Luo, H., Zhao, X., & Li, X. (2004). Clinical study on electro-acupuncture treatment for 30 cases of mental depression. *Journal of Traditional Chinese Medicine, 24,* 172–176.

Han, C., Li, X. W., & Luo, H. C. (2002). Comparative study of electro-acupuncture and maprotiline in treating depression. *Zhonggu Zhong Xi Yi Jie He Za Zhi, 22,* 512–514, 521.

Hanyu da zidian weiyuanhui (1995). Hanyu da zidian (Comprehensive Chinese Character Dictionary) , Wuhan: Hubei cishu chubanshe and Sichuan cishu chubanshe.

He, D., Medbø, J. I., & Høstmark, A.T. (2001). Effect of acupuncture on smoking cessation or reduction: An 8-month and 5-year follow-up study. *Preventive Medicine, 33,* 364–372.

Holland, A. (2000). *Voices of Qi: An introductory guide to traditional Chinese medicine* (Subsequent edition). North Atlantic Books.

Hollifield, M., Sinclair-Lian, N., Warner, T. D., & Hammerschlag, R. (2007). Acupuncture for Posttraumatic stress disorder, A randomized controlled pilot trial. *Journal of Nervous and Mental Disease, 195,* 504–513.

Holstege, G., Bandler, R., & Saper, C. B. (1996). The emotional motor system. In G. Holstege, R. Bandler, C. B. Saper (Eds.), *The emotional motor system.* Amsterdam, Netherlands, Elsevier Inc., pp. 3–6.

Hsu, E. (2007). *Innovation in Chinese medicine*. Needham Research Institute Studies (No. 3). Cambridge University Press.

Huang, Y., Li, D. J., Tang, A. .W., Li, Q. S., Xia, D. B., Xie, Y. N., Gong, W., & Chen, J. (2005). Effect of scalp acupuncture on glucose metabolism in brain of patients with depression. *Zhongguo Zhong Xi Yi Jie He Za Zhi, 25,* 119–122.

Huangdi Neijing Suwen (1956). *People's health press*. Beijing, China (Chinese).

Jeon S-W (1998). *A history of science in Korea*. Jimoondang, Seoul: Jimoondang International.

Kalavapalli, R., & Singareddy, R. (2007), Role of acupuncture in the treatment of insomnia: A comprehensive review. *Complementary Therapies in Clinical Practice, 13,* 184–193.

Kaptchuck, T. (2000). *The web that has no weaver*. McGraw-Hill Companies.

Karst, M., Winterhalter, M., Münte, S., Francki, B., Hondronikos, A., Eckardt, A., et al. (2007). Auricular acupuncture for dental anxiety: A randomized controlled trial. *Anesthesia and Analgesia, 104,* 295–300.

Kim, Y. H., Schiff, E. I., Waalen, J., & Hovell, M. (2005). Efficacy of acupuncture for treating cocaine addiction: A review paper. *Journal of Addictive Diseases, 24,* 115–132.

Kunz, S., Schulz, M., Lewitzky, M., Driessen, M., & Rau, H. (2007). Ear acupuncture for alcohol withdrawal in comparison with aromatherapy: A randomized-controlled trial. *Alcoholism, Clinical and Experimental Research, 31,* 436–442.

Leo, R. J., Liqot, & J. S. Jr. (2007). A systematic review of randomized controlled trials of acupuncture in the treatment of depression. *Journal of Affective Disorders, 97,* 13–22.

Lewith, G. T., White, P. J., & Kaptchuk, T. J. (2006). Developing a research strategy for acupuncture. *Clinical Journal of Pain, 22,* 632–638.

Li, X. D. (2006). *Who can invent Chinese medicine? Decoding Huang Di Nei Jing* (2nd edn), Beijing, China: China Changan Press.

Li, Y. F., Zeng, D. Y., & Zhuang, L. X. (2006). Analysis on the composing law of "Jin's 3-needle. *Journal of Clinical Acupuncture and Moxibustion, 22,* 35–36.

Lin, H., Li, G. Q., Zhou, Z. B., & Liu, J. X. (2005). Observation on therapeutic effect of combination of acupuncture with drug on depression.*Zhongguo Zhen Jiu, 25,* 27–29.

Linde, K., Jonas, W. B., Melchart, D., & Willich, S. (2001). The methodological quality of randomized clinical trials in homeopathy, herbal medicine and acupuncture. *International Journal of Epidemiology, 30,* 526–531.

Linde, K., Streng, A., Jurgens, S., Hoppe, A., Brinkhaus, B., Witt, C., et al. (2005). Acupuncture for patients with migraine: A randomized controlled trial. *Journal of the American Medical Association, 293,* 2118–2125.

Linde, K., Streng, A., Hoppe, A., Weidenhammer, W., Wagenpfeil, S., & Melchart, D. (2007). Randomized trial vs. observational study of acupuncture for migraine found that patient characteristics differed but outcomes were similar. *Journal of Clinical Epidemiology, 60,* 280–287.

Luo, H., Meng, F., Jia, Y., & Zhao, X. (1998). Clinical research on the therapeutic effect of the electro-acupuncture treatment in patients with depression. *Psychiatry and Clinical Neurosciences*, (52 Suppl), S338–40.

Luo, W. Z., Liu, H. J., & Mei, S. Y. (2007). Clinical study on "jin's three-needling" in treatment of generalized anxiety disorder. *Zhongguo Zhong Xi Yi Jie He Za Zhi*, *27*, 201–203.

Liu, T. (2007). Role of acupuncturists in Acupuncture treatment. *Evidence-Based Complementary and Alternative Medicine*, *4*, 3–6.

Lundeberg, T., Lund, I., & Näslund, J. (2007). Acupuncture—self-appraisal and the reward system. *Acupuncture in Medicine*, *25*, 87–99.

Ma, X.-S. (2004). Neurobiology of acupuncture: Toward CAM. *Evidence-Based Complementary and Alternative Medicine*, *1*, 41–47.

Maciocia, G. (1989). *The foundations of Chinese medicine: A comprehensive text for acupuncturists and herbalists*. New York: Churchill Livingstone.

MacPherson, H., Thorpe, L., Thomas, K., & Geddes, D. (2004). Acupuncture for depression: First steps toward a clinical evaluation. *Journal of Alternative and Complementary Medicine*, *10*, 1083–1091.

Manber, R., Schnyer, R., Allen, J., Rush, A., & Blasey, C. (2004). Acupuncture: A promising treatment for depression during pregnancy. *Journal of Affective Disorders*, *83*, 89–95.

Margolin, A., Kleber, H. D., Avants, S. K., Konefal, J., Gawin, F., Stark, E., et al. (2002). The treatment of cocaine addiction: A randomized controlled trial. *Journal of the American Medical Association*, *287*, 55–63.

McEwen, B. S. (2003). Interacting mediators of allostasis and allostatic load: Towards an understanding of resilience in aging. *Metabolism*, *52*, 10–16.

Monti, D., Gomella, L., Peterson, C., & Kunkel, E. (2007). Preliminary results from a novel psychosocial program for men with prostate cancer. 2007 Prostate Cancer Symposium, American Society of Clinical Oncology.

Mora, B., Iannuzzi, M., Lang, T., Steinlechner, B., Barker, R., Dobrovits, M., et al. (2007). Auricular acupressure as a treatment for anxiety before extracorporeal shock wave lithotripsy in the elderly. *Journal of Urology*, *178*, 160–164.

National Institute of Health Consensus Conference (1998). Acupuncture. *Journal of the American Medical Association*, *280*, 1518–1524.

Ong, C. K., Bodeker, G., Grundy, C., Burford, G., & Shein, K. (2005). *WHO Global Atlas of Traditional, Complementary and Alternative Medicine*, WHO Kobe Centre.

Park, H. J., Chae, Y., Jang, J., Shim, I., Lee, H., & Lim, S. (2005). The effect of acupuncture on anxiety and neuropeptide Y expression in the basolateral amygdala of maternally separated rats. *Neuroscience Letters*, *4*, 377, 179–184.

Park, H. J., Kim, S. T., Yoon, D. H., Jin, S. H., Lee, S. J., Lee, H. J., et al. (2005). The association between the DRD2 TaqI A polymorphism and smoking cessation in response to acupuncture in Koreans. *Journal of Alternative Complementary Medicine*, *11*, 401–405.

Paterson, C., & Dieppe, P. (2005). Characteristic and incidental (placebo) effects in complex interventions such as acupuncture. *British Medical Journal*, *330*, 1202–1205.

Pearson, S., Colbert, A. P., McNames, J., Baumgartner, M., & Hammerschlag, R. (2007). Electrical skin impedance at acupuncture points. *Journal of Alternative and Complementary Medicine, 13,* 409–418.

Pilkington, K., Kirkwood, G., Rampes, H., Cummings, M., & Richardson, J. (2007). Acupuncture for anxiety and anxiety disorders—a systematic literature review. *Acupuncture in Medicine, 25,* 1–10.

Qu, F., & Zhou, J. (2007). Electro-acupuncture in relieving labor pain. *Evidence-based Complementary and Alternative Medicine, 4,* 125–130.

Rathbone, J., & Xia, J. (2005). Acupuncture for schizophrenia. *Cochrane Database of Systematic Reviews,* Issue 4. Art. No., CD005475.

Rathbone, J., Zhang, L., Zhang, M., Xia, J., Liu, X., Yang, Y., et al. (2007). Chinese herbal medicine for schizophrenia—cochrane systematic review of randomized trials. *British Journal of Psychiatry, 190,* 379–384.

Riet, G. T., Kleijnen, J., & Knipschild, P. (1990). A meta-analysis of studies into the effect of acupuncture on addiction. *British Journal of General Practice, 40,* 379–382.

Rister, R. (1999). *Japanese herbal medicine: The healing art of Kampo.* New York: Avery.

Röschke, J., Wolf, C., Müller, M. J., Wagner, P., Mann, K., Grözinger, M., et al. (2000). The benefit from whole body acupuncture in major depression. *Journal of Affective Disorders, 57,* 73–81.

Sakatani, K. (2007). Concept of mind and brain in traditional Chinese medicine. *Data Science Journal* (6 Suppl), S220–S224.

Sandberg, M., Lundeberg, T., Lindberg, L. G., & Gerdle, B. (2003). Effects of acupuncture on skin and muscle blood flow in healthy subjects. *European Journal of Applied Physiology, 90,* 114–119.

Scheid, V. (2002). *Chinese medicine in contemporary China: Plurality and synthesis.* Durham, NC: Duke University Press.

Schlebusch, K., Maric-Oehler, W., & Popp, F.-A. (2005). Biophotonics in the infrared spectral range reveal acupuncture meridian structure of the body. *Journal of Alternative and Complementary Medicine, 11,* 171–173.

Schnyer, R. N., & Allen, J. J. B. (2002). Bridging the gap in complementary and alternative medicine research: Manualization as a means of promoting standardization and flexibility of treatment in clinical trials of acupuncture. *Journal of Alternative and Complementary Medicine, 8,* 623–634.

Shen, X. Y., Wei, J. Z., Zhang, Y. H., Ding, G. H., Wang, C. H., Zhang, H. M., et al. (2006). Study on volt–ampere (V-A) characteristics of human acupoints. *Zhongguo Zhen Jiu, 26,* 267–271.

Song, Y., Zhou, D., Fan, J., Luo, H., & Halbreich, U. (2007). Effects of electroacupuncture and fluoxetine on the density of GTP-binding-proteins in platelet membrane in patients with major depressive disorder. *Journal of Affective Disorders, 98,* 253–257.

Spence, D. W., Kayumov. L., Chen, A., Lowe, A., Jain, U., Katzman, M. A., et al. (2004). Acupuncture increases nocturnal melatonin secretion and reduces insomnia and anxiety: A preliminary report. *Journal of Neuropsychiatry & Clinical Neuroscience, 1,* 19–28.

Tan, S., Tillisch, K., & Mayer, E. (2004). Functional somatic syndromes: Emerging bio-medical models and traditional Chinese medicine. *Evidence-Based Complementary and Alternative Medicine, 1,* 35–40.

Tsuchiya, M., Sato, E. F., Inoue, M., & Asada, A. (2007). Acupuncture enhances generation of nitric oxide and increases local circulation. *Anesthesia and Analgesia, 104,* 301–307.

Tsumura, A. (1991). *Kampo: How the Japanese updated traditional herbal medicine.* Japan Publications.

Ulett, G. A., Han, S., & Han, J. S. (1998). Electro acupuncture: Mechanisms and clinical application. *Biological Psychiatry, 44,* 129–138.

Unschuld, P. U. (2003). *Huang Di Nei Jing Su Wen: Nature, knowledge, imagery in an ancient Chinese medical text.* Berkeley and Los Angeles, CA: University of California Press.

Usichenko, T. I., Kuchling, S., Witstruck, T., Pavlovic, D., Zach, M., Hofer, A., et al. (2007). Auricular acupuncture for pain relief after ambulatory knee surgery: A randomized trial. *Canadian Medical Association Journal, 176,* 179–183.

Usichenko, T. I., Lysenyuk, V. P., Groth, M. H., & Pavlovic, D. (2003). Detection of ear acupuncture points by measuring the electrical skin resistance in patients before, during and after orthopedic surgery performed under general anesthesia. *Acupuncture Electro-therapeutics Research, 28,* 167–173.

Vincent, C. A. (1989). A controlled trial of the treatment of migraine by acupuncture. *Clinical Journal of Pain, 5,* 305–312.

Wang, J., Jiang, J. F., & Wang, L. L. (2006). Clinical observation on governor vessel Daoqi method for treatment of dyssomnia in the patient of depression. *Zhongguo Zhen Jiu, 26,* 328–330.

Wang, S. M., Punjala, M., Weiss, D., Anderson, K., & Kain, Z. N. (2007). Acupuncture as an adjunct for sedation during lithotripsy. *Journal of Alternative and Complementary Medicine, 13,* 241–246.

Weyer, R. V. D. (1997). *Huang Di: The balance of Yin and Yang.* Tandem Library.

White, A. R., Moody, R. C., & Campbell, J. L. (2007). Acupressure for smoking cessation—a pilot study. BMC *Complementary and Alternative Medicine, 7,* 8.

Wick, F., Wick, N., & Wick, M. C. (2007). Morphological analysis of human acupuncture points through immunohistochemistry. *American Journal of Physical Medicine & Rehabilitation, 86,* 7–11.

Wong, J. Y. (1999). *A manual of neuro-anatomical acupuncture. Volume I: Musculo-skeletal disorders.* Toronto, ON: The Toronto Pain and Stress Clinic Inc.

Yang, X., Liu, X., Luo, H., & Jia, Y. (1994). Clinical observation on needling extra-channel points in treating mental depression. *Journal of Traditional Chinese Medicine, 14,* 14–18.

Yoo, S. S., Teh, E. K., Blinder, R. A., & Jolesz, F. A. (2004). Modulation of cerebellar activities by acupuncture stimulation: Evidence from fMRI study. *NeuroImage, 22,* 932–940.

Yu, J., Liu, Q., Wang, Y. Q., Wang, J., Li, X. Y., Cao, X. D., et al. (2007). Electroacupuncture combined with clomipramine enhances antidepressant effect in rodents. *Neuroscience Letters, 421,* 5–9.

Zhang, G. J., Shi, Z. Y., Liu, S., Gong, S. H., Liu, J. Q., & Liu, J. S. (2007). Clinical observation. *Chinese Journal of Integrative Medicine*, 13, 228–230.

Zhang, Q. G., Gu, K. W., Wang, D., & Zahng, H. J. (2004).Treatment of tobacco dependence with wrist-ankle acupuncture: A report of 30 cases. *Chinese Journal of Integrative Medicine*, 2, 444, 480.

Zhang, Z., & Lu, W. (2002), A clinical analysis on treatment of depression by electroacupuncture combined with Paroxetine of the electroacupuncture treatment of obsessive compulsive disorders. *Si Chuan Zhong Yi (The Journal of Si Chuan Chinese Medicine)*, 1, 75–76.

8

The Role of Chiropractic in Mind–Body Health

HENRY POLLARD

Introduction

Chiropractic is a dynamic profession that is sometimes defined as a first-line medical intervention, but mostly described as a complementary therapy (Keating, 1992; Scalena, 2007; Wardwell, 1994). Most recognize chiropractic as a manipulation-based therapy for the spine (Pollard et al., 2007), although chiropractic philosophy incorporates elements of holism, and the profession has maintained from the beginning that chiropractic treatments affect more than just the physical aspects of spine-based, mechanical musculoskeletal disorders (Hoskins, McHardy, Pollard, Windsham, & Onley, 2006; McHardy, Hoskins, Pollard, Onley, & Windsham, 2008; Palmer, 1910). The current evidence suggests that chiropractic may have a role in maintaining overall mind–body health, supporting stress reduction and improving health-related quality of life.

This chapter will present an overview of the foundations and evolution of the chiropractic profession and how it is morphing into a unique evidence-based health approach. Chiropractic models and paradigms will be presented in brief, with a particular emphasis on chiropractic's emerging role in the field of integrative medicine.

Historical Overview

The chiropractic profession was born in 1895, when Daniel David Palmer (1845–1913) effected the first chiropractic treatment. Palmer held great interest in and fascination with developments in anatomy and physiology and pursued the philosophies of magnetic healing and spiritualism common to the day (Palmer, 1910).

When working as a magnetic healer, Palmer was presented with a deaf janitor who it is said to have had a lump on his back. After questioning the janitor as to the origin of the lump, Palmer concluded that the onset of the deafness and the lump appeared to coincide. He then reasoned that, if he could reduce the lump, the hearing might return. After performing a manipulative procedure on the janitor, the lump reduced with a restoration of the hearing (Palmer, 1910). This later became known as the first chiropractic *adjustment*.

"Adjustment" is a term preferred by some in the profession to represent the type of manipulation done by a chiropractor. A chiropractic adjustment is a manipulation that has intent, focus, direction, and skillful application of force, rather than the more general application of force typical of the early Cyriax school of medical manipulators who performed manipulation mostly under anaesthesia (Cyriax, 1951, 1964).

Important in the initial philosophical offering from Palmer is the quote that "chiropractors of the future will address the frame, poisons and autosuggestion" (Palmer, 1910). This quote and the mindset it represents is important, as they position chiropractic at its inception as a healthcare approach that is concerned with the whole body, and certainly much more than the spine-centric musculo-skeletal viewpoint that typically prevails today.

However, under the guidance of his son Bartlett Joshua Palmer, the profession morphed into a reductionist approach to spinal manipulative therapy, largely due to the constant battles that Bartlett J. Palmer faced for practicing medicine without a license. The detail of this battle and the strategies that B. J. Palmer took to neutralize his critics are beyond the scope of this chapter, and the reader is referred to W. H. Quigley's book (1995) for a more in-depth discussion.

The evolution of the profession continued with various schools forming over the next 50 years, which propagated the reductionist view favoured out of necessity by B. J. Palmer and strongly disliked by the founder, D. D. Palmer.

The second half of the twentieth century saw chiropractic develop into two distinct subgroups, the philosophy-driven traditionalists and the science-driven modernists (Keating, 1992). These two groups are frequently referred to as "straights" and "mixers," respectively (Nelson et al., 2005; Villaneuva-Russel, 2005).

As some promoted the traditional philosophical values born out of the B. J. Palmer era (the straights), so the other group (the mixers) embraced the doctrine of science. To this day, the two groups remain distinct. However, it is likely that the true nature of the profession is probably better represented by a bell-shaped curve, with straight philosophically driven chiropractors at one end and evidence-based chiropractors at the other end of the curve (Keating, 1994, 1992). Within this model, it is likely that the majority of chiropractors are located in the middle and provide management that is multimodal in nature—largely spine-based and driven by a philosophy that the spine is important for the maintenance of overall health (Keating, 1994; Keating & Hansen, 1992).

Chiropractic Practice

Most chiropractors are primarily concerned with the management of mechanical musculoskeletal spinal disorders (Coulter et al., 2002), with chiropractic interns demonstrating good competence in musculoskeletal diagnosis (Humphreys, Sulkowski, McIntyre, Kasiban, & Patrick, 2007). Chiropractors use spinal manipulative therapy (SMT) or "adjustments" mainly for the management of musculoskeletal conditions to cause reduction in pain, improvement in joint range of motion, and reduction of muscle spasm (Alcantara, Plaugher, Thornton, & Salem, 2001; Pincus et al., 2007; Zhu, Haldeman, Hsieh, Wu, & Starr, 2000). This approach is similar to the way many osteopaths practice.

Chiropractic practice is not limited to muscluloskeletal scope of practice (Hawk, Long, & Boulanger, 2001); however, chiropractors use SMT to improve non-musculoskeletal conditions in a less predictable manner than that of the musculoskeletal conditions. Chiropractors also render various ancillary management modalities including soft tissue therapy, rehabilitation, electrotherapy, dietary advice, exercise prescription, and health counseling (Hawk, Long, Perillo, & Boulanger, 2004). The average chiropractic practitioner is likely to have a broad musculoskeletal, multimodal management approach (Lamm, Wegner, & Collard, 1995; Mootz et al., 2005). Recent systematic reviews confirm the broad based nature of chiropractic practices (Hoskins et al., 2006; McHardy et al., 2008).

The majority of patients presenting to chiropractors have chronic musculoskeletal conditions (Hartvigsen, Bolding-Jensen, Hviid, & Grunnet-Nilsson, 2003; Rubinstein, Pfeifle, van Tulder, & Assendelft, 2000). The most common of these is low back pain and the most common form of low back pain is chronic non-specific (mechanical) sprain/strain form of low back pain (Walker, Muller, & Grant, 2004). Yet, most of the evidence in support of chiropractic is based on acute pain syndromes (Sorensen, Stochkendahl, Hartvigsen, & Nilsson, 2006).

Much research has investigated chronic low back pain, and this literature has raised to the level of multiple randomized control trials and systematic reviews (Furlan, Tomlinson, Jadad, & Bombardier, 2008). A considerable amount of research supports the use of manipulation for acute pain, neck pain, migraine (Haas et al., 2004; Santilli, Beghi, & Finucci, 2006; Tuchin, Pollard, & Bonello, 2000), and a moderate level of evidence supports the use of manipulation in multimodal applications in common musculoskeletal conditions of the upper and lower extremities, conditions such as rotator cuff, epiconylittis, carpal tunnel, meniscal and retropatellar conditions of the knee, and lateral ankle sprain (Hoskins et al., 2006; McHardy et al., 2008) and acute disc presentations with sciatica (Santilli et al., 2006).

There is long-standing controversy regarding the risks of chiropractic manipulations/adjustments (Gouveia et al., 2007; Haneline, Croft, & Frishberg, 2003; Kier & McCarthy 2006; Rubinstein et al., 2007). A particular concern is vertebrobasilar insufficiency (VBI), although the prevalence appears to be quite low. Reasonable working estimates put the risk in the range of 1 in 400,000 to 1 in 1,000,000 (Dvoriak & Orelli, 1985; Jaskoviak, 1980). More up-to-date assessments of risk are needed.

Overall, more high-quality randomized, controlled trials are needed to further investigate treatment outcomes and cost-effectiveness.

Also needed are reliability studies to examine the usefulness of existing and emerging diagnostic approaches used, and to determine whether they demonstrate the degree of reliability to a criterion standard that would warrant their use in the field (Sackett, Rosenberg, Gray, Haynes, & Richardson, 2007).

CHRONIC PAIN PROBLEMS

Chiropractors are frequently consulted for a myriad of pain-related issues. Pain has been defined by the International Association for the Study of Pain as "an unpleasant sensory and emotional experience which is primarily associated with tissue damage or described in terms of such damage, or both" (Merskey & Bogduk, 1994). It is a multidimensional sensory and behavioural phenomenon that frequently requires multimodal treatment strategies to resolve.

Important to any discussion of chronic pain is the knowledge that most pain is associated with psychosocial co-morbidity (Webb et al., 2003). Whether acute and associated with anxiety based co-morbidities or chronic and associated with depressive type co-morbidities (Leeuw et al., 2007; Sloan, Gupta, Zhang, & Walsh, 2008), pain has been associated with many non-sensory components (Martin, McGrath, Brown, & Katz, 2007; Thomas, France, Sha, & Wiele, 2008). The chronic pain literature is full of research that aligns pain to various psychosocial phenomena, and a summary of this phenomena may be found in Tables 8.1 and 8.2.

A recent study highlights that the predictors of outcome of chronic pain in a workers' compensation setting are based more on psychosocial variables than physical ones (van Wijk et al., 2008). Although the population in that study is complex, the results reflect a growing literature on the multidimensional aspects of pain, as well as the need to have approaches to pain that consider the different contributors to pain sensation and the experience of suffering (Scascighini & Sprott, 2008).

Table 8.1. Psychological Factors of Pain and Psychological Factors
of Neck and Back Pain.

Psychological Factors of Pain	Psychological Factors in Neck and Back Pain
1) The reciprocal nature of psychological factors and spinal pain	1) Psychosocial variables **
	2) Cognitive factors: attitudes, beliefs
2) A variety of views on how psychological factors influence pain	3) Emotions: depression, anxiety
	4) Psychological factors: reported at onset
3) The temporal aspect of pain development, as factors may have different effects at different points of time.	5) Self-perceived poor health
	6) Sexual and/or physical abuse *
	7) Personality and traits *
	8) Psychosocial factors: predictors for chronic pain development *

Notes: Factors that are not noted were discussed as "associated with pain and disability," while factors noted with * were discussed as "may be related to pain and disability." Factors that are noted with ** were discussed as having more impact than biomedical or biomechanical factors on back and neck pain.

Source: Adapted from Linton (2000).

Table 8.2. Determinants of Chronic Disability.

Determinants of Chronic Disability	
Medical factors	Diagnosis, results of clinical tests, previous history.
Work-related	Physically demanding tasks, subjective appraisal of difficulty of tasks, work satisfaction, stress, monotony.
Psychological-related	Perceived pain, personality, cognitive variables, coping strategies, ability to perform tasks, dissatisfaction with work.
Sociodemographic	Age, sex, education, ethnic background. Financial compensation → influences chronic disability.

Based on the known case mix of the average chiropractor, it was apparent early on that a purely tissue-based model could not adequately address the complexity of many chronic pain issues. Complicating this view was a more traditional B. J. Palmer reductionist viewpoint that adapted the biomedical model of medicine into a biomedical model for chiropractic. The chiropractic incarnation of this model came to be known as the "subluxation," a term with various definitions that are based on articular lesions of the spine that are not a dislocation and can only be remedied through the application of the spinal adjustment (Cramer, Budgell, Henderson, Khalsa, & Pickar, 2006; Ernst, 2008; Homola, 2006).However, the subluxation model has been difficult to prove (Keating et al., 2005), and newer models are being considered (Cramer et al., 2006; Pollard, 2006).

The Traditional Chiropractic Model of Care

Chiropractors provide care in two key ways, and each form of care has different goals. The first type is a pain-based care that has the primary goal of improving joint mobility, reduction of muscle spasm, and reduction of pain (Axén et al., 2008; Leboeuf-Yde, & Hestbæk, 2008). Other goals include the improvement of non-musculoskeletal function, as well as various brain functions. In addition, many chiropractors aim to prevent pain, disability, and disease with a preventative regimen of therapy referred to as "wellness care" (Axén et al., 2008; Leboeuf-Yde, & Hestbæk, 2008). Wellness care is preventative in nature and can be referred to as "maintenance care." This second form of care is not primarily concerned with symptoms and aims to maximize the health potential of the patient. Maintenance care is provided infrequently on a regular basis and differs from care associated with acute pain, which is provided more frequently for a fixed (typically short) period of time.

Chiropractors traditionally have used manipulation (or adjustment) to effect change in their patients. The manipulative adjustment has been associated with various potential effects at a local or spinal level, particularly the reduction in pain and muscle spasm (Cassidy, Lopes, & Yong-Hing, 1992; Cleland et al., 2007; Giles & Muller, 2003). However, recent studies suggest that the mechanism of action of a manipulation may involve more than the somatic-based reflexes typically discussed. Brain-based (supraspinal) reflexes associated with more than just spinal based somatovisceral reflexes appear to play a role in generating symptoms (Cagnie et al., 2005; Haavik-Taylor & Murphy, 2007; Hill, Bateman, & Shaffie, 1998). A recent systematic review by our group (Lystad & Pollard, in press) concludes that the theory of manipulation affecting supraspinal function to be largely without evidence. Such work is in its infancy, and further research is needed to provide support for this view.

Another controversial theory is the notion that the manipulation affects somatovisceral reflexes that mediate visceral and nervous system functioning (Nansel & Szlazak, 1995). The limited support for this theory comes from single case reports and a few small, uncontrolled, and methodologically weak, studies that suggest manipulation can affect various non- musculoskeletal conditions.

Research shows that the stimulation of the somatovisceral reflex results in a change in the reflex of a millisecond duration (Coote & Dowman, 1966; Sato, 1995; Yoshimura & Nishi, 1982). The short-term nature of the reflex complicates the role given to it by many chiropractors, as such a stimulus would likely be insufficient to lead to pathology, let alone reverse it, through the action of a manipulative therapy (Pollard, 2004).

Chiropractic and the Biopsychosocial Model

As the profession evolved in the latter part of the twentieth century, chiropractic programs became science-based and presented a much broader view of health care. At the same time, medicine was noting limitations in its prevailing model of disease, the biomedical model (Weiner, 2007).

In 1977, George Engel published a landmark paper describing a new model, the biopsychosocial model (Engel, 1977). This new model contained elements of the traditional model but also recognized the role of mind, behaviour, and social influences on the formation, propagation, and resolution of ill health (Weiner, 2008).

This model helped explain the multidimensional character of chronic pain syndromes and the psychosocial influences on health in general (Friedmann et al., 2006; Spiller et al., 2007). In fact, modern medicine has noted the association of psychosocial influences on health conditions previously described solely in terms of tissue damage (see Table 8.3).

Psychosocial stress plays an important role in this new model. The detrimental effects of stress on any number of illness states have been reported, including psychiatric disorders such as depression and substance abuse (Meyer, Chrousos, & Gold, 2001; Spencer, & Hutchinson, 1999); cardiovascular disorders such as hypertension, atherosclerosis, and cardiovascular disease (Hemingway & Marmot, 1999); metabolic diseases, such as insulin resistance / metabolic X syndrome and obesity (Sapolsky, Romero, & Munck, 2000); and immune disorders that include chronic inflammatory processes and autoimmune diseases (McEwan, 1998; McEwen, 2000).

Stress can affect pain levels and degree of suffering in chronic pain patients (Melzack, 1999), particularly those with neuromusculoskeletal conditions (Pollard, 2004). Since the mechanism for the demonstrated positive effects of chiropractic adjustments on acute pain is largely pain-based, it is plausible that a contributing factor is a stress-reduction effect, presumably via autonomic nervous system modulation. Such an effect is described for manipulation

Table 8.3. Some Non-musculoskeletal Conditions that Medicine is Recognizing to Be Associated with Supraspinal Influences.

Condition	Author(s)
Gastroesophageal Reflux Disease	Bradley & Richter (1996)
Chronic Functional Abdominal Pain	Bonaz (2003) Sternberg, Chrousos, Wilder, & Gold (1992) Kellow & Phillips (1987) Whitehead, Engel, & Schuster (1980)
Crohn's Disease	Drossman et al. (1991)
Coronary artery disease	Carney et al. (1988) Carney et al. (1987)
Psychoneuroimmunology	Camara & Danao (1989)
SLE	Ader & Cohen (1982) Kiecolt-Glaser & Glaser (1989)
Coronary-prone behavior and hostility	Blumenthal, Williams, Kong, Schanberg, & Thompson (1978) Rosenman et al. (1975)

(Williams et al., 2007) and other body-based therapies, such as massage (Garner et al., 2008).

The biopsychosocial model also describes the need for chiropractors to be aware of contributing factors to pain, in addition to tissue irritation. This perspective and accompanying supportive data for it has bridged some of the long-standing philosophical divide in the chiropractic profession (Hardy & Pollard, 2006). For example, there is more general acceptance among mechanistically minded practitioners that a "whole person" approach to chronic problems is often necessary to achieve positive results.

Embracing the biopsychosocial model allows the potential for integrating different philosophies and healing approaches with standard elements of chiropractic care. It also has allowed chiropractors to investigate multiple levels of treatment effect. For example, there is a growing literature on the effects of chiropractic care on quality of life, which includes parameters such as mood and function (Williams et al., 2007).

Surveys have shown that the public seek care from chiropractors for the management of conditions such as depression (Bablis & Pollard, 2009; Wu et al., 2007); other research has shown that the utilization of alternative therapy practitioners (including chiropractic) for persons reporting mental conditions is high (Druss & Rosenheck, 2000). Thus, the public are seeking care from chiropractic practitioners for a variety of syndromes, and chiropractic is adapting to fulfill the need. Despite this apparent broadening of the chiropractic scope of practice, what evidence exists to support such practices?

Spinal manipulation has been shown to decrease emotional arousal in phobic subjects exposed to a threat stimulus (Petersen, 1997), to improve mental rotation reaction time (Kelly, Murphy, & Backhouse, 2000), tension type headache (Fernández-de-Las-Peñas, Alonso-Blanco, Cuadrado, & Pareja, 2005), mechanical neck pain (Vernon, Humphreys, & Hagino, 2007), migraine, migraine-related stress (Tuchin et al., 2000), and sleep disturbance (Haines & Haines, 2000). Disability is often associated with chronic pain syndromes, and recent work has suggested that exercise after a course of manipulation improves the self-reported outcomes over exercise alone (Marshall & Murphy 2008).

Patient satisfaction with chiropractic management is typically high in a Canadian military setting (Boudreau, Busse, & McBride, 2006), a Wisconsin non-Medicaid health cooperative (Hansen & Futch, 1997), in a U.S.-managed care organization (Hertzman-Miller et al., 2002). Satisfaction rates of patients are important predictors of outcome in the short- and longer-term, as they have been shown to be associated with short- and long-term clinical benefit (Hurwitz, Morgenstern, & Yu, 2005).

Long-term outcomes of low back pain treatment have been associated with the baseline levels of these psychosocial factors (Burton, McClune, Clarke, & Main, 2004). It is currently unknown whether chiropractic (or manipulative therapy in general) can alter the outcomes noted in pain-related behaviours, such as fear avoidance and catastrophisation. However, it is known that fear avoidance beliefs predict the success of manipulative techniques (George, Fritz, Childs, & Brennan, 2006). In addition, the provision of information through education of patients, and the reconfiguration of patient perceptions of their condition, have been associated with positive outcomes to treatment (Breen & Breen, 2003). Jamison (1997) has suggested after a survey investigation that the patient satisfaction noted in various studies (Gaumer, 2006; Nyiendo, Haas, Goldberg, & Sexton, 2001) could be used to enhance chiropractic care. She suggested that the higher satisfaction ratings were achieved by enhancing the verbal and nonverbal communication between the patient and practitioners to create an environment that was conducive to healing by reducing anxiety. This finding was echoed by the conclusion of the Gaumer review, which suggested that, besides communication, predictors of satisfaction to chiropractic care were inconsistent (Gaumer, 2006). Myers et al. (2008) suggest that patient expectations have a large role to play in patient outcomes. Such expectation is one of the factors that Jamison was referring to when she suggested that adopting such practices could be used by the practitioner to enhance the patient practitioner interaction for the benefit of the patient.

Predicting those who will improve with manipulative therapy is important in the absence of other research. Flynn et al. (2002) have shown in a cohort of nonradicular low back pain sufferers that the presence of four of the five (symptom duration, fear-avoidance beliefs, lumbar hypomobility, hip internal rotation range of motion, and no symptoms distal to the knee) increases the probablility of success with treatment from 45% to 95%. Investigation of these and other outcomes with subgroup analysis is a high priority for future research.

With such encouraging data, the chiropractic profession has further delved into the mind–body aspects of health issues. For example, the chiropractically based Neuro-Emotional Technique (NET), is a multimodal approach that addresses biological, emotional, and social contributors to various health complaints (Bablis, Pollard, & Monti, 2006).

NET was developed by chiropractor Scott Walker with the initial goals of achieving more complete and longer lasting effects from chiropractic care (Walker, 1990). The intervention is based on the observation that chiropractic treatments for symptoms of injuries have better outcomes when the adjustments are done while the patient is consciously thinking about the injurious event (Bablis, Pollard, & Bonello, 2008). The proposed theory is that emotional and cognitive distress related to the physical trauma is decreased when paired with the neurological relaxation of the adjustment (Walker, 1990; Bablis, Pollard, & Monti, 2006). Other factors are interwoven into this 15-step intervention process (Walker, 1990).

To date there has been a small but growing evidence base of supporting preliminary research. Research has investigated the reliability of key components of the multistep process, as well as describing select treatment observations and outcomes.

These studies include inter- and intra-examiner reliability studies of core procedures reported in various peer-reviewed journals (Cuthbert & Goodheart, 2007; Monti, Sinnott, Marchese, Kunkel, & Greeson, 1999; Petersen, 1996; Pollard, Bablis, & Bonello, 2006; Pollard, Lakay, Tucker, Watson, & Bablis, 2005).

In addition, the preliminary research includes descriptive studies of practitioner perceptions (Walker, Bablis, Pollard, & McHardy, 2005), the effects of a contemplated stressful event in hypercholesterolemic subjects (Petersen, 1995), and the intensity of arousal in phobic subjects (Petersen, 1997).

Observational studies have also been completed. These include case report/series in hypothyroidism (Bablis & Pollard, 2004), polycystic ovarian syndrome (Bablis, Pollard, & McHardy, 2006), annovulation infertility (Bablis,

Pollard, & Monti, 2006), reduction of trigger points in chronic neck pain (Bablis et al., 2008), and adolescent separation anxiety disorder (Karpouzis, Pollard, & Bonello, 2008).

More recently, Walker modified the original intervention to create a version that does not require a chiropractic adjustment. This version has recently been tested by a team of mental health professionals, showing high success in a case series of cancer patients with traumatic stress (Monti, Stoner, Zivin, & Schlesinger, 2007; Monti, Sufian, & Peterson, 2008).

Whilst still preliminary, the early evidence is encouraging of a significant effect for this new form of therapy in a variety of common conditions. Further research is needed to validate the conditions and situations that are most appropriate for this intriguing health intervention.

Conclusions

Chiropractic is an evolving healthcare paradigm that offers a unique and promising perspective of integrated health management. Although chiropractic has endured a rather challenging political development, its embrace of scientific methods in the last 20 years has enhanced its acceptance as a healthcare discipline. More research is needed on mechanisms of action involved with symptom relief from chiropractic adjustments, as well as mediators and moderators of treatment effect. Recent advances in neuro-imaging and biochemical analyses may offer exciting opportunities for further elucidation of the effects of chiropractic care. Newer multimodal approaches to management, such as the neuroemotional technique and others, have begun to expand the bounds of chiropractic care and enhance the possibilities for overall improved quality of life.

REFERENCES

Ader, R., & Cohen, N. (1982). Behaviorally conditioned immunosuppression and murine systemic lupus erythematosus. *Science, 19, 215*(4539), 1534–1536.

Alcantara, J., Plaugher, G., Thornton, R. E., & Salem, C. (2001). Chiropractic care of a patient with vertebral subluxations and unsuccessful surgery of the cervical spine. *Journal of Manipulative Physiological Therapy, 24*(7), 477–482.

Axén, I., Rosenbaum, A., Eklund, A., Halasz, L., Jørgensen, K., Lövgren, P. W., et al. (2008). The Nordic maintenance care program – case management of chiropractic patients with low back pain: A survey of Swedish chiropractors. *Chiropractic & Osteopathy, 16*: 6.

Bablis, P., & Pollard, H. (2004). Hypothyroidism: A new model for conservative management in two cases. *Chiropractic Journal of Australia, 34*, 11–18.

Bablis, P., & Pollard, H. (2009). Anxiety and depression profile of new patients presenting to a neuro emotional technique (NET) practitioner. *Journal of Alternative and Complementary Medicine*, 15(2), 121–127.

Bablis, P., Pollard, H., & Bonello, R. (2008). Neuro emotional technique for the treatment of trigger point sensitivity in chronic neck pain sufferers: A controlled clinical trial. *Chiropractic & Osteopathy*, 16: 4.

Bablis, P., Pollard, H., & McHardy, A. (2006). Two reports of resolution of polycystic ovary syndrome induced anovulation in females receiving nero emotional technique. *Chiropractic Journal of Australia*, 36, 2–8.

Bablis, P., Pollard, H., & Monti, D. (2006). Resolution of anovulation infertility using neuro emotional technique: A report of 3 cases. *Journal of Chiropractic Medicine*, 5(1), 13–21.

Blumenthal. J. A., Williams, R. B. Jr., Kong, Y., Schanberg, S. M., & Thompson, L. W. (1978). Type A behavior pattern and coronary atherosclerosis. *Circulation*, 58(4), 634–639.

Bogduk, N., & Merskey, H. (Eds). (1994). *Classification of chronic pain* (2nd edn). Seattle, WA: IASP Task Force on Taxonomy. IASP Press, pp. 209–214.

Brennan, P. C., Graham, M. A., Triano, J. J., Hondras, M. A., & Anderson, R. J. (1994). Lymphocyte profiles in patients with chronic low back pain enrolled in a clinical trial. *Journal of Manipulative and Physiological Therapeutics*, 17(4), 219–227.

Bonaz, B. (2003). Visceral sensitivity perturbation integration in the brain-gut axis in functional digestive disorders. *Journal of Physiology and Pharmacology*, 54(Suppl 4), 27–42.

Boudreau, L. A., Busse, J. W., & McBride, G. (2006). Chiropractic services in the Canadian Armed Forces: A pilot project. *Military Medicine*, 171(6), 572–576.

Breen, A., & Breen. R. (2003). Back pain and satisfaction with chiropractic treatment: What role does the physical outcome play? *Clinical Journal of Pain*, 19(4), 263–268.

Burton, A. K,, McClune, T. D., Clarke, R. D., & Main, C. J. (2004). Long-term follow-up of patients with low back pain attending for manipulative care: Outcomes and predictors. *Manual Therapy*, 9(1), 30–35.

Cagnie, B., Jacobs, F., Barbaix, E., Vinck, E., Dierckx, R., & Cambier, D. (2005). Changes in cerebellar blood flow after manipulation of the cervical spine using Technetium 99m-ethyl cysteinate dimer. *Journal of Manipulative and Physiological Therapeutics*, 28(2), 103–107.

Camara, E. G., & Danao, T. C. (1989). The brain and the immune system: A psychosomatic network. *Psychosomatics*, 30(2), 140–146.

Carney, R. M, Rich, M. W., Freedland, K. E., Saini, J., teVelde, A., Simeone, C., & Clark, K. (1988). Major depressive disorder predicts cardiac events in patients with coronary artery disease. *Psychosomatic Medicine*, 50(6), 627–633.

Carney, R. M., Rich, M. W., Tevelde, A., Saini, J., Clark, K., & Jaffe, A. S. (1987). Major depressive disorder in coronary artery disease. *American Journal of Cardiology*, 60(16), 1273–1275.

Cassidy, J. D., Lopes, A. A., & Yong-Hing, K. (1992). The immediate effect of manipulation versus mobilization on pain and range of motion in the cervical spine: A randomized controlled trial. *Journal of Manipulative and Physiological Therapeutics*, 15(9), 570–575.

Cleland, J. A., Glynn, P., Whitman, J. M., Eberhart, S. L., MacDonald, C., & Childs, J. D. (2007). Short-term effects of thrust versus nonthrust mobilization/manipulation directed at the thoracic spine in patients with neck pain: A randomized clinical trial. *Physical Therapy*, 87(4), 431–440.

Coote, J. H., & Downman, C. B. (1966). Central pathways of some autonomic reflex discharges. *Journal of Physiology*, 183(3), 714–729.

Coulter, I.D., Hurwitz, E.L., Adams, A.H., Genovese, B.J., Hays, R., & Shekelle, P.G. (2002). Patients using chiropractors in North America: Who are they, and why are they in chiropractic care? *Spine*, 27, 291–296.

Cramer, G., Budgell, B., Henderson, C., Khalsa, P., & Pickar, J. (2006). Basic science research related to chiropractic spinal adjusting: The state of the art and recommendations revisited. *Journal of Manipulative and Physiological Therapeutics*, 29(9), 726–761.

Cuthbert, S. C., & Goodheart, G. J., Jr. (2007). On the reliability and validity of manual muscle testing: A literature review. *Chiropractic & Osteopathy*, 15: 4.

Cyriax, J. (1951). Manipulation and the physiotherapist. *Medicine Illustrated.*, 5(7), 321–327.

Cyriax J. (1964). The pros and cons of manipulation. *Lancet*, 1(7333), 571–573.

Drossman, D. A,, Leserman, J., Li, Z. M., Mitchell, C. M., Zagami, E. A., & Patrick, D. L. (1991). The rating form of IBD patient concerns: A new measure of health status. *Psychosomatic Medicine*, 53(6), 701–712.

Druss, B. G., & Rosenheck, R. A. (2000). Use of practitioner-based complementary therapies by persons reporting mental conditions in the United States. *Archives of General Psychiatry*, 57(7), 708–714.

Engel, G. L. (1977). The need for a new medical model: A challenge for biomedicine. *Science*, 196(4286), 129–136.

Ernst, E. (2008). Chiropractic: A critical evaluation. *Journal of Pain Symptom Management*, 35(5), 544–562.

Fernández-de-Las-Peñas, C., Alonso-Blanco, C., Cuadrado, M. L., & Pareja, J. A. (2005). Spinal manipulative therapy in the management of cervicogenic headache. *Headache*, 45(9), 1260–1263.

Friedmann, E., Thomas, S. A., Liu, F., Morton, P. G., Chapa, D., & Gottlieb, S. S. (2006). Sudden cardiac death in Heart Failure Trial Investigators. Relationship of depression, anxiety, and social isolation to chronic heart failure outpatient mortality. *American Heart Journal*, 152(5), 940.e1–8.

Furlan, A. D., Tomlinson, G., Jadad, A. A., & Bombardier, C. (2008). Examining heterogeneity in meta-analysis: Comparing results of randomized trials and nonrandomized studies of interventions for low back pain. *Spine*, 33(3), 339–348.

Flynn, T., Fritz, J., Whitman, J., Wainner, R., Magel, J., Rendeiro, D., et al. (2002). Clinical prediction rule for classifying patients with low back pain who demonstrate short-term improvement with spinal manipulation. *Spine*, 27(24), 2835–2843.

Garner, B., Phillips, L. J., Schmidt, H. M., Markulev, C., O'Connor, J., Wood, S. J., et al. (2008). Pilot study evaluating the effect of massage therapy on stress, anxiety and aggression in a young adult psychiatric inpatient unit. *Australian and New Zealand Journal of Psychiatry, 42*(5), 414–422.

Gaumer, G. (2006). Factors associated with patient satisfaction with chiropractic care: Survey and review of the literature. *Journal of Manipulative and Physiological Therapeutics, 29*(6), 455–462.

George, S. Z., Fritz, J. M., Childs, J. D., & Brennan, G. P. (2006). Sex differences in predictors of outcome in selected physical therapy interventions for acute low back pain. *Journal of Orthopaedic and Sports Physical Therapy, 36*(6), 354–363.

Giles, L. G., & Muller, R. (2003). Chronic spinal pain: A randomized clinical trial comparing medication, acupuncture, and spinal manipulation. *Spine, 28*(14), 1490–50.

Gouveia, L. O., Castanho, P., Ferreira, J. J., Guedes, M. M., Falcão, F., & e Melo, T. P. (2007). Chiropractic manipulation: reasons for concern? *Clinical Neurology and Neurosurgery, 109*(10), 922–925.

Haas, M., Groupp, E., Aickin, M., Fairweather, A., Ganger, B., Attwood, M., et al. (2004). Dose response for chiropractic care of chronic cervicogenic headache and associated neck pain: A randomized pilot study. *Journal of Manipulative and Physiological Therapeutics., 27*(9), 547–553.

Haavik-Taylor, H., & Murphy, B. (2007). Cervical spine manipulation alters sensorimotor integration: A somatosensory evoked potential study. *Clinical Neurophysiology, 118*(2), 391–402.

Hains, G., & Hains, F. (2000). A combined ischemic compression and spinal manipulation in the treatment of fibromyalgia: A preliminary estimate of dose and efficacy. *Journal of Manipulative and Physiological Therapeutics, 23*(4), 225–230.

Haneline, M. T., Croft, A. C., & Frishberg, B. M. (2003). Association of internal carotid artery dissection and chiropractic manipulation. *Neurologist, 9*(1), 35–44.

Hansen, J. P., & Futch, D. B. (1997). Chiropractic services in a staff model HMO: Utilization and satisfaction. *HMO Practice, 11*(1), 39–42.

Hardy, K., & Pollard, H. (2006). The organisation of the stress response, and its relevance to chiropractors: A commentary. *Chiropractic & Osteopathy, 14*: 25.

Hartvigsen, J., Bolding-Jensen, O., Hviid, H., & Grunnet-Nilsson, N. (2003). Danish chiropractic patients then and now—a comparison between 1962 and 1999. *Journal of Manipulative and Physiological Therapeutics, 26*, 65–69.

Hawk, C., Long, C. R., & Boulanger, K. T. (2001). Prevalence of nonmusculoskeletal complaints in chiropractic practice: Report from a practice-based research program. *Journal of Manipulative and Physiological Therapeutics, 24*, 157–169.

Hawk, C., Long, C. R., Perillo, M., & Boulanger, K. T. (2004). A survey of US chiropractors on clinical preventive services. *Journal of Manipulative and Physiological Therapeutics, 27*(5), 287–298.

Hemingway, H., & Marmot, M. (1999). Psychosocial factors in the aetiology and prognosis of coronary heart disease: Systematic review of prospective cohort studies. *British Medical Journal, 318*, 1460–1467.

Hertzman-Miller, R. P., Morgenstern, H., Hurwitz, E. L., Yu, F., Adams, A. H., Harber, P., et al. (2002). Comparing the satisfaction of low back pain patients randomized to receive medical or chiropractic care: Results from the UCLA low-back pain study. *American Journal of Public Health, 92*(10), 1628–1633.

Hill, F., Bateman, C., & Shaffie, M. (1998). Changes in brain function after manipulation of the cervical spine. *Journal of Manipulative and Physiological Therapeutics, 21*(4), 304.

Homola, S. (2006). Chiropractic: History and overview of theories and methods. *Clinical Orthopaedics and Related Research, 444*, 236–242.

Hoskins, W., McHardy, A., Pollard, H., Windsham, R., & Onley, R. (2006). Chiropractic treatment of lower extremity conditions: A literature review. *Journal of Manipulative and Physiological Therapeutics, 29*(8), 658–671.

Humphreys, B. K., Sulkowski, A., McIntyre, K., Kasiban, M., & Patrick, A. N. (2007). An examination of musculoskeletal cognitive competency in chiropractic interns. *Journal of Manipulative and Physiological Therapeutics, 30*(1), 44–49.

Hurwitz, E. L., Morgenstern, H., & Yu, F. (2005). Satisfaction as a predictor of clinical outcomes among chiropractic and medical patients enrolled in the UCLA low back pain study. *Spine, 30*(19), 2121–2128.

Jamison, J. R. (1997). An interactive model of chiropractic practice: Reconstructing clinical reality. *Journal of Manipulative and Physiological Therapeutics, 20*(6), 382–388.

Karpouzis, F., Pollard, H., & Bonello, R. (2008). Adolescent Separation Anxiety Disorder managed by the Neuro Emotional Technique—a new biopsychosocial intervention: A case study. *Journal of Chiropractic Medicine, 31*(2), 146–159.

Keating, J. C., Jr. (1992). Shades of straight: Diversity among the purists. *Journal of Manipulative and Physiological Therapeutics, 15*(3), 203–209.

Keating, J. C., Jr. (1994). Metaphysics, rationality and science. *Journal of Manipulative & Physiological Therapeutics, 17*(6), 411–413.

Keating, J. C., Jr., Charlton, K. H., Grod, J. P., Perle, S. M., Sikorski, D., & Winterstein, J. F. (2005). Subluxation: Dogma or science? *Chiropractic & Osteopathy, 13*, 17.

Keating, J. C., Jr., & Hansen, D. T. (1992). Quackery vs. accountability in the marketing of chiropractic. *Journal of Manipulative and Physiological Therapeutics, 15*(7), 459–470.

Kellow, J. E., & Phillips, S. F. (1987). Altered small bowel motility in irritable bowel syndrome is correlated with symptoms. *Gastroenterology, 92*(6), 1885–1893.

Kelly, D. D., Murphy, B. A., & Backhouse, D. P. (2000). Use of a mental rotation reaction-time paradigm to measure the effects of upper cervical adjustments on cortical processing: A pilot study. *Jounal of Manipulative and Physiological Therapeutics, 23*(4), 246–251.

Kiecolt-Glaser, J. K., & Galser, R. (1989). Psychoneuroimmunology: Past, present, and future. *Health Psychology, 8*(6), 677–678.

Lamm, L. C., Wegner, E., & Collord, D. (1995). Chiropractic scope of practice: What the law allows—update 1993. *Journal of Manipulative & Physiological Therapeutics, 18*(1), 16–20.

Leboeuf-Yde, C., & Hestbæk, L. (2008). Maintenance care in chiropractic—what do we know? *Chiropractic & Osteopathy, 16*: 3.

Leeuw, M., Goossens, M. E., Linton, S. J., Crombez, G., Boersma, K., & Vlaeyen, J. W. (2007). The fear-avoidance model of musculoskeletal pain: Current state of scientific evidence. *Journal of Behavioral Medicine, 30*(1), 77–94.

Linton, S. J. (2000). A review of psychological risk factors in back and neck pain. *Spine, 25*(9), 1148–1156.

Martin, A. L., McGrath, P. A., Brown, S. C., & Katz, J. (2007). Anxiety sensitivity, fear of pain and pain-related disability in children and adolescents with chronic pain. *Pain Research & Management, 12*(4), 267–272.

Marshall, P., & Murphy, B. (2008). Self-report measures best explain changes in disability compared with physical measures after exercise rehabilitation for chronic low back pain. *Spine, 33*(3), 326–338.

McEwen, B. S. (1998). Stress, adaptation, and disease. Allostasis and allostatic load. *Annals of the New York Academy of Sciences, 840,* 33–44.

McEwen, B. S. (2000). The neurobiology of stress: From serendipity to clinical relevance. *Brain Research, 886,* 172–189.

McHardy, A., Hoskins, W., Pollard, H., Onley, R., & Windsham, R. (2008). Chiropractic treatment of upper extremity conditions: A systematic review. *Journal of Manipulative and Physiological Therapeutics, 31*(2), 145–146.

Melzack, R. (1999). Pain and stress: A new perspective. In R. C. Gatchel and D. C. Turk (Eds.), *Psychosocial factors in pain: Critical perspectives.* New York: Guilford Press, pp. 89–106.

Meyer, S. E., Chrousos, G. P., & Gold, P. W. (2001). Major depression and the stress system: A life span perspective. *Development and Psychopathology, 13,* 564–580.

Myers, S. S., Phillips, R. S., Davis, R. B., Cherkin, D. C., Legedza, A., Kaptchuk, T. J., et al. (2008). Patient expectations as predictors of outcome in patients with acute low back pain. *Journal of General Internal Medicine, 3*(2), 148–153.

Monti, D. A., Sinnott, J., Marchese, M., Kunkel, E. J., & Greeson, J. M. (1999). Muscle test comparisons of congruent and incongruent self-referential statements. *Perceptual and Motor Skills, 88*(3 Pt 1), 1019–1028.

Monti, D. A., Sufian, M., & Peterson, C. (2008). Potential role of mind–body therapies in cancer survivorship. *Cancer,* Apr 21.

Monti, D. A., Stoner, M., Zivin, G., & Schlesinger, M. (2007). Short term correlates of the neuro emotional technique for cancer-related traumatic stress symptoms: A pilot case series. *Journal of Cancer Survivorship, 1,* 161–166.

Mootz, R. D., Cherkin, D. C., Odegard, C. E., Eisenberg, D. M., Barassi, J. P., & Deyo, R. A. (2005). Characteristics of chiropractic practitioners, patients, and encounters in Massachusetts and Arizona. *Journal of Manipulative and Physiological Therapeutics, 28*(9), 645–653.

Nelson, C. F., Lawrence, D. J., Triano, J. J., Bronfort, G., Perle, S. M., Metz, R. D., et al. (2005). Chiropractic as spine care: A model for the profession. *Chiropractic & Osteopathy, 13:* 9.

Nyiendo, J., Haas, M., Goldberg, B., & Sexton, G. (2001). Pain, disability, and satisfaction outcomes and predictors of outcomes: A practice-based study of chronic low back pain patients attending primary care and chiropractic physicians. *Journal of Manipulative and Physiological and Therapeutics*, 24(7), 433–439.

Palmer, D. D. (1910). *The chiropractor's adjuster: The science, art, and philosophy of chiropractic*. Portland, OR: Portland Printing House.

Peterson, K. (1995). Two cases of spinal manipulation performed while the patient contemplated an associated stress event: The effect of the manipulation/contemplation on serum cholesterol levels in hypercholesterolemic subjects. *Chiropractic Technique*, 7, 55–59.

Peterson, K. B. (1996). A preliminary enquiry into manual muscle testing response in phobic and control subjects exposed to threatening stimuli. *Journal of Manipulative and Physiological Therapeutics*, 19(5), 310–316.

Peterson, K. B. (1997). The effects of spinal manipulation on the intensity of emotional arousal in phobic subjects exposed to a threat stimulus: A randomized, controlled, double-blind clinical trial. *Journal of Manipulative Physiological Therapeutics*, 20(9), 602–606.

Pincus, T., Foster, N. E., Vogel, S., Santos, R., Breen, A., & Underwood, M. (2007). Attitudes to back pain amongst musculoskeletal practitioners: A comparison of professional groups and practice settings using the ABS-mp. *Manual Therapy*, 12(2), 167–175.

Pollard, H. (2004). The somatovisceral reflex: How important for the type "O" condition? *Chiropractic Journal of Australia*, 34, 93–102.

Pollard, H., & Bablis, P. (2004). Hypothyroidism: A new model for Conservative Management in two cases. *Chiropractic Journal of Australia*, 34(1), 11–18.

Pollard, H., Bablis, P., & Bonello, R. (2006). Can the Ileocecal Valve Point Predict Low Back Pain Using Manual Muscle Testing? *Chiropractic Journal of Australia*, 36, 58–62.

Pollard, H., Hardy, K., & Curtin, D. (2006). Biopsychosocial Model of Pain and Its Relevance to Chiropractors. *Chiropractic Journal of Australia*, 36(3), 92–96.

Pollard, H., Hoskins, W., McHardy, A., Bonello, R., Garbutt, P., Swain, M., et al. (2007). Australian chiropractic sports medicine: half way there or living on a prayer? *BMC Chiropractic & Osteopathy*, 15: 14.

Pollard, H., Lakay, B., Tucker, F., Watson, B., & Bablis, P. (2005). Interexaminer reliability of the deltoid and psoas muscle test. *Journal of Manipulative Physiological Therapeutics*, 28(1), 52–56.

Quigley, W. H. (1995). Bartlett Joshua Palmer: Toward an understanding of the man, 1881–1961. *Chiropractic History*, 15(2), 30–35.

Richter, J. E., & Bradley, L. C. (1996). Psychophysiological interactions in esophageal diseases. *Seminars in Gastrointestinal Disease*, 7(4), 169–184.

Rosenman, R. H., Brand, R. J., Jenkins, D., Friedman, M., Straus, R., & Wurm, M. (1975). Coronary heart disease in Western Collaborative Group Study. Final follow-up experience of 8 1/2 years. *Journal of American Medical Association*, 233(8), 872–877.

Rubinstein, S., Pfeifle, C. E., van Tulder, M. W., & Assendelft, W. (2000). Chiropractic patients in the Netherlands: A descriptive study. *Journal of Manipulative and Physiological Therapeutics*, 23, 557–563.

Rubinstein, S. M,, Leboeuf-Yde, C., Knol, D. L., de Koekkoek, T. E., Pfeifle, C. E., & van Tulder, M. W. (2007). The benefits outweigh the risks for patients undergoing chiropractic care for neck pain: a prospective, multicenter, cohort study. *Journal of Manipulative Physiological Therapeutics, 30*(6), 408–418.

Sackett, D. L., Rosenberg, W. M., Gray, J. A., Haynes, R. B., & Richardson, W. S. (2007). Evidence based medicine: What it is and what it isn't. 1996. *Clinical Orthopaedics and Related Research, 455,* 3–5.

Santilli, V., Beghi, E., & Finucci, S. (2006). Chiropractic manipulation in the treatment of acute back pain and sciatica with disc protrusion: A randomized double-blind clinical trial of active and simulated spinal manipulations. *Spine Journal, 6*(2), 131–137.

Sapolsky, R. M., Romero, L. M., & Munck, A. U. (2000). How do glucocorticoids influence stress responses? Integrating permissive, suppressive, stimulatory, and preparative actions. *Endocrine Reviews, 21,* 55–89.

Sato, A. (1995). Somatovisceral reflexes. *Journal of Manipulative Physiological Therapeutics, 18*(9), 597–602.

Scalena, A. (2006). Defining Quackery: An examination of the Manitoba Medical Profession and the early development of professional unity. *Journal of the Canadian Chiropractic Association, 50*(3), 209–218.

Scascighini, L., & Sprott, H. (2008). Chronic nonmalignant pain: A challenge for patients and clinicians. *Nature Clinical Practice. Rheumatology, 4*(2), 74–81.

Sloan, T. J., Gupta, R., Zhang, W., & Walsh, D. A. (2008). Beliefs about the causes and consequences of pain in patients with chronic inflammatory or noninflammatory low back pain and in pain-free individuals. *Spine, 33*(9), 966–972.

Sorensen, L. P., Stochkendahl, M. J., Hartvigsen, J., & Nilsson, N. G. (2006). Chiropractic patients in Denmark 2002: An expanded description and comparison with 1999 survey. *Journal of Manipulative and Physiological Therapeutics, 29*(6), 419–424.

Spencer, R. I., & Hutchinson, K. E. (1999). Alcohol, aging, and the stress response. *Alcohol Research & Health, 23,* 272–283.

Spiller, R., Aziz, Q., Creed, F., Emmanuel, A., Houghton, L., Hungin, P., et al. (2007). Clinical Services Committee of The British Society of Gastroenterology. Guidelines on the irritable bowel syndrome: Mechanisms and practical management. *Gut, 56*(12), 1770–1798.

Sternberg, E. M., Chrousos, G. P., Wilder, R. L., & Gold, P. W. (1992). The stress response and the regulation of inflammatory disease. *Annals of Internal Medicine, 15,* 117(10), 854–866.

Thomas, J. S., France, C. R., Sha, D., & Wiele, N. V. (2008). The influence of pain-related fear on peak muscle activity and force generation during maximal isometric trunk exertions. *Spine, 33*(11), E342–E348.

Tuchin, P. J., Pollard, H., & Bonello, R. (2000). A randomized controlled trial of chiropractic spinal manipulative therapy for migraine. *Journal of Manipulative and Physiological Therapeutics, 23*(2), 91–95.

van Wijk, R. M., Geurts, J. W., Lousberg, R., Wynne, H. J., Hammink, E., Knape, J. T., et al. (2008). Psychological predictors of substantial pain reduction after minimally invasive radiofrequency and injection treatments for chronic low back pain. *Pain Medicine, 9*(2), 212–221.

Vernon, H., Humphreys, K., & Hagino, C. (2007). Chronic mechanical neck pain in adults treated by manual therapy: A systematic review of change scores in randomized clinical trials. *Journal of Manipulative and Physiological Therapeutics, 30*(3), 215–227.

Villanueva-Russell, Y. (2005). Evidence-based medicine and its implications for the profession of chiropractic. *Social Science & Medicine, 60*(3), 545–561.

Walker, S. *Neuro Emotional Technique: N.E.T basic manual.* Encinitas, CA: N.E.T Inc, 1996.

Walker, S. (1990). The triangle of health: Once more with feeling. *Digest of Chiropractic Economics,* May/June, 16–25.

Walker, S., Bablis, P., Pollard, H., & McHardy, A. (2005). Practitioner perceptions of emotions associated with pain: A survey. *Journal of Chiropractic Medicine, 4*, 8–11.

Walker, B. F., Muller, R., & Grant, W. D. (2004). Low back pain in Australian adults. Health provider utilization and care seeking. *Journal of Manipulative and Physiological Therapeutics, 27*(5), 327–335.

Wardwell, W. I. (1994). Alternative medicine in the United States. *Social Science & Medicine, 38*(8), 1061–1068.

Webb, R., Brammah, T., Lunt, M., Urwin, M., Allison, T., & Symmons, D. (2003). Prevalence and predictors of intense, chronic, and disabling neck and back pain in the UK general population. *Spine, 28*(11), 1195–1202.

Weiner, B. K. (2007). Difficult medical problems: On explanatory models and a pragmatic alternative. *Medical Hypotheses, 68*(3), 474–479.

Whitehead, W. E., Engel, B. T., & Schuster, M. M. (1980). Irritable bowel syndrome: Physiological and psychological differences between diarrhea-predominant and constipation-predominant patients. *Digestive Diseases and Sciences, 25*(6), 404–413.

Williams, N. H., Hendry, M., Lewis, R., Russell, I., Westmoreland, A., & Wilkinson, C. (2007). Psychological response in spinal manipulation (PRISM): A systematic review of psychological outcomes in randomised controlled trials. *Complementary Therapies in Medicine, 15*(4), 271–283.

World Health Organization (WHO). (2006). *Draft guidelines on basic training and safety in osteopathy.* World Health Organization, February.

Wu, P., Fuller, C., Liu, X., Lee, H. C., Fan, B., Hoven, C. W., et al. (2007). Use of complementary and alternative medicine among women with depression: Results of a national survey. *Psychiatric Services, 58*(3), 349–56.

Yoshimura, M., & Nishi, S. (1982). Intracellular recordings from lateral horn cells for the spinal cord in vitro. *Journal of the Autonomic Nervous System, 6*(1), 5–11.

Zhu, Y., Haldeman, S., Hsieh, C.Y., Wu, P., & Starr, A. (2000). Do cerebral potentials to magnetic stimulation of paraspinal muscles reflect changes in palpable muscle spasm, low back pain, and activity scores? *Journal of Manipulative and Physiological Therapeutics, 23*(7), 458–464.

9

Homeopathy and Psychiatry

BERNARDO A. MERIZALDE

Introduction

Homeopathy is a complementary and alternative medicine (CAM) system of health that has had a controversial history which continues today. In the early nineteenth century, it was a treatment approach that was in high favor in the United States among influential individuals, but later it was largely discounted, particularly after publication of the Flexner report (King, 1984). Yet, homeopathic training and investigation continued outside the dominant health system, and there is currently a substantial subset of health professionals practicing homeopathy and large numbers of patients utilizing it throughout the world. It is estimated that homeopathic rose 500% between 1996 and 2003, and sales of homeopathic medicines grew 39.5% between 2003 and 2005 (Jonas, Kaptchuk, & Linde, 2003; Spins, 2006). The literature base on homeopathy has grown since its early days; however, the wide variations in study designs and results leave as many questions as answers. Nonetheless, popularity of homeopathy continues to grow, and there are proposed applications for psychiatric treatment among its practitioners. The purpose of this chapter is to review some of the salient history and philosophical constructs of this health care approach, as well as the available data on its use in psychiatric care.

Brief History of Homeopathy

Samuel Hahnemann (1755–1843) was a German physician who became dissatisfied with the medical practices of his time, which included bloodletting, purging, vomiting, and the corporal punishment of persons with mental illness. He turned to translating medical texts for income, which inadvertently led to his developing homeopathy. While translating Cullen's *Materia Medica* section on Cinchona (Peruvian Bark), which was used to treat malaria, he noticed that Cinchona's secondary effects resembled the symptoms of malaria itself. This led to Hahnemann's concept of treating diseases with substances capable of producing pathological conditions similar to the patient's complaints, which he tested on 99 substances across the domains of mineral, vegetable, and animal. Hippocrates had previously postulated this therapeutic approach (Haehl, 1922). Hahnemann referred to his testing process as "proving," which he did initially in substantial doses of one to four grains (a grain equals approximately 62 mg). Hahnemann changed the practical application of his theory during his career, and later he prepared the medicines by serially diluting the solutions in flasks that were forcefully shaken and struck against a hard surface; the dilutions could go up to one part in 100^{-30}, a quinquillionth. This dilution would be then labeled "30C." Although these dilutions are well beyond Avogadro's number and are expected to have no atoms of the original substance, Hahnemann postulated that some essence of the substance remained. Dilution of a given remedy can vary widely. In homeopathy the dilution process is referred to as "potentization"; hence, the more dilute a preparation is, the more "potent" it is said to be. The phenomenon of a dose–response phenomenon characterized by low-dose stimulation and high-dose inhibition has been observed in pharmacology in both in vitro and in vivo experiments and is referred to as *hormesis* (Calabrese & Blain, 2004; Merizalde, 2005). However, in the non-homeopathic literature, the phenomenon describes the reactions of substances that have a measurable amount.

In Hahnemann's early investigations, preparations were ingested by "healthy" individuals in a semicontrolled manner, with close observation of the symptoms elicited. To participate in a proving, an individual had to be free from any evident pathology, so that the symptoms could get recorded accurately. The *Materia Medica* is the reference database, with an alphabetical inclusion of the medicinal substances including all symptoms elicited in the provings. Homeopaths decide dilution strengths based upon numerous variables related to the examination of the patient and the nature of symptoms presented (Dunham, 1984).

Although the philosophical concepts that define homeopathy are elusive, there are interesting parallel concepts in conventional biomedical science. For example, sleep deprivation or insomnia (a symptom of depression), taken to the extreme, can be a treatment for depression (Post & Weiss, 1992). Likewise, the model of time-dependent sensitization (TDS) indicates that exposure to a strong compound sensitizes an organism to a smaller dose of the same compound, which results in an amplified response. This type of effect has relevance to kindling phenomena, and also overlaps conceptually with hormesis (Antelman, 1988).

Like several other CAM modalities, there are no "one size fits all" treatment protocols for a given diagnosis or set of symptoms, such as generalized anxiety.

This can make doing and interpreting homeopathic research a challenge. Some investigators have chosen to use a number of different remedies (four to eight) that may suit a majority of patients with a diagnosis. There are also consistency issues with potencies chosen and amounts of the remedies given.

Research in Homeopathy

Although there are substantial numbers of documented provings, they are essentially case reports with the inherent limitations thereof. Numerous objective studies have been attempted, but most are wrought with methodological limitations with wide variations in results. One extensive review of the homeopathic literature concluded that, in spite of a great deal of experimental and clinical work, there is only a little scientific evidence to suggest that homeopathy could be effective. This is largely because of poor design, execution, reporting, or failure to repeat experimental work. The authors did conclude that there was sufficient evidence to warrant the execution of well-designed, carefully controlled experiments (Scofield, 1984). A well-known study by Linde et al. reviewed the available literature and concluded that homeopathy seemed to have a therapeutic effect, despite its implausibility (Linde et al., 1997). Another study, sponsored by the European Commission Homeopathic Medicine Research Advisory Group, came to very similar conclusions, using only randomized controlled studies with concrete, predefined, outcome measures (Cucherat, Haugh, Gooch, & Boissel, 2000). However, in a recent comparative review of homeopathic, controlled clinical trials, the authors concluded that the clinical effects of homoeopathy are placebo effects (Shang et al., 2005). It has been counterargued that the methodology of this review was flawed and unfairly biased against homeopathy (Fisher, 2006).

Unfortunately, the subset of literature that is psychiatrically based is no less ambiguous. Below is a discussion of some relevant studies that focus on mental illness. Although definitive conclusions cannot be drawn, it is hoped that this review will inform the practicing psychiatrist sufficiently to discuss with interested patients what is and is not known about the subject matter.

Homeopathy and Psychiatry

The first homeopathic hospital for the mentally ill was founded in Middletown, New York, in May 1874. One prominent physician who used homeopathy at the time to treat the mentally ill was Charles Frederick Menninger, founder of the Menninger Clinic, which is still in operation but no longer uses homeopathy.

Menninger was an active member of the American Institute of Homeopathy and is quoted as saying,

> Homeopathy is wholly capable of satisfying the therapeutic demands of this age better than any other system or school of medicine...it is imperative that we exhaust the homeopathic healing art before resorting to any other mode of treatment, if we wish to accomplish the greatest success possible. (Menninger, 1897)

Few studies on the use of homeopathy in mental health have been published that follow good scientific methodology, though some meta-analysis of the studies that exist have suggested overall positive effects that warrant further research. In one review, 8 of 10 reasonably high-quality studies on the treatment of mental or psychological problems, including depression, insomnia, nervous tension, agitation, aphasia, and behavior problems in children, showed positive effects from homeopathic treatment. Although none of those studies has been replicated, they cumulatively suggest potential value and the need for further exploration of homeopathic treatments (Kleijnen, Knipschild, & ter Riet, 1991; Linde et al., 1997).

Some interesting studies worthy of mention have been publshed since that review. One study suggested that homeopathy may be useful in the treatment of some patients with anxiety or depression, either as an adjunctive or sole treatment, in patients who specifically request it (Davidson, Morrison, Shore, Davidson, & Bedayn, 1997). Of course, such selection bias of the intervention can influence the placebo effect. In addition, the authors noted several limitations to this study, concluding that only larger, double-blind, controlled trials can provide answers to the questions that arise when using homeopathy in the treatment of disease, in general, and in psychiatry in particular.

Chapman et al. performed a randomized, double-blind, placebo-controlled study on 60 patients with persistent mild traumatic brain injury. Their results suggested that homeopathy alone, or used concurrently with conventional pharmacological and rehabilitation therapies, may be effective in treating patients with persistent mild traumatic brain injury, a condition for which there are limited treatment options (Chapman, Weintraub, Milburn, Pirozzi, & Woo, 1999).

Lamont performed a double-blind, placebo-controlled study on the treatment of 43 children with a diagnosis of Attention Deficit Hyperactivity Disorder, showing statistically significant improvement in the homeopathy group as compared to the control, supporting the notion that homeopathic treatment is superior to placebo (Lamont, 1997).

Another set of studies also address the treatment of Attention Deficit Hyperactivity Disorder. One double-blind, placebo-controlled study of 115 children in Switzerland found positive results from a course of homeopathic treatment over a period of 3 months. These children were treated according to a more classical homeopathic approach, in which the remedy selection was individualized to the particular patient's symptoms. (Frei & Thurneysen, 2001) This same research group decided to do a "crossover" phase of the study and stopped the remedies. They found that the children who had improved with homeopathy deteriorated when the placebo was given and then responded again when the remedy was reinstated (Frei et al., 2005).

Hundreds of case reports were published in homeopathic journals during the nineteenth and twentieth centuries about patients suffering from mental disorders who were treated with homeopathy. Even though some of the cases inadequately present the diagnoses, many of these patients would have met criteria for a mental disorder according to the DSM-IV and would have been candidates for conventional pharmacotherapy in the present day.

Below is a brief overview of some case reports that have relatively clear and thorough descriptions of the disorders and treatment effect. They are mainly provided as a reference for those who would like more in-depth examples of the homeopathic process. Although case reports are not the gold standard of investigational inquiry in conventional biomedicine, some CAM modalities such as homeopathy consider case descriptions and outcomes crucial because of the individualized treatment approach of the intervention. Also, some feel that detailed case reports in the homeopathic literature are important and relevant to establishing its evidence base (Slonim & White, 1983).

Detinis presented six interesting cases of patients suffering from depression with suicidal ideation, chronic pain, sleep disorder, premenstrual syndrome, and anxiety disorder treated homeopathically (Detinis, 1994). Bodman presents a series of cases of depression, anxiety, sleep disorder, phobias, neurosis, cerebral sequelae from a stroke, Menniere's disease, migraines, and other conditions treated successfully with homeopathy (Bodman, 1990). Boltz (1968) and Phalnikar (1962) presented cases of patients with acute psychosis; Saine (1997) presented a series of cases of patients with psychosis, manic-depressive disorder, obsessions, and neurosis. Shevin (1989) presented several cases of patients with dissociative disorders, character pathology, and posttraumatic stress disorder treated homeopathically. Gallavardin (1960, 1990) published a series of cases of patients treated for alcoholism, and Grazyna and Trzebiatowska-Trzeciak (1993) presented a series of 30 men treated for alcohol withdrawal.

Some authors have presented cases of children with various cognitive handicaps, including traumatic brain injury (Haidvogl, Lehner, & Resch, 1993).

One case series of twenty children with enuresis and behavioral problems reported 50% improvement in both symptoms. Unfortunately, this investigation was not done as a controlled study, making it difficult to evaluate (Cortina, 1994).

The Process of Homeopathic Treatment

After the homeopath takes a complete case history, a comprehensive set of symptoms are selected based on their importance, severity, and the predominant characteristics and peculiarities that are unusual or out of the ordinary; for example, preferring cold wraps for headaches, while being chilly in the rest of the body. Such peculiarities help with the choice of one remedy over another for a patient with a particular illness. For example, if the above-mentioned chilly patient also has depression, he or she may need Phosphorus, while a depressed patient who tends to be hot may need a different remedy such as Pulsatilla.

Hahnemann used the term "constitution" to refer to those distinguishing characteristics of an individual present at birth, along with such intrinsic factors as climate, education, diet, morals, customs, and habits that will contribute to the manifestation of chronic diseases. He advised that physicians have to consider a patient's physical constitution, their affective and intellectual character, lifestyle, social position, family relations, age, sexual life, and so on in order to determine the best treatment for the patient (Hahnemann, 1842). Assessment of constitution continues to be part of the homeopathic evaluation. Within this context, it is the person's particular constitution with its corresponding susceptibilities that will determine responsiveness to particular remedies. By identifying a person's constitutional makeup, the homeopath identifies the best-suited remedies for that patient.

Homeopathic researchers have developed a Constitutional Type Questionnaire (CTQ) that tests the validity and reliability of 20 common homeopathic constitutional, broad spectrum acting remedies in a patient population. The goal of this instrument is to help the homeopath screen individuals for provings, as well as to help select remedies for patients (Davidson, Fisher, Van Haselen, Woodbury, & Connor, 2001; Van Haselen, Cinar, Fisher, & Davidson, 2001).

One study (Bell, Baldwin, Schwartz, & Davidson, 2002) examined the association between the CTQ and scores on standardized psychological and medical measures. The scales included were the chemical intolerance index (CII) for environmental sensitivity, the NEO (Neuroticism-Extraversion-Openness) personality inventory, the Marlowe-Crowne Social Desirability Scale (MCSD) for defensiveness, the Harvard Parental Caring Scale (HPCS) for perceived mother and father traits, the Profile of Mood State (POMS) scale, the Pannebaker Symptom Checklist (PSC), and a global health rating scale.

The majority of CTQ constitutional-type scores correlated significantly with greater neuroticism, lower MCSD defensiveness, and greater psychological distress on the POMS subscales. NEO extraversion and Openness subscales correlated with specific CTQ scores in directions consistent with clinical remedy pictures. They also found confirmation of traditional homeopathic views for specific remedies with scores from standardized conventional scales.

Homeopathic remedies are generally safe and nontoxic. Lower potency remedies commonly are found in health food stores, usually in dilutions of 6X, 6C, and 12C. Recommended frequency of the dosage varies depending on the acuity of the symptoms: if they are acute, the remedy can be repeated every 2–4 hours; if they are moderate, every 6–8 hours; if they are mild, once per day.

It is considered that a remedy is effective if the patient improves after three to four dosages. If there is no improvement, it is an indication that a different remedy or potency may be needed.

Homeopathic training is rather involved, and it can take several years to learn the nuances of remedy selection and follow up, as well as the knowledge of the homeopathic materia medica and the repertory—the dictionary of symptoms with the corresponding remedies. Homeopaths use various remedies with apparently different biological actions. Some induce symptoms acutely, such as Belladona, Hyosciamus, Stramonium, and Veratrum album. Other, so-called slow acting remedies, like Natrum Muriaticum (Sodium Chloride), Silica, Phosphorus, or Sepia (Cuttlefish Tincture) take a longer time and repeated dosages to manifest their particular symptom picture. The selection of the remedies is always based on the totality of symptoms of the patient and considering her or his peculiar or characteristic qualities (Hahnemann, 1842/1996).

There are about 39 remedies cited by Guernsey, with their characteristic symptoms for the treatment of mental illness. Besides the mental symptoms, the characteristics of local (in what segment of the body), organic (which particular organ), and pathology are matched with the clinical pictures observed during the proving in order to select the correct remedy (Boericke, 1927; Guernsey, 1866).

The clinical picture, supposedly elicited in some published proving, is described in such a way as to resemble clinical syndromes found in conventional nosology. The narrative of the proving of Aurum Metallicum (gold) reports: "hopeless, despondent and great desire to commit suicide, disgust of life, feeling of self-condemnation and utter worthlessness" (Guernsey, 1866). For more information about specific remedies, the largest reservoir of data and the main tools of any practicing homeopath are the homeopathic materia medica and the homeopathic repertory (see Table 9.1) (Neatby & Stonham, 1948/1987; Schroyens, 2004).

Table 9.1. Homeopathic Remedies in Psychiatry.

Remedy	Indications	Characteristic Symptoms
Aconite	Anxiety, apprehension, palpitations.	Pulsations, fear of death, ailments from fright and shock, flushing
Arnica	Traumas, concussions, post-surgical recovery	Sore, achy, pain; sore muscles and soft tissues from contusive/concussive trauma, traumatic extravasations
Coffea	Sleep Disorders	Hyperactive mind, sleepless from overactivation and thinking
Ignatia	Grief, loss, mortification	Shortness of breath, constriction of the throat, sensation of a ball rising from the stomach to the esophagus.
Natrum Muriaticum	Chronic Grief; Coryza; Rhinitis	Persistent thoughts, stoicism, reserved character, dislikes consolation; sad but unable to cry
Nux Vomica	Irritability, grouchiness, substance abuse withdrawal, cramps.	Hurried, rushing, contrary, quarrelsome, twitching, craving for stimulants
Phosphoric Acid	Fatigue, physical and mental	Ailments from overwork, physical and/or mental.
Staphysagria	Ailments from abuse, suppressed anger from mortification. Neonuptial cystitis.	Recurrent urinary tract infections, styes.

Conclusions

Homeopathy is an alternative system of health that at one time was in high favor among physicians, but is no longer part of mainstream Western medicine. Most of the premises behind homeopathy are unproven, although there are some homeopathic principles that have interesting correlates with accepted scientific principles. The available data on the treatment effectiveness for homeopathy is inadequate, inconsistent, and controversial, and it is particularly limited in the mental health arena. The current evidence is insufficient to support the use of homeopathy as a primary psychiatric treatment. Nonetheless, there continues to be significant interest in homeopathy among clinicians and patients throughout the world, likely because of the wide breadth of positive anecdotal accounts.

BIBLIOGRAPHY

AIH. (2007). *Homeopathy up to date.* Retrieved December 8, 2007, from American Institute of Homeopathy: www.homeopathyusa.org

Alarcon, R., & Franceshini, J. (1984). Hypoparathyroidism and paranoid psychosis: Case report and review of the literature. *British Journal of Psychiatry, 145,* 477–486.

Ames, B., Elson-Schwab, I., & Silver, E. (2002). High-dose vitamin therapy stimulates variant enzymes with decreased coenzyme binding affinity (increased Km): Relevance to genetic disease and polymorphisms. *American Journal of Clinical Nutrition, 75,* 616–658.

Ananth, J., & Ruskin, R. (1974). Treatment of intractable depression. *International Pharmacopsychiatry, 9(4),* 218–229.

Antelman, S. M. (1988). Time-dependent sensitisation as the cornerstone for a new approach to pharmacotherapy: Drug as a foreign/stressful stimuli. *Drug Development Research, 14,* 1–30.

Audhya, T., & McGinnis, W. (2004). Nutrient, toxin and enzyme profile of autistic children. *International Meeting for Autism Research,* Sacramento, CA: May 7–8, p. 74.

Bell, I. R., Baldwin, C. M., Schwartz, G. E., & Davidson, J. R. T. (2002). Homeopathic constitutional type questionnaire correlates of conventional psychological and physical health scales: Individual difference characteristics of young adults. *Homeopathy, 91,* 53–74.

Bodman, F. (1990). *Insights into homeopathy.* Beaconsfield Press, England: Davies and Pinsent Editors.

Boericke, G. (1965). Tranquilizing drugs used homeopathically and homeopathic tranquilizers. *Journal of the American Institute of Homeopathy,* Jan-Feb , pp. 20–23.

Boericke, W. (1927). *Materia medica and repertory* (9th edn). Philadelphia, PA: Boericke and Runyon.

Bolon, R., Yeragani, V., & Pohl, R. (1988). Relative hypophophatemia in patients with panic disorders. *Archives of General Psychiatry, 45,* 294–295.

Boltz, O. (1968). Some original investigations on the treatment of schizophrenia and associated symptoms due to a functional disturbance of integration in the diencephalon using the principle of Similia Similibus Curantur. *Journal of the American Institute of Homeopathy, 61(4),* 219–234.

Borrell-Carrio, F., Suchman, A. L., & Epstein, R. M. (2004). The biopsychosocial model 25 years later, Principles, practice, and scientific inquiry. *Annals of Family Medicine, 2(6),* 576–582.

Calabrese, E. J., & Blain, R. (2004). The hormesis database: An overview. *Toxicology and Applied Pharmacology, 202(3),* 289–300.

CDC. (2004). www.cdc.gov/pcd/issues/2004/apr/04_0006.htm.

Chapman, E. H., Weintraub, R. J., Milburn, M. A., Pirozzi, T. O., & Woo, E. (1999). Homeopathic treatment of mild traumatic brain injury: A randomized, double-blind, placebo-controlled clinical trial. *Journal of Head Trauma Rehabilitation, 14*(6), 521–542.

Cortina, J. (1994). Enuresis and its homeopathic treatment: Study of 20 cases treated with ilex paraguenses. *British Homeopathic Journal, 83*(4), 220–222.

Crothers, D. (1980). Mental illness and homeopathy. *Northwest Academy of Preventive Medicine Newsletter, 7*(4).

Cucherat, M., Haugh, M. C., Gooch, M., & Boissel, J. P. (2000). Evidence of clinical efficacy of homeopathy: A meta-analysis of clinical trials. *European Journal of Clinical Pharmacology, 56,* 27–33.

Davidson, J. (1994). Psychiatry and homeopathy. *British Homeopathic Journal, 83*(2), 78–83.

Davidson, J., Fisher, R., Van Haselen, R., Woodbury, M., & Connor, K. (2001). Do constitutional types exist? A further study using grade of membership analysis. *British Homeopathic Journal, 90,* 138–147.

Davidson, J., Morrison, R., Shore, J., Davidson, R. T., & Bedayn, G. (1997). Homeopathic treatment of depression and anxiety. *Alternative Therapies, 3*(1), 46–49.

Detinis, L. (1994). *Mental symptoms in homeopathy.* London, England: Beaconsfield Pubs.

Detre, T. P., & Jarecki, H. G. (1971). *Modern psychiatric treatment.* Philadelphia, PA: J. P. Lippincott, pp. 53–54.

Dunham, C., (1984). *Homeopathy: The science of therapeutics,* B. New Delhi, India: Jain Publishers.

Eisenberg, D. M., Davis, R. B., Ettner, S. L., Appel, S., Wilkey, S., Van Rompay, M., et al. (1998). Trends in alternative medicine use in the United States, 1990–1997: Results of a follow-up national survey. *Journal of American Medical Association, 280*(18), 1569–1575.

Feskanich, D., Singh, V., Willett, W. C., & Colditz, G. A. (2002). Vitamin A intake and hip fractures among postmenopausal woman. *Journal of American Medical Association, 287,* 47–54.

Fisher, P. (2006). Scientific Research on Homeopathic Medicine, Proving and Improving the Efficacy. 1st Joint American Homeopathic Conference. NCH26-320. www.conferencerecordings.com.

Frass, M., Linkesch, M., Banyai, S., Resch, G., Dielacher, C., Löbl, T. et al. (2005) Adjunctive homeopathic treatment in patients with severe sepsis: A randomized, double-blind, placebo-controlled trial in an intensive care unit. *Homeopathy, 94,* 75–80.

Frei, H., Everts, R., von Ammon, K., Kaufmann, F., Walther, D., Hsu-Schmitz, S. F., et al. (2005). Homeopathic treatment of children with attention deficit hyperactivity disorder, a randomised, double blind, placebo controlled crossover trial. *European Journal of Pediatrics, 164,* 758–767.

Frei, H., & Thurneysen, A. (2001). Treatment for hyperactive children: Homeopathy and methylphenidate compared in a family setting. *British Homeopathic Journal, 90,* 183–188.

Gallavardin, J. (1960/90). *Psychism and homeopathy.* New Delhi, India: B. Jain Publishers.

Gaylord, S., & Davidson, J. (1998). The constitution: Views from homeopathy and psychiatry. *British Homeopathic Journal, 87*, 148–153.

Geyman, J. (1998). Evidence based medicine in primary care: An overview. *Journal of the American Board of Family Practice*, 11: 46–56.

Gibson, D., & Lond, B. (1953). Some observations on homeopathy in relations to psychoneurosis. *British Journal of Homeopathy, 43*(3).

Gray, W. (1981). Anorexia Nervosa: Case report presented at the Homeopathic Conference in San Francisco.

Grazyna, M., & Trzebiatowska-Trzeciak, O. (1993). Homeopathic treatment of alcohol withdrawal. *British Homeopathic Journal with Simile, 82*(4), 249–251.

Griggs, W. (1968). Normalizing abnormal children. *Journal of the American Institute of Homeopathy*, Oct–Dec., 235–238.

Guernsey, H. (1866). Hysteria. *Hahnemannian Monthly, 1*(11), 387–404.

Haehl, R. (1922). *Hahnemann, his life and work*. London: London Homeopathic Pub.Co.

Hahnemann, S. (1842/1996). *Organon of medicine, 6th Ed. Trans. Brewster-O'Reilly, W.* Redmond, WA: Birdcage Books.

Haidvogl, M., Lehner, E., & Resch, D. (1993). Homeopathic treatment of handicapped children. *British Homeopathic Journal, 82*(4), 227–236.

Harbour, R., & Miller, J. (2001). A new system for grading recommendations in evidence based guidelines. *British Medical Journal, 323*: 334–336.

Herscu, P. (2002). *Provings—an annotated selection of historic & contemporary writings.* Amherst, MA: The New England School of Homeopathy Press.

Jonas, W. B., Kaptchuk, T. J., & Linde, K. (2003). A critical overview of homeopathy. *Annals of Internal Medicine, 138*(5), 393–399.

Kaptchuck, T. (1998). Intentional ignorance: A history of blind assessment in medicine. *Bulletin of the History of Medicine, 73*(3), 389–433.

Keith, E. L. (1899). Progress of the year in regard to state hospital work. *Transactions of the American Institute of Homeopathy*, 566–568.

Kent, J. (1900/1979). *Lectures on homeopathic philosophy.* Berkeley, CA: North Atlantic Books.

King, L. S. (1984). The Flexner report of 1910. *Journal of the American Medical Association, 251*(8): 1079–1086.

Kleijnen, J., Knipschild, P., & terRiet, G. (1991). Clinical trials of homeopathy. *British Medical Journal, 302*(6782), 316–323.

Krohn, J., & Taylor, F. (2000). *Natural detoxification, a practical encyclopedia*, (2nd edn). Pt. Roberts, WA: Hartley & Marks Publishers.

Lamont, J. (1997). Homeopathic treatment of attention deficit hyperactivity disorder—a controlled study. *British Homeopathic Journal, 86*, 196–200.

Linde, K., Clausius, N., Ramirez, G., Melchart, D., Eitel, F., Hedges, L. V., et al. (1997). Are the clinical effects of homeopathy placebo effects? A meta-analysis of placebo-controlled trials. *Lancet, 359*(9081), 834–43.

Menninger, C. (1897). Some reflections relative to the symptomatology and materia medica of typhoid fever. *Transactions of American Institute of Homeopathy*, 430.

Merizalde, B. (2003–2004). Bipolar disorder: A presentation of three cases. *American Journal of Homeopathic Medicine, 96*(4), 300–315.

Merizalde, B. (2008). Homeopathic medicine and psychiatry. *Journal of the American Institute of Homeopathy*, in press.

Merizalde, B. (2005). Samuel Hahnemann: Hormesis and a probably mechanism of action of homeopathic remedies. *American Journal of Homeopathic Medicine*, 98(4), 249–254.

Miller, L. (2000). Herbal Medicinals: Selective clinical considerations focusing on known or potential drug–herb interactions. In P. E. Fontanarosa (Ed.), *Alternative medicine: An objective assessment*. Chicago, IL: American Medical Association.

Mock, D. M. (1989). Biotin. In M. Brown (Ed.), *Present knowledge in nutrition* (6th edn). Wahington, DC: International Life Sciences Institute, pp. 2047–2052.

Motoyama, T., Sano, H., & Fukusaki, H. (1989). Oral magnesium supplementation in patients with essential hypertension. *Hypertension*, 13, 227–232.

Muller, W., Singer, A., Wonnemann, M., Hafner, U., Rolli, M., & Schäfer, C. (1998). Hyperforin represents the neurotransmitter reuptake inhibiting constituent of hypericum extract. *Pharmacopsychiatry*, 31(1), 16–21.

Murray, M. (1996). *Encyclopedia of nutritional supplements*. Rocklin, CA: Prima Publishing.

Murray, M., & Pizzorno, J. (1998). *Encyclopedia of natural medicine* (2nd edn). Rocklin, CA: Prima Publishing.

Neatby, E., & Stonham, T. (1948/1987). *Manual of homeo-therapeutics* (Indian edition). India: Jain Publishers.

Ness, R. (2000). Is depression and adaptation? *Archives of General Psychiatry*, 57, 14.

Post, R. M., & Weiss, S. R. B. (1992). Endogenous biochemical abnormalities in affective illness: Therapeutic versus pathogenic. *Biological Psychiatry*, 32, 469–484.

Priestman, K. (1951). Fears. *British Journal of Homeopathy*, 41(2), 93–100.

Reichenberg-Ullman, J., & R. U. (1996). *Ritalin free kids: Safe and effective homeopathic medicine for ADD and other behavioral and learning problems*. Roseville, CA: Prima Publishing, Random House.

Reichenberg-Ullman, J., & Ullman, R. (1999). *Prozac free: Homeopathic medicine for depression, anxiety and other mental and emotional problems*. Roseville, CA: Prima Publishing, Random House.

Reichenberg-Ullman, J., & Ullman, R. (1999). *Rage free kids: Homeopathic medicine for defiant, aggressive and violent children*. Roseville, CA: Prima Publishing, Random House.

Saine, A. (1997). *Psychiatric Patients: Back to the Roots: Steps in case taking*. Eindhoven, Netherlands: Lutra Services.

Schroyens, F. (2004). *Synthesis repertory (Synthesis Repertorium Homeopathicum Syntheticum)*, (9.1 edn). London, England: Homeopathic Book Publishers.

Scofield, A.M. (1984). Experimental research in homeopathy—a critical review. *British Homeopathic Journal*, 73(3 and 4), July and October, 161–180, 211–226.

Shang, A., Huwiler-Müntener, K., Nartey, L., Jüni, P., Dörig, S., Sterne, J. A. C., et al. (2005). Are the clinical effects of homeopathy placebo effects?: Comparative study of placebo-controlled trials of homeopathy and allopathy. *Lancet*, 366, 726–32.

Shevin, W. (1989). Case presentations. *Journal of the American Institute of Homeopathy*, 77(2): 59–66.

Slonim, D., & White, K. (1983). Homeopathy and psychiatry. *Journal of Mind and Behavior, 4* (3): 401–410.

Spinella, M. (2001, Jan/Feb). Psychoactive herbal medicatons: How do we know they work? *Skeptical Inquirer*, 43–49.

Spins, Information and Services to Grow the Natural Products Industry (2006). Homeopathic medicines are growing at double-digit rates, A. C. Nielsen ScanTrack, 52 W ending 12/31/2005.

Steinberg, S., Annable, L., Young, S. N., & Liyanage, N. (1999). A placebo-controlled clinical trial of L-Tryptophan in premenstrual dysphoria. *Biological Psychiatry, 45*(3), 313–320.

Steinsbekk, A., Bentzen, N., Fonnebo, V., & Lewith, G. (2005) Self-treatment with one of 3 self-selected ultramolecular homeopathic medicines for the prevention of upper respiratory tract infections in children. A double blind-randomized controlled trial. *British Journal of Clinical Pharmacology, 59*, 447–455.

Stevens, L., Zentall, S., Deck, J., Abate, M., Watkins, B., Lipp, S., et al. (1995). Essential fatty acids metabolism in boys with attention deficit disorder. *American Journal of Clinical Nutrition, 62*(4), 761–768.

Stevinson, C., Devaraj, V. S., Fountain-Barber, A., Hawkins, S., & Ernst, E. (2003). Homeopathic arnica for prevention of pain and bruising: Randomized placebo-controlled trial in hand surgery. *Journal of the Royal Society of Medicine, 96*, 60–65.

Stiles, H. (1875). Homeopathic treatment of insanity cases. *Transactions of the Homeopathic Medical Society of the State of New York*.

Talcott, S. (1891). The curability of mental and nervous diseases under homeopathic medication. *Transactions of the American Institute of Homeopathy*, 875–886.

Van Haselen, R. A., Cinar, S., Fisher, P., & Davidson, J. R. T. (2001). The constitutional type questionnaire: Validation in a patient population of the Royal Homeopathic Hospital. *British Homeopathic Journal, 90*, 131–137.

Vasquez, A., Manso, G., & Cannell, J. (2004). The clinical importance of vitamin D (cholecalciferol): A paradigm shift with implications for all healthcare providers. *Alternative Therapies in Health and Medicine, 10*, 28–36.

Weel, C., & Knottnerus, J. (1999). Evidence-based interventions and comprehensive treatment. *Lancet, 353*, 916–918.

Weil, A. (1997). *8 Weeks to optimum health*. New York: Alfred A. Knopf.

Weil, A. (1995). *Spontaneous healing*. New York: The Ballantine Publishing Company.

White, A., Slade, P., Hunt, C., Hart, A., & Ernst, E. (2003). Individualised homeopathy as an adjunct in the treatment of childhood asthma: A randomised placebo controlled trial. *Thorax, 58*, 317–321.

Whitmont, E. (1980). *Psyche and substance: Essays on homeopathy in the light of Jungian psychology*. Richmond, CA: North Atlantic Books.

Williams, R. (1956). *Biochemical individuality*. New York: John Wiley and Sons.

Williams, R. (1971). *Nutrition against disease*. New York: Pitman Publishing Corporation.

Williams, R. D. G. (1967). Individuality in vitamin C need. *Proceedings of National Academy of Sciences, 67*, 1638–1641.

Wood, R., Kubena, K., O'Brien, B. et al. (1991). Lack of dose response by dietary n-3 fatty acids at a constant ratio of n-3 to n-6 fatty acids in suppressing eicosanoid biosynthesis from arachidonic acid. *American Journal of Clinical Nutrition, 54* (1), 111–117.

Wright-Hubbard, E. (1965). Results with the potentized simillimum in retarded children. *Journal of the American Institute of Homeopathy,* Nov-Dec, 338–342.

Wu, J., & Bunney, W. E. (1990). The biological basis of an antidepressant response to sleep deprivation and relapse: Review and hypothesis. *American Journal of Psychiatry, 147,* 14–21.

PART III

PROBLEMS

10

Sleep and Sleep Disorders

KARL DOGHRAMJI, GEORGE BRAINARD, AND JOHN M. BALAICUIS

KEY CONCEPTS

- Sleep is not simply the absence of wakefulness; it is the product of active brain processes that produce changes throughout the mind and body
- Many underlying causes of insomnia are to be identified first, using logs, serum tests, and polysomnography
- A variety of disorders can be responsible for the complaints of insomnia and excessive daytime somnolence; the optimal clinical approach to these complaints is, therefore, the initial identification of the underlying causes
- Identification of the cause of sleep disturbances may necessitate inventories, logs, serum tests, and polysomnography
- Complementary and alternative medicines have popular appeal; however, the database supporting their use in clinical settings is scant
- Bright light treatment has applications in a wide variety of sleep disorders, most commonly circadian rhythm disorders
- Aging is associated with decrements of deep, slow wave sleep, and increases in shallow, stage 1 sleep, and increases in arousals and awakenings
- Excessive daytime somnolence is associated with significant impairments, including decrements in performance, breaches in interpersonal relationships, and accidents
- Although insomnia is often a product of psychiatric illness, the emergence of insomnia in otherwise healthy individuals, and its persistence, strongly predict the emergence of future psychiatric disorders, including depression, anxiety disorders, and substance use disorders

Now I will tell you how the waves of quiet
Flow through the mind in sleep and release it from care;
I will make the verses sweet and not too many
For the swan's little song is better than all the clamour
Of cranes blowing about in the clouds from the south.

—Lucretius (circa 99–55 BCE) De Rerum Natura IV
(translated by C. H. Sisson)

Introduction

Sleep plays an important part in the life of every human being, indeed in the life of every living thing. This regular nocturnal experience, which has been called everything from "the little death" (Arabic) and "the arms of Morpheus" (Greek) to "the land of Nod" (English), has fascinated man throughout recorded history, and likely before. Approximately one-third of the life of a human being is spent asleep. It is natural that sleep would attract attention, interest, and speculation throughout history.

Sleep Medicine as a field of study and specific research, however, has existed for fewer than 50 years, and it was only in 1996 that Sleep Medicine was recognized as a medical specialty by the American Medical Association. Much has come to be understood about sleep in the past century, particularly the latter half. To understand and treat disorders of sleep, it is necessary to understand the structure of normal sleep, as well as its components and complex underlying processes. Before this, a bit of history is in order.

Normal Sleep

HISTORICAL INTRODUCTION

There have been many ideas throughout history as to the nature and purpose of sleep. In his work *On Sleep and Sleeplessness* (circa 350 BCE), Aristotle proposed that sleep was a "natural recoil" of accumulated bodily heat obtained primarily from food and wine, and that a sleeper awoke when digestion was complete (TICA, 2000). Sleep was seen as restorative. In 1862 Alfred Maury—the French scholar of history, medicine, and law—stated that, "insomnia or the privation of sleep, irrespective of its cause, conduces to madness, because the cerebro-spinal system is then forced to provide an unending supply of nervous energy that is not replenished" (Stone, 1997). Throughout the centuries, however, sleep was not a focus of scientific exploration until the advent of Sigmund Freud, neurologist and psychiatrist, who, in his 1900 book *The Interpretation of Dreams*, advanced the notion that dreams are a window into the mysteries of the mind (Freud, 1900). Freud's primary interest was the understanding of the thoughts and feelings that reside in the unconscious mind and motivate human behavior and lead to psychic conflict. However, Freud's interests led him to advance a number of theoretical formulations regarding the psychological processes that govern dream production and sleep maintenance. He also recognized the importance of sleep paralysis, which prevented the sleeper from acting out his dreams.

Hans Berger, a German psychiatrist, was the first to record and describe human electroencephalographic waveforms in 1924. This established the technological foundation for the milestone discovery of rapid eye movement (REM) sleep by Aesrinsky and Kleitman in 1953. The subsequent surge in research into electrophysiological sleep formed the foundation upon which much of the field of sleep medicine, as we know it today, is based (Dement, 2005).

Once sleep began to be studied with more specific focus, there was a controversy as to whether sleep was a general brain state or a generated process that could be anatomically localized. Even through the 1800s, most researchers rejected the notion of a localized sleep center in the brain, believing that wakefulness was simply a condition maintained by ongoing sensory stimulation of the brain. But in 1929, Austrian neurologist Constantin Von Economo suggested that a site for the regulation of sleep existed, after noting that patients who were suffering from encephalitis lethargica (which caused somnolence or coma) all had lesions in the posterior hypothalamus and rostral midbrain, whereas those with profound insomnia had anterior hypothalamic injury (Triarhou, 2006; Von Economo, 1930). Subsequent work by others further supported the conclusion that different brain regions were involved in sleep regulation and helped identify involved structures and pathways.

Harvard psychiatrist and sleep investigator J. Allan Hobson stated (1989), "More has been learned about sleep in the past 60 years than in the preceding 6,000". Research in the area of neuroanatomy and neurochemistry is pushing ever outward the frontiers of our knowledge of brain pathways and neurotransmitters, and giving us a better understanding of this third of our lives, which has been shrouded in mystery for the vast majority of human history.

ARCHITECTURE AND STAGES

Normal sleep is broadly divided into two categories: non-REM sleep and REM sleep. Non-REM sleep is further divided into four stages: stage 1, stage 2, stage 3, and stage 4. An individual falling asleep passes through stages 1–4 and REM, and this cycle (termed *ultradian*) is repeated throughout the night, usually four or five times, each cycle lasting roughly 90 minutes (Figure 10.1). While the time spent in each stage may vary, this aspect of sleep appears to be conserved across mammalian species. It has been reported that alternating slow-wave and REM sleep patterns can be observed in all placental and marsupial mammals, with the notable exception being the Australian monotreme, the echidna (Winson, 1990).

Stage 1 is experienced as a superficial, light sleep that is transitional to deeper levels. It makes up only 5%–10% of the night's sleep in young adults. In this stage, voluntary muscle activity begins to decrease, and the eyes demonstrate a slow-rolling pattern of movement. If awakened from this transition stage, the sleeper often reports fragmented imagery and may deny that he was asleep, or might doze yet remain somewhat aware of his surroundings and be easily roused.

As the person enters stage 2 sleep, eye movements begin to taper off and brainwave patterns show marked slowing on electroencephalogram (EEG).

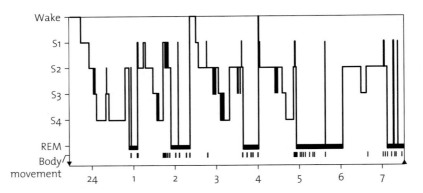

FIGURE 10.1. The progression of sleep stages across a single night in a normal young adult volunteer is illustrated in this sleep histogram. The text describes the "ideal" or "average" pattern. This histogram was drawn on the basis of a continuous overnight recording of electroencephalogram, electrooculogram, and electromyogram in a normal 19-year-old man. The record was assessed in 30-second epochs for the various sleep stages (S = Stage, REM = rapid eye movement). From Carskadon and Dement, (2005) © 2005 Elsevier, printed with permission.

Short, rapid bursts of electrical activity from the thalamus appear, presenting a pattern called "sleep spindles." These—along with occasional isolated slower waves called "K complexes"—are the characteristic markers of stage 2. In young adults, approximately 50% of the night is spent in stage 2.

Slower waves, called delta waves, eventually begin to appear. When these make up 20% or more of a 30 second segment (termed an "epoch") of a poly-somnographic recording. (termed an "epoch") stage 3 has been reached. Stage 4 is defined as over 50% of an epoch, consisting of delta waves. Stages 3 and 4 are referred to as "delta wave sleep," "slow wave sleep," or "deep sleep." [1] Slow wave sleep (SWS) is referred to as "deep" sleep, since the threshold for arousal from auditory stimuli is highest during this stage. It has also been thought of as the most refreshing and restorative sleep, although this is an area of controversy (Chokroverty, Thomas, & Bhatt, 2005; Neckelmann & Ursin, 1993).

Stage REM—characterized by rapid eye movements from which its name is derived, along with a general paralysis of all non-respiratory voluntary muscles—is entered next. Contrary to common expectation, this is not a deeper level of sleep; rather, the response to auditory stimuli is highly variable during this stage. The EEG actually shows faster waves, similar to stage 2, but without the spindles or K complexes characteristic to that stage. REM comprises approx-imately 20% of the night's sleep in young adults. Stage REM is a comparatively active period, as reflected by the rapid frequencies on the EEG. Additionally, the brain expends a considerable amount of metabolic energy during this stage (Siegel, 2005). REM sleep assumes two distinct patterns. During *tonic* REM, changes occur continuously over prolonged periods of time and are evident in the background during the entire sleep stage; examples include muscle ato-nia and desynchronized EEG. During *phasic* REM, changes are episodic and transient and are superimposed on tonic changes; they include isolated skeletal muscle twitches, bursts of rapid eye movements, and irregularities of respira-tion and heart rate, which are thought to be manifestations of ponto-geniculo-occipital (PGO) waves.

NEUROANATOMY

Wakefulness is a highly regulated process involving diverse brain structures and pathways. Von Economo's (1930) observations pointed him towards

---

[1] The American Academy of Sleep Medicine has recently recommended some changes in terminology. Beginning in January 2008, stage 3 and stage 4 sleep will be considered together and simply referred to as "slow wave sleep" or "delta wave sleep," although the terms "stage 3" and "stage 4" will still be used for research purposes (AASM 2007).

anterior hypothalamic neurons as sleep-promoting, and neurons near the hypothalamic-midbrain junction as wakefulness-promoting. Others focusing on this area demonstrated that stimulation of the reticular formation in the brainstem—a collection of neurons extending from the caudal medulla through the core of the mid-brain—changed EEG activity from sleep to wakefulness (Moruzzi & Magoun, 1949). Neurons from the reticular formation receive input from numerous sensory systems and forward excitatory impulses to the basal forebrain, thalamus, and hypothalamus (España & Scammell, 2004), and it is known that activation of the projection to the thalamus is needed for the thalamocortical activation responsible for producing high-frequency, low amplitude EEG signals indicative of wakefulness.

Multiple brain systems and pathways are also involved in the regulation of sleep. Acetylcholine, norepinephrine, histamine, serotonin, dopamine, and orexin/hypocretin all play a role. Details of structures and neurotransmitters involved in wakefulness and sleep can be seen in Figure 10.2 and Figure 10.3.

NEUROPHYSIOLOGY AND ENDOCRINE FUNCTION DURING SLEEP

Sleep is not limited to the brain; rather, a variety of peripheral physiological processes are coordinated by the neuroanatomical structures involved in sleep initiation and maintenance. Parasympathetic drive increases with the onset of sleep and peaks during NREM and tonic REM sleep; sympathetic drive dominates during phasic REM (Parmeggiani, 2005). Body temperature is maintained at a lower set point in NREM than in wakefulness, yet thermoregulation through shivering and sweating is absent during REM sleep, and body temperature approaches ambient temperature during REM. In general, respiratory and cardiovascular processes during NREM sleep are regular and monotonous. However, they are highly irregular during REM sleep. These irregularities are associated with an increased risk of cardiovascular events such as dysrhythmias and myocardial infarctions during REM sleep in vulnerable individuals (Table 10.1).

Slow wave sleep is associated with a peak in growth hormone secretion (Chokroverty et al., 2005), and the decrease in growth hormone production associated with middle and late life correlates with the normal age-associated decrease in SWS (Van Cauter, Leproult, & Plat, 2000). More recent work has shown that children who do not get enough sleep are more likely to be overweight (Lumeng et al., 2007). While this outcome may be influenced by factors such as increased consumption of food and decreased exercise secondary to tiredness and irritability, it is also possible that decreased sleep has an effect on appetite and metabolism, mediated through hormones such as leptin and insulin.

A

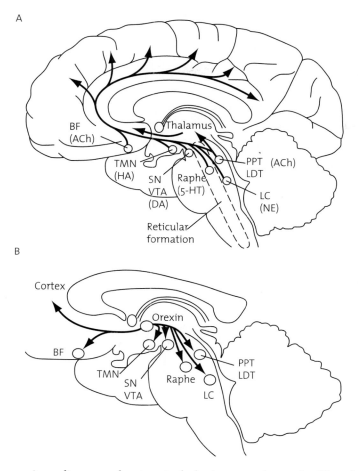

B

FIGURE 10.2. Ascending arousal systems in the brainstem and posterior. Hypothalamus sends projections throughout the forebrain. (A) Cholinergic neurons in the pedunculopontine and laterodorsal tegmental areas (PPT/LDT) activate many forebrain targets, including the thalamus. Neurons in the locus coeruleus (LC), dorsal and median raphe, tuberomammillary nucleus (TMN), substantia nigra and ventral tegmental area (SN/VTA), and basal forebrain (BF) excite many cortical and subcortical targets. The reticular formation projects to the thalamus, hypothalamus, and basal forebrain. (B) Orexin neurons in the lateral hypothalamic area innervate all of the ascending arousal systems, as well as the cerebral cortex. ACh refers to acetylcholine; HA, histamine; DA, dopamine; 5-HT, serotonin; NE, norepinephrine. From España, R. A., & Scammell, T. E. (2004). Sleep neurobiology for the clinician. *Sleep*, *27*(4), 811–820. ©Associated Professional Sleep Societies, LLC.

NREM sleep

REM sleep

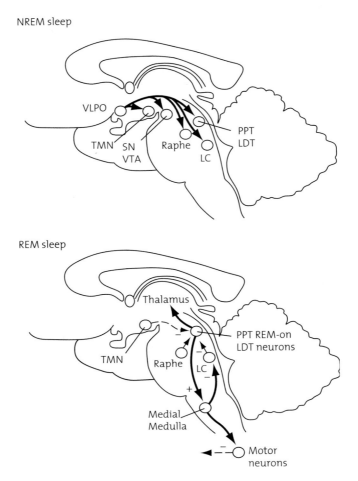

FIGURE 10.3. Non-rapid eye movement (NREM) and rapid eye movement (REM) sleep pathways. Neurons of the ventrolateral preoptic area (VLPO) produce γ-aminoybutyric acid (GABA) and galanin and inhibit all the arousal systems during NREM sleep. Many of these cells are active during REM sleep as well. REM sleep is driven by a distinct population of cholinergic pedunculopontine and laterodorsal tegmental areas (PPT/LDT) neurons. During wakefulness and NREM sleep, these cells are inhibited by norepinephrine, serotonin, and histamine, but during REM sleep, the aminergic neurons fall silent, thus disinhibiting the LDT/PPT REM-generating neurons. These cholinergic neurons also produce the atonia of REM sleep by activating the medial medulla, which inhibits motor neurons. The medial medulla also reduces excitatory signals from the locus coeruleus (LC), which normally increase motor tone. SN/VTA refers to the substantia nigra and ventral tegmental area; TMN, tuberomammillary nucleus. From España, R. A. & Scammell, T. E. (2004). Sleep neurobiology for the clinician. *Sleep, 27*(4), 811–820. ©Associated Professional Sleep Societies, LLC.

Table 10.1. Physiological Changes During Sleep.

Parameter	NREM	REM
Heart rate	Decreased	Irregular with increases and decreases
Blood pressure	Unchanged and stable	Irregular with increases and decreases
Respiratory rate	Decreased	Irregular in phasic REM
Ventilation	Decreased tidal volume and hypoxic response	Decreased tidal volume in phasic REM; decreased hypoxic response
Upper airway muscle tone	Decreased	Further decreased
Temperature	Preserved thermoregulation	Increased temperature and poikilothermia
Pupils	Constricted	Constricted in tonic REM; dilated in phasic REM
Gastrointestinal	Decreased acid secretion inhibition; prolonged acid clearance	Further prolonged acid clearance
Nocturnal penile tumescence and clitoral engorgement	Infrequent	Frequent

Source: Markov and Goldman (2007). © 2007 Elsevier. Printed with permission.

DREAMING

Dreams have intrigued man throughout the ages. Philosophers, priests, and poets have theorized regarding dreams and their meaning throughout history. The Greek physician Hippocrates (500–428 BCE) saw dreams as the mind's attending to internal needs, and Artemidorus of Ephesus in the first century AD compiled a list of 130 dreams symbols and their purported significance to the dreamer (Stone, 1997). In the Middle Ages, dreams were viewed with suspicion by the religious community, but after the writings of Albertus Magnus, teacher of Thomas Aquinas, dreaming came to be seen more as a matter of the body or the mind than of the spirit. Centuries later, Freud expressed his belief that dreams have meaning, that manifest dream content is produced by, and is an expression of, psychic conflict whose latent content is not readily available to the conscious mind while awake, and he popularized the idea that dreams serve as an instrument for the understanding of the unconscious mind and for implementing psychological change in therapeutic settings (Freud, 1900).

More recently some have proposed that dreams are formed by physiological brain activity and that they are, at least in their formation, devoid of psychic meaning, mere random firings of pontine neurons during sleep, ultimately given meaning by the dreamer as discharges reach higher cortical centers (Hobson & McCarley, 1977). Yet others have pointed to animal studies, which show that REM and dreaming reflect a pivotal aspect of the processing of memory, perhaps reflecting a basic mammalian memory process by which strategies for survival and current experience are evaluated (Winson, 1990). While dreaming can occur in non-REM sleep, dreams during REM appear to be more frequent, longer, more bizarre, more visual, more animated, and more emotional than their non-REM counterparts (Hobson, Pace-Schott, & Stickgold, 2000). Recent studies have suggested that dreaming acts to process the emotional content of a person's life events (Rothbaum & Mellman, 2001; Stickgold, 2002).

While there is a considerable body of knowledge in the field of dreaming, gaps in knowledge remain. There is no accepted understanding of the biological basis of dreaming, its physiology, or its mechanism or function. There is not even a consensus among researchers on definition, leading some to use the term "sleep mentation" (Stickgold, 2005).

ONTOGENY AND AGE-RELATED EFFECTS

Although sleep is a basic human need, sleep needs change with aging. During the first 2 years of life, more time is spent asleep than awake, leading many to conclude that sleep is an important aspect of early human development (Mindell & Owens, 2003). From age 2–5 years, a child spends about 50% of the time asleep, and this only drops to 40% by adolescence. Normal sleep length for a young adult is 7–8 hours per night (around 30%). This tends to decrease with age, with normal sleep after age 60 tapering down below 25%.

Paralleling changes in sleep quantity are changes in sleep quality (see Figure 10.4). In fact, age is the strongest and most consistent factor affecting the pattern of sleep stages across the night. Changes occur in the sleep cycle length: for example, in newborns the ultradian cycle has a period of just 50–60 minutes, as compared with 90 minutes in adults. The proportion of sleep stages also changes with age. Time spent in stage 1 sleep increases throughout adulthood, and stage 2 sleep increases from childhood until old age (Ohayon et al., 2004). While SWS is not present until age 2–6 months, the portion of the night devoted to SWS is at its highest point in young children, and thereafter decreases steadily throughout life, becoming almost nonexistent in old age (Markov & Goldman, 2006).

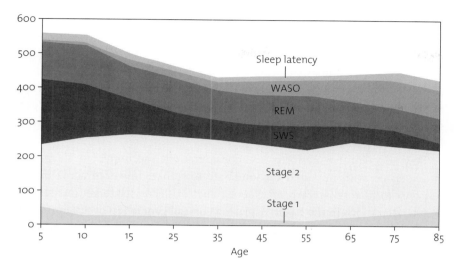

FIGURE 10.4. Changes in sleep with age. Time (in minutes) for sleep latency and wake time after sleep onset (WASO) and for rapid eye movement (REM) sleep and NREM sleep stages 1, 2, and slow wave sleep (SWS). Summary values are given for ages 5 to 85 years. From Carskadon & Dement (2005) © 2005 Elsevier, printed with permission.

REM sleep is quantitatively at its highest in the first year of life, but by age 3 it comprises only 20%–25% of the night, and remains at that level until decreasing further after age 60. After 60 years of age, sleep efficiency continues to steadily decrease, but all other sleep parameters remain relatively unchanged.

SLEEP NEEDS AND SLEEP DEPRIVATION

While quality and quantity of sleep may change throughout the lifecycle, what does not change is the need for sleep. A recent study revealed a mean sleep duration of 7.5 hours for men and 7.1 hours for women; mode durations were 8 hours (range 7.5–8.4 hours) and 7 hours (6.5–7.4), respectively (Tamakoshi & Ohno, 2004). Episodic and habitual restriction of sleep for social, vocational, or recreational reasons can lead to decreased cognitive performance (Belenky et al., 2003). Changes in daytime tests for alertness show changes with as little as 1.5 hours of reduction in baseline sleep times, and tests of vigilance and reaction time show significant impairment following the loss of as little as one night of sleep (Sheldon, Ferber, & Kryger, 2005). Cumulative effects of insufficient sleep are also noted, as chronic restriction of sleep to 6 hours per night for 14 consecutive nights produces deficits on tasks of cognitive performance roughly equivalent to complete sleep deprivation of 2 nights (Van Dongen,

Maislin, Mullington, & Dinges, 2003). Subjects of sleep deprivation begin to experience "micro sleeps"—brief periods of disorientation, misperception, and lapse in vigilance, sometimes only seconds long—which become more frequent as deprivation continues (Kales et al., 1970). Sufferers are often not aware of these lapses, despite the presence of obvious impairment. Following periods of prolonged sleep deprivation, EEG patterns consistent with stage 1 NREM sleep begin to predominate in subjects who are in fact behaviorally awake (Armington & Mitnick, 1959).

Beyond cognitive performance considerations, accumulated sleep debt is associated with impaired carbohydrate tolerance, impaired acute insulin response to glucose (an early marker of diabetes), decreased secretion of thyrotropin, alterations in the 24-hour plasma cortisol profile (Spiegel, Leproult, & Van Cauter, 1999), and compromise in immune response; sleep restriction to a period of 4 hours per night for 6 nights, or 1 night of complete sleep deprivation, were associated with reductions in immune response to vaccination when compared to no sleep restriction or deprivation conditions (Lange, Perras, Fehm, & Born, 2003; Spiegel, Sheridan, & Van Cauter, 2002).

EXCESSIVE SLEEPINESS

Sleepiness is defined as the tendency to fall asleep during the day, and excessive daytime sleepiness is the propensity to fall asleep at inappropriate times and under inappropriate conditions. Most individuals are familiar with the feeling of fatigue, a subjective state of anergy, tiredness, or exhaustion. Excessive sleepiness is to be distinguished from fatigue in that it is defined as the state of actually falling asleep. Interestingly, excessively sleepy individuals may fall asleep under dangerous situations yet not be aware of premonitory fatigue.

One of the most important contributors to daytime sleepiness is insufficient sleep. Average sleep durations have decreased from 9 hours per night in 1910 to 5–7 hours in more current times (Spiegel et al., 1999). This curtailment has been largely self-imposed to provide maximum time for work and recreation. Additionally, shift-work—a hallmark of modern society—has been increasing at a rate of about 3% per year since 1986, with recent reports indicating that 26% of men and 18% of women in the American workforce are engaged in some type of shift-work (Bliwise, 1996). Daytime sleepiness is also produced by factors that interfere with the quantity or quality of sleep, discussed more extensively below, such as pain, medical conditions, medication effects, and certain sleep disorders.

Daytime sleepiness is a public health concern. A national study reported that 60% of adult drivers—about 168 million people—say they have driven a vehicle while feeling drowsy in the past year, with more than one-third (37% or 103 million people) actually reporting falling asleep at the wheel. Approximately 11 million drivers admit to having had an accident or near accident because driving while drowsy (National Sleep Foundation, 2005). The National Highway Traffic Safety Administration's current statistics show that 100,000 police-reported crashes, 71,000 injuries, and 1,550 deaths occur each year in the United States due to accidents caused by drowsy drivers. Resultant monetary losses are estimated at $12.5 billion. Additionally, it is believed that these data significantly underestimate the extent of this problem due to the lack of data collection codes within many police crash report forms and the lack of specific training of police officers in this area (National Sleep Foundation, 2007). In data from European nations, all of whom have more consistent crash reporting procedures than the United States, drowsy driving is a factor in 10%–30% of all motor vehicle crashes.

REGULATION: HOMEOSTATIC AND CIRCADIAN PROCESSES

Sleep is regulated through the interplay of homeostatic and circadian processes, which run independently, yet in a complementary fashion (Edgar et al., 1993). Sleep deprivation leads to an increase in the duration and depth of subsequent sleep, reflecting a build-up of "sleep pressure" or homeostatic process. This also normally accumulates during periods of wakefulness and decreases during periods of compensatory sleep. The circadian process is a biological cycle approximately 24 hours in length (*circa*, "about;" *diem*, "a day") that regulates many bodily functions, such as hormone secretion, but most notably sleep. This clock is internally regulated, but maintained in its entrainment by external cues, most notably environmental light. The combined effects of Process S (homeostatic regulation) and Process C (circadian rhythm) are illustrated in Figure 10.5.

Biological Rhythms

The word "rhythm" refers to a regularly repeated event that has a waveform with a particular period length as measured from one peak to the next peak or from one trough to the next trough. Biological rhythms can have a wide variability in periodicity. As examples, some neurons can exhibit regular peaks of electrical activity every 100 milliseconds, whereas the fur return of a lynx occurs every 10 years (Stenseth et al., 1998). Circarhythms are classes of rhythms that are capable of free-running in constant conditions with periods approximating the environmental cycle to which they are normally synchronized. There are four major

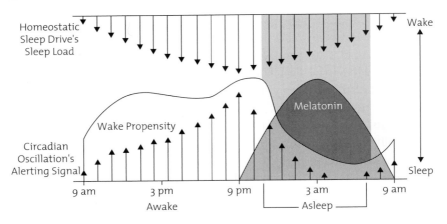

FIGURE 10.5. The two-process model of sleep regulation. From Richardson (2005) © 2005 Physicians Postgraduate Press.

classes of circarhythms. Circatidal rhythms are about one tidal cycle or approximately 12 hours long; circadian rhythms are about one day or approximately 24 hours long; circalunar rhythms are about one lunar cycle or approximately 28.5 days long; and circannual rhythms or seasonal rhythms are about 1 year or 365 days long (Aschoff, 1981; CIE, 2004; USCOTA, 1991). While all are of importance, circadian rhythms are most important to human sleep physiology.

The human environment is highly rhythmic, with predictable changes in surrounding conditions occurring on a daily (day/night) basis. To adapt to the periodically changing environment, humans, like most vertebrate species, have evolved internal circadian clocks that drive rhythms in physiology and behavior in order to anticipate daily environmental time cues. These endogenous clocks coordinate physiological and behavioral events externally with the environmental cycle, as well as internally, with each other. This synchronization both increases the chances of survival and ensures metabolic, physiologic, and behavioral efficiency in terms of varying needs of the body over the 24-hour day.

The endogenous human circadian clock, or pacemaker, does not run at exactly 24 hours (Czeisler et al., 1999). Thus, for the circadian pacemaker to appropriately time physiology and behavior with the outside world, environmental time cues must be able to reset this internal clock. Cycles of 24-hour environmental light and darkness provide the principle time cues to reset or phase-shift circadian rhythms (Czeisler & Wright, 1999). Thus, environmental light synchronizes, or entrains, the circadian system and consequently human physiology and behavior. Not all light stimuli are effective in entraining or resetting the phase of the circadian system. Specific characteristics of light, including its quantity, spectrum, duration, and timing, can influence the capacity of light to elicit a phase shift response or support entrainment. Other time cues, such as exercise, food intake, social interactions, and sleep may also affect the pacemaker to some extent in humans (Barger, Wright, Hughes, & Czeisler, 2004; Buxton, Lee, L'Hermite-Baleriaux, Turek, & Van Cauter, 2003; Danilenko, Cajochen, & Wirz-Justice, 2003; Klerman et al., 1998; Krauchi, Cajochen, Werth, & Wirz-Justice, 2002). Those nonphotic cues, however, are generally much weaker stimuli for maintaining circadian entrainment or evoking a circadian phase-shift.

LIGHT REGULATION OF CIRCADIAN AND NEUROBEHAVIORAL SYSTEMS

It is well known that environmental light stimulates the human retina and supports the sensory capacity of vision. In addition, nonvisual information about light is detected by the eyes and transmitted by the retinohypothalamic tract (RHT), a neural pathway which projects to the suprachiasmatic nuclei (SCN) in the hypothalamus (Aschoff, 1981; CIE, 2004; Gooley, Lu, Fischer, & Saper, 2003; Klein, Moore, & Reppert, 1991; Morin, 1994). The SCN serve as the primary central circadian oscillators in the human brain that regulate daily rhythms, such as the sleep/wake cycle, circadian secretory patterns of hormones, and body temperature rhythms. As illustrated in Figure 10.6, the RHT provides information about environmental light to a variety of nonvisual regions of the central nervous system for regulation of diverse circadian, neuroendocrine, and neurobehavioral responses (Brainard & Provencio, 2006; Gooley et al., 2003; Klein et al., 1991; Morin, 1994).

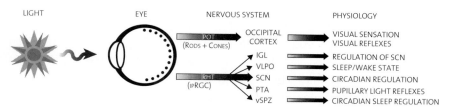

FIGURE 10.6. This illustration provides a simplified schematic of the neuroanatomy responsible for mediating both the sensory capacity of the visual system and the nonvisual regulation of circadian, neuroendocrine and neurobehavioral functions (Gooley et al., 2003). Abbreviations: POT — primary optic tract; RHT — retinohypothalamic tract; ipRGC — intrinsically photosensitive retinal ganglion cells; IGL — intergeniculate leaflets; VLPO — ventrolateral preoptic nuclei; SCN — suprachiasmatic nuclei; PTA — pretectal areas; vSPZ — ventral subparaventricular zones. This figure and legend were modified from an earlier publication. From Brainard & Provencio (2006).

Although the RHT is anatomically distinct from the visual system, there is a functional connection between the primary visual pathway and the circadian neuroanatomy by way of a projection from the intergeniculate leaflet to the SCN (Gooley et al., 2003; Klein et al., 1991; Morin, 1994). The most investigated circadian pathway extends from the SCN in the hypothalamus to the pineal gland, with sequential synaptic connections in the paraventricular hypothalamus, the upper thoracic intermediolateral cell column, and the superior cervical ganglion (Klein et al., 1991; Morin, 1994). By way of this pathway, the ambient light-dark cycle entrains the circadian synthesis and secretion of pineal melatonin, with high levels of melatonin secreted during the night and low levels secreted during the day (Arendt, 1998; Reiter, 1991). In addition to entraining melatonin circadian rhythms, light at night can elicit an acute suppression of the high nocturnal levels of this hormone. This light-induced suppression of melatonin has been consistently observed in humans as well as diverse other species, and has been used as a tool in many studies to examine the ocular, neural, and biochemical physiology of melatonin regulation and circadian rhythms (Brainard, Rollag, & Hanifin, 1997; Klein et al., 1991; Lewy, Wehr, Goodwin, Newsome, & Markey, 1980).

PHOTORECEPTION FOR CIRCADIAN AND NEUROBEHAVIORAL REGULATION

Recently, there has been an upheaval in the understanding of photoreceptive input to the circadian, neuroendocrine, and neurobehavioral systems of humans and other mammalian species. Multiple lines of evidence show that a novel photoreceptor is primarily responsible for transduction of photic stimuli for this physiology. Animal studies supporting involvement of a novel photoreceptor include circadian phase-shifting and melatonin suppression by light in rodless-coneless transgenic mice (Freedman et al., 1999; Lucas, Freedman, Munoz, Garcia-Fernandez, & Foster, 1999). This was quite surprising, given that tests demonstrated that these animals were completely visually blind. At the time, rods and cones were the only known ocular photoreceptors, leading to the paradox of photoreception occurring in an eye without photoreceptors. Similar to the findings in rodents, circadian entrainment and melatonin suppression studies in completely blind humans, partially blind humans, and humans with color vision deficiencies also suggested that a novel non-rod, non-cone photoreceptor was primarily responsible for circadian regulation in humans (Czeisler et al., 1995; Klerman et al., 2002; Lockley et al., 1997; Ruberg et al., 1996; Zaidi et al., 2007).

Separate from studies on blind animals and humans, a study on healthy, sighted men and women confirmed that the three-cone system that mediates human photopic vision is not the primary photoreceptor system that transduces light stimuli for nocturnal melatonin suppression (Brainard et al., 2001b). That discovery was rapidly followed by two separate wavelength studies in healthy human subjects that identified the blue portion of the visible spectrum as the most potent wavelength region for melatonin suppression (Brainard et al., 2001a; Thapan, Arendt, & Skene, 2001). Those wavelength data provided strong evidence that a novel photosensory system, distinct from the classical visual rods and cones, is primarily responsible for regulating melatonin in humans. Since then, ten published studies in rodents, monkeys, and humans have shown various biological and behavioral responses to light have a peak sensitivity to blue light between 446 nm and 484 nm (for review: Brainard & Hanifin, 2005; Gamlin et al., 2007; Ziadi et al., 2007).

Studies using both animal and human models are elucidating the neuroanatomy and neurophysiology of the human circadian photosensory system. In 1998, a new opsin-based photopigment, named melanopsin, was identified and has been localized both in the retinas of rodents and humans (Provencio, Jiang, De Grip, Hayes, & Rollag, 1998; Provencio, Rodriguez, Jiang, Hayes, Moreira, & Rollag, 2000). More specifically, melanopsin is found in a subtype of intrinsically photoreceptive retinal ganglion cells (ipRGCs) (Berson, Dunn, & Takao, 2002; Gooley, Lu, Chou, Scammell, & Saper, 2001; Hattar, Liao, Takao, Berson, & Yau, 2002). These unique ipRGCs comprise a 1%–3% subset of all retinal ganglion cells, are evenly distributed across the retina, and have an expansive dendritic net that is filled with the melanopsin photopigment (Gooley et al., 2003; Hannibal, Hindersson, Knudsen, Georg, & Fahrenkrug, 2002; Hattar et al., 2002; Provencio, Rollag, & Castrucci, 2002). As illustrated in Figure 10.6, these unique photosensory cells project to the SCN for circadian regulation, as well as to the ventral lateral preoptic nuclei (VLPO) that are involved in sleep/wake state, and the ventral subparaventricular zones (svPVZf) that are involved in circadian regulation of sleep and locomotor activity (Gooley et al., 2003; Hannibal et al., 2002; Hattar et al., 2002; Provencio et al., 2002). Three studies have provided compelling evidence that melanopsin mediates ipRGC light sensitivity. Specifically, when cells not sensitive to light—such as mouse neurons, frog oocytes, or human kidney cells—are transfected with the human melanopsin gene, they become directly photosensitive (Melyan, Tarttelin, Bellingham, Lucas, & Hankins, 2005; Panda et al., 2005; Qiu et al., 2005).

Despite abundant evidence that the melanopsin-containing ipRGCs provide primary input for circadian, neuroendocrine, and neurobehavioral phototransduction, the classical rod and cone photoreceptors still play a role in this physiology. Both animal and human studies show that the visual rods and cones normally provide input for these biological and behavioral responses

(Aggelopoulos & Meissl, 2000; Dkhissi-Benyahya, Gronfier, De Vanssay, Flamant, & Cooper, 2007; Figueiro, Bullough, Parsons, & Rea, 2004; Hattar et al., 2003; Jasser, Hanifin, Rollag, & Brainard, 2006; Panda et al., 2003; Smith, Schoen, & Czeisler, 2004). The exact role and degree of this input from rods and cones is currently under investigation. The seminal discoveries of melanopsin and the ipRGCs have been crowning achievements in modern neuroscience, and open the door to a better understanding of how circadian regulation by light and darkness influence normal human sleep.

Sleep Disorders and Their Treatments

In their 2005 poll of Sleep in America, the National Sleep Foundation notes an upward trend in the prevalence of sleep problems—defined as having difficulty falling asleep, waking a lot during the night, waking up too early and not being able to get back to sleep, waking up feeling unrefreshed, snoring, unpleasant feelings in the legs, and/or experiencing pauses in breathing—since 1999 (National Sleep Foundation, 2005). The two main symptoms of sleep disorders are insomnia and excessive daytime somnolence (EDS).

INSOMNIA AND RELATED DISORDERS

Insomnia—defined as difficulty initiating and/or maintaining sleep (American Academy of Sleep Medicine, 2005)—is the most frequent sleep-related complaint in adults. In the National Sleep Foundation's 2005 survey of Sleep in America, which polled 1,506 adults, over half of all respondents (54%) reported experiencing "at least one symptom of insomnia at least a few nights a week over the past year," with one-third (33%) reporting "at least one symptom every night or almost every night" (National Sleep Foundation, 2005). Insomnia is associated with daytime fatigue, mood disturbances, difficulties with concentration, and memory impairment. Studies have also shown that patients with insomnia make significantly more medical and psychiatric visits than those without such complaint, placing a greater burden on the health care system and employers (Edinger & Means, 2005).

Insomnia can be a primary sleep disorder, or a symptom and disorder that is secondary to (or comorbid with) other medical conditions (Sheldon et al., 2005). A primary sleep disorder that can be associated with insomnia is periodic limb movement disorder (PLMD)—a condition in which repetitive muscle twitching occurs in the limbs during sleep. Patients are not typically aware of these movements, but report daytime somnolence, an inability to maintain sleep, or both. Closely related in etiology is restless legs syndrome (RLS), which is characterized by an irresistible urge to move the lower and/or upper extremities, with unusual feelings in the limbs that occur mostly at rest and at bedtime, and which are temporarily relieved by voluntary activity. A significant percentage of patients with RLS also have PLMD (Montplaisir, Allen, Walters, & Ferini-Strambi, 2005), yet only a minority of patients with PLMD have RLS. Many psychiatric disorders—notably major depression, bipolar disorder, schizophrenia, post-traumatic stress disorder—have sleep disturbance clearly identified as a major component of the symptomology. Sleep disturbances are also commonly present in cases of substance use and abuse. Alcohol, for example, is probably the most frequently used sleeping aid in the general population, and while taking a "night cap" before bed is indisputably soporific, the metabolic consequences of alcohol consumption lead to shallow, disrupted sleep with an overall net result of decreased quality and quantity of sleep (Gillin, Drummond, Clark, & Moore, 2005). Sleep disturbance can be a common side effect of many medications, even when appropriately used. Table 10.2 lists conditions associated with insomnia.

Table 10.2. Conditions Associated with Insomnia and Excessive Daytime Somnolence.

Disorder	Insomnia	Excessive Daytime Somnolence
Primary insomnia	*	
Inadequate sleep hygiene	*	*
Medical and psychiatric sleep disorders	*	*
Insufficient sleep		*
Drug-dependent and drug-induced sleep disorders	*	*
Obstructive sleep apnea syndrome		*
Central sleep apnea syndrome	*	
Circadian rhythm sleep disorders	*	*
Narcolepsy		*
Periodic limb movement disorder	*	*
Restless legs syndrome	*	

* Present.

Source: Excerpted from International Classification of Sleep Disorders (2005).

THE MANAGEMENT OF INSOMNIA

Prior to resorting to symptomatic management, underlying causes of insomnia should be uncovered and managed. If treatment of insomnia itself is desired, a number of pharmacological, psychotherapeutic, and behavioral approaches are available (NIH, 2005).

Nonpharmacological Treatments

Nonpharmacological treatments for insomnia are listed in Tables 10.3 and 10.4 (Bootzin & Perlis, 1992). These methods can be used individually or in combination, and usually include sleep hygiene education as one of the components. Meta-analyses indicate that nonpharmacological therapies for chronic insomnia have clinically significant benefit in typical measures of hypnotic efficacy, including (in order of decreasing effect size) sleep latency, wake after sleep onset, and total sleep time (Morin, Culbert, & Schwartz, 1994). The magnitude of their effect is on par with traditional hypnotic medications; however, they have greater durability of benefit, shown to have sustained durability over the course of 2 years following the termination of treatment (Morin, Colecchi, Stone, Sood, Brink, 1999).

Table 10.3. Nonpharmacological Treatments for Insomnia.

Techniques	Method
Stimulus control therapy	If unable to fall asleep within 20 minutes, get out of bed and repeat as necessary
Relaxation therapies	Biofeedback, progressive muscle relaxation
Restriction of time in bed (sleep restriction)	Decrease time in bed to equal time actually asleep and increase as sleep efficiency improves
Cognitive therapy	Talk therapy to dispel unrealistic and exaggerated notions about sleep
Paradoxic intention	Try to stay awake
Sleep hygiene education	Promote habits that help sleep; eliminate habits that interfere with sleep
Cognitive-behavioral therapy	Combines sleep restriction, stimulus control, and sleep hygiene education with cognitive therapy

Table 10.4. Sleep Hygiene Measures.

The Do's of Sleep Hygiene	• Increase exposure to bright light during the day
	• Establish a daily activity routine
	• Exercise regularly in the morning and/or afternoon
	• Set aside a worry time
	• Establish a comfortable sleep environment
	• Do something relaxing prior to bedtime
	• Try a warm bath
The Don't's of Sleep Hygiene (Things to Avoid)	• Alcohol
	• Caffeine, nicotine, and other stimulants
	• Exposure to bright light during the night
	• Exercise within 3 hours of bedtime
	• Heavy meals or drinking within 3 hours of bedtime
	• Using your bed for things other than sleep (or sexual activity)
	• Napping (unless a shift-worker)
	• Watching the clock
	• Trying to sleep
	• Noise
	• Excessive heat/cold in room

Nonpharmacological treatments have not been associated with adverse effects. Their limitations include delayed onset of clinical effects; the need for ample time per session and multiple sessions for their implementation, which limits their applicability in primary care settings; cost; and the paucity of trained practitioners.

Complementary and Alternative Medicines

Complementary and alternative medicines (CAM), including melatonin, valerian, kava-kava, chamomilla, passiflora, avena sativa, and humulus lupulus, have widespread appeal, owing to a variety of factors, including their ready availability; relatively low cost compared to traditional medications; the popular belief that they are free of side effects; the perception that their "natural" status imparts them with greater biological and psychological harmony; and the notion that they have a low abuse risk. However, concerns have been raised regarding their lack of regulation by the U.S. Food and Drug Administration; inadequacy of studies evaluating their efficacy; lack of clarity regarding optimal dosing and safety, particularly when combined with other substances; and questions regarding purity and co-mingling of preparations with other active ingredients.

A recent review of 33 randomized controlled trials of various CAM treatments (e.g., acupuncture/pressure, light therapy, relaxation therapy, vitamins, Tai Chi, traditional Chinese medicine) noted that 67% of these studies yielded "positive results" in addressing a constellation of symptoms, including late-life depression, anxiety, and sleep disturbance. However, a "positive" finding was defined as a statistically significant difference between the active treatment and control groups, and the study did not evaluate efficacy results on the basis of clinical significance. Additionally, specific treatments and sleep-related findings were not separately evaluated, and the study did not examine the data in a meta-analytic fashion (Meeks, Wetherell, Irwin, Redwine, & Jeste, 2007). Adverse effects were also not systematically explored.

Melatonin is the most commonly utilized CAM for insomnia. The basic mechanism by which melatonin induces sleepiness in humans is unclear, although three main hypotheses have been proposed: the mechanism may involve a phase-shift of the endogenous circadian pacemaker, a reduction in core body temperature, and/or a direct action on somnogenic structures of the brain (Buscemi et al., 2005). A recent meta-analysis of 14 randomized, controlled trials encompassing 279 participants utilizing melatonin in the treatment of primary sleep disorders indicated that melatonin reduced sleep onset latency by 11.7 minutes (95% CI: −18.2, −5.2) with substantial heterogeneity among studies, and the effect was deemed to be "clinically unimportant." Additional measures, which are typically utilized to assess hypnotic efficacy, such as wakefulness after sleep onset and total sleep time, did not differ between melatonin and placebo groups. It was noteworthy, however, that melatonin's reduction in sleep latency was more prominent, and clinically relevant, in individuals with delayed sleep phase syndrome (−38.8 minutes; 95% CI: −50.3, −27.3; $n = 2$) compared to people with primary insomnia (−7.2 minutes; 95% CI: −12.0, −2.4; $n = 12$), suggesting that the effects of melatonin are mediated by a direct resetting of the endogenous circadian pacemaker, rather than via a direct action on somnogenic structures of the brain. Other studies seem to verify that short-term use of melatonin is not effective in treating most primary sleep disorders (Brzezinski et al., 2005; Meeks et al., 2007). A meta-analysis of 10 studies encompassing 222 participants, which have systematically assessed the safety of melatonin (Buscemi et al., 2005) when utilized over the course of 3 months or less, indicated that melatonin has few adverse events. The most common ones were headaches, dizziness, nausea, and drowsiness; yet the frequency of these events did not differ between melatonin and placebo. Clearly, further research is required to determine the safety and efficacy of melatonin in both short-term and long-term use.

Valerian extracts of the root of *Valeriana officinalis* have long been advocated and used for promoting sleep. A recent study indicated that valerian and valerenic acid may be selective agonists of the dopamine 5-HT$_{5a}$ receptor (Dietz, Mahady, Pauli, & Farnsworth, 2005), although possible sleep-promoting mechanisms are not clear. Valerian products often contain other agents, such as hops and diphenhydramine (Morin, Koetter, Bastien, Ware, & Wooten, 2005). Typical dosages are 400 to 450 mg *Valerian officinalis* root prior to bedtime. A recent review of nine randomized, controlled trials noted that the data on valerian monotherapy were inconclusive due to their contradictory nature and great inconsistency between trials in terms of patients, experimental design, procedures, and methodological quality (Stevinson & Ernst, 2000). Systematically derived data on the side effects of valerian are not available.

L-tryptophan is an endogenous amino acid. Evidence for its efficacy and safety in insomnia is limited and based on studies with small numbers of subjects (National Institutes of Health, 2005). Furthermore, there are concerns about its possible toxic effects, specifically eosinophila-myalgia syndrome. Many etiologic agents alone or in combination with L-tryptophan and various impurities, may be responsible for the tissue pathologic response resulting in the clinical syndrome of eosinophilia, myalgias, and fasciitis (Sternberg, 1996).

Kava-kava is a product of the root of *Piper methysticum*. Its use in insomnia has not been systematically explored. There are also recent reports of serious hepatotoxicity with it, resulting in its being banned in many countries and the issuance of a Consumer Advisory by the FDA (Center for Food Safety and Applied Nutrition, U.S. Food and Drug Administration, 2002).

Over-the-Counter Agents

Twenty-three percent of all insomniacs utilize over-the-counter medications for sleep, and 40% utilize these in combination with alcohol (Ancoli-Israel & Roth, 1999). These are comprised primarily of sedating antihistamines, primarily the H$_1$ receptor antagonists diphenhydramine and doxylamine. The former agent is well absorbed and widely distributed throughout the body, including the central nervous system. The peak serum concentration is about 8 hours and the elimination half-life is approximately 8 hours, making those who take it vulnerable to daytime effects. There is only scant evidence for this agent in the management of insomnia (Rickels et al., 1983), and it is associated with the rapid development of tolerance (Richardson et al., 2002). Its risks include residual daytime sedation, diminished cognitive function, and delirium, particularly in the elderly (Agostini et al., 2001). Other adverse effects include dry mouth, blurred vision, urinary retention, constipation, and risk of increased intraocular pressure in individuals with narrow angle glaucoma.

Sedating Antidepressants

Agents in this class are utilized as hypnotics but not indicated for this use by the Food and Drug Administration (FDA). Nevertheless, they are extensively utilized for insomnia, owing to their low abuse liability, availability of large dose ranges, and low cost. Although these agents may have been studied for their effects on sleep in other conditions complicated by insomnia, only information relative to primary insomnia will be reviewed here.

The use of these agents for insomnia is a common practice despite the fact that this practice has received little scientific evaluation. In 2002, the most commonly prescribed agent for insomnia was the sedating antidepressant trazodone. Sedating antidepressants are typically utilized at doses that are considered to be subtherapeutic for the treatment of depression or anxiety disorders. Trazodone is a heterocyclic antidepressant that has an elimination half-life of 5 to 12 hours (James & Mendelson, 2004). A recent 14-day controlled evaluation of trazodone—50 mg, zolpidem—10 mg, and placebo in primary insomniacs (Walsh et al., 1998) suggested that, during the first week, both active drugs reduced subjective sleep latency, although trazodone was significantly less effective than zolpidem. Neither medication affected total sleep time. By the second week, trazodone's effects were no different than placebo. Trazodone has also shown benefit, at low doses, for subjective sleep variables in post-traumatic stress disorder and major depression. There are virtually no dose–response data for trazodone in insomnia. Concerns have been raised regarding the high rates of daytime residual sedation, significant dropout rates, induction of arrhythmias (especially QT prolongation and polymorphous ventricular tachycardia when given with amiodarone), primarily in patients with histories of cardiac disease, and priapism, which has an estimated rate of 1 in 6,000 (James & Mendelson, 2004).

Doxepin, a tricyclic antidepressant, was examined for 4 weeks in a controlled study at dosages of 25 mg and 50 mg, and demonstrated an improvement in total sleep time but not in sleep latency (Hajak et al., 2001). Withdrawal insomnia was evident following abrupt discontinuation. As in other antidepressant agents, the use of doxepin can be complicated by daytime sedation and cognitive impairment, anticholinergic effects, weight gain, and drug–drug interactions. The tricyclic antidepressants are also potentially fatal in an overdose. A recent NIH state-of-the-science conference concluded that "evidence supports the efficacy of cognitive-behavioral therapy and benzodiazepine receptor agonists in the treatment of this disorder. Very little evidence supports the efficacy of other treatments, despite their widespread use" (National Institutes of Health, 2005).

Hypnotic Agents

Most of the prescribed hypnotic agents approved by the FDA are benzodiazepine receptor agonists (BzRAs), with the exception of ramelteon, which is a melatonin receptor agonist. All agents in the former class bind to benzodiazepine recognition site of the γ-aminobutyric acid type A (GABA-A) receptor complex and augment the effects of GABA, an inhibitory neurotransmitter in the central nervous system that mediates various clinical effects, including anxiety, cognition, vigilance, memory, and learning, among others (Sieghart & Sperk, 2002). Melatonin receptor agonists act at the MT_1 and MT_2 receptors of the suprachiasmatic nucleus. In so doing, they are thought to mute the wakefulness force of the SCN, thus allowing the homeostatic factor to dominate, resulting in sleep (Johnson, Suess, & Griffiths, 2006) (see Figure 10.5).

The hypnotic agents that are most commonly utilized are listed in Table 10.5 (Thomson Micromedex, 2008). The first group of BzRAs represents agents that have a benzodiazepine molecular structure. The second group represents agents that are nonbenzodiazepines in structure, and are also selective BzRAs. Melatonin receptor agonists are limited to ramelteon. The efficacy of these agents has been well established in studies utilizing both subjective and objective measures of sleep. As a group, they diminish sleep latency (time to fall asleep), wake after sleep onset (WASO, total time spent awake after falling asleep, a measure of sleep continuity), and increase total sleep time (TST). Within the overall group, however, specific agents may differ in their efficacy profile (Doghramji & Doghramji, 2006). For example, only zolpidem ER and eszopiclone have been shown to diminish WASO and thus to have particular utility in cases of sleep discontinuity. All agents diminish sleep latency. The only two agents with relatively long-term controlled studies (6 months) demonstrating continued efficacy are zolpidem ER and eszopiclone.

Adverse effects of the BzRAs include daytime sedation and psychomotor and cognitive impairment. These, as well as the risk of tolerance and rebound, can be

Table 10.5. Hypnotic Agents.

Medication	Dosage Range (mg)	Onset of Action	Half-life (h)	Schedule IV
BzRAs: Benzodiazepines				
Estazolam	0.5–2	Rapid	10–24	Yes
Flurazepam	15–30	Rapid	47–100	Yes
Quazepam	7.5–15	Rapid	39–100	Yes
Temazepam	7.5–15	Slow-Intermediate	9.5–12.4	Yes
Triazolam	0.25–0.50	Rapid	1.5–5.5	Yes
BzRAs: Non-Benzodiazepines				
Zolpidem	5–10	Rapid	2.5	Yes
Zolpidem ER	6.25–12.5	Rapid	2.8	Yes
Zaleplon	5–20	Rapid	1	Yes
Eszopiclone	1–3	Rapid	6	Yes
Melatonin Receptor Agonists				
Ramelteon	8	Rapid	1–5	No

minimized by utilizing the lowest effective dosage and shortest half-life agents. They also carry the small risk of respiratory depression in chronic obstructive pulmonary disease and obstructive sleep apnea syndrome and the potential for abuse liability in vulnerable populations. Adverse events of the melatonin receptor agonist ramelteon include headache, somnolence, fatigue, and dizziness. It is not recommended for use with fluvoxamine due to a CYP 1A2 interaction. A mild elevation in prolactin levels to within the normal range has been noted in a small number of females, and testosterone elevation has been noted in elderly males, yet the clinical relevance of these changes remains unclear. Possibly owing to its lack of activity at the GABA receptor, ramelteon does not demonstrate respiratory depression with mild to moderate COPD and obstructive sleep apnea syndrome. It does not carry the risk of abuse liability and is DEA unscheduled.

EXCESSIVE DAYTIME SOMNOLENCE AND RELATED DISORDERS

Conditions associated with excessive daytime somnolence (EDS) are listed in Table 10.2. EDS can be secondary to a number of sleep-specific causes, which include insufficient sleep, disorders of circadian rhythm, obstructive sleep apnea syndrome, narcolepsy, idiopathic hypersomnia, and periodic limb movement disorder. A detailed description of each of these disorders is beyond the scope of this chapter. In the general population this is most often caused by insufficient sleep, but medical or psychiatric illnesses, as well as medication side effects, are also common causes (Leibowitz, Brooks, & Black, 2006).

CIRCADIAN RHYTHM SLEEP DISORDERS

These disorders feature a disturbance in the coordination between the timing of internal circadian sleep/wake cycle and the environmental light–dark cycle. In all of the disorders discussed below, core symptoms include insomnia, excessive daytime somnolence, or both (American Academy of Sleep Medicine, 2005).

Jet Lag Syndrome

This is caused by rapid travel across two or more time zones. While the body readjusts its biological clock to a new time zone, many people experience symptoms whose severity is related to the direction of travel (eastward) and number of time zones crossed (more than two). These include insomnia, daytime sleepiness, gastrointestinal distress, irritability, mild depression, and confusion (Boulos et al., 1995; CIE, 2006; Lam, 1996; Wetterberg, 1993). Symptoms are thought to arise from the resulting mismatch between the sleep/wake schedules of the new environment and endogenous rhythms, and the consequent resulting desynchronization between internal body rhythms with respect to one another. Travel-specific factors can also be involved, such as discomfort on the aircraft, poor diet, use of caffeinated and alcoholic beverages, all of which result in curtailed sleep length and poor sleep quality.

The average period of readjustment may range from 3 to 12 days, depending on the direction of travel and the number of time zones that have been spanned (Boulos et al., 1995). Jet lag countermeasures include adherence to proper sleep hygiene measures. Maximizing exposure to daylight at the new locale can hasten the synchronization of circadian rhythms to the environmental light-dark cycle and to one another. Individuals should also be urged to shift their sleep/wake schedules gradually in the direction of the destination time zone prior to travel. If these methods are not effective or only minimally effective, treatment can be augmented with short-acting hypnotics and with stimulants for a brief period following arrival in the new locale.

While the benefit of light in alleviating jet lag seems likely, the best way to use light for minimizing symptoms is being evaluated. If timed properly, bright light should accelerate re-entrainment of the circadian rhythm. For example, a controlled field study tested light treatment of jet lag following a westward flight across six time zones (Zurich to New York). The data showed that a 3-hour exposure to a bright white light of 3,000 lux from a head-mounted visor during the first two evenings at the New York destination accelerated circadian re-entrainment (Boulos et al., 2002). Further studies, however, are still needed in order to determine how to best use light for this malady.

Shift Work Sleep Disorder

Shift work entails a job that involves any type of nonstandard schedule and may include night or evening work, rotating shifts with constantly changing hours, split shifts, and extended duty (usually over 12 hours). Most problematic is variable shift work, in which shifts are rotated or changed frequently; sleep times typically must be changed accordingly. The severity of symptoms is proportional to the frequency with which shifts are changed, the magnitude of each change, and the frequency of counterclockwise (phase-advancing) changes. However, even fixed shift workers who must sleep during the day experience difficulties, since daytime noise and light can interfere with the quality of their sleep and since they often change their sleep times for social or family events.

An estimated 20% of workers in industrialized nations are employed in some form of shift work (Eastman, Boulos, Terman, Campbell, Dijk, & Lewy, 1995; Moore-Ede, 1993; USCOTA, 1991). Selected industries, such as military, police, health care, and telecommunications, require 24-hours a day, 7 days a week of constant operation. Further, many companies have strong economic incentives for incorporating shift work into their schedule and progressing towards continuous operation.

Core symptoms of shift work sleep disorder are insomnia and daytime somnolence. Shift workers also have a higher incidence of cardiovascular disease and gastrointestinal distress, as well as cognitive and psychological problems (Eastman et al., 1995; Metlaine, Leger, & Choudat, 2005; Moore-Ede, 1993; USCOTA, 1991). Many researchers hypothesize that these ailments are caused, in part, by difficulty adjusting to a night shift or rotating schedules. Shift work also affects perception of sleepiness, thereby causing misperception of sleep needs. Research has shown that despite subjective reports of adequate sleep, shift workers sleep 5–7 hours less per week than their nonshift working counterparts (Leibowitz et al., 2006). In addition, there is a potential link to breast and colon cancer in women who are exposed to light at night, as is often the case with shift workers (Blask et al., 2005; Davis, Mirick, & Stevens, 2001; Schernhammer et al., 2001, 2003; Stevens, 1987; Stevens et al., 2007). Disruption of the diurnal rhythm of sleep and wakefulness, by both shorter sleep times and by doing shift work, is emerging as a potential contributor to obesity, diabetes, and hypertension (Pickering, 2006). In addition, recent work has shown night-shift work to be related to cancer risk (Straif et al., 2007), and the International Agency for Research on Cancer (the cancer arm of the World Health Organization), now lists overnight shift work as a "probable carcinogen," with the American Cancer Society expected to follow at the time of this writing. Shift work can also lead to problems of increased accidents and decreased productivity. The elderly are more profoundly affected by rapidly changing shifts.

Shift workers should be advised to maximize their exposure to sunlight at times when they should be awake and to ensure that the bedroom is as dark and quiet as possible when they are asleep, which is often during the day. A number of studies have shown that properly timed exposure to light and darkness may enhance workers' circadian systems to adapt to shift schedules (Czeisler et al., 1990; Dawson & Campbell, 1991; Dumont & Beaulieu, 2006; Lam, 1996; Minors, Waterhouse, & Wirz-Justice, 1991; Moore-Ede, 1993; Wetterberg, 1993). The use of light treatment and scheduled exposure to darkness for shift work problems, however, is complex and requires further investigation. If symptoms are not responsive to conventional countermeasures, it may be necessary to devise more rational shift schedules.

Studies have shown that rotating shift work is associated with higher rates of depression, divorce, and substance abuse. Additionally, such work increased cardiovascular risk more than smoking one pack of cigarettes per day (Whitehead, Thomas, & Slapper, 1992).

Delayed Sleep Phase Syndrome

Sufferers fall asleep later than normal nighttime bedtime hours, regardless of how early they go to bed, and awaken later than desired, often extending their bedtimes well into the afternoon. These are usually young adults who present for treatment because of diminished school performance resulting from daytime sleepiness or missed morning classes. Prior history reveals a tendency for individuals to be "night owls." They can be distinguished from people who stay up late by choice because of social or occupational needs in that they cannot fall asleep earlier even if they were to try.

Attempts to advance the sleep/wake cycle by retiring earlier are uniformly unsuccessful. Instead, it is more productive to delay bedtimes even further by increments of 3 hours a day, until the desired sleep/wake schedule is reached (chronotherapy: Weitzman et al., 1981). An alternative method (Rosenthal et al., 1990) is to administer bright light therapy for 2 hours early in the morning, with melatonin administration at bedtime, which can result in a phase advance of biological rhythms on subsequent nights and progressively earlier sleep times.

Advanced Sleep Phase Syndrome

Sleep/wake times are advanced in relationship to socially desired schedules. The disorder is more common in the elderly and is responsive to treatment with bright lights when administered in the evening, and goggles to prevent light exposure in the morning.

LIGHT THERAPY

Following the discovery that bright white light exposure could suppress melatonin released from the pineal glands of healthy humans (Lewy et al., 1980), researchers quickly determined that bright light could be used therapeutically to treat Seasonal Affective Disorder (SAD or winter depression). Among other symptoms, patients with SAD have hypersomnia. Light therapy has proven to be an effective therapeutic intervention for SAD, and its subclinical variant, sSAD, in numerous controlled, clinical trials (Golden et al., 2005; Lam & Levitt, 1999; Terman, Terman, Lo, & Cooper, 2001). A variety of light treatment devices have been tested for treating these affective disorders, including light boxes, dawn simulators, and light visors. Although there is not a current consensus about the etiology and pathophysiology of SAD, some investigators postulate that there is a circadian component related to this disorder. The current standard practice is for patients to have a trial of 10,000 lux white fluorescent light for 30–60 minutes in the morning upon awakening (Golden et al., 2005; Lam & Levitt, 1999; Terman et al., 2001). As with many medical disorders, patients vary in their responsiveness to light therapy. Although a majority of clinical trials employing light therapy have been concerned with the treatment of SAD, additional clinical applications have been explored, including light treatment of non-seasonal depression, selected sleep disorders, menstrual cycle related problems, bulimia nervosa, and problems associated with senile dementia (CIE, 2004, 2006; Golden et al., 2005; Kripke, 1993; Lam, Goldner, Solyom, & Remick, 1994; Mishima, Okawa, Hozumi, & Hishikawa, 2000; Parry, Berga, Mostofi, Klauber, & Resnick, 1997; Terman et al., 1995; Tuunainen, Kripke, & Endo, 2004; Van Someren, Kessler, Mirmiran, & Swaab, 1997).

In addition to the treatment of clinical disorders discussed above, the utility of light therapy for resolving problems associated with intercontinental jet travel, shift work, and space flight is being studied. For more than 15 years, light has been studied as a countermeasure for disruption of circadian rhythms and sleep/wake patterns in astronauts during space flight. Disturbed circadian rhythms and altered sleep/wake patterns are major risk factors for the safety and health of astronauts (Longnecker & Molins, 2005). Associated behavioral changes include decreased alertness, performance decrements, and diminished concentration, all of which can compromise the safety of personnel and the objectives of space missions. Studies of astronauts have shown light treatment to be an effective tool for supporting circadian entrainment, while ground-based studies continue to investigate the optimization of light as a countermeasure for circadian and sleep disruption in space flight missions (Czeisler, Chiasera, & Duffy, 1991; Dijk et al., 2001; Fucci et al., 2005; Stewart, Hayes, & Eastman, 1995; Whitson, Putcha, Chen, & Baker, 1995; Wright, Hughes, Kronauer, Dijk, & Czeisler, 2001). The aerospace community is evaluating how lighting can be engineered properly for supporting vision, circadian regulation, and optimum sleep of astronauts in advanced human environments, such as the International Space Station and planned lunar habitats. This research is likely to be relevant both to objectives in space exploration as well as to general architectural lighting design on earth for civilians with specific clinical disorders and problems associated with shift work and jet lag.

PARASOMNIAS

Parasomnias are abnormal and disturbing events associated with sleep. They are broadly divided into those that occur in non-REM sleep (e.g., confusional arousals, sleepwalking, sleep terrors) and those that occur in REM (e.g., REM sleep behavior disorders, sleep paralysis, nightmare disorder), although there are a number that do not fit neatly into either category (e.g., catathrenia, sleep related eating disorder, sleep enuresis) (American Academy of Sleep Medicine, 2005). The sleep stage in which they occur can also influence the portion of the night in which they are likely present. Somnambulism and night terrors, for example, usually occur during SWS, so they may be expected more often in the first third of the night when SWS predominates, whereas parasomnias that occur during REM (e.g., nightmare disorder) tend to be more common in the latter portion of the night (Carney, Berry, & Geyer, 2005).

Treatment of parasomnias starts with education and reassurance. It is important for the treating physician to teach the patient about the disorder, which many times has seemed bizarre to the patient and has been quite frightening. The next part of education involves teaching the patient to establish a safe sleeping environment. Since many parasomnias may involve unpleasant emotions or behaviors in the night, frequently not under voluntary control, precautions are important. There have been reports, for example, of patients with REM sleep behavior disorder or sleepwalking disorder causing significant, even fatal, injuries to themselves or others during sleep (Pressman, 2007; Schenck & Mahowald, 1995).

No medications are approved by the U.S. FDA for use in the parasomnias. However, while often requiring no other treatment than education and safety precautions, non-REM and REM parasomnias have both been treated with benzodiazepines, tricyclic antidepressants (TCAs), and selective serotonin reuptake inhibitors (SSRIs) (Chokoverty, 2000), although there is more clinical support for such treatment than there are controlled trials (Plante & Winkelman, 2006). Cognitive psychotherapies may also be of benefit in a supporting role, particularly for patients with those parasomnias that have a more affective component (e.g., nightmare disorder). Some of the salient clinical features of selected parasomnias are listed in Table 10.6.

Table 10.6. Selected Parasomnias.

Parasomnia	Clinical Features	Polysomnographic Findings	Treatment
Sleep Terror	Intense vocalization during sleep, with autonomic hyperarousal	Usually unrevealing; if positive, shows behaviors emerging from slow wave sleep	Reassurance of parents Psychiatric evaluation for adults
Sleepwalking	Walking during sleep, usually during the first third of night Difficulty in awakening the sufferer during an episode Amnesia for the event the following day Usually affects adolescents	Usually unrevealing; if positive, shows sleepwalking emerging from slow wave sleep	Removal of sharp objects from the bedside and sleeping on floor mattress Psychiatric evaluation for adults Benzodiazepines
Nightmares	Recall of disturbing dream content Usually occur in latter half of night	Abrupt awakening from REM Tachycardia and tachypnea during episode	Psychotherapy Hypnosis
Bruxism	Tooth grinding during sleep	Bursts of masseter EMG activity	Dental examination Mouth guards Relaxation training Psychotherapy
REM sleep behavior disorder	Violent or injurious behaviors during REM sleep Dreams are enacted while they occur Most cases idiopathic	Loss of REM EMG atonia	Protective measures Clonazepam Psychotherapy

Source: Based upon information from American Academy of Sleep Medicine 2005.

Evaluation of Sleep Disorders

Complaints—such as insomnia, EDS, and disturbing events during sleep—warrant a thorough evaluation; steps in this process are outlined in Table 10.7. The first step in the evaluation of a sleep disorder is taking a detailed sleep history. Questionnaires and inventories can also be useful, including the Epworth Sleepiness Scale (Table 10.8), which is useful for the quantification of the extent of daytime somnolence (Johns, 1991). Scores above 10 are generally considered significant. Serial administration over time also provides a way of monitoring efficacy of treatment.

A nocturnal polysomnogram (PSG) is appropriate if the office-based evaluation raises the possibility of primary sleep disorders, such as sleep apnea syndrome, narcolepsy, periodic limb movement disorder, or sleep-related epilepsy;

Table 10.7. The Clinical Evaluation of Sleep Disorders.

1. Interview

   a. Chief complaint: insomnia, EDS, or parasomnia?

   b. History of present illness

   c. Sleep/wake habit history

   d. Sleep hygiene history: meal and exercise times, ambient noise, light and temperature, etc.

   e. Pattern of consumption of recreational substances (especially caffeine and alcohol) and medications

   f. Medications

   g. General medical, psychiatric, and surgical history

2. Sleep diary

3. Inventories for daytime sleepiness/ alertness

4. Psychological inventories

5. Bed partner interview

6. Physical and mental status examination

7. Serum laboratory tests

8. Polysomnography

Table 10.8. The Epworth Sleepiness Scale.

How likely are you to doze off or fall asleep under the following situations? Use the following scale to choose the most appropriate number for each situation:

0 = would never doze

1 = slight chance of dozing

2 = moderate chance of dozing

3 = high chance of dozing

Sitting and reading	0	1	2	3
Watching TV	0	1	2	3
Sitting, inactive, in a public place	0	1	2	3
Passenger in a car for an hour without a break	0	1	2	3
Lying down to rest in the afternoon	0	1	2	3
Sitting and talking to someone	0	1	2	3
Sitting quietly after a lunch with no alcohol	0	1	2	3
In a car, while stopped for a few minutes in traffic	0	1	2	3

Total

Source: Johns (1991).

when the clinician is confronted with potentially dangerous behaviors during sleep; when there is severe daytime somnolence; and to assess response to treatment for various sleep disorders. Polysomnography involves the recording of multiple physiological measures during sleep, including the electroencephalogram, electrooculogram, electromyogram of various muscle groups, electrocardiogram, respiration, and oxyhemoglobin saturation, among others. In cases of suspected narcolepsy, daytime variations of the PSG (specifically multiple sleep latency testing [MSLT]) is used. To quantify the extent of daytime somnolence, the maintenance of wakefulness testing (MWT) can be used. Once a specific sleep disorder has been diagnosed, treatment can be tailored.

Summary

Sleep is an active process that involves the interplay of an array of brain processes and structures, as well as an orderly progression of changes throughout all body systems. Complaints regarding sleep and wakefulness are common, and can be caused by medical, psychiatric, and intrinsic sleep disorders. Once the causes of the complaints have been identified, treatment modalities can be integrated to produce optimal benefit. A variety of treatments are available, including cognitive-behavioral therapy, bright light therapy, and pharmacotherapy. In the last category, the only therapeutic agents that have been extensively evaluated for safety and efficacy, and that have been approved for use for insomnia by the FDA, are the benzodiazepine receptor agonists and the melatonin receptor agonists. Over-the-counter agents and sedating antidepressants are utilized, yet their efficacy and safety profile is in question. Complementary and alternative medicines have great allure. Nevertheless, further research is needed to answer key questions regarding these agents, such as efficacy, safety, and optimal dosages with these promising agents.

Acknowledgments

The authors gratefully acknowledge the dedicated support of Benjamin Warfield for development of Figure 10.6 and John Hanifin for assistance with references. With permission from the CIE, portions of this manuscript, including Figure 10.6, were adapted and updated from an earlier CIE report (Brainard and Provencio, 2006). The work was supported, in part, by a grant from NSBRI under NASA Cooperative Agreement NCC 9–58.

REFERENCES

Aggelopoulos, N. C., & Meissl, H. (2000). Responses of neurones of the rat suprachiasmatic nucleus to retinal illumination under photopic and scotopic conditions. *Journal of Physiology, 523,* 211–222.

Agostini, J. V., Leo-Summers, L. S., & Inouye, S. K. (2001). Cognitive and other adverse effects of diphenhydramine use in hospitalized older patients. *Archives of Internal Medicine, 161,* 2091–2097.

American Academy of Sleep Medicine (2005). *International classification of sleep disorders: Diagnostic and coding manual* (2nd edn). Westchester, IL: American Academy of Sleep Medicine.

American Academy of Sleep Medicine (2007). *The AASM manual for the scoring of sleep and associated events: Rules, terminology and technical specification.* Westchester, IL: American Academy of Sleep Medicine.

American Cancer Society. Available online at: http://www.cancer.org

Ancoli-Israel, S., & Roth, T. (1991). Characteristics of insomnia in the United States: Results of the 1991 National Sleep Foundation Survey. I. *Sleep, 22*(suppl 2), S347–S353.

Arendt, J. (1998). Melatonin and the pineal gland: Influence on mammalian seasonal and circadian physiology. *Reviews of Reproduction, 3*, 13–22.

Armington, J. C., & Mitnick, L. L. (1959). Electroencephalogram and sleep deprivation. *Journal of Applied Physiology, 14*, 247–250.

Aschoff, J. (Ed.) (1981). *Handbook of behavioral neurobiology, biological rhythms.* New York: Plenum Press.

Barger, L. K., Wright, K. P., Hughes, R. J., & Czeisler, C. A. (2004). Daily exercise facilitates phase delays of circadian melatonin rhythm in very dim light. *American Journal of Physiology—Regulatory Integrative & Comparative Physiology, 286*, R1077–R1084.

Belenky, G., Wesensten, N. J., Thorne, D. R., Thomas, M. L., Sing, H. C., Redmond, D. P., et al. (2003). Patterns of performance degradation and restoration during sleep restriction and subsequent recovery: A sleep dose–response study. *Journal of Sleep Research, 12*, 1–12.

Berson, D. M., Dunn, F. A., & Takao, M. (2002). Phototransduction by retinal ganglion cells that set the circadian clock. *Science, 295*, 1070–1073.

Blask, D. E., Brainard, G. C., Dauchy, R. T., Hanifin, J. P., Davidson, L. K., Krause, J. A., et al. (2005). Melatonin-depleted blood from premenopausal women exposed to light at night stimulates growth of human breast cancer xenografts in nude rats. *Cancer Research, 65*, 11174–11184.

Bliwise, D. L. (1996). Historical change in the report of daytime fatigue. *Sleep, 19*(6), 462–464.

Bootzin, R. R., & Perlis, M. L. (1992). Nonpharmacologic treatments of insomnia. *Journal of Clinical Psychiatry,* (53 Suppl), 37–41.

Boulos, Z., Campbell, S. S., Lewy, A. J., Terman, M., Dijk, D.-J., & Eastman, C. I. (1995). Light treatment for sleep disorders: Consensus report. VII. jet lag. *Journal of Biological Rhythms, 10*, 167–176.

Boulos, Z., Macchi, M. M., Stürchler, M. P., Stewart, K. T., Brainard, G. C., Suhner, A., et al. (2002). Light visor treatment for jet lag after westward travel across six time zones. *Aviation Space and Environmental Medicine, 73*, 953–963.

Brainard, G. C., & Hanifin, J. P. (2005). Photons, clocks and consciousness. *Journal of Biological Rhythms, 20*, 314–325.

Brainard, G. C., Hanifin, J. P., Greeson, J. M., Byrne, B., Glickman, G., Gerner, E., et al. (2001a). Action spectrum for melatonin regulation in humans: Evidence for a novel circadian photoreceptor. *Journal of Neuroscience, 21*, 6405–6412.

Brainard, G. C., Hanifin, J. P., Rollag, M. D., Greeson, J., Byrne, B., Glickman, G., et al. (2001b). Human melatonin regulation is not mediated by the three cone photopic visual system. *Journal of Clinical Endocrinology and Metabolism, 86*, 433–436.

Brainard, G. C., & Provencio, I. (2006). Photoreception for the neurobehavioral effects of light in humans. In *Proceedings of the 2nd CIE Expert Symposium on Light and Health,* pp. 6–21, CIE x031:2006, Vienna.

Brainard, G. C., Rollag, M. D., & Hanifin, J. P. (1997). Photic regulation of melatonin in humans: Ocular and neural signal transduction. *Journal of Biological Rhythms, 12*, 537–546.

Brzezinski, A., Vangel, M. G., Wurtman, R. J., Norrie, G., Zhdanova, I., Ben-Shushan, A., et al. (2005). Effects of exogenous melatonin on sleep: A meta-analysis. *Sleep Medicine Reviews, 9,* 41–50.

Buscemi, N., Vandermeer, B., Hooton, N., Pandya, R., Tjosvold, L., Hartling, L., et al. (2005). The efficacy and safety of exogenous melatonin for primary sleep disorders: A meta-analysis. *Journal of General Internal Medicine, 20,* 1151–1158.

Buxton, O. M., Lee, C. W., L'Hermite-Baleriaux, M., Turek, F. W., & Van Cauter, E. (2003). Exercise elicits phase shifts and acute alterations of melatonin that vary with circadian phase. *American Journal of Physiology—Regulatory Integrative & Comparative Physiology, 284,* R714–R724.

Carney, P. R., Berry, R. B., & Geyer, J. D. (Eds.) (2005). *Clinical sleep disorders.* Philadelphia, PA: Lippincott Williams & Wilkins.

Carskadon, M. A. & Dement, W. C. (2005). Normal human sleep: An overview. In M. H. Kryger, T. Roth, & W. C. Dement (Eds.), *Principles and practice of sleep medicine* (4th edn). Philadelphia, PA, Elsevier Saunders Inc., pp. 13–23.

Center for Food Safety and Applied Nutrition, U.S. Food and Drug Administration (2002). Kava-containing dietary supplements may be associated with severe liver injury. FDA Consumer Advisory, March 25, 2002. Available at: http://www.cfsan.fda.gov/~dms/addskava.html. Accessed 05/03/08.

Chokroverty, S. (2000). *Clinical companion to sleep disorders medicine* (2nd edn). Woburn, MA: Butterworth-Heinemann.

Chokroverty, S., Thomas, R. J., & Bhatt, M. (2005). *Atlas of sleep medicine.* Philadelphia, PA: Elsevier Saunders Inc.

Commission Internationale de l'Eclairage (2004). Ocular lighting effects on human physiology and behaviour, Commission Internationale de l'Eclairage, Technical Report 158, Vienna.

Commission Internationale de l'Eclairage (2006). *Proceedings of the 2nd CIE Expert Symposium on Light and Health,* CIE x031:2006, Vienna.

Czeisler, C. A., Chiasera, A. J., & Duffy, J. F. (1991). Research on sleep, circadian rhythms and aging: Applications to manned spaceflight. *Experimental Gerontology, 26,* 217–232.

Czeisler, C. A., Duffy, J. F., Shanahan, T. L., Brown, E. N., Mitchell, J. F., Rimmer, D. W., et al. (1999). Stability, precision, and near-24-hour period of the human circadian pacemaker. *Science, 284,* 2177–2181.

Czeisler, C. A., Johnson, M. P., Duffy, J. F., Brown, E. N., Ronda, J. M., & Kronauer, R. E. (1990). Exposure to bright light and darkness to treat physiologic maladaptation to night work. *New England Journal of Medicine, 322,* 1253–1259.

Czeisler, C. A., Shanahan, T. L., Klerman, E. B., Martens, H., Brotman, D. J., Emens, J. S., et al. (1995). Suppression of melatonin secretion in some blind patients by exposure to bright light. *New England Journal of Medicine, 332,* 6–11.

Czeisler, C. A., & Wright, K. P. (1999). Influence of light on circadian rhythmicity in humans. In F. W. Turek, & P. C. Zee (Eds.), *Regulation of sleep and circadian rhythms.* New York: Marcel Dekker, pp. 149–180.

Danilenko, K. V., Cajochen, C., & Wirz-Justice, A. (2003). Is sleep per se a Zeitgeber in humans? *Journal of Biological Rhythms, 18,* 170–178.

Davis, S., Mirick, D. K. & Stevens, R. G. (2001). Night shift work, light at night, and risk of breast cancer. *Journal of the National Cancer Institute, 93*, 1557–1562.

Dawson, D., & Campbell, S. S. (1991). Timed exposure to bright light improves sleep and alertness during simulated night shifts. *Sleep, 14*, 511–516.

Dement, W. C. (2005). History of sleep physiology and medicine. In M. H. Kryger, T. Roth, & W. C. Dement (Eds.), *Principles and practice of sleep medicine* (4th edn). Philadelphia, PA: Elsevier Saunders Inc., pp. 1–12.

Dietz, B. M., Mahady, G. B., Pauli, G. F., & Farnsworth, N. R. (2005). Valerian extract and valerenic acid are partial agonists of the 5-HT5a receptor in vitro. *Brain Research. Molecular Brain Research, 138*, 191–197.

Dijk, D. J., Neri, D. F., Wyatt, J. K., Ronda, J. M., Riel, E., Ritz-De Cecco, A., et al. (2001). Sleep, performance, circadian rhythms, and light-dark cycles during two space shuttle flights. *American Journal of Physiology, 281*, R1647–R1664.

Dkhissi-Benyahya, O., Gronfier, C., De Vanssay, W., Flamant, F., & Cooper, H. M. (2007). Modeling the role of mid-wavelength cones in circadian responses to light. *Neuron, 53*, 677–687.

Doghramji, K., & Doghramji, P. (2006). *Clinical management of insomnia.* West Islip, NY: Professional Communications, Inc.

Dumont, M., & Beaulieu, C. (2006). Effects of dim and bright work environments on circadian functions. In *Proceedings of the 2nd CIE Expert Symposium on Light and Health*, pp. 46–49, CIE x031:2006, Vienna.

Eastman, C. I., Boulos, Z., Terman, M., Campbell, S. S., Dijk, D.-J., & Lewy, A. J. (1995). Light treatment for sleep disorders: Consensus report. VI. shift work. *Journal of Biological Rhythms, 10*, 157–164.

Edgar, D. M., Dement, W. C. & Fuller, C. A. (1993). Effect of SCN lesions on sleep in squirrel monkeys: Evidence for opponent processes in sleep–wake regulation. *Journal of Neuroscience, 13*, 1065–1079.

Edinger, J. D., & Means, M. K. (2005). Overview of insomnia: Definitions, epidemiology, differential diagnosis, and assessment. In M. H. Kryger, T. Roth, & W. C. Dement (Eds.), *Principles and practice of sleep medicine* (4th edn). Philadelphia, PA: Elsevier Saunders Inc., pp. 702–713.

España, R. A., & Scammell, T. E. (2004). Sleep neurobiology for the clinician. *Sleep, 27*(4), 811–820.

Figueiro, M. G., Bullough, J. D., Parsons, R. H., & Rea, M. S. (2004). Preliminary evidence for spectral opponency in the suppression of melatonin by light in humans. *Neuroreport, 15*, 313–316.

Freedman, M. S., Lucas, R. J., Soni, B., von Schantz, M., Munoz, M., David-Gray, Z., et al. (1999). Regulation of mammalian circadian behavior by non-rod, non-cone, ocular photoreceptors. *Science, 284*, 502–504.

Freud, S. (1900). (1965 edition, translation by James Strachey). *The interpretation of dreams.* New York: Basic Books, Inc.

Fucci, R. L., Gardner, J., Hanifin, J. P., Jasser, S., Byrne, B., Gerner, E., et al. (2005). Toward optimizing lighting as a countermeasure to sleep and circadian disruption in space flight. *Acta Astronautica, 56*, 1017–1024.

Gamlin, P. D. R., McDougal, D. H., Pokorny, J., Smith, V. C., Yau, K.-W., & Dacey, D. M. (2007). Human and macaque pupil responses driven by melanopsin-containing retinal ganglion cells. *Vision Research, 47,* 946–954.

Gillin, J. C., Drummond, S. P. A., Clark, C. P., & Moore, P. (2005). Medication and substance abuse. In M. H. Kryger, T. Roth, & W. C. Dement (Eds.), *Principles and practice of sleep medicine* (4th edn). Philadelphia, PA: Elsevier Saunders Inc., pp. 1345–1358.

Golden, R. N., Gaynes, B. N., Ekstrom, R. D., Hamer, R. M., Jacobsen, F. M., Suppes, T., et al. (2005). The efficacy of light therapy in the treatment of mood disorders: A review and meta-analysis of the evidence. *American Journal of Psychiatry, 162,* 656–662.

Gooley, J. J., Lu, J., Chou, T. C., Scammell, T. E., & Saper, C. B. (2001). Melanopsin in cell of origin of the retinohypothalamic tract. *Nature Neuroscience, 4,* 1165.

Gooley, J. J., Lu, J., Fischer, D., & Saper, C.B. (2003). A broad role for melanopsin in nonvisual photoreception. *Journal of Neuroscience, 23,* 7093–7106.

Hajak, G., Rodenbeck, A., Voderholzer, U., Riemann, D., Cohrs, S., Hohagen, F., et al. (2001). Doxepin in the treatment of primary insomnia: A placebo-controlled, double-blind, polysomnographic study. *Journal of Clinical Psychiatry, 62,* 453–463.

Hannibal, J., Hindersson, P., Knudsen, S. M., Georg, B., & Fahrenkrug, J. (2002). The photopigment melanopsin is exclusively present in pituitary adenylate cyclase-activating polypeptide-containing retinal ganglion cells of the retinohypothalamic tract. *Journal of Neuroscience, 22,* 1–7.

Hattar, S., Liao, H.-W., Takao, M., Berson, D. M., & Yau, K.-W. (2002). Melanopsin-containing retinal ganglion cells: Architecture, projections, and intrinsic photosensitivity. *Science, 295,* 1065–1070.

Hattar, S., Lucas, R. J., Mrosovsky, N., Thompson, S., Douglas, R. H., Hankins, M. W., et al. (2003). Melanopsin and rod–cone photoreceptive systems account for all major accessory visual functions in mice. *Nature, 424,* 76–81.

Hobson, J. A. (1989). *Sleep.* New York: Scientific American Library.

Hobson, J. A., & McCarley, R. W. (1977). The brain as a dream state generator: An activation-synthesis hypothesis of the dream process. *American Journal of Psychology, 134*(12), 1335–1348.

Hobson, J. A., Pace-Schott, E. F., & Stickgold, R. (2000). Dreaming and the brain: Toward a cognitive neuroscience of conscious states. *Behavioral & Brain Sciences, 23*(6), 793–842.

International Agency for Research on Cancer. Available online at: http://www.iarc.fr

James, S. P., & Mendelson, W. B. (2004). The use of trazodone as a hypnotic: A critical review. *Journal of Clinical Psychiatry, 65,* 752–755.

Jasser, S. A., Hanifin, J. P., Rollag, M. D., & Brainard, G. C. (2006). Dim light adaptation attenuates acute melatonin suppression in humans. *Journal of Biological Rhythms, 21,* 394–404.

Johns, M. W. (1991). A new method for measuring daytime sleepiness: The Epworth sleepiness scale. *Sleep, 14*(6), 540–545.

Johnson, M. W., Suess, P. E., & Griffiths, R. R. (2006). Ramelteon. A novel hypnotic lacking abuse liability and sedative adverse effects. *Archives of General Psychiatry, 63,* 1149–1157.

Kales, A., Tan, T.L., Kollar, E. J., Naitoh, P., Preston, T. A., & Malmstrom, E. J. (1970). Sleep patterns following 205 hours of sleep deprivation. *Psychosomatic Medicine, 32*, 189–200.

Klein, D. C., Moore, R. Y., & Reppert, S. M. (Eds.) (1991). *Suprachiasmatic nucleus: The mind's clock.* Oxford: Oxford University Press.

Klerman, E. B., Rimmer, D. W., Dijk, D. J., Kronauer, R. E., Rizzo, J. F., & Czeisler, C. A. (1998). Nonphotic entrainment of the human circadian pacemaker. *American Journal of Physiology, 274*, R991–R996.

Klerman, E. B., Shanahan, T. L., Brotman, D. J., Rimmer, D. W., Emens, J. S., Rizzo, J. F., et al. (2002). Photic resetting of the human circadian pacemaker in the absence of conscious vision. *Journal of Biological Rhythms, 17*, 548–555.

Krauchi, K., Cajochen, C., Werth, E., & Wirz-Justice, A. (2002). Alteration of internal circadian phase relationships after morning versus evening carbohydrate-rich meals in humans. *Journal of Biological Rhythms, 17*, 364–376.

Kripke, D. F. (1993). Light regulation of the menstrual cycle. In L. Wetterberg (Ed.), *Light and biological rhythms in man.* Stockholm, Sweden: Pergamon Press, pp. 305–312.

Lam, R. W. (1996). *Beyond seasonal affective disorder: Light treatment for SAD and non-SAD disorders.* Washington, DC: American Psychiatric Press, Inc.

Lam, R. W., Goldner, E. M., Solyom, L., & Remick, R. A. (1994). A controlled study of light therapy for bulimia nervosa. *American Journal of Psychiatry, 151*, 744–750.

Lam, R. W., & Levitt, A. J. (Eds.) (1999). *Canadian consensus guidelines for the treatment of seasonal affective disorder.* Vancouver, British Columbia: Clinical and Academic Publishing.

Lange, T., Perras, B., Fehm, H. L., & Born, J. (2003). Sleep enhances the human antibody response to hepatitis A vaccination. *Psychosomatic Medicine, 65*, 831–835.

Leibowitz, S. M., Brooks, S. N., & Black, J. E. (2006). Excessive daytime sleepiness: Considerations for the psychiatrist. In K. Doghramji (Ed.), *The sleep-psychiatry interface. Psychiatry clinics of North America, 29*(4), 921–945.

Lewy, A. J., Wehr, T. A., Goodwin, F. K., Newsome, D. A., & Markey, S. P. (1980). Light suppresses melatonin secretion in humans. *Science, 210*, 1267–1269.

Lockley, S. W., Skene, D. J., Arendt, J., Tabandeh, H., Bird, A. C., & Defrace, R. (1997). Relationship between melatonin rhythms and visual loss in the blind. *Journal of Clinical Endocrinology and Metabolism, 82*, 3763–3770.

Longnecker, D., & Molins, R. (Eds.) (2005). *Bioastronautics: A risk reduction strategy for human exploration of space.* National Research Council, Committee on Review of NASA's Bioastronautics Roadmap.

Lucas, R. J., Freedman, M. S., Munoz, M., Garcia-Fernandez, J. M., & Foster, R. G. (1999). Regulation of the mammalian pineal by non-rod, non-cone, ocular photoreceptors. *Science, 284*, 505–507.

Lumeng, J. C., Somashekar, D., Appugliese, D., Kaciroti, N., Corwyn, R. F., & Bradley, R. H. (2007). Shorter sleep duration is associated with increased risk for being overweight at ages 9 to 12 years. *Pediatrics, 120*(5), 1020–1029.

Markov, D., & Goldman, M. (2006). Normal sleep and circadian rhythms: Neurobiologic mechanisms underlying sleep and wakefulness. In K. Doghramji (Ed.), *The sleep–psychiatry interface. Psychiatry Clinics of North America, 29*(4), 841–853.

Meeks, T. W., Wetherell, J. L., Irwin, M. R., Redwine, L. S., & Jeste, D. V. (2007). Complementary and alternative treatments for late-life depression, anxiety and sleep disturbance: A review of randomized controlled trials. *Journal of Clinical Psychiatry, 68*(10), 1461–1471.

Melyan, Z., Tarttelin, E. E., Bellingham, J., Lucas, R. J., & Hankins, M. W. (2005). Addition of human melanopsin renders mammalian cells photoresponsive. *Nature, 433,* 741–745.

Metlaine, A., Leger, D., & Choudat, D. (2005). Socioeconomic impact of insomnia in working populations. *Industrial Health, 43*(1), 11–19.

Mindell, J. A., & Owens, J. A. (2003). *A clinical guide to pediatric sleep medicine: Diagnosis and management of sleep problems.* Philadelphia, PA: Lippincott Williams & Wilkins.

Minors, D. S., Waterhouse, J. M., & Wirz-Justice, A. (1991). A human phase-response curve to light. *Neuroscience Letters, 133,* 36–40.

Mishima, K., Okawa, M., Hozumi, S., & Hishikawa, Y. (2000). Supplementary administration of artificial bright light and melatonin as potent treatment for disorganized circadian rest-activity and dysfunctional autonomic and neuroendocrine systems in institutionalized demented elderly persons. *Chronobiology International, 17,* 419–432.

Montplaisir, J., Allen, R. P., Walters, A. S., & Ferini-Strambi, L. (2005). Restless legs syndrome and periodic limb movements during sleep. In M. H. Kryger, T. Roth, & W. C. Dement (Eds.), *Principles and practice of sleep medicine* (4th edn). Philadelphia, PA: Elsevier Saunders Inc., pp. 839–852.

Moore-Ede, M. C. (1993). *The twenty-four hour society: Understanding a world that never stops.* New York: Addison-Wesley Publishing Company.

Morin, C. M., Colecchi, C., Stone, J., Sood, R., & Brink, D. (1999). Behavioral and pharmacological therapies for late-life insomnia. *JAMA, 281,* 991–999.

Morin, C. M., Culbert, J. P., & Schwartz, S. M. (1994). Nonpharmacological interventions for insomnia: A meta-analysis of treatment efficacy. *American Journal of Psychiatry, 151,* 1172–1180.

Morin, L. P. (1994). The circadian visual system. *Brain Research Brain Research Reviews, 19,* 102–127.

Morin, C. M., Koetter, U., Bastien, C., Ware, J. C., & Wooten, V. (2005). Valerian-hops combination and diphenhydramine for treating insomnia: A randomized placebo-controlled clinical trial. *Sleep, 28*(11), 1465–1471.

Moruzzi, G., & Magoun, H. W. (1949). Brain stem reticular formation and activation of the EEG. *Electroencephalography & Clinical Neurophysiology, 1,* 455–473.

National Institutes of Health. (2005). Manifestations and management of chronic insomnia in adults. State-of-the-Science Conference Statement, June 13–15, 2005 (Final Statement: August 18, 2005), 1–18.

National Sleep Foundation. (2005). Sleep in America poll. March 29, 2005. Available online at: http://www.sleepfoundation.org

National Sleep Foundation (2007). State of the states report on drowsy driving. November 5, 2007. Available online at: http://www.drowsydriving.org

Neckelmann, D., & Ursin, R. (1993). Sleep stages and EEG power spectrum in relation to acoustical stimulus arousal threshold in the rat. Sleep, 16(5), 467–477.

Ohayon, M. M., Carskadon, M. A., Guilleminault, C., & Vitiello, M. V. (2004). Meta-analysis of quantitative sleep parameters from childhood to old age in healthy individuals: Developing normative sleep values across the human lifespan. Sleep, 27, 1255–1273.

Panda, S., Nayak, S. K., Campo, B., Walker, J. R., Hogenesch, J. B., & Jegla, T. (2005). Illumination of melanopsin signaling pathway. Science, 307, 600–604.

Panda, S., Provencio, I., Tu, D. C., Pires, S. S., Rollag, M. D., Castrucci, A. M., et al. (2003). Melanopsin is required for non-image-forming photic responses in blind mice. Science, 301, 525–527.

Parmeggiani, P. L. (2005). Physiologic regulation in sleep. In M. H. Kryger, T. Roth, & W. C. Dement (Eds.), Principles and practice of sleep medicine (4th edn). Philadelphia, PA: Elsevier Saunders Inc., pp. 185–191.

Parry, B. L., Berga, S. L., Mostofi, N., Klauber, M. R., & Resnick, A. (1997). Plasma melatonin circadian rhythms during the menstrual cycle and after light therapy in premenstrual dysphoric disorder and normal control subjects. Journal of Biological Rhythms, 12, 47–64.

Pickering, T. G. (2006). Could hypertension be a consequence of the 24/7 society? The effects of sleep deprivation and shift work. Journal of Clinical Hypertension, 8(11), 819–822.

Plante, D. T., & Winkelman, J. W. (2006). Parasomnias. In K. Doghramji (Ed.), The Sleep-Psychiatry Interface. Psychiatry Clinics of North America, 29(4), 969–987.

Pressman, M. R. (2007). Disorders of arousal from sleep and violent behavior: The role of physical contact and proximity. Sleep, 30(8), 1039–1047.

Provencio, I., Jiang, G., De Grip, W. J., Hayes, W. P., & Rollag, M. D. (1998). Melanopsin: An opsin in melanophores, brain, and eye. Proceedings of the National Academy of Sciences of the United States of America, 95, 340–345.

Provencio, I., Rodriguez, I. R., Jiang, G., Hayes, W. P., Moreira, E. F., & Rollag, M. D. (2000). A novel human opsin in the inner retina. Journal of Neuroscience, 20, 600–605.

Provencio, I., Rollag, M. D., & Castrucci, A. M. (2002). Photoreceptive net in the mammalian retina. Nature, 415, 493.

Qiu, X., Kumbalasiri, T., Carlson, S. M., Wong, K. Y., Krishna, V., Provencio, I., et al. (2005). Induction of photosensitivity by heterologous expression of melanopsin. Nature, 433, 745–749.

Reiter, R. J. (1991). Pineal gland: Interface between the photoperiodic environment and the endocrine system. Trends in Endocrinology and Metabolism, 2, 13–19.

Richardson, G. S. (2005). The human circadian system in normal and disordered sleep. Journal of Clinical Psychiatry, 66(Suppl 9), 3–9.

Richardson, G. S., Roehrs, T. A., Rosenthal, L., Koshorek, G., & Roth, T. (2002). Tolerance to daytime sedative effects of H1 antihistamines. *Journal of Clinical Psychopharmacology, 22,* 511–5.

Rickels, K., Morris, R. J., Newman, H., Rosenfeld, H., Schiller, H., & Weinstock, R. (1983). Diphenhydramine in insomniac family practice patients: A double-blind study. *Journal of Clinical Pharmacology, 23,* 234–242.

Rosenthal, N. E., Joseph-Vanderpool, J. R., Levendosky, A. A., Johnston, S. H., Allen, R., Kelly, K. A., et al. (1990). Phase-shifting effects of bright morning light as treatment for delayed sleep phase syndrome. *Sleep, 13,* 354–361.

Rothbaum, B. O., & Mellman, T. A. (2001). Dreams and exposure therapy in PTSD. *Journal of Traumatic Stress, 14*(3), 481–90.

Ruberg, F. L., Skene, D. J., Hanifin, J. P., Rollag, M. D., English, J., Arendt, J., et al. (1996). Melatonin regulation in humans with color vision deficiencies. *Journal of Clinical Endocrinology and Metabolism, 81,* 2980–2985.

Schenck, C. H., & Mahowald, M. W. (1995). A polysomnographically documented case of adult somnambulism with long-distance automobile driving and frequent nocturnal violence: Parasomnia with continuing danger as a noninsane automatism? *Sleep, 18*(9), 765–772.

Schernhammer, E. S., Laden, F., Speizer, F. E., Willett, W. C., Hunter, D. J., Kawachi, I., et al. (2001). Rotating night shifts and risk of breast cancer in women participating in the nurses' health study. *Journal of the National Cancer Institute, 93,* 1563–1568.

Schernhammer, E. S., Laden, F., Speizer, F. E., Willett, W. C., Hunter, D. J., Kawachi, I., et al. (2003). Night-shift work and risk of colorectal cancer in the nurses' health study. *Journal of the National Cancer Institute, 95,* 825–828.

Sheldon, S. H., Ferber, R., & Kryger, M. H. (2005). *Principles and practice of pediatric sleep medicine.* Philadelphia, PA: Elsevier Inc.

Siegel, J. M. (2005). REM sleep. In M. H. Kryger, T. Roth, & W. C. Dement (Eds.), *Principles and practice of sleep medicine* (4th edn). Philadelphia, PA: Elsevier Saunders Inc., pp. 120–135.

Sieghart, W., & Sperk, G. (2002). Subunit composition, distribution and function of GABA(A) receptor subtypes. *Current Topics in Medicinal Chemistry, 2,* 795–816.

Smith, K. A., Schoen, M. W., & Czeisler, C. A. (2004). Adaptation of human pineal melatonin suppression by recent photic history. *Journal of Clinical Endocrinology and Metabolism, 89,* 3610–3614.

Spiegel, K., Leproult, R., & Van Cauter, E. (1999). Impact of sleep debt on metabolic and endocrine function. *The Lancet, 354,* 1435–1439.

Spiegel, K., Sheridan, J. F., & Van Cauter, E. (2002). Effect of sleep deprivation on response to immunization. *Journal of American Medical Association, 288,* 1471–1472.

Stenseth, N. C., Falck, W., Chan, K.-S., Bjornstad, O. N., O'Donoghue, M., Tong, H., et al. (1998). From patterns to processes: Phase and density dependencies in the Canadian lynx cycle. *Proceedings of the National Academy of Sciences of the United States of America, 95,* 15430–15435.

Sternberg, E. M. (1996). Pathogenesis of L-tryptophan eosinophilia myalgia syndrome. *Advances in Experimental Medical Biology, 398,* 325–30.

Stevens, R. G. (1987). Electric power use and breast cancer: A hypothesis. *American Journal of Epidemiology, 125*, 556–561.

Stevens, R. G., Blask, D. E., Brainard, G. C., Hansen, J., Lockley, S. W., Provencio, I., et al. (2007). Meeting report: The role of environmental lighting and circadian disruption in cancer and other diseases. *Environmental Health Perspectives, 115*, 1357–1362.

Stevinson, C., & Ernst, E. (2000). Valerian for insomnia: A systematic review of randomized clinical trials. *Sleep Medicine, 1*, 91–99.

Stewart, K. T., Hayes, B. C., & Eastman, C. I. (1995). Light treatment for NASA shiftworkers. *Chronobiology International, 12*, 141–151.

Stickgold, R. (2002) EMDR: A putative neurobiological mechanism of action. *Journal of Clinical Psychology, 58*(1), 61–75.

Stickgold, R. (2005). Introduction to dreams and their pathology. In M. H. Kryger, T. Roth, & W. C. Dement (Eds.) *Principles and practice of sleep medicine* (4th edn). Philadelphia, PA: Elsevier Saunders Inc., pp. 519–521.

Stone, M. H. (1997). *Healing the mind: A history of psychiatry from antiquity to the present.* New York: W. W. Norton & Company.

Straif, K., Baan, R., Grosse, Y., Secretan, B., El Ghissassi, F., Bouvard, V., et al. (2007). Carcinogenicity of shift-work, painting, and fire-fighting. *Lancet Oncology, 8*, 1065–1066.

Tamakoshi, A., & Ohno, Y. (2004). Self-reported sleep duration as a predictor of all-cause mortality: Results from the JACC study, Japan. *Sleep, 27*(1), 51–54.

Terman, J. S., Terman, M., Lo, E. S., & Cooper, T. B. (2001). Circadian time of morning light administration and therapeutic response in winter depression. *Archives of General Psychiatry, 58*, 69–75.

Terman, M., Lewy, A. J., Dijk, D.-J., Boulos, Z., Eastman, C. I., & Campbell, S. S. (1995). Light treatment for sleep disorders: Consensus report IV sleep phase and duration disturbances. *Journal of Biological Rhythms, 10*, 135–147.

Thapan, K., Arendt, J., & Skene, D. J. (2001). An action spectrum for melatonin suppression: Evidence for a novel non-rod, non-cone photoreceptor system in humans. *Journal of Physiology, 535*, 261–267.

The Internet Classics Archive (2000). *On sleep and sleeplessness by Aristotle.* Available online at: http://classics.mit.edu/Aristotle/sleep.html.

Thomson Micromedex (2008). Available online at http://www-thomsonhc-com.proxy1.lib.tju.edu:2048/hcs/librarian

Triarhou, L. C. (2006). The percipient observations of Constantin von Economo on encephalitis lethargica and sleep disruption and their lasting impact on contemporary sleep research. *Brain Research Bulletin, 69*(3), 244–258.

Tuunainen, A., Kripke, D. F., & Endo, T. (2004). Light therapy for non-seasonal depression. *Cochrane Database of Systemic Reviews, 2*, 1–83.

United States Congress Office of Technology Assessment. (1991). *Biological Rhythms: Implications for the Worker.* # OTA-BA-463, U.S. Government Printing Office.

Van Cauter, E., Leproult, R., & Plat, L. (2000). Age-related changes in slow wave sleep and REM sleep and relationship with growth hormone and cortisol levels in healthy men. *JAMA, 284*, 861–868.

Van Dongen, H. P., Maislin, G., Mullington, J. M., & Dinges, D. F. (2003). The cumulative cost of additional wakefulness: Dose–response effects on neurobehavioral functions and sleep physiology from chronic sleep restriction and total sleep deprivation. *Sleep, 26*(2), 117–126.

Van Someren, E. J. W., Kessler, A., Mirmiran, M., & Swaab, D. F. (1997). Indirect bright light improves circadian rest-activity rhythm disturbances in demented patients. *Biological Psychiatry, 41*, 955–963.

Von Economo, C. (1930). Sleep as a problem of localization. *Journal of Nervous and Mental Disease, 71*, 249–259.

Walsh, J. K. (2004). Drugs used to treat insomnia in 2002: Regulatory-based rather than evidence-based medicine. *Sleep, 27*, 1441–1442.

Walsh, J. K., Erman, M., Erwin, C. W., Jamieson, A., Mahowald, M., Regestein, Q., et al. (1998). Subjective hypnotic efficacy of trazodone and zolpidem in DSMIII-R primary insomnia. *Human Psychopharmacology, 13*(3), 191–198.

Washington, P. (Ed.) (2004). *Poems of sleep and dreams.* New York: Alfred A. Knopf / Random House, Inc.

Weitzman, E. D., Czeisler, C. A., Coleman, R. M., Spielman, A. J., Zimmerman, J. C., Dement, W., et al. (1981). Delayed sleep phase syndrome. A chronobiological disorder with sleep-onset insomnia. *Archive of General Psychiatry, 38*, 737–746.

Wetterberg, L. (Ed.) (1993). *Light and biological rhythms in man.* Stockholm, Sweden: Pergamon Press.

Whitehead, D. C., Thomas, H., & Slapper, D. R. (1992). A rational approach to shift work in emergency medicine. *Annals of Emergency Medicine, 21*, 1250–1258.

Whitson, P. A., Putcha, L., Chen, Y. M., & Baker, E. (1995). Melatonin and cortisol assessment of circadian shifts in astronauts before flight. *Journal of Pineal Research, 18*, 141–147.

Winson, J. (1990). The meaning of dreams. *Scientific American, 236*, 86–96.

Wright, K. P., Hughes, R. J., Kronauer, R. E., Dijk. D.-J., & Czeisler, C. A. (2001). Intrinsic near-24-hour pacemaker period determines limits of circadian entrainment to a weak synchronizer in humans. *Proceedings of the National Academy of Sciences of the United States of America, 98*, 14027–14032.

Zaidi, F. H., Hull, J. T., Peirson, S. N., Wulff, K., Aeschbach, D., Gooley, J. J., et al. (2007). Short-wavelength light sensitivity of circadian, pupillary, and visual awareness in humans lacking an outer retina. *Current Biology, 17*, 2122–2128.

11

Integrative Approaches to the Management of Chronic Pain

LYNETTE MENEFEE PUJOL AND BETTINA HERBERT

The Problem of Pain

Pain is a common human experience. According to a World Health Organization report, 22% of primary care patients in Asia, Africa, Europe, and the United States described the presence of persistent pain with a duration of at least 6 months that is severe enough to lead to health care consultation, medication use, or impairment of daily functioning (Gureje, Von Korff, Simon, & Gater, 1998). One in ten adults in the United States describes pain lasting a year or more, and one in four describes a pain lasting 1 day in the past month (National Center for Health Statistics, 2006). Sources of chronic pain include back and neck conditions, arthritis, myofacial pain, Complex Regional Pain Syndrome (CRPS), headaches, phantom limb pain, headache, and other conditions. In a recent review, cancer pain was not lower than 14% in any single study and was as high as 100% (Goudas, Bloch, Gialeli-Goudas, Lau, & Carr, 2005). Increasing numbers of survivors of cancer now report chronic pain resulting from cancer treatments such as surgery, radiotherapy, and/or chemotherapy (Alfano & Rowland, 2006; Institute of Medicine of the National Accademy Report, 2006).

Chronic pain results in alarming human and economic costs (Pai & Sundaram, 2004). Take back pain as one example. The annual costs of back pain in the United States range from $20 to $50 billion (Deyo, 1998). Back pain is the leading cause of disability for individuals younger than 45 and is the most expensive health care problem for individuals aged 30–50 (Bigos et al., 1994). It is one of three physical factors that increase disease burden in older Americans (Cooper & Kohlmann, 2001). Further, the risks for back pain and disability are rising with the increase in age and obesity in the U.S. population (Fries & McShane, 1998; Lake, Power, & Cole, 2000).

Individuals with chronic pain are often undertreated. Awareness of undertreatment and the rising need for pain management led the U.S. Congress to name 2001–2010 as the Decade of Pain Control and Research. Additionally, the Joint Commission on Accreditation of Healthcare Organizations (JCAHO) instituted review procedures for physicians that include that pain be considered the fifth vital sign (Gatchel, BoPeng, Peters, Fuchs, & Turk, 2007).

The Biopsychosocial Model and Integrative Medicine

Pain theory and neuroscience have largely dispensed with the idea that pain is in the mind or in the body. Now thought to be an interaction among complex factors that involve the body, mind, and social environment, the biopsychosocial model includes each perspective for chronic pain (Turk & Monarch, 2002). Since multidisciplinary care is the "gold standard" for pain management, this model serves as a useful heuristic in describing the physiological, psychological, and social factors that are a part of the pain experience.

Integrative medicine adds to the understanding and treatment of chronic pain by providing a holistic view of the person with pain, an integrated treatment team approach, and modalities that are complementary or alternative. Complementary and alternative medicine (CAM) modalities have been applied to chronic pain. CAM is "a group of diverse medical and health care systems, practices and products that are not presently considered to be a part of conventional medicine," according to the The National Center for Complementary and Alternative Medicine (NCCAM), a division of the National Institutes of Health (NCCAM, 2002). Complementary medicine is defined as practices used with conventional medicine, such as the use of meditation added to a conventional medical treatment plan for low back pain. Alternative medicine is defined as practices that are used instead of conventional medicine, such as use of herbal preparations for rheumatoid arthritis instead of conventional medications. Major domains of CAM are alternative medicine systems, mind–body interventions, biologically based treatments, manipulative and body-based treatments, and energy therapies.

Grouping treatment modalities into more traditional biopsychosocial modalities and integrative modalities poses some difficulties, since some are dually classified by different authors. Further, some treatments thought of as integrative in the past (e.g., biofeedback and acupuncture) have become more common, perhaps due to the empirical support they have received and/or the positive experiences of clinicians with their efficacy. A spiritual component of coping with pain, often included in integrative approaches to care, is notably absent from the biopsychosocial model.

One of the key difficulties for patients with chronic pain is the loss of control, both over their pain and important aspects of their lives. The overall goal of this chapter is to expand the number of tools available to psychiatrists to provide avenues for regaining perceived higher self-efficacy and self-regulation and to reduce the impact of pain and suffering. In the following sections, selected integrative medicine modalities for the treatment of chronic nonmalignant pain will be reviewed. Modalities were selected primarily because of empirical support, although some reviewed here are promising areas of treatment or research. A few basic concepts of pain medicine, as well as the psychological and psychiatric difficulties encountered by people with pain will be presented.

The Definition of Pain

Pain is defined as "an unpleasant sensory and emotional experience associated with actual or potential tissue damage, or described in terms of such damage" (Merskey and Bugduk, 1994). Pain is generally considered to become chronic when it has persisted over a period of 3 to 6 months, or beyond the time when healing was expected to have occurred (Hadjistavropoulos & Clark, 2001). Chronic pain is often constant, called baseline pain, with intermittent exacerbations, called breakthrough pain.

Patients describe pain using descriptors that relate to physical sensations (e.g., burning, throbbing), emotional consequences (e.g., agonizing, terrifying), and temporal characteristics, (e.g., constant, flaring). At times, they describe pain using graphic images, such as hundreds of needles sticking them repeatedly in a single place or of being burned with a hot poker. People with pain may communicate pain behaviorally, grimacing, wincing, or holding the affected body part. They experience a variety of consequences of pain in their daily lives, including changes in physical, emotional, and social functioning. For survivors of cancer, ongoing pain may evoke existential concerns involving life and death.

Although pain may be defined and described, it is a private experience, different for each individual. This aspect of pain means that believing the patient's report of pain is the best source of information about how it affects him or her, regardless of the clinician's assessment of what should be "normal" pain experience.

How is Pain Perceived?

Research on pain perception has moved the science far from the days when peripheral input was interpreted cortically as pain. The Gate Control Theory (Melzack & Casey, 1968) was proposed as a way to explain the multidimensional aspects of pain, along with the neuroanatomy and physiology. These investigators proposed a "gate" mechanism, located in the dorsal horn of the spinal cord, that weighs input from ascending peripheral neural tracts and from neural tracts descending from the cortex. The resulting modulation leads to pain perception (Melzack & Casey, 1968). This theory accounted for variations in pain experience by proposing the "opening" and "closing" of the gate by various factors, including prior experience with painful sensation, emotion, and cognition. Further refinement of this theory led to the Neuromatrix Theory of Pain (Melzack, 2001, 2005). The neuromatrix is a widely distributed brain neural network, called the "body-self neuromatrix," that involves cognitive-evaluative, sensory-discriminative, and motivational-affective components of pain (Melzack, 2001, 2005). Central to the neuromatrix theory is the idea that homeostatic, behavioral, and perceptual systems are engaged in response to injury and chronic stress.

Long-term changes in dorsal horn neurons have recently been noted. This phenomenon is called neuronal plasticity (Woolf, 2004). The changes in dorsal horn neurons over time may explain exaggerated or prolonged pain to noxious stimuli (hyperalgesia/hyperpathia) and pain experienced from normally innocuous stimuli (allodynia) (Woolf, 2004). These symptoms may be present in neuropathic pain syndromes, such as post herpetic neuralgia, phantom limb pain, or Complex Regional Pain Syndrome-I (formerly known as Reflex Sympathetic Dystrophy). The process of peripheral stimuli causing long-term changes is called "central sensitization" and is an active area of research.

Recently, Chapman, Tuckett, and Woo Song (2008) have proposed a psychophysiological systems view of pain, in which an initial injury generates a complex stress response in an interdependent nervous, endocrine, and immune "supersystem." Responses to injury, in addition to social stressors, are thought to disregulate homeostatic systems of the individual. The authors posit that some chronic pain conditions and multisymptom disorders (e.g., sleep, emotion regulation) are the result of disregulation. Individual variability is explained by interactions of genetic, epigenetic, social, and environmental factors and the past experiences of the person with pain (Chapman, Tuckett, & Woo Song, 2008).

Theories and research on the development of chronic pain and pain perception point to targets for intervention and the consequences of untreated pain. Since pain modulation is affected by modulation from the cortex, psychological and psychosocial experiences become important. Beliefs about pain, past experience with pain, motivation to escape pain, thoughts and emotions, stress and life circumstances combine to "open" or "close" the dorsal horn "gate" and affect the modulation and perception of pain. Inasmuch as psychological and psychosocial factors affect pain perception, they become targets for intervention. In addition, central sensitization, whereby repeated noxious stimuli at the dorsal horn causes hypersensitivity, is reason to treat pain aggressively to alleviate pain and suffering (Miakowski et al., 2005).

Assessment of Pain

A thorough assessment of pain should precede and guide treatment planning. Conventional assessment involves a physical and a detailed musculoskeletal, neurologic, and mental status evaluation (Pujol, Katz, & Zacharoff, 2007). Pain intensity is generally measured in the clinical setting using a Numerical Rating Scale (e.g., Cleeland & Ryan, 1994) ranging from 0 (no pain) to 10 (pain as bad as it can be). Common time points for measurement are the patient's current pain, and the most and least pain experienced during a 1-week period prior to the assessment. The following aspects of the pain experience are important to assess: the frequency and description of pain; patterns of pain; alleviating and exacerbating factors; previous treatments and their efficacy; current treatments and their efficacy; current physical, social, emotional, and occupational functioning; current coping techniques; and expectations for treatment (Menefee, 2005). Standardized instruments for the measurement of pain, mood, and functioning may also supplement the evaluation.

Assessment from an integrative medicine perspective includes standard assessment, as well as a whole person assessment. Some evaluations for integrative modalities are dependent on the treatment for which the person is evaluated. For example, traditional Chinese acupuncture involves a system of belief whereby energy is moved along meridians in the body. Therefore, assessment from this perspective would include an evaluation for blocked energy and a recommendation for its movement.

Psychological & Psychiatric Aspects of Pain Experience

The person with pain will bring his or her whole being to treatment. Traditionally, these perspectives might be defined and described in terms of disease models or diagnostic categories. Integrative medicine focuses on creating resourcefulness and well-being in mind, body, and spirit, and applying a wide range of practices toward these ends. In this section, common psychological and psychiatric difficulties associated with chronic pain are described.

THE ROLE OF NEGATIVE EMOTIONS

Psychological concomitants of chronic pain are well documented in the literature. This should not be surprising given that the definition of pain includes that it is always *unpleasant* and *an emotional experience* (Merskey and Bugduk, 1994). In addition to the constant unpleasant physical and emotional sensations, individuals with chronic pain often undergo dramatic changes in their psychosocial lives. These changes may include significant losses, such as of employment, avocational activities, and significant relationships.

Depressive symptoms and disorders have been documented in 40%–50% of patients with chronic pain conditions (Banks & Kerns, 1996; Dersh, Gatchel, Mayer, Polatin, & Temple, 2006). Whether pain precedes depression or vice versa is a subject of research, with some reviews finding depressive disorders in people with pain after, but not before, the onset of pain (e.g., Brown, 1990; Katz, 2005). However, Jarvik et al. (2005) found that the level of depression predicted back pain 3 years after the initial assessment for depression. In this study, back pain was 2.3 times more likely for patients with depression compared to patients without depression (Jarvik et al., 2005).

Other negative emotions commonly reported by people with pain are anxiety and anger (Gatchel et al., 2007). Anxious reactions to physical symptoms and/or pain-related anxiety can lead to avoidance of activities. Avoidance is then reinforced though reduced pain and physical activity. Over time, avoidance becomes a maladaptive response to pain (McCracken, Gross, Sorg, & Edmands, 1993). Anger has been studied less frequently compared to depression and anxiety, but it is a common clinical complaint. Suppressed anger accounts for significant variance in pain intensity, interference in life activities, and pain behaviors (Kerns, Rosenberg, & Jacob, 1994). Persons with chronic pain are often angry because a "cause" of pain hasn't been found, and/or that pain treatment has not alleviated or resolved painful sensations. Additionally, patients may express anger toward insurance companies, significant others, treatment providers, employers, and attorneys (Okifuji, Turk, & Curran, 1999).

THE ROLE OF COGNITIONS

The role of cognitions in chronic pain has been widely studied. Gatchel et al. (2007) reviewed several of the most studied cognitive factors, including appraisal and belief, catastrophizing and fear-avoidance, and perceived control and self-efficacy. Beliefs about pain can impact affective and behavioral responses. Beliefs of pain as something to be avoided—as a signal of damage, as uncontrollable, and a permanent condition—are associated with poor outcomes (Jensen, Turner, Romano, & Lawler, 1994; Turner, 2000).

Catastrophizing is an exaggerated negative reaction to pain, such as, "This pain is horrible. I can't stand it. It will never go away." Catastrophizing is positively related to depressive symptoms, and is associated with increased pain

(Bishop & Warr, 2003), decreased physical functioning (Bishop & Warr, 2003), risk of death by suicide (Tang & Crane, 2006), and interpersonal distress (Lackner & Gurtman, 2004). Physiologic markers, such as cortical responses to pain (Seminowicz & Davis, 2006) and inflammatory disease activity (Edwards, Bingham, Bathon, & Haythornthwaite, 2006), may also be related to catastrophizing.

Perceived control and self-efficacy refer to the degree to which painful stimuli (e.g., pain frequency, duration, intensity, and unpleasantness) can be controlled and the degree to which an individual believes in his or her ability to exert such control (Gatchel et al., 2007). Improvements in self-efficacy following self-management interventions and cognitive-behavioral therapy are associated with reduced pain and increases in functional and psychological status (Keefe, Rumble, Scipio, Giordano, & Perri, 2004).

THE ROLE OF PERSONALITY

Similar to any medical condition, chronic pain is present in some proportion of individuals with psychiatric disorders. Persons with chronic pain are most often diagnosed with depression, anxiety, and substance-use disorders (Dersh, Polatin, & Gatchel, 2002). However, the prevalence of personality disorders in patients with chronic pain is higher than that of other medical populations, ranging between 31% and 59% (Weisberg, Vittengl, Clark, Gatchel, & Gorin, 2000). The diathesis-stress model was proposed as one mechanism by which these percentages are higher than those in the general population (Paris, 1998). That is, the stress of an ongoing aversive sensation may activate an underlying vulnerability and lead to the development of maladaptive personality patterns.

Individuals with pain may be labeled "somatizers" or "drug-seekers" by practitioners who may not know or regularly apply formal diagnostic criteria for these terms. Among the criteria for somatization disorder are multiple somatic symptoms, lasting over significant periods of time, which occurred starting before age 30 and cause significant social or occupational distress. Unexplained somatic symptoms may be present in people with chronic pain, but somatization disorder is rare (Sullivan & Turk, 2001). Undifferentiated somatoform disorder requires one or more physical complaints that cannot be explained by a general medical condition. Keep in mind that diagnostic testing for chronic pain is limited and "objective" radiologic evidence may or may not be evident. Additionally, "drug-seeking" may have a variety of meanings, including that the person's quite legitimate pain condition is not being adequately controlled by the medicine and other interventions designed to treat it.

Careful assessment of persons with pain should be made prior to diagnosis of a personality disorder or psychiatric difficulty. Avoiding dualism (e.g., pain is in the mind or in the body) is a first step toward assessing individuals with chronic pain conditions (Pujol, Katz, & Zacharoff, 2007). The experience of pain is distressing, and some emotional or behavioral expressions may be a "cry for help" versus the manifestation of a psychiatric disorder. Additionally, cultural considerations concerning the expression of pain should be considered in the assessment of individuals with pain, since overt expressions of pain and distress are more common in some cultures than others.

Mind–Body Interventions

Mind–body interventions are probably best known and most used by psychiatrists. In addition to more conventional therapies, integrative approaches that may be considered as a part of the treatment plan are reviewed.

PSYCHOPHYSIOLOGIC INTERVENTIONS

Diaphragmatic breathing, progressive and autogenic relaxation, and biofeedback are modalities that involve helping the patient become aware of the ability to exert control over physiologic processes of which they are not normally aware (e.g., skin temperature, muscle tension, respiration). Progressive muscle relaxation involves tensing and relaxing various muscle groups (Jacobson, 1974). Autogenic relaxation involves sensing tension or tightness in various muscle groups and mentally "letting go" of the tension while engaging in diaphragmatic breathing. Biofeedback uses a device or computer to give information about these functions. Psychophysiologic interventions are critical for patients with pain, since patients tend to hold muscles tight around the pain site, bracing against painful sensations. This bracing produces increased muscle tension and pain. These techniques can also aid in sleep and reducing emotional reactivity. Outcomes for relaxation and biofeedback are generally positive for patients with chronic pain conditions. A recent review of relaxation strategies for acute and chronic pain found a significant, positive effect on pain in 8 of 15 studies reviewed (Kwekkeboom & Gretasdottir, 2006). A dose–response relationship occurred, with more studies showing effectiveness when relaxation was taught and practiced over several sessions (Kwekkeboom & Gretasdottir, 2006). When combined with relaxation training, individuals with migraine and or tension-type headaches show a 50%–55% success rate in reducing pain (Arena & Blanchard, 2001). A review of mind–body therapies found that relaxation and thermal biofeedback are effective for recurrent migraine headaches and relaxation and electromyography biofeedback are effective for recurrent tension headache (Astin, 2004). Other reviews of randomized controlled trials found biofeedback and relaxation effective for chronic low back pain, headache, and rheumatologic pain (NIH, 1996).

GUIDED IMAGERY

Guided imagery may be paired with diaphragmatic breathing and/or autogenic relaxation techniques. Imagery may be distracting in nature (e.g., a beach or meadow); focused (e.g., imagining white blood cells destroying cancer cells); or as a form of mental rehearsal (e.g., performing physical therapy exercises) (Barrows & Jacobs, 2002; Monroe & Greco, 2007). In a meta-analytic review, imagery techniques were shown to be helpful in reducing painful sensations and had the highest rates of efficacy among 12 placebo-controlled trials of other cognitive interventions (Fernandaz & Turk, 1989). Guided imagery studies with older adults show good preliminary results when paired with relaxation (Baird & Sands, 2004) or alone (Lewandowski, 2004).

HYPNOSIS

Hypnosis is defined as "a state of inner absorption, concentration and focused attention" by the American Society of Clinical Hypnosis. Hypnosis for pain generally involves the suggestion of pain reduction, but may also involve a variety of positive outcomes (e.g., increased activity). A National Institutes of Health Technology Panel found strong support for hypnosis in the reduction of pain (NIH, 1996). Hypnosis has been found to improve recovery time after surgery when it is learned and performed preoperatively and to improve postsurgical pain (Astin, 2004). A review and a meta-analysis found that hypnosis was an effective analgesic for many types of experimental and clinical pain conditions (Montgomery, Duhamel, & Redd, 2000), including chronic pain from headache, cancer, fibromyalgia, osteoarthritis, low back pain, tempromandibular pain disorder, disability-related pain, and mixed chronic pain problems (Jensen & Patterson, 2006). When hypnosis was compared with relaxation therapy for osteoarthritis, both groups improved, but the hypnosis group was the only one that maintained improvement at 3 months (Gay, Philippot, and Luminet, 2002). No differences were found at the 6-month mark.

MINDFULNESS MEDITATION

Mindfulness meditation involves paying attention to the present moment with a nonjudgmental attitude and fosters disengagement from strong attachments to thoughts and emotions (Ludwig & Kabet-Zinn, 2008). Mindfulness meditation has been studied as a part of the Mindfulness-Based Stress Reduction (MBSR) program, an 8-week group that teaches the technique. MBSR has been found to be helpful for patients with a variety of chronic pain conditions (Kabat-Zinn, Lipworth, & Burney, 1985), with a 4-year follow-up showing pain improvement in 60%–72% of participants (Kabat-Zinn, Lipworth, & Burney, 1987). Two reviews of MBSR found that MBSR has positive outcomes in stress, anxiety, depression, and pain (Baer, 2003; Grossman Neimann, Schmidt, and Walach, 2004). MBSR was recently studied for a group of older adults with chronic low back pain. Compared to a wait-list control group, participants in the 8-week program had significant improvement in pain acceptance and in physical functioning, although the groups did not differ in pain ratings (Monroe, Greco, & Weiner, 2008).

Mindfulness-Based Art Therapy (MBAT) is a relatively new intervention that combines MBSR with art therapy. This program has been shown to be successful with women with breast cancer in decreasing psychological distress and enhancing quality of life (Monti & Peterson, 2004; Monti et al., 2006). Although no studies to date have implemented MBAT for persons with chronic pain, this therapy remains a promising one for this population.

SPIRITUAL APPROACHES

Faith-based practices may be an important source of social support and coping for patients with chronic pain. Surveys of the literature on religious and spiritual practices found that prayer was either the first or second most used coping strategy to deal with physical pain (Koenig, 2001; Rippentrop, 2005). Positive associations between prayer and pain were found in four of six cross sectional studies surveyed by Koenig (2001), indicating that prayer was used during exacerbations of pain. A 30-day diary study with patients with rheumatoid arthritis found that coping efficacy, positive mood, and higher levels of emotional and social support were found on days participants endorsed the ability to control pain using positive religious or spiritual coping (Keefe et al., 2001). Survivors of cancer may have questions about the afterlife that are best directed to a leader of their faith practice (Pujol et al., 2007). Although physicians may not understand the patient's faith beliefs, seeking to understand how they affect the patient's understanding of pain and meaning in life is important.

Few studies have focused on spiritual or religious beliefs and chronic pain. One recent study investigated positive spiritual practices (e.g., seeking spiritual support from a higher power, problem solving with God, helping others) and negative spiritual coping (e.g., feeling abandoned by God, blaming God for difficulties) (Rippentrop, Altmaier, Chen, Found, & Keffala, 2005). These investigators found that for patients in an orthopedic practice: (1) poorer physical health was related to private spiritual practices; (2) pain duration was associated with less forgiveness and less support from a religious or spiritual community; (3) poorer mental health was related to lack of forgiveness, feeling punished, and abandoned by God, lack of daily spiritual experiences, little support from a religious community, and not being religious or spiritual; and (4) pain and interference due to pain were not related to higher levels of religion or spirituality (Rippentrop et al., 2005). The authors hypothesized that individuals who are doing the worst physically may be more likely to turn to private religious activities to cope with pain. Alternatively, increased negative religious coping may be an impediment to healthy emotional functioning (Rippentrop et al., 2005).

The experience of chronic pain may bring individuals in closer touch with their faith, providing comfort, or alternatively, lead to demoralization and negative attributions toward religion. A recent review suggests three ways that religion and spiritual beliefs might be effective for people with pain (Wachholtz, Pearce, and Koenig, 2007). One is through the modeling of positive historical religious or spiritual figures (e.g., Jesus, prophets, Buddha), who may form a basis on which to frame the experience of pain. The second is by increasing one's feelings of self control and self-efficacy through religious and spiritual coping. The third is that daily spiritual practices (e.g., prayer, meditation, reading spiritual texts) may serve as a distraction from pain (Wachholtz et al., 2007).

COGNITIVE BEHAVIORAL THERAPY

Cognitive Behavioral Therapy (CBT) is the term used to describe a broad array of cognitive and behavioral techniques that derive from different therapeutic models. Cognitive Therapy (Beck, 1976) posits that automatic thoughts, underlying dysfunctional assumptions, cognitive distortions, and emotion interact in a reinforcing cycle that leads to psychopathology (Freeman, Pretzer, Fleming, & Simon, 1990). These thoughts influence mood and behavior. For example, a person with pain might wake up noticing increased pain. An automatic thought might be, "It's going to be a bad pain day." This thought can lead to negative mood and increasingly negative cognitions, such as, "I'm going to have to cancel everything today. I can't do anything any more." The cycle perpetuates increased negative emotion and potentially maladaptive behavior (e.g., staying in bed all day).

Behavioral treatment methods for pain grew from operant research. Fordyce (1976) described the application to pain, focusing on pain behaviors, such as guarding, limping, taking medication, and resting. Fordyce (1976) posited that contingencies in the environment maintained pain behaviors, and that changing reinforcement would change attention to painful experiences. For example, an overly solicitous spouse might be taught to give less attention to pain behaviors and more attention to times of increased physical activity, thereby decreasing the frequency of pain behavior and increasing the frequency of more adaptive strategies.

A number of cognitive and behavioral strategies are combined in CBT. Behavioral strategies, such as helping a patient learn to pace activities and teaching relaxation techniques, are common. Numerous studies have found CBT effective for patients with chronic pain. A meta-analysis of 25 randomized controlled trials of CBT compared to wait-list control conditions found improved pain, mood, coping, pain behavior, and social interactions. When compared to alternative treatments, CBT participants had greater improvements in pain, coping, and pain behavior (Morley, Eccleston, and Williams, 1999).

CBT with patients with pain conditions is an active therapy that is generally short term (usually 6–12 weeks). It has demonstrated effectiveness with pain, as well as with depression and anxiety, both of which may affect people with pain. Patients are expected to be active participants in therapy and are often assigned "homework" to facilitate accomplishing therapeutic goals (Freeman et al., 1990). Therapeutic goals might be reducing pain, depression, anxiety or stress, and/or increasing daily activity, sleep, pain-coping skills, and purpose in life. Difficulties in relationships caused by changes brought on by pain may also be the focus of intervention. Identifying and changing maladaptive thoughts, emotions, and behaviors are central to the process of change in CBT.

CONTEXTUAL COGNITIVE BEHAVIORAL THERAPY

A newer approach to working with patients with pain is Contextual Cognitive Behavioral Therapy (CCBT; McCracken, 2005). The therapy addresses a criticism of CBT, namely that thinking about thoughts or physical sensations and trying not to focus on them only makes them stronger. Avoidance is conceptualized as potentially helpful in the short-term, but ultimately ineffective. A common application for people with pain conditions is physical exercise or activity; that is, avoiding activity can reduce painful sensations and reinforce inactivity, ultimately producing a maladaptive response to painful sensations.

CCBT aims to help patients with pain by moving away from attempts to manage or control pain and toward acceptance of the present reality of thoughts, emotions, behaviors, and physical sensations. First steps involve helping the person review historical efforts to control or manage painful sensations. Awareness of responses by significant others is also discussed. Mindful awareness and exercises that introduce the concept of noticing in the present moment are central to the process of defusing cognitions (McCracken, 2005). Through the course of therapy, patients practice experiencing emotions without need for a response. Additionally, the therapy includes a values-based action component in which the person with pain clarifies his or her values and begins to make value-based life choices (McCracken, 2005).

PAIN-COPING STRATEGIES

There is a large literature on the use of pain-coping strategies, which are assessed by several coping measures. Some ways of coping with pain are guarding the affected painful part, resting, taking medication, ignoring painful sensations, using coping self-statements (e.g., "I can handle the pain"), praying and hoping the pain will be better, increasing activities, diverting attention from the pain, and catastrophizing. Coping has been linked to some pain treatment outcomes, but not strongly to others, such as exercise (Jensen, Turner, & Romano, 2001). A recent follow-up study compared scores on coping and belief measures at posttreatment, and 1 year following treatment in a multidisciplinary pain treatment program. The investigators found that increasing disability and depression at follow-up was positively associated with increased use of resting, guarding, and asking for assistance, catastrophizing, and the belief that one is disabled by pain (Jensen, Turner, & Romano, 2007).

Body-Mind Therapies

The Platonic-Cartesian mind–body duality model, with separate specialties to treat one entity, has shaped the biomedical profession. Most mental health professionals do not touch their patients, and most physical medicine specialists, such as osteopathic physicians, chiropractors, physical therapists, and other hands-on care providers do not provide counseling. The patient must know enough to consult both, separately, for what is essentially a unified issue. In day-to-day practice, the two specialists often do not confer or collaborate, even though it is now well-known that pain is a physical and psychological event, as reviewed above. Within the integrative model, mind and body are inseparable, which is why addressing psychological distress is almost universal to any integrative medicine treatment plan. In regard to pain issues, there are therapeutic approaches under the umbrella of CAM that address body and mind primarily through manual manipulation of the physical structure; i.e., manipulative and body-based therapies, and we review a few that have particular relevance to integrative medicine.

OSTEOPATHIC MANIPULATIVE TREATMENT

For patients with one or multiple chronic neuromusculoskeletal or visceral conditions (osteoarthritis, cervicalgia, osteoporosis, low back pain, irritable bowel syndrome, neurodegenerative disease), consulting an osteopathic physician trained in osteopathic manipulative treatment (OMT) may be a useful approach. In the United States, but not in Canada or Great Britain, osteopaths (DOs) have the same medical training as allopaths (MDs) with an additional emphasis on anatomical structure, physiology, and manipulation. There are some philosophical distinctions; for example, osteopathy contends that a body's structure affects its function, and, given proper alignment, the body will heal itself as much as possible. Good body biomechanics is integral to maintaining health. It is noted that OMT is not a component of many osteopathic physician practices, most of which now resemble allopathy more than classic osteopathic practice.

The emotional component of pain is part of osteopathic philosophy, and some manipulative techniques may produce cathartic emotional releases (Kuchera, 2007). OMT provides many soft tissue (fascial) techniques that aim to effect changes that may be deep and long lasting. Manipulation, as part of a whole treatment approach, may be delivered either directly, up to and through tissue or joint restriction, or indirectly, following the direction of ease. The latter approach gradually allows the body (fascia, joint, muscle, bone, organ, spine) to release. Some of the most frequently used techniques include the following:

- Myofascial release–a technique designed that uses continual palpatory feedback to release myofascial tissues (ECOP, 2006)
- Strain/ counterstrain–a system of diagnosis and indirect treatment in which somatic dysfunction is associated with a myofascial tenderpoint and treated by use of a passive position (ECOP, 2006)
- Cranial osteopathy/ craniosacral therapy–a system of diagnosis and treatment that involves the primary respiratory system and balanced membranous tension

- Visceral manipulation–a technique for releasing restrictions and adhesions in fascia suspending specific organs
- Positional release–a technique that uses leverage, ventilatory movement, and a fulcrum to mobilize a dysfunctional segment (ECOP, 2006)
- Functional technique–an indirect treatment that involves finding a dynamic balance point and applying a force, holding the postion or adding compression to allow for readjustment (ECOP, 2006)
- High velocity low amplitude (thrust)–taking a joint up to its functional barrier and adding a slight force to restore range of motion (ECOP, 2006)

Osteopathic manipulative treatment has been found to be a useful modality for chronic pain. Three randomized trials of OMT have been conducted in the United States for individuals with chronic low back pain (Andersson et al., 1999; Hoehler, Tobis, & Buerger, 1981; Licciardone et al., 2003). Control groups generally received sham manipulation (e.g., Hoehler et al., 1981; Licciardone et al., 2003) or usual care (e.g., Andersson et al., 1999). Licciardone (2004) made three generalizations about these studies: (1) OMT appeared to reduce the use of other treatment modalities, such as medication and physical therapy; (2) OMT appeared more effective when compared to no-intervention controls and compared to sham manipulation control groups; and (3) clinical relevance of OMT may have been attenuated in these studies due to the relatively small number of subjects.

MASSAGE

Therapeutic massage has been found to decrease pain, improve sleep, reduce muscle tension, and provide a sense of relaxation (Field, 1998). Massage can soften musculature and increase blood flow, promote restful sleep, release endorphins, and affect levels of catecholamines (Monti & Yang, 2005). It is especially effective for pain relief when combined with exercise or physical therapy.

Massage has been tested in several randomized clinical trials, but all suffer from methodologic weaknesses (Ernst, 2000, 2004). A pilot study comparing Mindfulness-Based Stress Reduction or massage therapy to a standard care group for musculoskeletal pain found reduced pain unpleasantness and increased mental health status at 8 weeks (Plews-Ogan, Owens, Goodman, Wolfe, & Schorling, 2005). Improved longer-term mental health status was found with MBSR compared to standard care. The authors concluded that massage was more effective at pain reduction and MBSR was more effective than massage in mood improvement (Plews-Ogan et al., 2005).

Contraindications for massage include deep vein thrombosis, burns, skin infections, eczema, open wounds, bone fractures, and advanced osteoporosis.

POSTURAL/MOVEMENT RE-EDUCATION THERAPIES

Western movement approaches are often utilized by patients with chronic pain. Many share the therapeutic combination of passive therapy and active integration of that therapy using group classes, verbal cues, and gentle home exercises. Only a few of the more commonly used ones will be discussed here.

The Feldenkrais Method consists of a large variety of very gentle, simple exercises to develop new movement habits that are pain-free. The work consists of two parts: group movement lessons (Awareness Through Movement) and individual, hands-on sessions. Limited studies of the Feldenkrais Method suggest that it may be useful for anxiety, neck and shoulder pain, and both disability and anxiety in multiple sclerosis patients (Lunblad, 1999).

The Alexander Technique, often used for chronic back and neck pain, uses verbal instructions and light touch to guide the patient to improve postural habits. Clinical trials are promising and small studies have also suggested benefits for reduction of both stress and chronic pain, enhanced relaxation as well as enhanced respiratory function (Ernst, 2003).

The Trager Psychophysical Integration approach also combines tablework and simple movement practices to release accumulated tension and help the patient learn ways of moving freely. Tablework consists of gentle movements to release restrictive holding patterns that create pain. Using "Mentastics," patients are taught to recreate the feelings of relaxation that they felt during the sessions. A recent study on the combination of the Trager Approach and acupuncture found that the treatment was effective in reducing shoulder pain in spinal cord injury patients (Dyson-Hudson, 2001). It may also be effective in other musculoskeletal problems.

The Hellerwork practitioner, again, uses hands-on soft tissue manipulation techniques and educates the client about how to sit, stand, and walk in a more relaxed and comfortable way. Dysfunctional muscular holding patterns and diminished breathing may be addressed using therapeutic dialogue to address any emotional contribution.

YOGA

Yoga is part of Ayurveda, an ancient medical system developed in India, that addresses the physical, mental, and spiritual aspects of the individual. There are many different forms of yoga practice, each of which emphasizes different skills, goals, and philosophies. For someone with pain, a very gentle type is recommended. Postures may be adjusted to meet the needs and physical conditions of the student. Therapeutic yoga is the performance of postures for treating medical disorders (Raub, 2002).

Though preliminary, there are a few studies that suggest useful applications of therapeutic yoga practice for low back pain (Sherman, 2005) and osteoarthritis of the knee (Kolasinski, 2005). Another pilot study in breast cancer patients notes improvements in affect and quality of life (Moadel, 2007) that indirectly influence the perception of pain. As such, it may be useful to consider it as part of an integrated approach.

NUTRITION

Nutrition is a cornerstone of wellness and is utilized in integrative approaches to chronic conditions. The daily diet of Americans is deficient in fruit and vegetable consumption and excessive in meat, refined grain products, and desserts (Seaman, 2002). It is proposed that the results of this diet cause a biochemical reaction which creates a diet-induced proinflammatory state (Seaman, 2002) and may contribute to inflammatory pain. Premature and accelerated atherosclerosis, thought to be related to chronic inflammation, has been found in patients with rheumatoid arthritis, increasing morbidity and mortality (Naranjo et al., 2008).

Several nutrient groups have been identified and validated as anti-inflammatory (Goldberg, 2007). Perhaps the best known is omega-3 fatty acids. Foods containing high levels of the anti-inflammatory omega-3 fatty acids include cold water oily fish such as wild caught salmon, herring, mackerel, and sardines as well as krill, walnuts, flax seeds, soybeans, seeds and nuts, and some dark green leafy vegetables. There is also evidence to support the anti-inflammatory effects of other foods, such as green and white teas, extra virgin olive oil, and many phytonutrients. A gluten-free vegan diet has been shown to reduce LDL and oxidized LDL and raise atheroprotective natural antibodies against phosphorylcholine in patients with rheumatoid arthritis (Elkan et al., 2008).

Dietary examination may be useful in pain conditions where there is an inflammatory component, including joint pain, headaches, low back pain, and neuroinflammation. An integrative nutritionist will help a patient identify what foods might exacerbate symptoms and which could be added to a diet that would, over time, act to quell some of the inflammation. Some patients may wish to try a food elimination diet, followed by food challenge (Drisko, 2006). Keeping a food and symptom diary is often an illuminating first step.

SUPPLEMENTS

The use of dietary supplements among individuals with chronic pain has risen dramatically as the popularity of other CAM interventions has grown (Cauffield, 2000; Fleming, Rabago, Mundt, & Fleming, 2007). Patients are generally reluctant to report taking herbal preparations and/or supplements to their doctors, even though research finds physicians more open than anticipated by patients (Cauffield, 2000).

A Cochrane Systematic Database review of herbal medicine for nonspecific low back pain (Gagnier, van Tulder, Berman, & Bombardier, 2008) found strong evidence for Harpagophytum Procumbens (Devil's Claw), with a daily dose of 50 mg or 100 mg to be better than placebo for short-term improvements in pain and rescue medications (Chrubasik, 1999). Another high quality trial reviewed found Harpagophytum Procumbens to be equivalent to 12.5 mg per day dose of rofecoxib (Vioxx: Chrubasik, Model, Black, & Pollak, 2003). Moderate evidence was found for Salix Alba (White Willow Bark) at daily doses of 120 mg or 240 mg compared to placebo for short-term improvements in pain and rescue medication, and for Capsicum Frutescens (Cayenne) compared to placebo and other topical preparations (Gagnier et al., 2008).

As many as one third of patients with osteoarthritis (OA) have used a supplement as a part of their treatment. Glucosamine sulfate has been shown to reduce symptoms and possibly slow disease progression (Bruyere & Reginster, 2007). Preliminary evidence shows chondroitin sulfate produces symptomatic relief and, possibly, structure-modifying effects, but it does not appear to have a significant benefit over that of glucosamine sulfate (Bruyere & Reginster, 2007; Gregory, Sperry, & Wilson, 2007). S-adenosylmethionine (SAMe) also decreases pain in osteoarthritis (Gregory et al., 2007). In addition to these, avocado soybean unsaponifiables show beneficial effects in OA according to a Cochrane systematic review (Little, Parsons, & Logan, 2008).

Most studies of nutraceuticals are performed with small numbers of subjects with standardized preparations, as opposed to those available over-the-counter (Clayton, 2007). More well-designed, prospective studies are necessary to determine the safety and efficacy of a variety of nutraceuticals. Still, some reasonable evidence exists for some of these compounds.

Energy Therapies

ACUPUNCTURE

One of the most studied CAM modalities for pain is acupuncture. Acupuncture is an ancient Chinese practice and philosophy that involves the movement of life force, qi (pronounced "chee"), around meridians of the body. Disease or dysfunction is thought to result from a disturbance of the flow of energy. Acupuncture involves the insertion of small-gauge needles at various places on the body (e.g., ear, muscles) to rebalance qi.

Evidence for the efficacy of acupuncture for pain is strong for postoperative pain (National Institutes of Health, 1998). A meta-analysis found efficacy of acupuncture for low back pain over sham acupuncture and no additional treatment (Manheimer, White, Berman, Forys, & Ernst, 2005). Acupuncture has also been found effective for neck pain (He, Veirsted, Hostmark, & Medbo, 2004); back pain (Manheimer et al., 2005; Weidenhammer, Linde, Streng, Hoppe, & Melchart, 2007); headache (Melchart, 2006); knee osteoarthritis (Manheimer et al., 2005); migraine (Vickers et al., 2004); and fibromyalgia (Deluze, Bosia, Zirbs, Chantraine, & Vischer, 1992; Targino, Imamura, Kaziyama, et al., 2002). However, Staud (2007) points out that many of these trials have not been replicated.

The quality of randomized controlled trials has been questioned. In a study of more than 50 such trials, two-thirds received low scores for quality (Ezzo et al., 2000). Part of the difficulty of conducting trials is that "sham" control groups do consistently better than inert placebo groups (Ezzo et al., 2000). Although the evidence for low back pain and OA of the knee are relatively strong, more research is needed to evaluate the effect of acupuncture for other pain conditions (Staud, 2007).

TAI CHI AND QI GONG

Both Tai Chi and Qi Gong are gentle movement practices that have been used for centuries in China. In addition to creating better balance with gentle exercise, they reduce stress and help relieve tension headaches (Abbott, 2007). When combined with education and relaxation training, they have also been shown to be effective for fibromyalgia (Chen, 2006), chronic low back pain (Gallagher, 2003), and osteoarthritis (Song, 2003).

PULSED ELECTROMAGNETIC THERAPY

Pulsed Electromagnetic Therapy ("PEMF") has been used for many years to aid in healing fractures. More recent data suggest pain reduction in rheumatoid arthritis, fibromyalgia (Shupack, 2006), and cervical and knee osteoarthritis (Hulme, 2007; Pepitone, 2001).

Summary

Chronic pain is a relentless, multifaceted condition that affects people physically, emotionally, psychologically, psychosocially, and spiritually. Multidisciplinary treatment is the gold standard for pain management. Integrative medicine provides additional perspectives to standard treatment and a whole person approach. Knowledge of the large array of treatment options, both conventional and complementary, may help reduce the suffering of people with chronic pain. An integrative medicine approach can expand treatment options and thereby facilitate the common goals of practitioner and patient—to lessen suffering, rekindle hope, and offer the opportunity for a more fulfilling life.

REFERENCES

Abbott, R., Hui, K., Hays, R., Li, M., Pan, T. (2007). A randomized controlled trial of Tai Chi for tension headaches. *Evidence-Based Complementary and Alternative Medicine*, 4(1), 107–113.

Alfano, C. M., & Rowland, J. H. (2006). Recovery issues in cancer survivorship: A new challenge for supportive care. *The Cancer Journal*, 12, 432–443.

American Society of Clinical Hypnosis. Definition of hypnosis. Available at: http://asch. net/genpubinfo.htm. Accessed February 22, 2008.

Andersson, G. B., Lucente, T., Davis, A. M., Kappler, R. E., Lipton, J. A., & Leurgans, S. (1999). A comparison of osteopathic spinal manipulation with standard of care for patients with low back pain. *New England Journal of Medicine*, 341, 1426–1431.

Arena, J. G., & Blanchard, E. (2001). Biofeedback therapy for chronic pain. In J. D. Loser, S. H. Butler, C. R. Chapman, & D. C. Turk (Eds.), *Bonica's management of pain* (3rd edn). Philadelphia, PA: Lippincott, Williams, & Wilkins, pp. 1759–1767.

Assendelft, W., Morton, S., Yu, E., Suttorp, M., & Shekelle, P. (2007). Spinal manipulative therapy for low-back pain. *EBM Reviews—Cochrane Database of Systematic Reviews*, 4.

Astin, J. A. (2004). Mind–body therapies for the management of pain. *Clinical Journal of Pain, 20*, 27–32.

Baer, R. A. (2003). Mindfulness training as a clinical intervention: A conceptual and empirical review. *Clinical Psychology Science and Practice, 10*, 125–143.

Baird, C. L., & Sands, L. (2004). A pilot study of the effectiveness of guided imagery with progressive muscle relaxation to reduce chronic pain and mobility difficulties of osteoarthritis. *Pain Management Nursing, 5*, 94–104.

Banks, S. M., & Kerns, R. D. (1996). Explaining high rates of depression in chronic pain: A diathesis-stress framework. *Psychological Bulletin, 119*, 95–110.

Barrows, K. A., & Jacobs, B. P. (2002). Mind–body medicine: An introduction and review of the literature. *Medical Clinics of North America, 86*, 1–15.

Beck, A. T. (1976). *Cognitive therapy and the emotional disorders.* New York: International Universities Press.

Berbert, A., Kondo, C., Almendra, L., Matsuo, T., & Dichi, I. (2005). Supplementation of fish oil and olive oil in patients with rheumatoid arthritis. *Nutrition, 21*(2), 131–136.

Bigos, S. J., Bowuer, O. R., Braen, G. R., Brown, K., Deyo, R., Haldemann, S., et al. (1994). Acute low back problems in adults. Clinical practice guideline no. 14 (AHCPR publication no. 95-0642). Rockville, MD: U.S. Department of Health and Human Services, Public Health Service, Agency for Health Care Policy and Research.

Bishop, S. R., & Warr, D. (2003). Coping, catastrophizing and chronic pain in breast cancer. *Journal of Behavioral Medicine, 26*, 265–281.

Brown, G. K. (1990). A casual analysis of chronic pain and depression. *Journal of Abnormal Psychology, 99*, 127–137.

Bruyere, O., & Reginster, J. Y. (2007). Glucosamine and condroitin sulfate as therapeutic agents for knee and hip osteoarthritis. *Drugs and Aging, 24*(7), 573–580.

Cauffield, J. S. (2000). The psychosocial aspects of complementary and alternative medicine. *Pharmacotherapy, 20*(11), 1289–1294.

Chapman, C. R., Tuckett, R. P., & Woo Song, C. (2008). Pain and stress in a systems perspective: Reciprocal neural, endocrine and immune interactions. *Journal of Pain, 9*(2), 122–145.

Chen, K., Hassett, A., Hou, F., Staller, J., & Lichtbroun, A. (2006). A pilot study of external Qigong therapy for patients with fibromyalgia. *Journal of Alternative Complementary Medicine, 12*(9), 851–856.

Chrubasik, S., Junck, H., Breitschwerdt, H., Conradt, C., & Zappe, H. (1999). Effectiveness of Harpagophytum extract WS 1531 in the treatment of exacerbation of low back pain: A randomized, placebo-controlled, double-blind study. *European Journal of Anaesthesiology, 16*, 118–129.

Chrubasik, S., Model, A., Black, A., & Pollak, S. (2003). A randomized double-blind pilot study comparing Doloteffin and Vioxx in the treatment of low back pain. *Rheumatology, 42*, 141–148.

Clayton, J. J. (2007). Nutraceuticals in the management of osteoarthritis. *Orthopedics, 30*(8), 624–629.

Cleeland, C. S., & Ryan, K. M. (1994). Pain assessment: Global use of the brief pain inventory. *Annals of the Academy of Medicine, 23*, 129–138.

Cooper, J. K., & Kohlmann T. (2001). Factors associated with health status of older Americans. *Age and Ageing, 30,* 495–501.

Deluze, C., Bosia, L., Zirbs, A., Chantraine, A., & Vischer, T. L. (1992). Electroacupuncture in fibromyalgia: results of a controlled trial. *British Medical Journal, 305,* 1249–1252.

Dersh, J., Gatchel, R. J., Mayer, T. G., Polatin, P. B., & Temple, O. W. (2006). Prevalence of psychiatric disorders in patients with chronic disabling occupational spinal disorders. *Spine, 31,* 1156–1162.

Dersh, J., Polatin, P., & Gatchel, R. (2002). Chronic pain and psychopathology: Research findings and theoretical considerations. *Psychosomatic Medicine, 64,* 773–786.

Deyo, R. A. (1998). Low-back pain. *Scientific American, 279,* 48–53.

Drisko, J., Bischoff, B., Hall, M., & McCallum, R. (2006). Treating irritable bowel syndrome with a food elimination diet followed by food challenge and probiotics. *Journal of the American College of Nutrition, 6,* 514–522.

Dyson-Hudson, T., Shiflett, S., Kirshblum, S., Bowen, J., & Druin, E. (2001). Acupuncture and trager psychophysical integration in the treatment of wheelchair user's shoulder pain in individuals with spinal cord injury. *Archives of Physical Medicine, 82*(8), 1038–1046.

Educational Council on Osteopathic Principles and the American Association of Colleges of Osteopathic Medicine. (2006). *Glossary of Osteopathic Terminology Usage Guide,* 11–13. http://www.aacom.org/people/councils/Documents/OsteopathicTerminologyGlossary.pdf .

Edwards, R. R., Bingham, C. O., III, Bathon, J., & Haythornthwaite, J. A. (2006). Catastrophizing and pain in arthritis, fibromyalgia, and other rheumatic diseases. *Archives and Rheumatism, 55,* 325–332.

Elkan A.C., Sjoberg, B., Kolsrud, B., Hafstrom, I., & Frostegard, J. (2008). Gluten-free vegan diet induces decreased LDL and oxidized LDL levels and raised atheroprotective natural antibodies against phosphorylcholine in patients with rheumatoid arthritis: A randomized study. *Arthritis Research and Therapy, 10,* R34 (doi:10.1186/ar2388).

Ernst, E. (2004).Musculoskeletal conditions and complementary/alternative medicine. *Best Practice & Research in Clinical Rheumatology, 18*(4), 539–556.

Ernst, E., & Canter, P. (2003). The Alexander technique: A systematic review of controlled clinical trials. *Forsch Komplementarmed Research in Complementary and Classical Natural Medicine, 10,* 325–329.

Ezzo, J., Berman, B., Hadhazy, V. A., Jadad, A. R., Lao, L., & Singh, B. B. (2000). Is acupuncture effective for the treatment of chronic pain? A systematic review. *Pain, 86,* 217–225.

Fernandez, E., & Turk, D. (1989). The utility of cognitive coping strategies for altering pain perception: A meta-analysis. *Pain, 38,* 123–135.

Field, T. M. (1998). Massage therapy effects. *American Psychologist, 53,* 1270–1281.

Fleming, S., Rabago, D. P., Mundt, M. P., Fleming, M. F. (2007). CAM therapies among primary care patients using opioid therapy for chronic pain. *BMC Complementary and Alternative Medicine, 7,* 15 (doi.10.1186/1472-6882-7-15).

Fordyce, W. E. (1976). *Behavioral methods for chronic pain and illness.* Saint Louis, MO: Mosby.

Freeman, A., Pretzer, J., Fleming, B., & Simon, K. M. (1990). *Clinical applications of cognitive therapy.* New York, Plenum Press.

Fries, J. F., & McShane, D. (1998). Reducine need and demand for medical services in high-risk persons. A health education approach. *Western Journal of Medicine, 169,* 201–207.

Furlan, A., Brosseau, L., Imamura, M., & Irvin, E. (2002). Massage for low-back pain. [update of *Cochrane Database Sys Rev.* 2000, (4):CD001929; PMID: 11034734] *Cochrane Database of Systematic Reviews,* (2), CD001929.

Gallagher, B. (2003). Tai Chi Chuan and Qigong: Physical and mental practice for functional mobility. *Topics in Geriatric Rehabilitation, 19*(3), 172–182.

Gagnier, J. J., vanTulder, M., Berman, B, & Bombardier, C. Herbal medicine for low back pain. (2008). *The Cochrane Database of Systematic Reviews, 1.*

Garrett, K., Basmadjian, G., Khan, I., Schaneberg, B., & Seale, T. (2003). Extracts of kava (*Piper methysticum*) induce acute anxiolytic-like behavioral changes in mice. *Psychopharmacology, 170*(1), 33–41.

Gatchel, R. J., BoPeng, Y., Peters, M. L., Fuchs, P. N., & T urk, D. C. (2007). The biopsychosocial approach to chronic pain: Scientific advances and future directions. *Psychological Bulletin, 133,* 581–624.

Gay, M. C., Philippot, P., & Luminet O. (2002). Differential effectiveness of psychological interventions for reducine osteoarthritis pain: A comparison of Erikson. *European Journal of Pain, 6,* 1–16. *Zeitschrift für Gastroenterologie,*

Goldberg, R. J., & Katz, J. (2007). Meta-analysis of the analgesic effects of omega-3 polyunsaturated fatty acid supplementation for inflammatory joint pain. *Pain, 129*(1-2), 210–223.

Goudas, L. C., Bloch, R., Gialeli-Goudas, M., Lau, J., & Carr, D. B. (2005). The epidemiology of cancer pain. *Cancer Investigation, 23,* 182–190.

Gregory, P. J., Sperry, M., & Wilson, A. F. (2007). Dietary supplements for osteoarthritis. *American Family Physician, 77*(2), 177–184.

Grossman, P., Neimann, L., Schmidt, S., & Walach, H. (2004). Mindfulness-based stress reduction and health benefits: A meta-analysis. *Journal of Psychosomatic Research, 54,* 35–43.

Gureje, O., Von Korff, M., Simon, G. E., & Gater, R. (1998). Persistent pain and well-being: A World Health Organization study in primary care. *JAMA, 280,* 147–151.

Hadjistavropoulos, H. D., & Clark, J. (2001).Using outcome evauations to assess interdisciplinary acute and chronic pain programs. *The Joint Commission Journal on Quality Improvement, 27*(7). Available at http://www.jcrinc.com/1249/. (Accessed February 1, 2008.)

He, D., Veirsted, K. B., Hostmark, A. T., & Medbo, J. L. (2004). Effects of acupuncture treatment on chronic neck and shoulder pain in sedentary female workers: A 6-month and 3-year follow-up study. *Pain, 109,* 299–307.

Hoehler, F. K., Tobis, J. S., & Buerger, A. A. (1981). Spinal manipulation for low back pain. *JAMA, 245,* 1835–1838.

Hulme, J. (2007). Electromagnetic fields for the treatment of osteoarthritis. *Cochrane Review Abstracts*.

Integration of Behavioral and Relaxation Approaches into the Treatment of Chronic Pain and Insomnia. NIH Technological Statement 1995, 1–34. Available at http://consensus.nih.gov/1995/1995BehaviorRelaxPainInsomniata017html.htm (accessed February 22, 2008).

Institute of Medicine of the National Academies Report, November 7, 2006. From cancer patient to cancer survivor: Lost in transition. Available at http://www.iom.edu/report.asp?id=30869. (accessed January 28, 2008).

Jacobson, E. (1974). *Progressive relaxation: A physiological and clinical investigation of muscular states and their significance in psychology and medical practice.* Chicago, IL: University of Chicago Press.

Jarvik, J. G., Hollingworth, W., Heagerty, P. J., Haynor, D. R., Boyco, E. J., & Deyo, R. A. (2005). Three-year incidence of low back pain in an initially asymptomatic cohort. Clinical and imaging risk factors. *Spine, 30*, 1541–1548.

Jensen, M., & Patterson, D. R. (2006). Hypnotic treatment of chronic pain. *Journal of Behavioral Medicine, 29*, 95–124.

Jensen, M. P., Turner, J. A., & Romano, J. M. (2001). Changes in beliefs, catastrophizing and coping are associated with improvement in multidisciplinary pain treatment. *Journal of Consulting and Clinical Psychology, 69*, 655–662.

Jensen, M.P., Turner, J. A., & Romano, J. M. (2007). Changes after multidisciplinary pain treatment in patient pain beliefs and coping are associated with concurrent changes in patient functioning. *Pain, 13*, 38–47.

Jensen, M. P., Turner, J. A., Romano, J. M., & Lawler, B. K. (1994). Relationship of pain-specific beliefs to chronic pain adjustment. *Pain, 57*, 301–309.

Kabat-Zinn, J., Lipworth, L., & Burney, R. (1985). The clinical use of mindfulness meditation for the self-regulation of chronic pain. *Journal of Behavioral Medicine, 8*, 163–190.

Kabat-Zinn, J., Lipworth, L., & Burney, R. (1987). Four year follow-up of a meditation-based program for the self-regulation of chronic pain: Treatment outcomes and compliance. *Clinical Journal of Pain, 2*, 157–173.

Katz, J., McDermott, M. P., Cooper, E. M., Walther, R. R., Sweeney, E. W., & Dworkin, R. H. (2005). Psychosocial risk factors for postherpetic neuralgia: A prospective study of patients with herpes zoster. *Journal of Pain, 6*, 782–790.

Keefe, F. J., Affleck, G., Lefebvre, J., Underwood, L., Caldwell, D. S., Drew, J., et al. (2001). Living with rheumatoid arthritis: The role of daily religious and spiritual coping. *Journal of Pain, 2*, 101–110.

Keefe, F. J., Rumble, M. E., Scipio, C. D., Giordano, L. A., & Perri, L. M. (2004). Psychological aspects of persistent pain: Current state of the science. *Journal of Pain, 5*, 195–211.

Kerns, R. D., Rosenberg, R., & Jacob, M. (1994). Anger expression and chronic pain. *Journal of Behavioral Medicine, 17*, 57–67.

Koenig, H.G. (2001). Religion and medicine IV: Religion, physical health, and clinical implications. *International Journal of Psychiatry in Medicine, 31*, 321–336.

Kolasinski, S. L., Garfinkel, M., Tsai, A. G., Matz, W., Van Dyke, A., & Schumacher, H. R. (2005). Iyengar yoga for treating symptoms of osteoarthritis of the knees: a pilot study. *Journal of Alternative & Complementary Medicine, 11*(4), 689–693.

Kuchera, M. L. (2007). Applying osteopathic principles to formulate treatment for patients with chronic pain. *Journal of the American Osteopathic Association, 107*(10 Suppl 6), ES28–ES38.

Kwekkeboom, K. L., & Gretarsdottir, E. (2006). Systematic review of relaxation interventions for pain. *Journal of Nursing Scholarship,* Third Quarter, 269–277.

Lackner, J. M., & Gertman, M. B. (2004). Pain catastrophizing and interpersonal problems: A circumplex analysis of the communal coping model. *Pain, 110,* 597–604.

Lake, J. K., Power, C., & Cole, T. J. (2000). Back pain and obesity in the 1958 British birth cohort. Cause or effect? *Journal of Clinical Epidemiology, 53,* 245–250.

Lewandowski, W. A. (2004). Patterning of pain and power with guided imagery. *Nursing Science Quarterly, 17,* 233–241.

Licciardone, J. C. (2004). The unique role of osteopathic physicians in treating patients with low back pain. *Journal of American Osteopathic Association, 104*(Supplement 8), S13–S18.

Licciardone, J. C., Stoll, S. T., Fulda, K. G., Russo, D. P., Siu, J., Winn, W., et al. (2003). Osteopathic manipulative treatment for chronic low back pain: a randomized controlled trial. *Spine, 28,* 1355–1362.

Little C. V., Parsons, T., & Logan, S. (2008). Herbal therapy for treating osteoarthritis. *The Cochrane Database of Systematic Reviews, 1.*

Ludwig, D. S., & Kabet-Zinn, J. (2008). Mindfulness in medicine. *JAMA, 300,* 1350–1352.

Lundblad, I., Elert, J., & Gerdle, B. (1999). Randomized controlled trial of physiotherapy and Feldenkrais interventions in female workers with neck-shoulder complaints. *Journal of Occupational Rehabilitation, 9*(3), 179–194.

Manheimer, E., White, A., Berman, B., Forys, K., & Ernst, E. (2005). Meta-analysis: Acupuncture for low back pain. *Annals of Internal Medicine, 142,* 651–663.

McCracken, L. M. (2005). *Contextual cognitive-behavioral therapy for chronic pain.* Seattle, WA: IASP Press.

McCracken, L. M., Gross, R. T., Sorg, P. J., & Edmands, T. A. (1993). Prediction of pain in patients with chronic low back pain: Effects of inaccurate prediction and pain-related anxiety. *Behavior Research and Therapy, 43,* 1335–1346.

Melchart, D., Weidenhammer, W., Streng, A., Hoppe, A., Pfaffenrath, V., & Linde, K. (2006). Acupuncture for chronic headaches—an epidemiological study. *Headache, 46,* 632–641.

Melzack, R. (2001). Pain and the neuromatrix in the brain. *Journal of Dental Education, 65,* 1378–1382.

Melzack, R. (2005). Evolution of the neuromatrix theory of pain. *Pain Practice, 5,* 85–94.

Melzack, R., & Casey, K. L. (1968). Sensory, motivational and central control determinants of pain: A new conceptual model. In D. Kenshalo (Ed.), *The skin senses.* Springfield, IL, Charles C. Thomas, pp. 423–443.

Menefee, L. A. (2005). Psychological evaluation of the patient with chronic pain (Chapter 16). In M. Pappagallo (Ed.), *The neurological basis of pain*. New York: McGraw Hill, pp. 219–223.

Merskey, H., & Bugduk, N. (1994). *Classification of chronic pain. Description of chronic pain syndromes and definitions of pain terms* (2nd edn). Seattle, WA: IASP Press.

Miakowski, C., Cleary, J., Burney, R., Coyne, P., Finley, R., Foster, R., et al. (2005). *Guideline for the management of cancer pain in adults and children*. APS Clinical Practice Guidelines Series, No 3. Glenview, IL: American Pain Society.

Moadel, A. B., Shah C., Wylie-Rosett, J., Harris, M. S., Patel, S. R., Hall, C, B., et al. (2007). Randomized controlled trial of yoga among a multiethnic sample of breast cancer patients: effects on quality of life. *Journal of Clinical Oncology, 25*(28), 4387–4395.

Montgomery, G. H., Duhamel, K. N., & Redd, W. H. (2000). A meta-analysis of hypnotically induced analgesia: How effective is hypnosis? *International Journal of Clinical and Experimental Hypnosis, 48*, 138–153.

Monroe, N. E., & Greco, C. M. (2007). Mind–body interventions for chronic pain in older adults: A structured review. *Pain Medicine, 8*, 359–375.

Monroe, N. E., Greco, C. M., & Weiner, D. K. (2008). Mindfulness meditation for the treatment of chronic low back pain in older adults: A randomized controlled pilot study. *Pain, 134*, 310–319.

Monti, D. A., & Peterson, C. (2004). Mindfulness-based art therapy: Results from a two year study. *Psychiatry Times, 21*, 63–66.

Monti, D. A., Peterson, C., Kunkel, E. J., Hauck, W. W., Pequignot, E., Rhodes, L., et al. (2006). A randomized controlled trial of mindfulness-based art therapy (MBAT) for women with cancer. *Psycho-Oncology, 15*, 363–373.

Monti, D. A., & Yang, J. (2005). Complementary medicine in chronic cancer care. *Seminars in Oncology, 32*, 225–231.

Morley, S., Eccleston, C., & Williams, A,C. (1999). Systematic review and meta-analysis of randomized adults, excluding headache. *Pain, 80*, 1–13.

National Center for Complementary and Alternative Medicine, National Institutes of Health. (2002). What is complementary and alternative medicine? NCCAM Publication no: D156. At http://nccam.nih.gov/health/whatiscam/. Accessed February 22, 2006.

National Center for Health Statistics. (2006). *Health, United States, 2006, with chartbook on trends in the health of Americans with special feature on pain*. Centers for Disease Control and Prevention(PHS), 1232.

National Institutes of Health Consensus Conference. (1998). Acupuncture. *Journal of American Medical Association, 280*, 1518–1524.

Naranjo A., Sokka, T., Descalzo, M.A., Calvo-Alen, J. Horslev-Petersen, K., Luukkainen, R. K., et al. (2008). Cardiovascular disease in patients with rheumatoid arthritis: results from the QUEST-RA study. *Arthritis Research & Therapy, 10*(2), R30 (doi:10.1186/ar2383).

Okifuji, A., Turk, D. C., & Curran, S. L. (1991). Anger in chronic pain: Investigations of anger targets and intensity. *Journal of Psychomatic Research, 61*, 771–780.

Pai, S., & Sundaram, L. J. (2004). Low back pain: An economic assessment in the United States. *Orthopedic Clinics of North America, 35*, 1–5.

Paris, J. (1998). Significance of biological research for a biopsychosocial model of the personality disorders. In K. Silk (Ed.), *Biology of personality disorders.* Washington, DC: American Psychiatric Press, pp. 17, 126–148.

Pipitone, N., & Scott, D. (2001). Magnetic pulse treatment for knee osteoarthritis: A randomized, double-blind, placebo-controlled study. *Current Medical Research Opinion, 17*(3), 190–196.

Plews-Ogan, M., Owens, J. E., Goodman, M., Wolfe, P., & Schorling, J. (2005). A pilot study investigating mindfulness-based stress reduction and massage for the management of chronic pain. *Journal of General Internal Medicine, 20*, 1136–1138.

Pujol, L. A. M., Katz, N. P., & Zacharoff, K. L. (2007). *PainEdu.org manual: A pocket guide to pain management,* (3rd edn). Newton, MA: Inflexxion.

Raub, J. (2002). Psychophysiologic effects of Hatha Yoga on musculoskeletal and cardiopulmonary function: A literature review. *Journal of Alternative Complementary Medicine, 8*(6), 797–812.

Rippentrop, A. E., Altmaier, E. M., Chen, J. J., Found, E. M., & Keffala, V. J. (2005). The relationship between religion/spirituality and physical health, mental health, and pain in a chronic pain population. *Pain, 116*, 311–321.

Seaman, D. R. (2002). The diet-induced proinflammatory state: A cause of chronic pain and other degenerative diseases? *Journal of Manipulative and Physiological Therapeutics, 25*(3), 168–179.

Seminowicz, D. A., & Davis, K. D. (2006). Cortical responses to pain in healthy individuals depends on pain catastrophizing. *Pain, 120*, 297–306.

Sherman, K., Cherkin, D., Erro, J., Miglioretti, D., & Deyo R. (2005). Comparing yoga, exercise, and a self-care book for chronic low back pain A randomized, controlled trial. *Annals of Internal Medicine,* Dec 20, *143*(12): 849–856.

Shupak, N., McKay, J., Nielson, W., Rollman, G., Prato, F., & Thomas, A. (2006). Exposure to a specific pulsed low-frequency magnetic field: A double-blind placebo-controlled study of effects on pain ratings in rheumatoid arthritis and fibromyalgia patients. *Pain Research Management.,* Summer, *11*(2), 85–90.

Song, R., Lee, E., Lam, P., & Bae, S. (2003). Effects of tai chi exercise on pain, balance, muscle strength, and perceived difficulties in physical functioning in older women with osteoarthritis: A randomized clinical trial. *Journal of Rheumatology, 30*(9), 2039–2044.

Staud, R. (2007). Mechanisms of acupuncture analgesia: Effective therapy for musculoskeletal pain? *Current Rheumatology Reports, 9*, 473–481.

Sullivan, M. D., & Turk, D. C. (2001). Psychiatric illness, depression, and psychogenic pain. In J. D. Loeser, S. H. Butler, C. R. Chapman & D. C. Turk (Eds.), *Bonica's management of pain* (483–500). Philadelphia: Lippincott.

Tang, N. K., & Crane, C. (2006). Suicidality in chronic pain: A review of the prevalence, risk factors and psychological links. *Psychological Medicine, 36*, 575–586.

Targino, R. A., Imamura, M., Kaziyama, H. H. Souza, L. P., Hsing, W. T., & Imamura S. T. (2002). Pain treatment with acupuncture for patients with fibromyalgia. *Current Pain Headache Reports, 6*, 679–383.

Turk, D. C., & Monarch, E. S. (2002). Biopsychosocial perspective on chronic pain. In: Turk, D.C., & Gatchel, R.J. (Eds.), *Psychological Approaches to Pain Management: A Practitioner's Handbook* (2nd edn), New York, NY, Guilford Press, pp. 3–29.

Turner, J. A., Jensen, M. P., & Romano, J. M. (2000). Do beliefs, coping and catastrophizing independently predict functioning in patients with chronic pain? *Pain, 85*, 115–125.

Vickers, A. J., Rees, R. W., Zollman, C. E., McCarney, R., Smith, C., Ellis, N., et al. (2004). Acupuncture of chronic headache disorders in primary care: Randomized controlled trial and economic analysis. *Health and Technology Assessment, 8*, 1–35.

Wachholtz, A. B., Pearce, M. J., & Koenig H. (2007). Exploring the relationship between spirituality, coping and pain. *Journal of Behavioral Medicine, 30*, 311–318.

Weidenhammer, W., Linde, K., Streng, A., Hoppe, A., & Melchart, D. (2007). Acupuncture for chronic low back pain in routine care—a multicenter observational study. *Clinical Journal of Pain, 23*, 128–135.

Weisberg, J. N., Vittengl, J. R., Clark, L. A., Gatchel, R. J., & Gorin, A. A. (2000). Personality and pain: Summary and future perspectives. In R. J. Gatchel & J. N. Weisberg (Eds.), *Personality characteristics of patients with pain.* Washington, DC: American Psychological Association, pp. 259–282.

Woolf, C. J. (2004). Dissecting out mechanisms responsible for peripheral neuropathic pain: Implications for diagnosis and therapy. *Life Science, 74*(21), 2605–2610.

12

Integrative Approaches to Brain Rehabilitation

DENISE E. MALKOWICZ, JOLENE ROSS, AND JAMES CAUNT

KEY CONCEPTS

- Until recently, brain injured patients and persons with some psychiatric disorders were thought to have poor prognoses for recovery. New insights into neuroplasticity and neurorehabilitation methods have significantly improved outcomes.
- Noninvasive therapies for brain retraining, based on normal progressive neurodevelopmental models, can be designed to stimulate and reconnect neural circuits.
- Quantitative Electroencephalography (QEEG)-Neurofeedback or Neurotherapy uses operant conditioning to reinforce desirable self-regulated EEG changes which help to reorganize neural networks.
- The sensorimotor rhythms (SMRs), 12–15 Hertz rhythms seen over sensory-motor cortex, C3 and C4 EEG electrodes, are associated with regulation of thalamocortical circuits. Neurotherapy reinforcing SMR is effective in facilitating recovery from brain injury, sleep disorders, epilepsy, and some psychiatric disorders.
- QEEG-Neurotherapy is under study for treatment of many neurological disorders, psychiatric conditions, behavioral problems, and cognitive dysfunction and seems to be able to predict outcomes in some disorders.

■

Introduction

R esearch into brain function, neuroplasticity, physiology, neurochemistry, brain imaging, and advanced technologies bring us insights into a number of disorders. This permits noninvasive rehabilitation by brain retraining, greatly improving outcomes in neurological and psychiatric disorders. Quantitative Electroencephalography (QEEG)-Neurotherapy, a powerful, noninvasive therapy, promotes reintegration of neural circuits and networks. Normalization of underlying physiology appears to be associated with the return of function. Scientific studies of QEEG-neurofeedback have been conducted since the 1960s. Advanced technology and recognition of brain neuroplasticity promoted opportunities to use such methods for diagnosis and treatment of psychiatric and neurological disorders. QEEG-Neurotherapy technologies, techniques, and treatment protocols are evolving. QEEG-neurotherapy requires an expert understanding of neurophysiology, EEG interpretation, operant conditioning, and neurological and psychiatric disorders.

Hippocrates stated, "Healing is a mater of time, but sometimes it is a matter of opportunity."

Neuroplasticity is the inherent ability of the brain to learn, change, reintegrate, and recover neurological and psychological function. Effective neurorehabilitation programs can influence the rate and amount of recovery. These noninvasive brain retraining approaches are based on operant conditioning.

Technique

In QEEG-Neurotherapy, the first step is acquisition of the EEG in a series of progressively activated awake states: eyes closed, eyes open, and during the performance of reading, math, or cognitive and behavioral tasks. Each condition places greater demand on brain integration of the neural circuits and neurophysiology underlying the electrophysiological function reflected on the EEG. Tasks requiring increased levels of brain activation can show abnormalities in the QEEG, while in specific areas and connections between brain areas, during less demanding tasks, EEG can appear normal. Artifact and other nonsignificant findings are removed from the raw digital EEG, which is processed with Fourier transform and other mathematical analysis. The resultant QEEG is compared statistically against age and state matched controls. QEEG data can be displayed in a variety of montage formats. QEEG can be displayed in a data mode or statistical mode, and data shown in spectral analysis, topometric maps, brain maps,

Brodman's area maps, comodulation and coherence neural network maps. Comodulation analyzes the relationship of wave magnitudes at sites of interest (Sterman & Kaiser, 2001). Coherence maps look at phase relationship between sites. QEEG can detect abnormalities not seen in raw EEG. Abnormal patterns that show up on various analytic displays and in statistic analysis increase the reliability of identifying areas of dysfunction guiding diagnosis and design of neurotherapy. (See Table 12.1.)

Neurotherapy uses operant conditioning. The subject receives visual and auditory rewards reinforcing desirable EEG changes in appropriate areas and within functional brain networks. QEEG-neurotherapy that uses training of the sensorimotor rhythm (SMR)—a 12–15 Hz rhythm seen over the sensorimotor cortex at C3 and C4—has been effective in helping to reintegrate thalamocortical circuits and has been studied in the treatment of brain injury stroke, epilepsy, sleep disorders, and of a number of cognitive, behavioural, and psychiatric conditions. Physiologically, training SMR seems to lead to long-term potentiation (LTP) in thalamocortical circuits. This is the area that underlies EEG generation. LTP is associated with learning and its associated physiological changes in the central nervous system. Research on SMR effects on LTP is seen in thalamocortical circuits and striatum (Sterman, 1986, 1996; Sterman & Friar, 1972). Neuronal protein synthesis, growth, and remodeling appear to occur. Changes appear durable and self-regenerating. Continuing physiological and clinical improvement can be seen months between sessions

Table 12.1. Data Acquisition.

Data Acquisition Procedures	
Minimizing EEG artifact:	**What is EEG Artifact?** EEG artifact is the portions of the EEG signal that are not true EEG. Artifact examples: muscle tension, EKG (electrocardiogram), eye movement, eye blink, head movements, EMI (see below)
Patient management	**Patient management factors**: adequate sleep, proper nutrition (prior to taking data), minimize movement during data acquisition, other coaching
Record length	**Optimum record length**: long enough to have statistically sufficient data, but not so long that subject becomes inattentive or drowsy
Preventing outside electrical interference	**Electromagnetic Interference (EMI)**: corrupts EEG signal, from sources such as fluorescent lights, power line spikes, cable movement, pacemakers, vagal nerve stimulators, etc.

or without further neurotherapy. Neurotherapy has been effective in recovery even years after brain injury, or for psychiatric disorders which had failed other interventions.

EEG and QEEG-Neurotherapy

QEEG-Neurofeedback or Neurotherapy is based on analysis of the mathematically processed and formatted EEG data obtained from subjects in awake and increasingly neurologically engaged states. Each recording is performed for 3 minutes with several repetitions. Sleep and routine activation procedures are not performed. A 19-channel digital EEG is recorded with electrodes placed according to the International 10-20 System. Reference electrodes—such as linked ear references, and ground electrodes—are also applied. Electrode impedances are kept at an optimal range of >1 kilo Ohm to <5 kilo Ohm to optimize EEG. The pre-training QEEG is analyzed and compared with normative databases for the various age, state task, and conditions. The "raw" EEG information is visually analyzed by an expert EEG reader to eliminate any artifact or benign variants. Artifacts can arise from physiological sources, such as muscle or eye movement, while nonphysiological artifact occurs from other electrical fields in the environment, such as equipment. Artifact can obscure true EEG or be interpreted falsely as true EEG activity. Artifact is eliminated prior to mathematical processing, such as Fourier transform, to avoid contamination of data with false frequencies, which can yield false analysis. EEG intepretation requires an expert clinician. It is too important to leave to an "artifact" button in the computer program or an to inexperienced reader. QEEG is analzed for normal and abnormal patterns. Scalp EEG records volume conducted excitatory and inhibitory postsynaptic potentials from cortical pyramidal neurons influenced by input from thalamocortical circuits. The EEG machine's common mode rejection detects potential electrical differences between electrode recording dipoles (positive-negative charge units). Dipoles closer to the surface electrodes are most easily seen on the EEG. Those farther away—such as deeper gray matter, sulci, fissures, mesial or basal areas of the brain—are less easily seen. Voltage or magnitude on is decreased by intervening stuctures of the CSF, meningies, skull, and scalp. Small areas of activity can be missed. Epileptiform features and intermittent activity may not be recorded on each EEG. Location, timing, and size matter.

The EEG machine's common mode rejection design eliminates potentials common to many electrodes, like artifact, but amplifies true brain potentials. Brain activity is localized by analysis of the field of distribution or the maximum voltage of the activity.

The QEEG is interpreted in the context of age and task, emphasizing waking background activity correlated with history and clinical factors. Artifacts can arise from physiologic sources, such as eye movement, muscle movement, chewing, swallowing, or cardiac activity.

A normal EEG has a rich mixture of appropriate background activities in all states and has reactivity. There are no focal or generalized abnormalities. EEG frequency is reported in Hertz (Hz); voltage or magnitude is reported in microvolts per millimeter (uV/mm). The term *power*, refers to magnitude squared, and is not used in QEEG-Neurotherapy described here. EEG frequencies range from delta, 0.5 < 4 Hz, theta >4 and <8, alpha >8 <13 Hz and beta >13 Hz. The SMR is a 12–15 Hz, seen at C3and C4 maximally, and is not abolished by contralateral limb movement like "mu" rhythm.

The Posterior Dominant Rhythm "PDR" is best seen in the occipital-parietal leads in relaxed wakefulness with eyes closed, blocks with eye opening, and with alerting. In adults it is normally 9.5 Hz, relatively constant over a lifetime including healthy old age.

EEG abnormalities can be diffuse or focal. White matter injury or dysfunction tends to manifest with focal or diffuse slowing, such as paroxysmal delta activity. Grey matter injury or dysfunction appears as a loss or slowing of normal expected frequencies, or reduction in their voltage. Epileptiform spike or sharp waves may be seen but do not necessarily signify epilepsy. The age and state of the patient, effects of medication or alcohol, or withdrawal states can alter background or cause paroxysmal activity. Normal EEQ looks different in individuals of different ages and in the same individual in different states. Abnormalities may be episodic and might not show up on each EEG.

QEEG-Neurotherapy and Neuroplasticity

Many important assumptions underlie the practice of neurotherapy, including concepts of brain neuroplasticity, operant conditioning, and the alteration of EEG rhythms reflecting alteration of neural circuitry, an example of EEG self-regulation and its behavioral associations (Sterman & Macdonald, 1978; Sterman, Mcdonald, & Stone, 1974). It is accomplished by QEEG analysis and well-designed neurotherapy (see Table 12.2, Protocol Development Considerations). Interpretation of QEEG data on spectral plots, Brodman's area maps, topometrics, brain mapping, comodulation, coherence, and other parameters are key to proper diagnosis and planning of neurotherapy. Spectral plots graph EEG frequency on the x axis, and magnitude on the y axis, for all 19 electrodes on a head diagram. Topometric Analysis displays 19 EEG sites on the x axis and frequencies on the y axis. It shows normal values and standard

Table 12.2. Protocol Development Considerations.

Close examination and interpretation of the raw EEG data. The raw EEG, which is the signal trace that is seen at each cortical location, contains an enormous amount of information to the trained eye. This information provides clues about both normal and abnormal brain function and can be correlated with further analysis of the EEG.

Identification of frequency bands of interest and their locations on the cortex. Bands of interest are those frequency bands that are elevated or reduced in magnitude, compared to other bands, or compared to a normative database

Examining changes in the EEG when the subject transitions from one brain state to another, such as changes between eyes closed and eyes open

Identifying left-right hemispheric magnitude asymmetries

Noting anterior-posterior relative band magnitude patterns

Choosing cortical locations to be trained simultaneously that will enhance connectivity between locations where connectivity is disrupted

deviations for age and state matched control data bases. Brain maps show a head diagram of all EEG sites with color-coded data for frequencies in magnitude and statistical views, and can also show brain network connectivity properties such as comodulation and coherence. The Brodman's maps display brain areas such as Broca's area and visual areas 17, 18, 19, etc. They can show QEEG frequencies and magnitudes for each area. Convergent information, compared to statistical databases, identifies dysfunction and leads to diagnosis and neurotherapy protocols designed to treat the issues. Neurotherapy parameters ,such as EEG frequencies, threshold, and networks connections must be set. The desirable EEG changes produced by the patient are rewarded and reinforced by operant conditioning with visual and auditory rewards. Progress is continuous with benifical changes noted during neurotherapy on the EEG. EEG is re-evaluated and the parameters changed within a session in response to training. This can shape or reinforce desirable activity. Studies have shown that changes take place in behavior with appropriately applied operant conditioning. Furthermore, ability to adapt, "learn," and reinforce these changes under proper conditions make lasting changes in the generation and regulation of selected brain neural circuits and thalamocortical loops underlying the activity that we record as EEG. Sterman's research showed that neurogenesis and regulation that appeared as learned control of a particular EEG rhythm, over the sensorimotor cortex that emerged above nonrhythmic low voltage background activity, was the SMR characterized on EEG by a rhythm with a special peak of around 12–14 Hz. Sterman applied operant condition methods, recorded EEG, and discovered that the experimental animal, the cat, could voluntarily produce SMR on EEG. Later, the cats that had taken part in SMR training were found to have a significantly elevated seizure thresholds, compared to the untrained cats, when exposed to a highly epileptogenic compound. The SMR constitutes the dominant "stand by" frequency of the integrated thalamocortical somatosensory and somatomotor pathways. Operant training of SMR improved control in over-excitation in this system with increased thresholds for excitation thought to underlie the clinical benefit of SMR training in epilepsy. This seems to be true in other disorders characterized by cortical and/or thalamocortical hyperexcitability, such as ADHD. Studies in children with ADHD using fMRI support the idea that those who improved significantly in cognitive tests, after neurofeedback training, have had an observed significant increase in metabolic activity in the striatum. Facilitation and/or regulation of SMR substrates alters motor output. This can set up reduced proprioceptive afferent input to the thalamus and suggests reorganization of motor and thalamic status accompanied by volleys of strong oscillating discharge to the cortex with each trained SMR response.

Neurotherapy training changes oscillatory activity influenced by neurotransmitter activity, such as cholinergic and monoaminergic neuromodulators that affect excitability levels. Changes in neuromodulator influences and cortical projections affect cellular depolarization and bursting patterns. Increased metabolic activity, noted in specific areas of the brain, include increased synaptic strength, increased protein synthesis, and insertion of new excitatory neurotransmitter channels at post synaptic receptor sites resulting in LTP. This increases synaptic sensitivity and the probability of future activity in neuronal circuits. Also, EEG oscillation with SMR conditioning is seen after reward delivery: the neurological reward for meeting EEG criteria is referred to as "Post Reinforcement Synchronization," (PSR), which produces a brief burst of EEG activity resulting in drive reduction and feelings of satisfaction and achievement. This is the neurological reward for meeting EEG criteria. This results in changing the EEG toward normalization. Neurotherapy seems to alter the neurophysiology of the brain in appropriate ways as changes occur to optimize the patient's underlying function. These changes have been seen in fMRI studies (Levesque, Beauregard, & Mensour, 2006).

QEEG-Neurotherapy in Epilepsy

A seizure is a paroxysmal, abnormal electrical discharge from cortical neurons. One category of seizure is the partial seizure, which arises from a discrete focus but can spread to involve other areas. The second category, generalized seizures, appears to involve the whole brain from the onset. The epilepsies are disorders of the brain with the tendency for recurrent unprovoked seizures. Treatment options for epilepsy include the use of anti-epilepsy medications, surgery, and vagal nerve stimulation. Not all people with epilepsy are candidates for such treatments, or therapies fail. Many patients have recurrent seizures that significantly alter their lives. An alternative approach for seizure control is QEEG-Neurotherapy. QEEG-Neurotherapy, based on operant conditioning and self modulation of of desirable frequency ranges EEG by the patient, is thought to train different EEG frequencies that result in seizure control (Monderer, 2002).

During neurotherapy the patient has electrodes placed over the areas of interest. Operant conditioning rewards occur when the goal EEG frequencies, duration, and threshold at the specific electrode sites are maintained, or certain brain areas fire together in a desired pattern. This reinforces desirable activity over time and is thought to reintegrate the involved thalamocortical circuits. The goal is to normalize the EEG by producing normal frequencies where there was a lack of normal activity, or in an area of abnormal activity. Reinforcing a frequency makes it more likely to occur and become permanent over time with multiple repetitions. One can also train down- or inhibit abnormal EEG activity by setting parameters that reward the patient for reducing or eliminating abnormal activity. EEG at training sites is displayed on two computer monitor screens. The patient sees the visual reward or part of the EEG linked to appropriate responses on their screen. The therapist sees the detailed simultaneous EEG displayed on a separate therapist's screen, allowing the therapist to make adjustments of parameters required to receive a reward. This is called "shaping" and enhances the ability to produce the desired responses. Site by site and session by session the desired neural circuitry is built and reinforced until the changes in EEG background are permanent and the desired behavior is achieved.

Research into neurofeedback is about 30 years old. Sterman (1996) and Sterman, Wyrwicka, and Roth (1969) demonstrated EEG operant conditioning. Sterman's studies investigated learned suppression of the production of EEG in cats (Roth, Sterman, & Clemente, 1967). A particular EEG rhythm over the sensorimotor cortex, with a spectral peak around 12–14 Hz, not unlike EEG sleep spindles with a spectral peak of around 12–14 Hz, has been referred to as the SMR (Roth et al., 1967). In experiments involving operant conditioning with a food reward, cats were trained to control SMR voluntarily. The EEG self-regulation and behavior associated with SMR production was one of corporal immobility, with SMR bursts regularly proceeded by a drop in muscle tone (Sterman et al., 1969; Wuricka & Sterman, 1968). Later, Sterman's experiments on seizures related to an epileptogenic compound demonstrated that cats having prior SMR conditioning training had significantly elevated epileptic thresholds compared with untrained cats. This suggested that SMR training had kept the SMR animal from experiencing seizures (Sterman et al., 1969). Sterman and others showed that the SMR rhythm originates from the thalamus in the ventrobasal nuclei (nVB) (Howe & Sterman, 1972). The nVB conducts afferent somatosensory information. During conditioned SMR production, nVB firing patterns shift from tonic, fast, and nonrhythmic discharges to systematic, rhythmic burst of discharge that, in turn, are associated with suppression of somatosensory information passage and reduction of muscle tone (Howe & Sterman, 1972, 1973; Sterman, 1973). Upon reduction of afferent somatosensory input, the cells in the nVB hyperpolarize. Instead of remaining at a stable level of inhibition, a gradual depolarization mediated by a slow calcium influx causes the neurons of the nVB to discharge a burst of spikes. These spikes are relayed to the sensorimotor cortex and to the neurons of the thalamic reticular nucleus (nRT). Stimulation of the nRT leads to a GABAergic inhibition of VB relay cells, returning them to a hyperpolarized state. This initiates a new cycle of slow depolarization. Thus the interplay between neuronal populations in the thalamic nVB, thalamic nRT, and the sensorimotor cortex results in rhythmic thalamocortical volley and consequent cortical EEG oscillations (Sterman & Egner, 2006). Several situations can affect SMR. Attenuation of efferent motor and afferent somatosensory activity can initiate SMR. The oscillatory activity is also largely influenced by nonspecific cholinergic and monoaminergic neuromodulation, which can affect excitability levels both in thalamic relay nuclei and in the cortical areas receiving the relay signals.

SMR constitutes the dominant frequency of the integrated thalamocortical, thalamosensory, and somatomotor pathway. Thus operant conditioning of SMR is assumed to result in improved control over-excitation in this system. Increased thresholds for excitation are thought to underlie the clinical benefits of SMR training in epilepsy (Sterman, 2006). There are many studies of QEEG-Neurofeedback and/or SMR training for the treatment of seizures. Patients with refractory partial seizures or generalized seizures were studied. Overall an 82 percent of 174 patients in various studies who had otherwise uncontrolled epilepsy showed significant improvement in seizure control with neurofeedback/SMR training (Sterman, 2000). This outcome is significantly better than that for most anti-epilepsy drugs or other therapies.

The Role of QEEG-Neurotherapy in Neuro-rehabilitation

Increased thresholds for excitation are thought to underlie the clinical benefits of SMR training in epilepsy and other disorders characterized by cortical and/or thalamocortical hyperexcitability. QEEG-neurofeedback assumes that the EEG is a reflection of the underlying neural physiological regulatory processes. Disruptions in these processes alter the EEG. Neurofeedback alters the EEG toward normalcy, as the underlying physiology normalizes. This can be an alternative for individuals who continue to have seizures that impact their life. Neurotherapy is designed to result in a functional change, increasing or reinforcing normal or favorable brain activity and decreasing or inhibiting abnormal activity. The neurotherapy, focusing on the areas of concern, may elevate seizure thresholds and reduce the tendency for seizures. Changes in EEG activity presumably reflect the neuroplasticity changes occurring in underlying neural circuitry. The treatment of seizure disorders with SMR is arguably the best established clinical application of EEG operant conditioning.

The neocortex receives information about the environment and the rest of the brain through pathways from the thalamus. The pathways have frequency-dependent properties that can strongly influence their effect on the neocortex.

This case example is of a 29-year-old man who had traumatic brain injury from a motor vehicle accident 10 years ago. His multiple neurological problems included refractory partial seizures with secondary generalization, with a post-ictal state lasting up to 10 days, during which his neurological function regressed. He had failed other therapies. His seizures and post-ictal state exacerbated his severe motor, coordination, and language difficulties. He was dependent in all activities of daily living. He underwent a comprehensive intensive rehabilitation with some success. However, his seizures and prolonged post-ictal state caused interruption in the program or regression. He was neurologically impaired, without significant improvement in function for 4 years.

He had severe Broca's aphasia, dysarthria, and swallowing difficulties. Severe motor dysfunction and incoordination was seen in trunk, and lower and upper extremities with no use of hands or fingers due to spasticity and weakness. A severe disorder of sleep disruption allowed him only 2 hours of sleep per night. QEEG studies were done pre-training, mid-training, and post-training. Neurofeedback was designed to address his seizures and neurological problems as assessed on neurological exam and QEEG. A cap EEG was done with 19 scalp electrodes placed according to the international 10–20 system using a Neuronavigator (J&J Engineering). The QEEG was analyzed using SKIL (Sterman Kaiser Imaging Lab)and the neurotherapy was done with a C2 Plus Neurofeedback Unit (J&J Engineering). A unique protocol was used for neurotherapy, with a patient reward screen linked to the clinician's computer monitor.

Pre-training QEEG showed Brodman's area maps, statistical brain maps, topometric displays, and spectral plots showed prominent delta up to 12 standard deviation above normal and theta in frontal, central temporal and parietal brain area without normal activity as seen on brain maps. The diffuse delta and theta maximum in frontal, central temporal, and parietal regions was consistent with white matter damage in the thalamocortical connections to cortex. Low voltage activity and lack of any normal frequencies suggested cortical gray matter dysfunction as well. MRI showed extensive cortical atrophy in the same areas with ventricular dilatation.

Neurotherapy started by reinforcing SMR at C3 and C4, increasing training time daily. Operant conditioning visual and auditory reward was linked to maintaining specific EEG activity at appropriate sites. The goal was to reintegrate the thalamocortical circuits, reduce slowing, and increase normal frequencies, such as SMR (12–15 Hz) and alpha, to reduce seizures, improve sleep and improve motor pathway connectivity. Adjacent frontal, temporal, and parietal areas were reinforced for 8.6 to 10.6 Hz activity to reactivate these areas and help inhibit seizure spread and increase function. Neurotherapy rewarded holding desired activity for 0.5 seconds at higher magnitudes, with multiple sites simultaneously interacting to increase connectivity. The reward was a pleasant sound and a picture that appeared on the computer screen along with EEG readout and threshold bars. Unlike most neurotherapy protocols, the patient underwent "intensive" neurotherapy. He trained every day for 3 weeks, rather than for 1 or 2 days a week, for 20–40 sessions. Due to distance, he could not return for 5 months.

During the first 3-week session, his strength, balance, motor coordination swallowing, and Broca's aphasia improved significantly. He could throw a ball and type 20–25 letters in 1 minute. Seizures frequency dropped from 12 at time, which caused post-ictal neurological impairment lasting up to 10 days to one partial seizure, from which he recovered in 1 day. His sleep improved from 2 to 8 hours in the first week (Sterman & Shouse, 1980).

He not only maintained these gains for a 5-month period between sessions without any further neurofeedback, but he made additional improvements in motor control, coordination, speech, swallowing, and seizure control without further neurotherapy during the 5-month interval. During the second training session, all of these parameters improved. He demonstrated increased attention, concentration, and responsiveness. Further gross and fine motor control was evidenced by his ability to type, play the guitar, walk independently, and dance. He was seizure free and off all medications. After the first 3-week session, his delta and theta showed reduction to 2 standard deviations on the topometric. After the second 3-week session, the delta and theta were at normal level, and there was increased normal activity throughout the QEEG. These results suggest that there is considerable neuroplasticity, even years after brain injury, and that QEEG-neurofeedback with SMR reinforcement can be an effective way to reintegrate thalamocortical circuits and regain neurological function, control seizures, and reintegrate sleep. It appears that once neural circuits and functional networks form, the results are durable and can continue to grow even without additional QEEG-neurofeedback. Neurotherapy is not the only way to stimulate neuroplasticity. In Cortical Visual Impairment (CVI)—bilateral visual loss due to severe injury of the visual areas of the brain—95% of 21 children recovered useful vision in an average of 6.9 months, using only light-dark and high contrast images in their environment (Malkowicz, Meyers, & Leisman, 2006). In another study, a large cohort of persons with CVI regained little or no vision over time, but had no visual stimulation (Hoyt, 2003; Morse, 1990).

QEEG-Neurotherapy for the Treatment of Psychiatric Disorders and Mood Disorders

The most satisfying moments in Neurotherapy work come from the improvements in the lives of patients reflected in pre- and post-treatment evaluations and EEG, and patients' descriptions of their positive changes. The following anecdotal cases are typical of a larger treatment population.

Neurotherapy treated the symptoms of Asperger's Disorder (Scolnick, 2005). The mother of an 11-year-old male filled out an assessment taken on the Adapted Australian Asperger's Scale, after 40 Neurotherapy sessions (Atwood, 1998). It showed a two-thirds improvement in post-treatment behavior (Ross & Caunt, 2003). The post-treatment EEG showed significant reductions in 6–9 Hz slow wave activity in the medial central and medial parietal regions with eyes open. Elevations in these medial locations are often seen in conjunction with obsessive behaviors that are characteristic of Asperger's Syndrome (American Psychiatric Association, 2000). The magnitude of 9–12 Hz activity in the parietal and occipital regions with eyes open, while reading and while performing math, was dramatically reduced. Magnitude reductions in the post-treatment EEG represent a greatly improved ability to engage the visual centers of the brain. Visual disturbances are deficits often seen in Asperger's Syndrome and can result in difficulty in reading, facial expressions, and other social cues, such as body posture and gestures (Klin & Volkmar, 1995). Asperger's can include difficulty in developing peer relations appropriate to developmental level. Asperger's individuals typically do not show clinically significant delay in cognitive development, curiosity about their environment in childhood, delay in language or in other age appropriate self-help skills (American Psychiatric Association, 2000).

Neurotherapy helps treat insomnia (Feinstein, Sterman, & MacDonald, 1974; Sterman, Howe, & Macdonald, 1970). Protocol is based on QEEG data. A 49-year-old female with insomnia increased her sleep onset from 61% to 97%, over a 7-month period of Neurotherapy treatment. Her ability to maintain sleep increased 43% to 61%, in scores from her sleep log. QEEG showed very low magnitudes across most frequency bands and disruptions in connectivity between anterior cortex. Treatment increased magnitudes in specific anterior locations (Moore, 2000), with simultaneous training of locations to improve connectivity.

An 11-year-old female with conduct disorder with aggressive outbursts, combined with attention deficit and hyperactivity and post-traumatic stress disorder, was treated using Neurotherapy. QEEG showed disruptions in connectivity between left and right frontal locations of the cortex, and between left anterior and posterior locations. QEEG also showed high amplitude slow wave activity and disruptions in the sensory motor cortex. An orphan adopted from Guatemala, she had experienced the violence of war, and poor nutrition and had little health care. She had preservative, obsessive behaviors, emotional meltdowns, conflicts with peers, a rigid need for fairness and justice, dissociations of perceptions and emotions, and other difficulties (Hammond, 2003). When she began neurotherapy, she was institutionalized, and after 30 sessions, she went to a special needs school and, living at home, continued neurotherapy.

Pre- and post-treatment evaluations and post-treatment EEGs are performed, and EEG changes are compared with the evaluations. EEG changes towards normalization are seen post- treatment, and correlating with changes in other pre- and post-treatment evaluations (Fernandez, Herrera et al., 2003; Sichel, Fehmi, & Goldstein, 1995).

Neurotherapy treatment in ADD/ADHD (Attention Deficit Disorder/ Attention Deficit Hyperactivity Disorder) results in remarkable improvements in symptoms in children and adults (Baydala, & Wikman, 2001; Linden, Habib, & Radojevic, 1996; Monastra, 2005; Rossiter, 2005; Xiong, Shi, & Xu, 2005). Improvements in some symptoms of ADHD equal or exceed those from medication (Fuchs, Birbaumer, Lutzenberger, Gruzelier, & Kaiser, 2003). Significantly improved attention, focus, behavior control, cognition, and comprehension, resulted in improved school or work performance, and a more fulfilling personal and family life. ADD/ADHD has various causes: genetic predisposition, head injury, difficult births, poor nutrition, early neglect, and environmental factors. The effects on brain function are cumulative. Common characteristics in ADD/ADHD are seen in the QEEG. Frontal lobe dysfunction, with abnormally high amplitude, low frequency EEG activity, is almost always seen. Frontal lobes are vulnerable to damage and can show disruptions in thalamocortical and left-right hemispheric connectivity. QEEG analysis reveals disruption of the sensory motor areas of the brain (primarily, the central region), resulting in an inability of the brain to modulate control of physical activity and movement, seen in the hyperactivity component of ADHD. QEEG sometimes reveals disruptions in visual, auditory, and memory activity, which contribute to attention and behavior difficulties.

QEEG reveals the specific locations of atypical EEG oscillatory frequencies, along with connectivity disruptions. The goal of Neurotherapy in ADD/ADHD is to normalize attention, focus, and behavior. Neurotherapy rewards changes in EEG activity towards normalization, which improves the function of the underlying neurological structures (Sterman, 2002). This results in the achievement of improved behavioral, cognitive, and physiological function and seizure activity, and improvements in emotional state. Frank Duffy, M.D. of Children's Hospital in Boston, MA, sums up the effectiveness of Neurotherapy as follows: "The literature, which lacks any negative study of substance, suggests that EBT (EEG Biofeedback Therapy, or Neurotherapy) should play a major therapeutic role in many difficult areas. "In my opinion, if any medication had demonstrated such a wide spectrum of efficacy it would be universally accepted and widely used" (Duffy, 2000).

Autistic Spectrum Disorder responds to Neurotherapy (Jarusiewicz, 2002; Sichel, Fehmi & Goldstein, 1995). EEG is characterized by extremely high amplitude, low frequency activity over large areas of the cortex, often highest in anterior locations. Frequencies are often lower than those seen in many other disorders. High amplitude, low frequency activity can bee seen in temporal regions and the midline. There are often disruptions in connectivity between frontal regions and large areas of the cortex. Symptoms can vary widely in type and severity, and often include disrupted and repetitive language, obsessive thoughts, defiant and sometimes violent behavior, uncontrolled anger, poor muscle tone and flapping, and a disconnection from others and their environment, essentially being within themselves (Jarusiewicz, 2002). Neurotherapy for Autistic Spectrum Disorder based upon QEEG is customized to fit the individual's analyzed EEG. Protocols for autism are designed to reward magnitude reductions and improvements in connectivity in specific cortical locations. Training cortical locations towards normalization affects thalamocortical relay circuits, improving function of deeper brain structures (Sterman, 1977). Neurotherapy treatment of Autistic Spectrum Disorder can provide dramatic improvements in behavior control, development of spontaneous language and conversation, recognition of others and of their environment, and improvement in attention, focus, and play activity in children, allowing greater educational gains. Other improvements include improved coordination, improved sleep, and reductions in anxiety (Jarusiewicz, 2002; Burti & Sicilian, 1983).

Neurotherapy can treat addiction disorders, such as alcoholism (Goldberg, Greenwood, & Taintor, 1977; Saxby, & Peniston, 1995; Trudeau, 2005; Watson, Herder, & Passini, 1978). Causes of addictive disorders can include genetic predisposition, the need to self medicate due to psychological stress, and head injury. A 19-year-old male, had multiple high fevers from age 3 months to 3 years due to chronic ear infections resulting in early childhood seizures. Alcohol abuse resulted in multiple head traumas due to fights. He abused multiple drugs with overdosing and attempted suicide. QEEG revealed patterns often seen in head injury, including frontal lobe dysfunction in the form of left-right hemispheric connectivity disruption, connectivity disruptions between prefrontal, frontal, and central (sensory motor) regions, and high amplitude, low frequency EEG activity in frontal locations and center of the cortex. Prefrontal-frontal and frontal-central connectivity disruptions, along with high amplitude, low frequency EEG activity, demonstrates an inability to activate and engage the frontal lobes, all of which interfere with judgment and behavior control (Duff, 2004). Neurotherapy consisted of training down the frontal and central high amplitude, low frequency EEG activity, and treating multiple frontal and central lobe locations simultaneously to improve connectivity. The patient had 20 Neurotherapy sessions. When he returned after 6 months for further treatment, he was no longer on probation, and had no further illegal or behavioral incidents. He had returned to college.

Summary

Advantages of QEEG-Neurotherapy are that it is noninvasive, self-regulated, and has no known side effects, or systemic or pharmacological interactions. It is effective across a wide range of conditions and age groups. Physiologically, training SMR seems to lead to long-term potentiation (LTP) in thalamocortical circuits. This is the area that underlies EEG generation. LTP is associated with learning. Research on SMR effects on LTP is seen in thalamocortical circuits and striatum. Neuronal protein synthesis, growth, and remodeling appear to occur. Changes appear to be durable and self-regenerating. Continuing physiological and clinical improvement can be seen months between sessions or without further Neurotherapy. Neuroplasticity mechanisms in the acute phase of therapy may include the reactivation of injured or inactive neurons, enhancement of transmitter release, initial reintegration of thalamocortical circuits and other projection areas. In long term and between training sessions, perhaps LTP sets off continued protein synthesis, elaborates connections and dendritic projections, and integrates other neuroprocesses, with continued improvements of initial circuits. Possibly improved neurotransmitter release and neurogenesis occur. These mechanisms may also be involved in therapeutic changes noted in some psychiatric disorders. Neurotransmitter regulation and reactivation of suppressed neural circuits could be positively effected by QEEG-neurotherapy. Research suggests regulation of over-excitation at various brain areas and in thalamocortical circuits. Neurotherapy has been effective in recovery even years after brain injury, or for psychiatric disorders that had failed. Continued research into technique and mechanism of action underlying the physiological changes in EEG are ongoing. It appears that healing occurs through the intrinsic properties of brain neuroplasticity. This may be enhanced by Neurotherapy, but other factors are also effective. Symptoms of disorders treated using neurotherapy can vary widely, and individual symptoms may overlap multiple diagnoses (Uhlmann & Froscher, 2001). Neurotherapy training protocol depends upon directly addressing the dysfunctional, atypical characteristics of the EEG. These characteristics are a reflection of disruptions in the underlying neurophysiologic regulatory processes. Therefore, if neurotherapy alters the EEG towards normalization, it must also normalize the underlying neurophysiology (Sterman, 2002; Fleischman & Othmer, 2005). Recovery is enhanced by combining Neurotherapy with other therapies. Behavior management helps replace old behaviors. Neurotherapy affects neurotransmitter modulation. Nutrition and lifestyle have a profound effect on brain function and neurotransmitters. Drug and dietary deficiencies can compromise brain function. Sufficient sleep and healthy lifestyle can enhance the effect of neurotherapy. Nutrition and lifestyle counseling are important. While QEEG-Neurotherapy is not the only way of promoting neuroplasticity or neurorehabilitation, it appears to have a promising role to enhance opportunity for healing along with other beneficial lifestyle choices.

REFERENCES

American Psychiatric Association (2000). Diagnostic criteria for 299.80 Asperger's Disorder (AD), *Diagnostic and Statistical Manual of Mental Disorders* (4th edn, text revision). Washington, DC: American Psychological Association.

Atwood, T. (1998). Australian Scale for Asperger's Syndrome (ASAS). In *Asperger's Syndrome: A Guide for Parents and Professionals.* London: Jessica Kingsley Publishers, pp. 16–20.

Baydala, L., & Wikman, E. (2001). The efficacy of neurofeedback in the management of children with attention deficit/hyperactivity disorder. *Paediatrics and Child Health,* 6(7), 451–455.

Burti, L., & Siciliani, O. (1983). Increase in alpha-rhythm in anxious subjects using biofeedback: A preliminary study. *Psichiatria Generale e del Età Evolutiva,* 21(2–4), 79–97.

Duff, J. (2004). The usefulness of quantitative EEG (QEEG) and neurotherapy in the assessment and treatment of post-concussion syndrome. *Clinical EEG & Neuroscience,* 35(4), 198–209.

Duffy, F. H. (2000). The state of EEG biofeedback therapy (EEG operant conditioning). *Clinical Electroencephalography,* 31(1), V–VII.

Feinstein, B., Sterman, M. B., & MacDonald, L. R. (1974). Effects of sensorimotor rhythm training on sleep. *Sleep Research, 3*, 134.

Fernandez, T., Herrera, W., Harmony, T., Diaz-Comas, L., Santiago, E., Sanchez, L., et al. (2003). EEG and behavioral changes following neurofeedback treatment in learning disabled children. *Clinical Electroencephalography, 34*(3), 145–150.

Fleischman, M. J., & Othmer, S. (2005). Case study: Improvements in IQ score and maintenance of gains following EEG biofeedback with mildly developmentally delayed twins. *Journal of Neurotherapy, 9*(4), 35–46.

Fuchs, T., Birbaumer, N., Lutzenberger, W., Gruzelier, J. H., & Kaiser, J. (2003). Neurofeedback treatment for attention-defecit/hyperactivity disorder in children: A comparison with methyphenidate. *Applied Psychophysiology and Biofeedback, 28*(1), 1–12.

Goldberg, R. J., Greenwood, J. C., & Taintor, Z. (1977). Alpha conditioning as an adjunct treatment for drug dependence: Part II. *International Journal of Addiction, 12*, 195–204.

Hammond, D. C. (2003). QEEG-guided neurofeedback in the treatment of obsessive compulsive disorder. *Journal of Neurotherapy, 7*(2), 25–52.

Howe, R. C., & Sterman, M. B. (1972). Cortical-subcortical correlates of suppressed motor behavior during sleep and waking in the cat. *Electroencephalography and Clinical Neurophysiology, 6*, 681–695.

Howe, R. C., & Sterman, M. B. (1973). Somatosensory system evoked potentials during waking behavior and in sleep in the cat. *Electroencephalography and Clinical Neurophysiology, 6*, 605–618.

Hoyt, C. S. (2003). Visual function in the brain injured child. *Eye, 17*, 369–384.

Jarusiewicz, B. (2002). Efficacy of neurofeedback for children in the autistic spectrum: A pilot study. *Journal of Neurotherapy, 6*(4), 39–49.

Klin, A., & Volkmar, F. (1995). Asperger's syndrome guidelines for assessment and diagnosis. Retrieved January 13, 2008, from Yale School of Medicine Web Site: http://info.med.yale.edu/chldstdy/autism/asdiagnosis.pdf

Levesque, J., Beauregard, M., & Mensour, B. (2006). Effect of neurofeedback training on the neural substrates of selective attention in children with attention-deficit/hyperactivity disorder: A functional magnetic resonance imaging study. *Neuroscience Letters, 394*(3), 216–221.

Linden, M., Habib, T., & Radojevic, V. (1996). A controlled study of the effects of EEG biofeedback on cognition and behavior of children with attention deficit disorder and learning disabilities. *Biofeedback & Self-Regulation, 21*(1), 35–49.

Malkowicz, D. E., Meyers, G., & Leisman, G. (2006). Rehabilation of cortical visual impairment in children. *International Journal of Neuroscience, 116*, 1015–1033.

Monastra, V. J., (2005). Electroencephalographic biofeedback (neurotherapy) as a treatment for attention deficit hyperactivity disorder: Rationale and empirical foundation. *Child & Adolescent Psychiatric Clinics of North America, 14*(1), 55–82.

Monderer, R. S., Harrison, D. M. & Hunt, S. R. (2002). Neurofeedback and Epilepsy. *Epilepsy and Behavior, 3*, 214–218.

Moore, N. C. (2000). A review of EEG biofeedback treatment of anxiety disorders. *Clinical Electroencephalography, 31*(1), 1–6.

Morse, M. (1990). Cortical visual impairment in young with multiple disabilities. *Journal of Visual Impairment and Blindness, 84,* 200–203.

Ross, J., & Caunt, J. (2003). QEEG characteristics in asperger's disorder [Abstract]. *Journal of Neurotherapy, 7*(1), 128–129.

Rossiter, T. R. (2005). The effectiveness of neurofeedback and stimulant drugs in treating AD/HD: Part II. Replication. *Applied Psychophysiology & Biofeedback, 29*(4), 233–243.

Roth, S. R., Sterman, M. B., & Clemente, C. C. (1967). Comparisons of EEG correlates of reinforcement, internal inhibition and sleep. *Electroencephalography and Clinical Neurophysiology, 23,* 509–520.

Saxby, E., & Peniston, E. G. (1995). Alpha-theta brainwave neurofeedback training: An effective treatment for male and female alcoholics with depressive symptoms. *Journal of Clinical Psychology, 51*(5), 685–693.

Scolnick, B. (2005). Effects of electroencephalogram biofeedback with Asperger's syndrome. *International Journal of Rehabilitation Research, 28*(2), 159–163.

Sichel, A. G., Fehmi, L. G., & Goldstein, D. M. (1995). Positive outcome with neurofeedback treatment of a case of mild autism. *Journal of Neurotherapy, 1*(1), 60–64.

Sterman, M. B. (1973). Neurophysiological and clinical studies of sensorimotor EEG biofeedback training: Some effects on epilepsy. *Seminars in Psychiatry, 5*(4), 507–525.

Sterman, M. B. (1977). Sensorimotor EEG operant conditioning: Experimental and clinical effects. *Pavlovian Journal of Biological Sciences, 12*(2), 6392.

Sterman, M. B. (1986). Epilepsy and its treatment with EEG feedback therapy. *Annals of Behavioral Medicine, 8,* 21–25.

Sterman, M. B. (1996). Physiological origins and and functional correlates of EEG rhythmic activies : Implications for self regulation. *Biological Psychology, 3,* 157–184.

Sterman, M. B. (2000). Basic concepts and clinical findings in the treatment of seizure disorders with EEG operant conditioning. *Clinical Electroencephalography, 31*(1), 45–55.

Sterman, M.B. (2002). *Physiology, Learning, Analysis, Nuance.* QEEG/Neurofeedback Training Course.

Sterman, M. B., & Egner, T. (2006). Foundation and practice of neurofeedback for the treatment of epilepsy. *Applied Psychophsiology and Biofeedback, 1,* 21–35.

Sterman, M. B., & Friar, L. (1972). Suppression of seizures in epileptics following sensorimotor EEG feedback training. *Electroencephalography & Clinical Neurophysiology, 33,* 89–95.

Sterman, M. B., Howe, R. D., & Macdonald, L. R. (1970). Facilitation of spindle-burst sleep by conditioning of electroencephalographic activity while awake. *Science, 167,* 1146–1148.

Sterman, M. B., & Kaiser, D. (2001). Comodulation: A new QEEG analysis metric for assessment of structural and functional disorders of the central nervous system. *Journal of Neurotherapy, 4*(3), 73–83.

Sterman, M. B., & Macdonald, L. R. (1978). Effects of central cortical EEG feedback training on incidence of poorly controlled seizures. *Epilepsia, 19*(3), 207–222.

Sterman, M. B., Macdonald, L. R., & Stone, R. K. (1974). Biofeedback training of the sensorimotor electroencephalogram rhythm in man: Effects on epilepsy. *Epilepsia, 15*(3), 395–416.

Sterman, M. B., & Shouse, M. N. (1980). Quantitative analysis of training, sleep EEG and clinical response to EEG operant conditioning in epileptics. *Electroencephalography & Clinical Neurophysiology, 49,* 558–576.

Sterman, M. B., Wyrwicka, W., & Roth, S. R. (1969). Electrophysiological correlates and neural substrates of alimentary behavior in the cat. *Annuals of the New York Academy of Science, 157,* 723–739.

Trudeau, D. L. (2005). Applicability of brain wave biofeedback to substance use disorder in adolescents. *Child & Adolescent Psychiatric Clinics of North America, 14*(1), 125–136.

Uhlmann, C., & Froscher, W. (2001). Biofeedback treatment in patients with refractory epilepsy: Changes in depression and control orientation. *Seizure, 10,* 34–38.

Watson, C. G., Herder, J., & Passini, F. T. (1978). Alpha biofeedback therapy in alcoholics: An 18-month follow-up. *Journal of Clinical Psychology, 34*(2), 765–769.

Wyrwicka, W. & Sterman, M. B. (1968). Instrumental conditioning of sensorimotor cortex EEG spindles in the waking cat. *Physiology and Behavior, 3,* 703–707.

Xiong, Z., Shi, S., & Xu, H. (2005). A controlled study of the effectiveness of EEG biofeedback training on children with attention deficit hyperactivity disorder. *Journal of Huazhong University of Science & Technology, 25*(3), 368–370.

PART IV

MIND

13

Mindfulness and Mindfulness-Based Stress Reduction

DONALD McCOWN AND DIANE REIBEL

KEY CONCEPTS

- Mindfulness-Based Stress Reduction (MBSR) and a range of newer mindfulness-based interventions (MBIs) are reaping the benefits of three decades of scientific research into mindfulness and are attaining status as evidence-based treatments.
- The flowering of mindfulness is intertwined with the history of the influence of Eastern thought on Western psychology and medicine—particularly since World War II.
- Mindfulness, expressed formally as meditative practice or informally in one's approach to life, can be described as paying attention on purpose, in the present moment, without judgment.
- MBSR is a nonpathologizing, education-based program, designed for delivery in a group setting; its curriculum includes formal and informal mindfulness practice, didactic modules on stress reactivity and physiology, and modules intended to contribute to participants' biopsychosocial well-being.
- The major factor in successful teaching in the MBIs is the teacher's capacity for "embodiment" of mindfulness; this suggests deep commitment to personal mindfulness practice and mindfulness teacher training before bringing these interventions to others.
- Integrative psychiatrists may choose to engage with MBSR and other MBIs by (1) referring patients to appropriate interventions; (2) beginning mindfulness practice themselves, which has been shown to enhance personal well-being of the practitioner as well as improve clinical outcomes; (3) undertaking the necessary practice and study to become an MBSR/MBI teacher.

■

Background: The Flourishing of Mindfulness-Based Interventions

Lately, there has been dramatic growth of interest by researchers, clinicians, and patients in mindfulness-based approaches to treating a wide range of conditions. At the time of writing this chapter, mindfulness-based interventions are being used or investigated for medical conditions such as asthma, breast cancer, prostate cancer, solid organ transplant, bone marrow transplant, fibromyalgia, chronic pain, hypertension, HIV, myocardial ischemia, type-2 diabetes, hot flashes, obesity, irritable bowel syndrome, immune response to human papillomavirus, rheumatoid arthritis, chronic obstructive pulmonary disease (COPD), lupus, and more (Clinical Trials, 2008); they are also in use and investigation for a range of psychiatric disorders, including anxiety disorders, depression, suicidality, personality disorders, eating disorders, drug abuse and dependence, posttraumatic stress disorder (PTSD), schizophrenia, delusional disorders, and others (Clinical Trials, 2008). The list of mindfulness-based and mindfulness-informed interventions has been growing with increasing velocity since the turn of the century, now including Mindfulness-Based Cognitive Therapy (MBCT), Mindfulness-Based Relationship Enhancement (MBRE), Mindfulness-Based Relapse Prevention (MBRP), Mindfulness-Based Eating Awareness Training (MB-EAT), and Mindfulness-Based Art Therapy (MBAT), as well as interventions with a significant mindfulness component, such as Acceptance and Commitment Therapy (ACT) and Dialectical Behavior Therapy (DBT). Amid the din of discourse on meditation, mindfulness, and their places in health care, there is an intervention that is salient for many reasons: Mindfulness-Based Stress Reduction (MBSR).

Introduction: The Importance of MBSR

Dryden and Still (2006) identify the year 1990 as a watershed, after which the use of the term "mindfulness" began burgeoning in the discourse of Western psychology and psychotherapy. This coincides with the publication of Jon Kabat-Zinn's *Full-Catastrophe Living*, a description and de facto manualization of the MBSR program that he and colleagues at the University of Massachusetts Medical Center had been developing since 1979. Its success and influence on

Mindfulness-Based Interventions and Health Benefits: Meta-analyses

Since its beginning, there has been an effort to develop an empirical evidence base for MBSR's efficacy. This effort has been part of all subsequent elaborations of the program, and is a feature, as well, of the other key mindfulness-based interventions. As a result, there is a significant literature, of mostly

Table Based on Baer (2003)

Variable	N	Mean Effect Size*
By Research Design		
Pre-post	8	0.71
Between group	10	0.69
By Population		
Chronic pain	4	0.37
Axis 1 (anxiety, depression)	4	0.96
Medical (fibromyalgia, cancer, psoriasis)	4	0.55
Nonclinical (medical students, healthy volunteers)	4	0.92
By Outcome Measure		
Pain	17	0.31
Anxiety	8	0.70
Depression	5	0.86
Medical symptoms (self-report)	11	0.44
Global psychological**	18	0.64
Medical symptoms (Objective)***	2	0.80

* At post-treatment.

** Profile of Mood States (POMS)—total mood disturbance, SCL-90 R Global severity index.

*** Urine and skin.

N = Number of studies included in the meta-analysis. Of the studies included in the analysis, two employed MBCT as the intervention, one employed listening to mindfulness tapes, and the remaining used MBSR or a variant of MBSR as the treatment intervention.

Table Based on Grossman et al. (2004)

Variables	N	Mean Effect Size*
Mental Health Variables		
Pre-post	18	0.50
Between groups	10	0.54
Physical Health Variables		
Pre-post	9	0.42
Between groups	5	0.53

*At post-treatment
N = Number of studies included in the meta-analysis.
Between Groups (controlled studies) include both wait-list controls (WLC) and active controls (AC). No difference in mean effect size noted between WLC and AC.

noncontrolled study designs, that has reinforced interest and most recently has engendered significant investment through government agencies and private foundations for clinical trials of mindfulness-based interventions for a range of medical and psychological conditions.

The two meta-analyses profiled in the tables above provide a snapshot of the state of the research on mindfulness-based interventions as interest began to surge. Both applied stringent criteria for selection of the studies to be analyzed. Conclusions may be characterized by this statement from Grossman, Niemann, Schmidt, and Walach (2004), "Thus far, the literature seems to clearly slant toward support for basic hypotheses concerning the effects of mindfulness on mental and physical well-being."

the development of other interventions incorporating mindfulness arise from its status as an "evidence-based practice," its immediate appeal as a transformative group experience for the participants *and* the teacher, and its position at the confluence of certain social and institutional factors, including the energy and charisma of its leadership, the need within academic medicine and psychology for "safe" new avenues of research, and the endorsement by powerful institutions in the academy and the popular media, including PBS, *Time,*

Newsweek, and *Business Week* (Dryden & Still, 2006; Hovanessian, 2003; Kalb, 2003; Moyers, 1993; Stein, 2003).

Given MBSR's position both as a culmination of a two-centuries-long dialogue between Eastern and Western culture, and as a highly influential template or touchstone for elaboration of other interventions incorporating mindfulness meditation practice, we have chosen to focus this chapter specifically on this singular intervention. The chapter is not designed primarily as a recounting of the evidence base for MBSR's efficacy, which is easily accessible and rapidly expanding, but rather as a view of the construction and delivery of the MBSR curriculum—from a teacher's perspective. We hope that this view will inspire further the adoption of MBSR and other mindfulness-based interventions within integrative medicine, and also will begin to help those interested to develop the necessary skills and capacities as teachers to incorporate mindfulness practices into other programs for the wellness of mind–body–spirit. Our intention is to facilitate the expansion of mindfulness practice into continually broadening medical and social contexts.

The chapter begins by situating MBSR in the history of East–West dialogue. We then turn to essential theoretical understandings that inform MBSR practice and pedagogy, including an attempt to define mindfulness as a process or mode of being, and to identify the mechanisms of action that may contribute to the improvement—even transformation—of participants. What follows next is more concrete: a description of the MBSR curriculum and an account of how participants' increasing abilities and understandings unfold from session to session. Focus then shifts to the teacher, in an attempt to identify the unique skills required in MBSR—educational, meditative, and clinical. Further reflection suggests that mindfulness teachers, regardless of the specific intervention they deliver, must embody mindfulness, not only in the class but also in the world, and we suggest three characteristics to be considered and cultivated. Finally, we consider ways in which the integrative psychiatrist might engage with mindfulness and MBSR, and suggest resources for training and development for those interested in teaching mindfulness—both inside and outside the MBSR context.

History: Meditation and Mindfulness in the Meeting of East and West

Early roots: The appeal of the mindfulness-based interventions runs deep into the historic rapprochement of Western and Eastern philosophical, religious, and medical thought over the past two centuries. In the United States, this first surfaced most clearly in the nineteenth century in the philosophical, aesthetic, and social expressions of the New England Transcendentalists. In writers such as Emerson and Thoreau the influence of Indian thought is evident (Brooks, 1936). Translations of the Vedas and Upanishads, as well as Buddhist texts, were becoming available in the West at that time. In fact, Thoreau was one of the first Americans to read Buddhist scripture, as he brought into English in 1844 a section of the Lotus Sutra, which had just been translated into French (Fields, 1981; Tweed, 1992). This engagement with the East also included East Asian culture, with Chinese, Korean, and Japanese arts, literature, and religion—including Buddhist practice—shaping the intellectual direction of the American and European avant-garde. For example, the thought of Ernest Fenollosa, American scholar of East Asian art and literature, and convert to Buddhism, as interpreted by Ezra Pound and other modern poets and thinkers, brought this spirit into wider intellectual discourse (Bevis, 1988; Brooks, 1962). Perhaps these few lines from Fenollosa's poem, "East and West," his Phi Beta Kappa address at Harvard in 1892, capture the yearning of modern Western consciousness. Addressing a Japanese mentor, Fenollosa says, "I've flown from my West/ Like a desolate bird from a broken nest/ To learn thy secret of joy and rest" (quoted in Brooks, 1962, p. 50).

About the last 60 years: According to Dryden and Still (2006), the influence of Eastern thought began developing greater momentum in post-World War II Japan, when Western physicians, scientists, and other intellectuals who held posts during the American occupation were exposed to Japanese culture, including the many manifestations of Zen Buddhism. In identifying direct influences on psychotherapeutic thought, Still (2006) points to the exposure of American military psychiatrists to the Zen-informed psychotherapy of Shoma Morita, "which reversed the Western medical approach of attacking the symptoms. Instead, he taught patients to accept symptoms, such as anxiety, with calm awareness, or mindfulness." This paradoxical orientation, rather than the specific techniques of Morita therapy, resonated with Western health care professionals, as Zen did with Westerners of other disciplines, and began to find cultural expression.

Zen had a double-barreled influence in the West, particularly in the postwar "Zen boom" years of the 1950s and 1960s. There was a powerful impact on Western intellectuals in spirituality, psychotherapy, and aesthetic practice, famously exemplified by the effects on Christian contemplative practice through the Trappist monk Thomas Merton, on psychoanalysis through the thought of Eric Fromm, and on contemporary art music through the composer John Cage, all of whom encountered the Zen scholar D.T. Suzuki (e.g., respectively, Merton, 1968; Suzuki, Fromm, & De Martino, 1960; Cage, 1966). There was an equally strong impact on the more popular levels of discourse, characterized by the small but growing counterculture, which took on the challenges of Zen and other esoteric disciplines in a more dramatic if less orderly fashion, making participation as much a statement of resistance to the social status quo as a personal practice of transformation, as described pithily in Alan Watts's *Beat Zen, Square Zen, and Zen* (1959). On both the substantive and popular levels, then, the market (so to speak) for Eastern and Eastern-inflected spiritual practices grew steadily. Through political dislocations, waves of immigration, and economic opportunity seeking, teachers from many of the Eastern traditions became available to offer instruction in the West. Some of those teachers began to "repackage" their practices for Western students, with the Maharishi Mahesh Yogi's repackaging of Hindu mantra meditation as Transcendental Meditation® (TM®) as perhaps the most well-known and influential example (Mahesh Yogi, 1968/1963).

In the 1960s, TM quickly captured the attention of the medical establishment through its high profile in popular culture and scientific research into its physical and psychological outcomes (e.g., Seeman, Nidich, & Banta, 1972; Wallace, 1970). The result was development of, and research on, medicalized versions, such as the Relaxation Response (Benson, 1975) and Clinical Standardized Meditation (Carrington, 1975/1998). The factors at work here—popular recognition, translation into Western language and settings, and adoption within scientific research in powerful institutions—all come into play later in the development of the discourse around mindfulness.

A necessary parsing of the various forms of meditation practice presented across the range of spiritual traditions, particularly Buddhism, was performed by Goleman (1977/1988), who describes meditation approaches of *concentration* and *insight*, and who in discussing insight meditation explicitly uses the term *mindfulness* in the way that it has entered current discourse. Concentration forms of meditation teach a focus on a single object of attention, such as the breath. Insight forms teach attention to all experiences arising in the sense perceptions and the domains of thought and emotion. Goleman explains the commonly exploited interrelation of these two forms, as concentration practice develops qualities of mind that support insight practice. Goleman's description of mindfulness is a concise foreshadowing of the current attempts in the scientific literature to define mindfulness and its mechanisms of action:

> Our natural tendency is to become habituated to the world around us, no longer to notice the familiar. We also substitute abstract names or preconceptions for the raw evidence of the senses. In mindfulness, the meditator methodically faces the bare facts of his experience, seeing each event as though occurring for the first time. (Goleman, 1988, p. 20)

Between two worlds: Rothwell (2006), Still (2006), and Martin (1997) all delineate two different intellectual environments that have influenced and contributed to the contemporary approaches to mindfulness in research and clinical applications. On the one hand, there is the discourse associated with the cognitive-behavioral therapies. Within these therapies, identifiable forms of mindfulness-based or informed intervention have arisen, which may or may not include meditation practice for cultivating mindfulness, and which predict outcomes based on cause and effect (Rothwell, 2006). Such interventions have found significant appeal within the dominant social and political discourses and practices of health care, particularly in the United States, where evidence-based practices have a preferred status. On the other hand, there are the more holistic approaches, associated with the basic insight of the meditative traditions, epitomized in the paradoxical turning toward one's symptoms, and with an appreciation of the religious roots and resonances of meditation practice that can be found within contemporary psychodynamic, humanistic, transpersonal, and postmodern streams of psychotherapy (e.g., respectively, Epstein, 1995; West, 2000; Boorstein, 1996; Norum, 2000). In this approach, interventions incorporate meditation and spiritual practices to cultivate ways of being, rather than specific outcomes (Rothwell, 2006). Such interventions are building their own evidence bases, strengthening their appeal within the social and cultural discourse that has allowed integrative medicine to grow and flourish. For example, consider the presence of explicit MBSR programs at five of the eight Bravewell Collaborative integrative medicine centers, and the presence of mindfulness-influenced programs at others (Bravewell Collaborative, 2008). It is apparent, then, that MBSR is situated on the fault line between these two intellectual environments, and directly feeds, offers inspiration to, and benefits from the research and development of mindfulness-based and mindfulness-informed interventions in both environments.

THEORY I: CONSTRUCTING A MODEL OF MINDFULNESS IN MBSR

The effort to develop a single, scientific account of mindfulness useful for both clinicians and researchers is admittedly difficult and complex (Allen, Blashki, & Gullone, 2006; Baer, 2003; Bishop et al., 2004; Brody & Park, 2004; Brown & Ryan, 2004; Claxton, 2006; Hayes & Feldman, 2004; Hayes & Shenk, 2004; Hayes & Wilson, 2003; Ivanovski & Malhi, 2007; Rothwell, 2006; Shapiro, Carlson, Astin, & Freedman, 2006). Reasons for this include the following:

1. Use of identical terms in significantly different outlooks and discourses, from Buddhist texts and their English translations in a variety of traditions to humanistic psychotherapy and to scientific psychology (Dryden & Still, 2006).

2. Confusion as to whether mindfulness is a practice, a process, an outcome, a transient state to be exploited, or a way of life to be cultivated (Hayes & Wilson, 2003).

3. Group contexts and inclusion of disparate didactic and experiential components in mindfulness-based interventions, providing many competing mechanisms of action (Bishop, 2002; Ivanovski & Malhi, 2007; Shapiro et al., 2006).

This chapter's exclusive focus on MBSR as an exemplary mindfulness-based intervention neatly sidesteps many of the above complications. We can take up a social constructionist perspective (e.g., Gergen, 1999) in which we accept that knowledge is not an objective reflection of what is "out there in the world" but rather is co-created within relationships. Thus, we need not posit one "true" definition or model of mindfulness in order to understand, apply, and research outcomes from MBSR. Instead, we can deeply examine the model of mindfulness, the practices that cultivate it, and the mechanisms of action that are implicit (and explicit) in the discourse of MBSR theory, pedagogy, and research. These have been (and continue to be) co-constructed in the professional dialogues in the MBSR community, fostered by the Center for Mindfulness and its programs, through which more than 9,000 MBSR researchers and teachers have developed their understanding of and capacity to teach MBSR, via trainings, conferences, and personal relationships (CFM, 2007a). The model of mindfulness, therefore, evolves when MBSR shifts to different leadership and institutional contexts. And, importantly, the model is co-created again and again, with infinite variations, by the communities of practice and learning defined by MBSR classes and their teachers.

The most commonly quoted definitions of mindfulness in the mindfulness-based intervention literature come, not surprisingly, from Jon Kabat-Zinn:

- ...paying attention in a particular way: on purpose, in the present moment, and non-judgmentally. (1994, p. 4)
- Mindfulness meditation is a consciousness discipline revolving around a particular way of paying attention in one's life. It can be most simply described as the intentional cultivation of nonjudgmental moment-to-moment awareness (1996)

Three key elements of the definition—intentionality, present-centeredness, and absence of judgment—are repeated and reinforced both in the ongoing scientific-research-oriented discussions of MBSR, and through MBSR teachers in hundreds of classes unfolding week by week around the world. These three key elements continue to shape the thinking, practice, and experience of an ever-changing and expanding MBSR community.

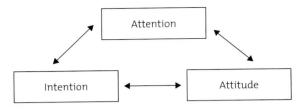

FIGURE 13.1 The three axioms of intention, attention, and attitude (IAA) are not sequential, but rather are engaged simultaneously in the process of mindfulness (Shapiro et al., 2006).

It is telling that the first attempt at developing an operational definition of mindfulness took place within the greater community of the many mindfulness-based and mindfulness-informed interventions, in which other ad hoc definitions are current, and that the result was a two-part definition that omitted the element of intention (Bishop et al., 2004). A "second generation" model uses the above quoted Kabat-Zinn texts as a touchstone, and proposes a model that is congruent with MBSR teaching and practice (Shapiro et al., 2006). This model, shown graphically in Figure 13.1, posits three axioms: intention, attention, and attitude (IAA), which are simultaneously manifesting elements of the moment-to-moment practice of mindfulness, whether formal or informal. Each axiom captures a part of the direct experience of a participant practicing in an MBSR class. As to the axiom of intention, Shapiro, et al., note that a personal vision or motivation for initiating mindfulness practice is not explicit in the "secular" construct of MBSR in the same way that it is found in its religious corollaries. The vision of each participant, then, is "personal" and has been shown to shift along a continuum "from self-regulation, to self-exploration, and finally to self-liberation" (Shapiro et al., 2006). As to the axiom of attention, this captures the different capacities involved in attending to one's moment-to-moment experience. Shapiro et al. (2006) suggest that the essential capacities are sustained focus and flexibility of focus. These are cultivated explicitly in the MBSR classes through the methods and order by which the formal mindfulness practices are introduced and assigned. As to the axiom of attitude, the nonjudgment that is called for is not an affect-free "bare awareness," but rather an accepting, open, and kind curiosity toward one's own experience (Shapiro et al., 2006).

THEORY II: IDENTIFYING MECHANISMS OF ACTION

In the descriptions of outcomes of mindfulness practice both inside and outside the MBSR community, a major emphasis is placed on a particular shift in the practitioner's relationship to self and experience—the awareness of an observing consciousness that is both *a part of* and *apart from* the experience. In MBSR classes, in the authors' experiences, such realization may be typically revealed in expressions by participants along the lines of, "I am not my thoughts," or "I am not this pain."

In many scientific accounts across the different investigating disciplines and the different approaches to meditation and mindfulness, this shift has been identified as a central mechanism. McCown (2004) reviewed early studies, pointing out that Deikman (1966) suggested a mechanism of "*de-automatization* of the psychological structures that organize, limit, select and interpret perceptual stimuli"; Linden (1973) and Pelletier (1974) noted the increased *field independence* of practiced meditators, evidenced by their ability to discern the hidden shapes in Embedded Figures Tests and, in pioneering EEG studies, Kasamatsu and Hirai (1973) noted a *de-habituation* to stimuli in Zen Masters that they described as "constant refreshing of perception of the moment." Martin (1997), reviewing later concepts, notes Deikman's *observing self* (1982); Safran and Segal's (1990) contribution of such terms as *deautomization*, in which habitual modes of perception are suspended, and *decentering*, in which a capacity to view experience from "outside" is cultivated; and Langer's (1989) concept of *mindfulness*, developed solely within the context of Western scientific psychology, which defines a cognitive process in which three mechanisms operate: creation of new categories, openness to new information, and awareness of more than one perspective.

Flowing from their MBSR-informed definition of mindfulness, Shapiro et al. (2006) propose a meta-mechanism that they call *reperceiving*, and that they define as "a rotation in consciousness in which what was previously 'subject' becomes 'object.'" They further suggest that this meta-mechanism is basic to human development, and, therefore, that mindfulness practice simply strengthens and accelerates the growth of this capacity. The statements quoted above from participants in the authors' MBSR classes illustrate this capacity to move from a position in which one is completely identified with one's experience to a position in which the experience becomes available for observation. It must be noted here that within MBSR pedagogical practice: (1) reperceiving does not create distance and disconnection from one's experience, but rather enables one to look, feel, and know more deeply; (2) the "observing self" is not reified, but rather is seen as a temporary platform for observation and questioning.

With one's experience thus available for reflection and inquiry, additional mechanisms may come into play. Shapiro et al. (2006) highlight four. One is *self-regulation and self-management*, where with reperceiving we can gain knowledge about experiences that may previously have been too challenging to explore in depth or over time, and we can identify and then choose to override habitual reactions and respond with more balance and greater skill. Second is *values clarification*, where reperceiving provides an opportunity to reflect on values that may have been adopted unquestioningly and to choose to adapt or adopt values more resonant with our current context. Third is *cognitive, emotional, and behavioral flexibility*, where the "objective" viewpoint inherent in reperceiving allows a more clear view of the thoughts, emotions, and (anticipated) actions of an emergent situation, from which may follow new, situation-specific responses. Fourth is *exposure*, where reperceiving's "objective," nonreactive character provides the space and time for intimate encounters with formerly disturbing emotions, thoughts, and body sensations, in which their capacity for disruption is reduced. As we shall see in the section on MBSR pedagogical theory and practice below, these kinds of mechanisms are not only implicit in the MBSR mindfulness meditations, but are also discovered, actuated, and elaborated through the group dialogues and individual teacher–participant exchanges that are at the core of the MBSR experience.

Mindfulness-Based Stress Reduction

MBSR was designed for a heterogeneous patient population, open to people with physical and/or psychological diagnoses or with simply a desire to alleviate the "stress" of the human condition. Rothwell (2006) points out that it is inherently holistic. It is nondualistic in its thinking about the body–mind complex. It is nonpathologizing in its insistence that "as long as you are breathing, there is more right with you than there is wrong" (Kabat-Zinn, 1990, p. 2). It is designed to train participants in formal and informal practices, as well as to actuate and accelerate the placebo effect, and to exploit the social factors of emotional support and caring (Kabat-Zinn, 1996). Further, it is not positioned as a clinical intervention at all, but rather as an educational program.

The structure of the MBSR program that is modeled as a template at the Center for Mindfulness is an 8-week, 9-session course that is educational, experiential, and patient centered. Participants attend 2-1/2 hour sessions once a week for 8 weeks, with a full-day (7-hours) class between the sixth and seventh sessions. Class time each week is divided between formal meditation practice, small and large group discussions, and inquiry with individuals into their present-moment experiences.

Formal practices include body scan, sitting meditation (with focus on the breath), mindful Hatha yoga, sitting meditation (moving from focus on the breath to an expanded awareness of other objects of attention, i.e., body sensations, hearing, thoughts, emotions, and ending with an open awareness of all that is arising in the present moment), walking meditation, and eating meditation. Class discussions focus on group members' experiences in the formal meditation practices and the application of mindfulness in day-to-day life. Home practice is an integral part of MBSR. In Kabat-Zinn's original program, participants are asked to commit to formal practice, supported by audio recordings of guided meditations, for 45 minutes a day, 6 days per week.

As they move from their training at the Center for Mindfulness out to their own locations and audiences, teachers often find that they are called to deliver MBSR programs to a wide variety of populations, in circumstances that may require adaptation of the template program. This is implicit in teacher training. In fact, in an article by Kabat-Zinn (1996) that is part of the literature provided in the "entry-level" training delivered by the Center for Mindfulness, he states:

> We emphasize that there are many different ways to structure and deliver mindfulness-based stress reduction programs. The optimal form of its delivery will depend critically on local factors and on the level of experience and understanding of the people undertaking the teaching. Rather than "clone" or "franchise" one cookie cutter approach, mindfulness ultimately requires effective use of the present moment as the core indicator of the appropriateness of particular choices.

For example, three areas of choice that have been studied are the length of the course, duration of class sessions, and duration of home practice sessions. Several studies report course lengths of four to ten weeks (Jain et al., 2007; Rosenzweig, Reibel, Greeson, Brainard, & Hojat, 2003), and class durations shorter than the model, ranging from 1-1/2 to 2 hours (Astin, 1997; Jain et al., 2007; Rosenzweig et al., 2003; Roth & Calle-Mesa, 2006). Formal home practice times shorter than the model range from 15 to 35 minutes (Jain et al., 2007; Reibel et al., 2001; Rosenzweig et al., 2003; Roth & Calle-Mesa, 2006). It is interesting to note that the average practice time reported by participants in the CFM model program, where 45-minute recordings are used, is found to be variable, depending upon the specific practice, from an average of 16 to 35 minutes per day (Carmody & Baer, 2008). There is no consensus on the relationship between home practice duration or frequency and health outcomes. Some reports do not show a correlation between formal home practice time and health outcomes (Astin, 1997; Carmody, Reed, Kristeller, & Merriam, 2008; Davidson et al., 2003) while others find correlations between practice time and specific health outcomes (Carmody & Baer, 2008; Speca, Carlson, Goodey, & Angen, 2000). For example, in Carmody and Baer (2008), practice time was correlated with improvement in psychological well being and perceived stress but not medical symptoms.

A TYPICAL MBSR CURRICULUM

The original MBSR curriculum undergoes a transformation based on local population, setting, and teacher factors. However, the integrity of the model is typically maintained through continuity of basic themes and practices. The outline below describes themes, learning objectives, and specific practices introduced in each session. The themes and practices are reinforced and built upon in each succeeding week.

Session One. *Theme*: There is more right with you than wrong with you, no matter what challenges you are facing. Problems can be worked with, and the MBSR program offers the opportunity to do this in a supportive environment. Present-moment awareness of body sensations, thoughts, and emotions is the foundation of this work, because it is only in the present that one can learn, grow, and change.

Practices introduced: Eating meditation, diaphragmatic breathing, body scan

Session Two. *Theme*: Perception and creative responding: How you see things, or do not see them, will determine how you will respond to them. It is not the events themselves but rather how you handle them that influences the effects on your body and mind.

Practice introduced: Sitting meditation (focus on awareness of breath)

Session Three. *Theme*: There is pleasure and power in being present. We miss many of our pleasant moments, perhaps by focusing only on the unpleasant ones (i.e., crisis or pain). You can have pleasant moments even when you a re-experiencing pain. Focus on the triangle of awareness: body sensation, thought, and emotion.

Practices introduced: Mindful yoga

Session Four. *Theme*: Awareness of being stuck in one's life and how to get unstuck. Cultivating mindfulness can reduce the negative effects of stress reactivity, as well as help develop more effective ways of responding positively and proactively to stressful situations and experiences.

Practices introduced: Sitting meditation (expanding focus from awareness of breath to body sensations and hearing)

Session Five. *Theme*: Reacting and responding to stress. The learning objective of this session is to connect mindfulness with perception, appraisal, and choice in the critical moment. Particular attention is paid to observing thoughts as events, and distinguishing events from content—"You are not your thought."

Practices introduced: Sitting meditation (expanding awareness beyond breath, body sensations, and hearing to observing thoughts, emotions, and whatever arises in the present moment)

Session Six. *Theme*: Mindful communication in stressful situations, including awareness of your needs in the present moment, and ways to express those needs effectively. The learning objective of this session is to learn how to maintain your center, recognize habitual patterns of relating, and discern skillful options in stressful interpersonal exchanges.

Practices introduced: Walking meditation

All-Day Session. *Theme*: Integrate mindfulness practices learned in the prior sessions. Deepen mindful awareness of experience by formally cultivating mindfulness over an extended period of time, fostering the possibility of greater self-knowledge and insight into the impermanence of body–mind states.

Practices: The full range of practices from prior sessions are reinforced, and two new practices are introduced—mountain or lake meditation and loving-kindness meditation

Session Seven. *Theme*: Cultivating kindness toward self and others. The learning objective of this session is to learn to cultivate a disposition of generosity in formal meditation practice so that it may arise more readily in our day-to-day life.

Practices introduced: Concentration meditations on kindness and compassion

Session Eight. *Theme*: "The eighth week is the rest of your life." The learning objectives are to help participants keep up the momentum and discipline they have developed over the past 7 weeks in mindfulness practice, both formal and informal, and to present a range of resources, such as books, tapes, advanced programs, and other opportunities for practice in the community, is reviewed to support continued practice. Meditations and opportunities for sharing with the group close the session and the course.

PARTICIPANT LEARNING OUTCOMES

The scheme presented in Figure 13.2 is just one of an infinite number of ways of framing the learning outcomes of MBSR, which can be seen from another angle as its intentions. At the moment of writing, this scheme serves the authors'

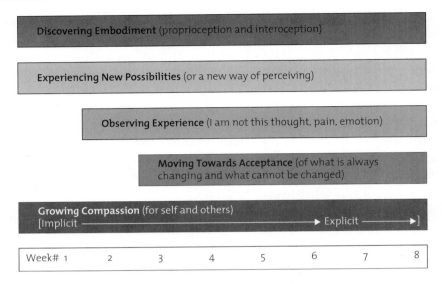

FIGURE 13.2 Participant learning outcomes over course duration.

purposes; we find it both explanatory and generative of insights and questions. Yet, we realize that at some point it will cease to be useful and, indeed,
will need to be jettisoned as fresh explanations and questions arise. We believe
that this "temporary truth" approach to theorizing reflects the MBSR values
of maintaining a present-moment focus, avoiding the reification of concepts,
and understanding the impermanence of experience.

   The outcomes presented are implicit throughout the course, and become
explicit in the curriculum as it develops across 8 weeks. Notice that the vertical
structure of Figure 13.2 places the unfolding of the outcomes of the course within
boundaries comprising, at the top, the experience of new possibilities, and, at
the bottom, the growth of compassion. This suggests the interdependence and
simultaneity of the three axioms of mindfulness in the IAA model (intention,
attention, and attitude) proposed by Shapiro et al. (2006). The horizontal structure suggests the incremental and experiential nature of the course, in which
knowledge is not added to participants, but rather, reflecting the Greek root of
the verb *to educate,* is "drawn out" of participants.

Experiencing New Possibilities

From the first moment of encounter with the MBSR curriculum, participants'
expectations are subverted; their habitual worldviews are slightly destabilized.

The heterogeneity of diagnoses of participants—indeed, the nonpathologizing nature of group construction—sends a message that is amplified by the often quoted statement that in MBSR, "as long as you are breathing, there is more right with you than there is wrong, no matter how ill or hopeless you may feel" (Kabat-Zinn, 1990, p. 2). One of the authors destabilizes the identity of MBSR as a typical educational course, through a reversal: "Maybe you signed up for a once-a-week class supported by homework assignments, but you may find it more useful to see it as eight weeks of homework supported by a once-a-week class."

This immediate subverting of expectations and destabilizing of familiar concepts can be seen through a number of different lenses that are more or less acknowledged as influences on the development of MBSR curriculum and pedagogy (Santorelli, 2004). The Buddhist lens is succinctly represented in Goleman's definition of mindfulness given in full above; in short, "In mindfulness, the meditator methodically faces the bare facts of his experience, seeing each event as though occurring for the first time" (1988, p. 20). This is made explicit as "beginner's mind," one of the "attitudinal foundations" in MBSR; as Kabat-Zinn (1990, p. 35) explains, "Too often we let our thinking and our beliefs about what we 'know' prevent us from seeing things as they really are." Another acknowledged lens is that of transformative learning, defined by its originator Jack Mezirow (2000, pp. 7–8), as one by which "we transform our taken-for-granted frames of reference (meaning-perspectives, habits of mind, mind-sets) to make them more inclusive, discriminating, open, emotionally capable of change, and reflective so that they may generate beliefs and opinions that will prove more true or justified to guide action." A lens that is highly useful though less pointedly acknowledged is the concept of reframing, most distinctly defined in the family therapy literature by Wátzlawick, Weakland, and Fisch (1974, p. 95), as meaning "to change the conceptual and/or emotional setting or viewpoint in relation to which a situation is experienced and to place it in another frame which fits the 'facts' of the same concrete situation equally well or even better, and thereby changes its entire meaning."

In the first class, the model curriculum emphasizes new possibilities in two particularly directed exercises (Kabat-Zinn, 1993). First is the mindful eating of a raisin. Through a guided encounter with one raisin at a time, participants are helped to suspend their "knowing" and to investigate the "facts" of the encounter in the present moment. By exploring the raisin with all the senses, new information destabilizes familiar ways of perceiving. As one example, when asked to "listen to" the raisin, an unconsidered dimension opens up; participants react with humor and real curiosity. Through such a contemplative approach to an ordinary undertaking, participants find they have challenged their understandings and habitual patterns. A participant in a recent class noted, "I've been eating raisins since I can remember, because I like sweet things and raisins are sweet. Now, I don't think I really like them. They are sweet, but I noticed the texture of the skin and the pulp... I don't find that particularly pleasant." The second exercise is the nine-dot problem (see box below: The nine dots), often given as homework after the first class. To struggle with the problem, and then to see the "out of the box" solution, can suggest the power of experiencing new possibilities. Coincidentally, Wátzlawick et al. (1974) discussed the nine dots in their work, and the continuing effect of seeing the solution: "Once somebody has explained to us the solution of the nine-dot problem, it is almost impossible to revert to our previous helplessness and especially our original hopelessness about the possibility of a solution" (p. 99) It is this reduction in helplessness and hopelessness that the "experiencing new possibilities" outcome emphasizes. Throughout the 8 weeks, and into postcourse life, we, as teachers, trust that new possibilities tremble at the edge of participants' experience, and that the potential for reframing experience moves from a guided offering by the teacher to a personal capacity within the participant.

The nine dots: A puzzle

. . .

. . .

. . .

Instructions: Without lifting the pencil from the paper, draw four lines so that all of the dots are connected by having a line passing through them.

The nine dots: An answer

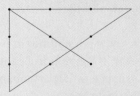

Solution: The "box" shape of the dots suggests that the solution is found inside the confines our boundaries of the dots. It is only when you see that you can move "outside the box" that solutions become possibilities.

Discovering Embodiment

Our contemporary culture in the West privileges the cognitive domain over the domains of affect and embodiment. Direct experience is "sicklied o'er with the pale cast of thought," in Hamlet's evocative phrase. Indeed, much of the discourse of academic and clinical psychology takes place in cognitive terms, and attempts made to explain mindfulness from within this discourse risk reducing embodied experiences to events in the mind (Drummond, 2006). In contrast, the co-created mindfulness of MBSR classes and the ongoing pedagogical practices in the classes reflect a holistic, nondual approach to the mind–body complex (Rothwell, 2006). This outcome of "discovering embodiment" points to a much closer relationship of MBSR to the humanistic tradition in psychology, with its interest in bodily experience (e.g., Gendlin, 1962; Perls, Hefferline, & Goodman, 1951/1969; Rogers, 1961), as well as to the expansion of interest to "embodied knowing" from "language-based knowing" in postmodern psychotherapy (e.g., Andersen, 2007; Hoffman, 2007).

Beginning with the first class, participants in MBSR are invited to "be with" or "be in" whatever experience is arising in the domain of body sensation, without judgment. This is as true of the exploration of the raisin as it is of the body scan. The body scan is, perhaps, a useful example. The teacher's guidance attempts to bring participants to their own experience of their bodies. The guidance provides permission for *any* experience to be present; for example, we begin at the top of the head, calling the participant's attention there, and offering language that names a range of experiences, from variations in temperature, to tingling, itching, pressure, to "nothing at all"—with an emphasis that "nothing at all" is a possible, acceptable experience. Further, initial guidance helps participants to parse immediate experience from stories *about* experience, to separate anticipation or opinion from the present-moment happening. Insights are often experienced at the pre-semantic level, and later revealed through such statements as, "I feel more connected to myself," and "I know that my back hurts, but I didn't know what that actually feels like until now." Insights may also be translatable into the cognitive domain, through concepts that can be generalized: "I thought it was going to be my right foot that started hurting, but it was my left!" The understanding of embodiment deepens as classes and practices unfold: the teacher's guidance helps make explicit the interoceptive information available in the body scan meditation ("noticing the sense of the lungs filling and emptying in the chest, and perhaps the presence of the heartbeat"); guidance points out the responsiveness of the breath to meditation posture and cognitive and affective states ("becoming curious about the quality of the breath"); fine-tuning the reception of proprioceptive information in mindful yoga or other movement ("Where are the arms in relationship to the ground and to the rest of the body in this moment?").

Movement, such as the mindful Hatha yoga presented in the model curriculum in our experience, is easily accessible as an embodiment practice. Participants make connections to their bodies quickly and in many cases joyfully. Central to the presentation of movement is the permissiveness with which it is presented. It is offered for the purpose of exploration of the interrelationship of body and mind, without expectations of meeting a standard of "performance." Participants who are physically challenged are encouraged to adapt the offered postures to their capabilities, or to practice through imagination—noticing the possibility for connection with the body in that way. Throughout the many co-creations of mindfulness in MBSR classes worldwide, forms of movement other than yoga are offered as well, including *Taijichuan* and *Qi Gong*, and simple experiments of sensory awareness—tuning in to the necessary processes of standing, sitting, lying down, and walking that arise within the context of the class. The teacher works best from her own deepest experience and training; for example, qualifications for MBSR teachers at the UMASS Center for Mindfulness are open, asking for experience in "Hatha yoga and/or body-centered awareness disciplines" (Santorelli & Kabat-Zinn, 2003, unpaginated).

The exploration of embodiment is a key to participant learning outcomes across the entire 8 weeks: steering participants away from the privileged cognitive domain and its confined conceptual and semantic explanations moves them toward the edge of new possibilities noted above. The ordinary is poised for reframing. The holistic relationship of the triangle of awareness becomes instrumental. For example, when a participant is experiencing strong affect, the teacher can invite her to drop the "story" in the cognitive domain, and simply be with/in the body sensations—exploring and describing these without judgment. Such an exploration of, say, anger, may lead to a discovery that the bodily sensations by themselves are energetic and even pleasurable, which in turn may gently prompt a reframing.

Cultivating the Observer

This is the realization of the IAA mindfulness model of Shapiro et al. (2006), through which class participants find they have the capacity to detect and actualize new possibilities *for themselves*. This realization begins in and grows through the formal exercises and meditations taught in class one and practiced at home the first week. It most often becomes explicit in week two, when the initial challenge of the MBSR approach has settled. Not coincidentally, this is also the week when sitting meditation is first introduced. In the formal practice of both the body scan and sitting meditation in class two, guidance assists participants to work *with* rather than *against* the "wandering mind" that leaves the focus of attention (body part or breath) and must be refocused. This practice of noticing when and where the mind has wandered points to the existence of the observing consciousness that does the noticing, and, thus, of the mechanism of reperceiving, "in which what was previously 'subject' becomes 'object'" (Shapiro et al., 2006). Using this "observer" as a temporary platform for investigation, one can open to immediate experience, and even choose to reframe it.

This capacity is developed and strengthened through adoption of the full range of formal and informal practices and in dialogue with the instructor as described in the "inquiry" section below.

Moving toward Acceptance

This is the actualization of the third of the IAA axioms of Shapiro et al.'s model—the *attitude* of mindfulness. In MBSR, this attitude points to a warmth that has its roots in nonjudgment and that flowers into "an affectionate, compassionate quality...a sense of openhearted, friendly presence and interest" (Kabat-Zinn, 2003, p. 145, quoted in Shapiro et al., 2006). This is revealed in the co-creation of mindfulness in MBSR in three interpenetrating sites of expression. First is the person of the teacher. The teacher's ability to build a safe, open, nonjudgmental class environment by embodying the warm qualities of mindfulness in MBSR is of paramount importance. Santorelli (2004) has discussed this as the capacity to create a "holding environment," a "potential space" characterized by trust and confidence, as described by Winnicott (1971). When the teacher is able to hold the class in this way, the class members form a second site of expression of mindfulness, and the group becomes a potential space for exploration. Statements such as "I feel safe here," and "This class is a refuge for me each week," and "I never thought I'd be saying this out loud," are common currency in MBSR classes in our experience.

Within this self-reinforcing teacher/group container, the individual participant, the third site of expression, often finds that she has the capacity to meet whatever may arise for her with clarity and affection. She finds that she can be with/in strong affect or challenging physical pain, that she can accept the condition of the moment. For example, a woman whose husband died a year before she took the course, and who had been avoiding and denying her grief, was able at last to sit still with her grief in class. Feeling the depth of her heartache, she said through her tears that she felt a tremendous relief, a realization that "I don't need to run away from my grief. I just need to give it room and let it be." Such movement toward acceptance is actualized and strengthened in the full range of formal and informal practices, and in one-on-one "inquiry" dialogues with the instructor, to which all class participants are empathic witnesses. In fact, it is important to note that as the class develops over the weeks, the format of inquiry shifts from teacher–participant dialogue to include sharing of personal experiences from around the group that help catalyze greater acceptance.

Growing Compassion

Compassion, rooted in the attitude of nonjudging, shifts from an implicit compassion directed mostly toward the self, to an explicit extension of compassion defined as loving-kindness directed mostly toward the other. In the early weeks of the class, as mindfulness is co-created in the group, the motion of compassion is centripetal—drawn into each participant's experience from the teacher's embodiment of and dialogues about mindfulness. As the mindfulness in the group makes participants more available to each other moment by moment, the motion of compassion becomes centrifugal, as well, moving outward to transform the class into a group that cares for its members.

Compassion, particularly its centripetal motion, is implicit in the formal and informal mindfulness practices introduced in the early weeks of the course. It is in teacher–participant inquiry, group dialogue, and participants' extra-group relationships that its centrifugal motion is enacted in those weeks. Then, in typical adaptations of the model curriculum, an explicit practice of loving-kindness is introduced somewhere between weeks 5 and 7, often during the all-day session. This practice of offering wishes for happiness, safety, well-being, and ease provides a link that helps many participants join their personal practice to the relational dimension. They discover the potential impact of their individual transformation on family, social circle, workplace, and political, social, and environmental awareness, as well as on their spirituality—and the centripetal and centrifugal motions become a single force.

Exactly how compassion-related practices should be integrated into a course devoted to development of mindfulness skills has been a subject of debate in the MBSR community. Kabat-Zinn (2005) notes that for pedagogical and practical reasons, he was reluctant to include such practices, as they are implicit and embodied in all of the practices and teaching, and as they may confuse participants just learning mindfulness practice by interjecting a sense of *doing*, by "invoking particular feelings and thoughts and generating desirable states of mind and heart" (p. 286). For him, limited introduction of loving-kindness practice is justified because, "on a deeper level, the instructions only *appear* [his italics] to be making something happen. Underneath, I have come to feel that they are revealing feelings we actually already have, but which are so buried that they need continual invitation and some exceptional sustaining to touch" (p. 286). Other MBSR teachers have not found such pedagogical dissonance, and thus have developed curriculum adaptations that include loving-kindness and other compassion-oriented practices from the earliest weeks of the course and/or include such practices in ongoing home practice for participants. In the authors' own adaptations, the four traditional Buddhist compassion-oriented practices—loving-kindness, compassion, sympathetic joy, and equanimity— may all be introduced, and such introduction happens at the all-day session or in later classes. To defuse any dissonance of doing versus being, the practices may be guided with recurring injunctions such as "noticing how it is with you right now, in the body, emotions, and thoughts," and " knowing that you can offer loving-kindness [for example] with all that you are in this moment— whether you're feeling loving-kindness, or anger, or sadness, or any other way of being." From such a perspective, participants can allow their own experiences, while touching in to the practice.

MBSR PEDAGOGICAL THEORY AND PRACTICE I: INTRODUCING A MYSTERY

There are clouds obscuring both the *who* and the *how* of the teaching of mindfulness-based interventions in general, and MBSR specifically. The dearth of published information about the person of the mindfulness teacher and the specific skills required in teaching mindfulness-based interventions stems from overarching systemic issues in the research and practice community— the tensions between the drive to elaborate a strong evidence base, which is located solidly within the current scientific/medical paradigm, and the need to refine the pedagogy of mindfulness, which in many of its dimensions lies outside that paradigm.

The person of the mindfulness teacher, her qualities of being, and her unique skill sets are obscured in the current literature for the same reasons that the person of the therapist is obscured in efficacy research in psychotherapy generally: the social and economic forces that have constructed and maintain the "gold standard" research model of medical randomized clinical trials. Substantive critiques of this issue (e.g., Beutler et al., 2004; Lebow, 2006; Wampold, 2001) are succinctly summarized by Blow, Sprenkle, and Davis (2007), who note that "A major implication of the medical model is that the specific ingredients of the treatment are what are important in therapy, *not* who delivers the ingredients." Blow et al. (2007) further suggest that this type of research is driven by the requirements of funding sources for adherence to the medical model, as well as by the demands of health care payors for evidence of efficacy of treatments to be presented within this model. Finally, Blow et al. (2007) note the pressure for development of manualized models and fidelity measures to control for therapist effects. This last is of particular importance in the direction that mindfulness research has taken, as reflected, for example, in the concern over control of treatment fidelity expressed in two highly influential meta-analyses of mindfulness-based interventions (Baer, 2003; Grossman et al., 2004). A poignant example of wishful or willful underestimation of the effect of the person of the teacher appears in a recent study (Jain et al., 2007), in which, "To determine whether warmth and affability of the teacher or surroundings could contribute to intervention efficacy, students were asked to rate the pleasantness of the room and the affability, knowledge, and caring of the teacher." Implicitly, then, the person of the teacher is of no greater importance than the health of the plant on the windowsill or the color of the carpet on the floor.

The general enterprise of building a strong evidence base for mindfulness-based interventions is both valuable and praiseworthy. At the same time, the resultant emphasis on defining and measuring the impact of the specific "ingredients" of the intervention at the expense of similar research on the person and skills of the teacher has helped to isolate the ongoing development and elaboration of pedagogical theory and practice from public description and debate. The following two sections are offered to help those interested in delivering MBSR or other mindfulness-meditation-based interventions to understand the true depth and breadth of the dimensions of being and knowing required for successful teaching. Much of the material below derives, appropriately, from the authors' own educations and personal transformations through participation in MBSR training programs offered by the Center for Mindfulness and in our experiences of developing and delivering professional trainings for potential teachers of mindfulness-meditation-based interventions. Just as the MBSR teacher's challenge is to translate what are essentially pre-semantic experiences of moment-to-moment presence into effective and affecting language for the wide range of individuals in a class, the challenge in public discussion of the pedagogy of mindfulness is likewise to bring the tacit characteristics and skills of the teacher into language and concepts that are open to continuing critique, revision, and improvement.

MBSR PEDAGOGICAL THEORY AND PRACTICE II: THE PERSON OF THE TEACHER

The person of the teacher is obscured in much current research because of at least four aspects of teacher training and development: (1) the ongoing personal transformation of the teacher holds a central place in training; (2) teacher-training courses are highly experiential; (3) the teacher–student relationship has a powerful role in communal healing; and (4) teacher-training programs have been reticent to limit a teacher's creativity. When explored, these aspects make salient many important characteristics of effective teachers.

1. The ongoing personal transformation of the teacher holds a central place in training. Commitment to a personal practice of mindfulness is crucial to the development required. Jon Kabat-Zinn (2003) notes that the MBSR program at the Center for Mindfulness "requires extensive grounding in mindfulness practice as one criterion in hiring new teachers." He asks,

> For how can one ask someone else to look deeply into his or her own mind and body and the nature of who he or she is in a systematic and disciplined way if one is unwilling (or too busy or not interested enough) to engage in this great and challenging adventure oneself, at least to the degree that one is asking it of one's patients or clients?

For example, Neil Rothwell (2006) compares his experiences teaching both Cognitive-Behavioral Therapy based groups and MBSR courses, and realizes that

> In MBSR, rather than being a teacher in a conventional sense, the leader's role feels much more like immersing oneself in a process or a way of being....The role of the teacher is mainly to engender mindfulness by bringing attention to the moment-to-moment awareness of participants whilst actually in the room. The main means of doing this is by being mindful oneself, which seems to provide the opportunity for experiential learning by the client.

Indeed, it would be difficult to exaggerate the importance of this point. As Kabat-Zinn (1999) characterizes it, "The attitude that the teacher brings into the room ... ultimately influences absolutely everything in the world. Once you make the commitment, as Kabir put it, 'To stand firm in that which you are,' to hold the central axis of your being human, the entire universe is different."

Commitment to regular formal mindfulness meditation practice is defined at minimum as practicing at least with the frequency and duration expected of students in the class (Kabat-Zinn, 2003). Further, prolonged periods of practice provide the developing teacher the opportunity for greater insight into the mind–body complex and into the practice itself. Therefore, a regular pattern of silent retreats of 5 days or more is required of teachers in the model MBSR program (Santorelli, 2001a), and of candidates for training beyond the foundational level through the Center for Mindfulness (2007). Retreats are not extensions of daily practice, not just "more of the same." There is a qualitative as well as a quantitative difference between what is revealed by formally cultivating mindfulness for, say, 1 hour, and seamless formal and informal practice for one's waking hours over, say, 10 consecutive days. The arising and dissolution of sensations, emotions, and thought in an hour might be considered metaphorically as a photograph of a natural scene, while the metaphor for a 10-day retreat might be a time-lapse movie of the same scene as seasons change: both are dense with potential for experience and insight, yet the movie reveals and opens for exploration dimensions only hinted at in the photo.

Mindfulness sitting meditation appears to be the preferred form of practice for MBSR teachers (McCown, Reibel, & Malcoun, 2007), and is the predominant form offered through the retreats in the Theravada Buddhist tradition that MBSR teachers are encouraged to attend (Center for Mindfulness, 2007). However, a second requirement of teachers in the UMASS model MBSR program and of teachers applying for advanced training at the Center for Mindfulness is ongoing involvement in body-centered disciplines, which includes but is not limited to Hatha yoga (Center for Mindfulness, 2007; Santorelli, 2001a). For the authors, such practice and training includes Hatha yoga, *Taijichuan, Qi Gong, Tsa Lung*, Eurythmy, and Sensory Awareness. The potential variety of practices implied by this list makes it evident that their power for personal transformation is not found in a striving for mastery—picture perfect postures, award-winning performances. Rather, the power is in the moment-by-moment opportunity to be in touch with the body–mind complex. This is profoundly expressed by the Sensory Awareness teacher Charlotte Selver (Selver & Brooks, 2007, p. 225):

Discoveries can happen anywhere.
The question is not what you do,
but how you do it.
You can't be in a higher state of being
than to be there for something.

A third requirement for teacher development, as defined by the Center for Mindfulness (2007), is continuing personal psychological development, characterized by "learning as much as possible about your own personality and patterns of relating" (p. 4). Certainly, this implies the experience of one's own psychotherapy, including the strengthening of one's capacity to recognize and work with one's own reactivity in the moment, and, failing that, to accept one's missteps and repair relationships as appropriate. Searching further in the expectations of the Center for Mindfulness (2007b), there is also an explicit linkage of psychological and *spiritual* development. In spiritual development, one's own mindfulness practice is central, especially work with mindfulness teachers on retreats and in one-to-one regular contact. Most likely, such teachers will have authority in some traditional Buddhist lineage. It is common in the authors' experiences that our teaching colleagues and teachers in training have an abiding interest in Buddhist philosophy and psychology, if not in Buddhist ritual practice. This does not imply, however, that MBSR teachers necessarily identify as Buddhist. In the authors' experiences, most teachers are sympathetic to the full range of theistic and nontheistic traditions. For example, while we have practiced and trained with teachers within several Buddhist traditions, we have also worked for many years with clergy and spiritual directors within our "home" traditions of Judaism and catholic Christianity, and we are informed about and interested in religious and spiritual expression across cultures and around the world. A useful definition of the kind of spiritual maturity required of an MBSR teacher comes from Fowler's (1981) elaboration of six "stages of faith": Stage 5 is characterized by *dialogical knowing*, in which knower and known enter an I–Thou relationship. Fowler assists in understanding the contributions of mindfulness practice in actualizing such maturity, noting, "What the mystics call 'detachment' characterizes Stage 5's willingness to let reality speak its word, regardless of the impact of that word on the security or self-esteem of the knower" (p. 185). The clinical value of mature spirituality in an MBSR teacher is clear in Fowler's (p. 198) statement that, "this stage is ready to spend and be spent for the cause of conserving and cultivating the possibility of others' generating identity and meaning."

2. Teacher-training courses are highly experiential. MBSR classes for patients are built around mindfulness practice inside and outside the class, and teacher-training parallels that emphasis. For example, two of the four key teacher education courses offered by the Center for Mindfulness (2007) are billed as "training/retreats." The content and conduct of the courses, in the authors' experiences, encourages both formal and informal cultivation of mindfulness, and challenges students to critical self-reflection. The preference in the majority of the training time is for *being* over *doing*, *process* over *content*. Santorelli (2001c) identifies three elements of pedagogy for professionals: (1) a knowledge base, (2) a reflective base, and (3) a contemplative base. This scheme suggests a two-to-one bias toward self-exploration over didactic content. Put another way, a recent (CFM, 2007a, p. 27) formulation of "The Way of Teaching" describes how "Teaching by heart calls on teachers to access all that we are rather than allowing learning to be dominated by knowledge acquired almost exclusively through the filters of objectivity and intellect", and notes that "learning dominated by these attributes can readily lead us, as teachers and students, to feel disconnected from the very sources of inquiry and creativity that fueled our passion to study and teach the subjects we love."

3. The teacher–student relationship has a powerful role in communal healing. As characterized by Santorelli (1999), the relationship between any health care provider and patient potentially is a "crucible for mutual transformation" (p. 15). He suggests that when both MBSR teacher and student, through the cultivation of mindfulness, are able to explore unflinchingly their own literal and metaphorical wounds, and to relate to each other based on what they learn and share, both can experience healing. Such an archetypal vision reveals not only how far from the medical model mindfulness can carry us, it reveals, as well, how important are the nearly indefinable factors that make a good teacher. As both Kabat-Zinn (2003) and Santorelli (2001c) have pointed out, and the authors' experience in the training of teachers supports, the most effective MBSR teacher is not simply the one with the longest history of mindfulness practice, rather it is the one best equipped to make and maintain compassionate connections. As Santorelli (2001c) describes it: "We have had teachers and interns with less meditation practice who have had strong academic and 'life' training that has created within them the possibility of understanding some things that you can't get any other way by being alive." The assumption is that the teacher has *chosen* to live mindfully, and that mindfulness practice, however short-lived, permeates the person. Observed through a more wide-angle lens, that of the common factors perspective in psychotherapy, the MBSR teacher epitomizes Simon's proposal (2003, 2006) that a therapist is most effective when using a model of therapy based on a worldview congruent with her own. He explains that in such a case clients do not experience the model so much as the person of the therapist, while the teacher's primary experience is her use of self. He concludes (2003, p. 11), "Therapy thus becomes what it always is at its best—an encounter between persons."

4. Teacher-training programs have been reticent to limit a teacher's creativity. MBSR, and, indeed, the full range of mindfulness-based interventions emerged as creative responses to the challenges in adapting each developer's personal experience of mindfulness practice to work within their own professional environment, targeting populations with whom they have significant experience and for whom they care deeply. As Santorelli (2001c) describes it, such was the genesis of MBSR: "In the beginning, no one gave Jon [Kabat-Zinn] curriculum or a blueprint for how to do this. It arose out of the situation itself; out of the life he was living and a longing he felt compelled to follow."

In that spirit, the Center for Mindfulness encouraged professionals to learn from MBSR *and* from their personal meditation practices, as well as to apply their unique professional and life experiences to create programs in the spirit of, though not to the letter of, the UMASS model. Santorelli (2001c) notes, "We didn't want to put the lid on creativity but instead to give it the space to unfold in a thousand and one ways that we couldn't possibly conceive of." As a result, there are now many mature MBSR and mindfulness-meditation-based programs in institutions around the world that have departed in certain ways from the UMASS model, and that nevertheless have been shown through empirical studies to be as effective as the UMASS model (Jain et al., 2007; Reibel, Greeson, Brainard, & Rosenzweig, 2001; Rosenzweig et al., 2003; Roth & Calle-Mesa, 2006). These programs are staffed by professionals who have received training through the Center for Mindfulness *and* from their home program's senior staff. Further, some of these mature programs have begun their own formal training programs for professionals considering the use of mindfulness-meditation-based interventions. The program at the Jefferson-Myrna Brind Center of Integrative Medicine is a case in point, with effective, empirically supported curriculum shifts (Reibel et al., 2001), and a staff trained through both the Center for Mindfulness and Jefferson-based internships and a practicum course—which is also open to other professionals, who in turn may elaborate, experiment, and evolve further curriculum shifts.

That the MBSR community incorporates such a spectrum of approaches highlights the importance of public dialogue about the person and skills of professional mindfulness teachers. The pedagogy of mindfulness is a co-creation of the entire community of its teachers, and is ipso facto the property of that community. It comes into being and shifts shapes moment-to-moment, context-to-context, class-to-class. Its lively, flowing quality, bounded only by the intimate grapplings of each teacher and class with the practice, is its ultimate value. The emerging enterprise of elaborating a pedagogical theory and practice must, therefore, be based on public, accessible ways to share, critique, and synthesize the new and effective methods and media that are always arising. Without continual dialogue that honors the inherent creativity of every teacher, the fate of such a pedagogy is like that of a rainbow trout, which, removed from the flowing stream, quickly loses its wondrous iridescence.

From Paradox to Definition

We have attempted to describe the person of the teacher by starting with the reasons that the scientific discourse of mindfulness makes such description difficult. What has emerged through this paradoxical endeavor, we hope, is a living picture of the complexity, vibrancy, and necessary uniqueness of each teacher. With such an appreciation established, we can attempt a definition of the person of the teacher that may in its simplicity be useful for self-reflection and clinical or supervisory application. This definition, based on the dimensions of *authenticity, authority,* and *friendship,* is elaborated in the box.

The person of the teacher

In both group and individual work in interventions incorporating mindfulness meditation, the mindful use of the person of the teacher is of central importance, and can be considered across three dimensions:

1. *Authenticity:* This is connected to the teacher's own mindfulness practice and the fruits of other psychological and spiritual work. Moment-to-moment, in relationship to the group or individual, the teacher *embodies* mindfulness, living the transformative realities of reperceiving, acceptance, and compassion.

2. *Authority:* This is not meant to imply power granted by position or profession. Rather, authority suggests that the teacher's knowledge, which is derived from personal practice, psychological and spiritual development, experience teaching mindfulness, and expertise in a professional discipline, is unique and *thoroughly* processed. When the teacher talks or acts from this material, her real or symbolic authorship of it is evident—both the person and the knowledge she reveals speak volumes.

3. *Friendship:* This is a term gleaned from the contemporary Buddhist theologian, Stephen Batchelor (1997). His description of friendship in the world of Buddhist practice and study fits the mindfulness teacher's role with a student: "Such a friend is someone whom we can trust to refine our understanding of what it means to live, who can guide us when we're lost and help us find our way along a path, who can assuage our anguish through the reassurance of his or her presence" (p. 50). It begins with the intention of meeting people "where they are," coming to any encounter *without* an agenda or intention to "fix" the other, and *with* a willingness to allow relationships and situations to unfold in a fresh way.

MBSR PEDAGOGICAL THEORY AND PRACTICE III: SUGGESTED SKILLS FOR A TEACHER

We have suggested that teachers teach first from their own experience, and that, therefore, the pedagogy of mindfulness is infinitely variable, flowing like water. Yet, at the same time, we also believe that there are general types of skills that teachers share. These could be seen as the banks and bends, chutes and falls through which the water flows—the *course* of the water, as it were—and through which each teacher uses similar skills to maneuver in unique ways. Each of the four skills described below has evolved from many sources. The pedagogy of mindfulness as exemplified in the trainings through the Center for Mindfulness is pragmatic and eclectic, making use of a wide range of medical, psychotherapeutic, educational, and anthropological–sociological insights and techniques. This material is not integrated theoretically; rather, it is integrated in the person of the teacher, through her embodiment of mindfulness. The descriptions of these skills come from the authors' experiences in our own ongoing training, from our own elaborations and explorations of these skills in the crucible of the classroom, and from witnessing the work of colleagues (relatively few, given the more than 9,000 people who have completed professional trainings through the Center for Mindfulness!). Necessarily, then, the sections below are more evocative than prescriptive. Where references to specific theories or literature have been made by the Center for Mindfulness, we have supplied citations for further exploration. We have also supplied citations for theories and techniques that have significantly influenced our own teaching styles.

1. Creating and maintaining a working group. Kabat-Zinn and Santorelli (2003) describe the necessary elements for this as "highly developed skills in group dynamics, interactive teaching, and a sensitivity for what it is that different people need in any moment in a class-like situation." Skill and experience in group development, conceptualized in any number of ways (e.g., Agazarian, 1997; Bion, 1961/1989; Tuckman & Jensen, 1977; Yalom, 1985), is valuable as a starting point. It is important to remember, however, that MBSR was conceived in an educational rather than a therapeutic model (Kabat-Zinn, 1996), and that in its ongoing refinement it has absorbed a wide range of influences. Santorelli (2004) enumerates four powerful influences on the running of the group: education for liberation (Freire, 1988), transformative education (Mezirow, 2000), the inner landscape of the teacher (Palmer, 1998), and Winnicott's concept of the holding environment (1971). In the early weeks of the MBSR course, in which the participants contract for and begin to build safety for one another, the contribution of Winnicott's work plays a significant role. At the start, the teacher must invoke her authority to provide much of the "holding" that allows students to withstand the challenges to their rigid conceptions of self. Simultaneously, however, the teacher is also potentiating development of a holding capacity within the group: using every opportunity to turn the students toward each other and encouraging supportive interaction, perhaps by using group formats that help control emotional reactivity, competition, and contradiction, such as Council Circle (Zimmerman & Coyle, 1996) or Systems Centered Theory (Agazarian, 1997; Ladden, 2007). Further relationship building is encouraged through extensive use of dyadic and small-group exercises, and through the group's direct experiences of the teacher's authenticity. Participants' experiences of the teacher include witnessing both rifts and repairs in her relationships with individuals and the group, making plain her imperfections and emphasizing that the group process is, indeed, a process.

All of this is essential prelude to and concomitant with the co-creation of mindfulness in the group, which brings its own intentions of safety and self-exploration, with shared attitudes of acceptance, nonjudgment, and compassion. The formal group practices of mindfulness meditations and attendant group dialogue and teacher–student inquiry, which are a major part of each week's class experience, seem to foster interpersonal connections and a capacity to "be with" the other participants with compassion and without judgment. A transcendent theme in participants' verbal comments to their group in the final session are continually echoed in this statement from a participant: "I'm not sure I even know everyone's name, but I have never felt so close to a group of people before in my life. It's like we know and care about each other in a whole different way."

2. Delivering didactic material. There are several modules within a typical MBSR curriculum that require a teacher to provide informational content that may not reside in the group: for example, a working definition of mindfulness, a working understanding of stress physiology, and information about particular models of group or individual communication. Authoritative skills in developing brief, clear, and memorable presentations that engage the triangle of awareness—thought, emotion, and sensation—are extremely helpful in facilitating common understandings of basic concepts and a common vocabulary among group members.

Individual teachers call on their unique "authority" for approaches that work for their specific populations. There are, however, two preferences that shape most teachers' styles. First is a preference for drawing as much of the material out of the group as possible. As Santorelli (2001b) describes it:

> Importantly, rather than "lecturing" to program participants, the attention and skill of the teacher should be directed towards listening to the rich, information laden insights and examples provided by program participants and then, in turn, to use as much as possible these participant-generated experiences as a starting point for "weaving" the more didactic material into the structure and fabric of each class.

Second is a preference for ways of knowing that go beyond the cognitive dimension. This is easily illustrated by the fact that a poem, a story, even a children's picture book may be the medium of choice for introducing or reinforcing an important idea. For example, in the first or second class, a teacher may choose to intensify the idea that our habitual ways of perceiving the world keep us from experiencing new possibilities by telling or reading a story, such as the very short one that follows from children's television icon Fred Rogers (2004, p. 187).

> When I was a boy and I would see scary things in the news, my mother would say to me, "Look for the helpers. You will always find people who are helping." To this day, especially in times of "disaster," I remember my mother's words, and I am always comforted by realizing that there are still so many helpers—so many caring people in this world.

The person of the narrator, the intimacy of the mother–child scene, the content of the story, and its social and historical resonances all contribute to an experience and a knowing that engages the whole person, not just the intellect.

3. Guiding formal meditations. The teacher guides the meditations "live" in the classroom where participants often have their eyes closed and are simply listening. The teacher's guidance is also heard via audio recordings supplied to class members for home practice. This implies how much the skill of guiding meditations depends on verbal communication. Effective meditation guidance requires control of performance in four interdependent dimensions: (a) languaging, (b) allowing, (c) orienting, and (d) embodying.

(a) *Languaging*. Jon Kabat-Zinn has masterfully analyzed the impact that language can have on clients' experiences of mindfulness practice, and his insights have shaped how MBSR teachers are trained through the Center for Mindfulness to guide meditation. Kabat-Zinn (2004) identifies four problems that can be introduced through verbal and nonverbal communication, and that can "generate resistance" in students, or "create more waves in the thought structure": (1) striving, as in "if you did this long enough, you'd be better;" (2) idealizing, as in "I know how to do this and I'm going to teach you;" (3) fixing, as in the implication that something is wrong with you that meditation is addressing; and (4) dualism, as in language that suggests that there is an observed and an observer. As to what kind of language to use, specifically, he states that nobody likes a command—that one should instead make suggestions. For example, rather than say "Breathe in," which can lead to a who-are-you-to-tell-me-what-to-do reaction, one could say, "When you're ready, *breathing* in...". The use of the present participle rather than the imperative minimizes the teacher–participant hierarchy, eliminates the subject–object distinction, emphasizes the present-moment experience, and possibly elicits inquiry into just who or what is breathing. One can also generate distance and space for exploration and reflection by using the definitive article rather than a possessive pronoun, saying "lifting *the* right leg" rather than "lifting *your* right leg." Kabat-Zinn (2004) advises that such rules should not be held too tightly, however, as too much use of the present participle can become distracting, while too much distancing through the definitive article may result in a he's-not-talking-to-me reaction.

(b) *Allowing.* Of central concern in the pedagogy of MBSR is ensuring that each participant feels free to have his or her own experience, not some "required" experience specified by the teacher or the group. This dimension is critical, because it encompasses a paradox for the teacher: when one can bring detail and specificity moment by moment into the guidance, participants connect well with the practice, yet each person will be having a unique experience. Teachers find balance by offering a range of choices, and by couching suggestions in tentative phrases. For instance, in guiding a body scan, the teacher may ask participants to focus on the forehead by saying, "Noticing any tightness or softness in the muscles...perhaps there's tingling, or maybe the sensation of the air moving in the room is available to you...or it may be that there's no sensation available at all—and that's OK; that's simply your experience in this moment...." Such a construction offers permission for whatever arises, encouragement for exploration beyond habitual responses, and unconditional acceptance of any outcome.

(c) *Orienting.* Here, again, the teacher faces a paradox. Mindfulness practice makes all of one's experience available as it arises moment by moment, which suggests that the search for organizing concepts or narrative runs counter to practice. Participants are urged to "drop the story" and return the attention to what is arising in the moment. And yet, in guiding mindfulness practices, particularly in the early classes, participants need to sense coherence and direction to feel safe enough to undertake an experience that destabilizes the mental constructs.

The teacher must find some form of organizing principle for the guidance to be acceptable. This may be easy. For example, the first formal practice, the body scan, engages sensations of the body sequentially, from head to foot or vice versa. Mindful movement practices such as Hatha Yoga or Qi Gong have inherent structures, both in the individual postures, and in potential sequencing. Sitting meditations may have a "narrative arc," as in an expanding awareness meditation that sequentially opens to experience in the domains of breath, body sensation, sound, thought, and emotion, leading to choiceless awareness of what arises in the present moment in any domain.

Other meditations may have no inherent organizing principle at all, such as a single focus on awareness of breathing, or the practice of choiceless awareness. Guiding such meditations requires an approach to language and performance that has coherence and integrity. It is essential to have an extemporaneous capacity to create purely verbal constructions that provide for participants a secure base from which they can explore. There are three basic strategies that can create this kind of coherence and safety, and that can be used to help integrate guidance of any type of practice. First is a simple refrain, a recurring construction that suggests some stability in the flow of experience. For example, in a choiceless awareness meditation, the question "Where is your attention in this moment?" will bring participants back to their direct experience. Second is the ongoing elaboration or blossoming of a concept. The teacher may introduce a useful principle for practice, and then, throughout the guidance of the meditation session, expand its definition and describe different times and reasons for bringing it into one's practice. For example, in an awareness of breath meditation, the teacher could introduce the principle of kindness toward oneself, and then elaborate the practice of cultivating a loving response toward one's own distractions throughout the guidance. Third is the incorporation of moment-to-moment events in the environment into the flow of the guidance. For example, in the large city, large institution context in which the authors teach, street-level tumult such as sirens or jackhammers, hallway happenings from rumbling carts to whispered conversations, even the undependability of heating and air conditioning can be noted and offered to the group—"What's happening within you as that siren sounds nearer and nearer?" These basic strategies can be combined creatively to improve guidance for any specific practice, for any specific group.

(d) *Embodying.* This is the most critical dimension of guidance: the connection of the teacher to her own practice while speaking. Guiding a meditation is not an empty performance; the teacher herself is engaged with the practice from moment-to-moment as she speaks. The verbal constructions she creates are thereby rooted in her experience. Her strategies of orienting are not abstract, but arise from experience; the blossoming of a term or concept is a description of the teacher's own observations, both immediate and remembered. She incorporates what arises in the shared environment, using herself as a sensing instrument, yet allowing for the infinite range of potential subjective experiences of the participants. The importance of embodying to effective guidance cannot be overstressed. In the authors' experiences in training and developing new teachers, it is quite easy to perceive whether a teacher is "dropped in" to the practice she is guiding; a felt sense of authenticity comes right through when the connection is there. Word choice, tone of voice, confidence of expression—all reflect authenticity when the teacher is embodying the practice, and all help to shape participants' experiences.

(4) Inquiring into participants' subjective experiences. Much of the transformative effect of MBSR may be potentiated by dialogic encounters in the classroom. Santorelli (2001b) states: "It is recommended that a significant amount of time in each class be dedicated to an exploration of the participants' experience of the formal and informal mindfulness practices and other weekly home assignments." The authors believe that this activity is an extremely important and dynamic element in participants' experiences of MBSR that has not been adequately addressed as part of the process in MBSR research.

As noted in the *Participant Learning Outcomes* section above, dialogue between participant and teacher in the group space can assist especially in enhancing the critical outcomes of "cultivating the observer" and "moving towards acceptance." Teacher–participant dialogue of this type is an "inquiry" into the participant's subjective experience—his or her pre-semantic knowing in the moment—with an intention to make more conscious meanings that are then available for further investigation. The skill of the teacher in such an undertaking is to be available to the other person, to be genuinely interested in the participant's experience.

Inquiry, then, is a meeting of two subjectivities in which neither assumes an expert position and both are able to work from a "not knowing" position to explore the fullness of possibilities for meaning. To be most helpful in inquiry with participants, an MBSR teacher works from (a) a philosophical approach to inquiry that supports a "not knowing" position, (b) an awareness of the cultural and individual resistances to inquiry that may be present, (c) a willingness to abandon language and return to experience and tacit knowing when dialogue ceases to generate meaning, and (d) a capacity to remain open to the outcome of any exchange with a participant or the group.

(a) *Philosophical approaches*. Batchelor's (1997) attempt to reimagine the Buddhist teacher for the contemporary West in terms of "friendship" provides a telling parallel to the role of the adult educator as described by Mezirow (2000). Both Buddhist thought and the discipline of transformative education have been major influences on the philosophy of MBSR pedagogy. Batchelor, from the student's perspective, imagines teachers this way (1997, pp. 50–51):

> These friends are teachers in the sense that they are skilled in the art of learning from every situation. We do not seek perfection in these friends but rather heartfelt acceptance of human imperfection. Nor omniscience but an ironic admission of ignorance.... For true friends seek not to coerce us, even gently and reasonably, into believing what we are unsure of. These friends are like midwives, who draw forth what is waiting to be born. Their task is not to make themselves indispensable but redundant.

Mezirow (2000, pp. 26–27), speaking from the teacher's perspective, uses the term "discourse" in much the same way we are using "inquiry" here:

> Discourse is the process in which we have an active dialogue with others to better understand the meaning of an experience.... Fostering discourse, with a determined effort to free participation from distortions by power and influence, is a long established priority of adult educators. The generally accepted model of adult education involves a transfer of authority from the educator to the learners; the successful educator works herself out of a job as educator and becomes a collaborative learner.

Both assert the importance of a nonhierarchical teacher–student relationship, the necessity of a shared stance of not knowing, the power of the action of "drawing out" the tacit knowing of the student, and the value of understanding the teacher's success as found, ultimately, in the diminishment of her status.

(b) *Cultural and individual resistances.* Given the dominant "banking" model of education, in which students are waiting for teachers to deposit knowledge into them, the initial encounters of inquiry may frustrate participants. There is security in the teacher as expert; there is fear in being one's own authority. Overcoming the attendant resistance to inquiry becomes an informal mindfulness practice for participants: they must become aware of, and transform, the habits of the banking model—working at staying open to their own insights.

The teacher's role in this is to bring compassionate curiosity and nonjudgment to the encounter, particularly a capacity to withstand the urges to "fix" or give advice and instead to stand with the participant in a space where meaning may unfold. As is so often true, what is required of the teacher is an embodiment of mindfulness. The teacher's authentic presence reciprocally supports participants' capacities to not know, to not fix, and to stand with/in their own experiences, which may lead to insights.

(c) *Language and experience.* It is often the case that an inquiry dialogue can help a participant bring their pre-semantic experience of formal or informal mindfulness practice increasingly into consciousness through language. The teacher's genuine curiosity and unassuming (having no assumptions) presence may be expressed in very simple questions about an experience, such as "What was it like for you?" This may generate a tentative response. Further open-ended exploration—"Can you say more about that?" or "Is there more that you've noticed?"—require reflection and an engagement with language that helps the participant toward greater understanding. For example, a participant described his experience with the body scan by saying, "I feel more connected somehow." The question from the teacher, "More connected to what?", provided the impetus and the space for deeper recognition: "More connected to myself and my family and other people," and then a long pause, followed by, "But mostly to myself. That's what's really different." In one way, perhaps that is simply a new shade of meaning; in another way, perhaps, it is a profound recognition of a gulf of experience never before bridged. During such an exchange, the other members of the group are both witnesses to one person's changing perspective and participants in their own reflections and recognitions. Inquiry is shared work.

It is also often the case that an inquiry dialogue leads to confusion rather than clarity. At such a point the teacher may suggest that the participant use formal mindfulness practice for further pre-semantic exploration of sensation, thought, and emotion. Such re-visiting, in the authors' experiences, often opens to greater emotional intensity and dialogue about personal material. Therefore, teachers proceed cautiously with the subject and the rest of the group, asking if the subject would like to work more in this way, and inviting the group both to witness the inquiry and participate in their own "inner" dialogue if that seems potentially useful for them. The toggling back and forth between pre-semantic experience and open dialogue with the teacher can clarify an experience and its meaning. What is required of the teacher in such encounters is a willingness to go only where the participant is willing to go, and a sensitivity to the needs of both the participant and the rest of the group.

(d) *Openness to outcome.* Inquiry is an invitation to the innate wisdom of the other to be known in experience and language. When this spirit of invitation is embodied by the teacher, it also may become a way of being for the participant (and all class members). Valuable dialogue may take place, yet the value is not simply in the particular insight or construction of experience in language. The value is in loosening the grip of habits of thought, patterns of reaction, and rigid self-concepts.

The potential of inquiry is a new capacity for freedom that is well described in Carse's (1986) metaphor of finite and infinite games. Finite games have specific rules, so that we know what the game is and how to win by defeating others. Infinite games have ever-changing rules, so that we can continue play indefinitely without zero-sum outcomes. At its best, inquiry takes the teacher, participant, and class into the realm of continual play, which can result in epiphanies that may be ongoing, or in planting seeds that may grow in later classes (or years), or in simply going nowhere while maintaining play. No one fails, everyone benefits.

Further, the teacher has no fixed role in the infinite version of the inquiry game. Particularly as the classes move into the later weeks, it may be possible for the group members to inquire on their own, either in "internal" dialogue, or with one another.

Mindfulness and MBSR in Integrative Psychiatry Practice

The integrative psychiatrist may choose to engage with MBSR or other mindfulness-based interventions at any or all of three different levels: (1) by referring patients to MBSR or other appropriate courses, (2) by undertaking mindfulness training and cultivating a personal practice, (3) by incorporating mindfulness teaching into clinical practice.

Referring patients. As suggested at the outset, there is growing empirical support for the efficacy of MBSR. Because MBSR is holistic, nonpathologizing, and offered (most often) to a heterogeneous patient population, a wide range of psychiatric patients may benefit. The main caveat is that their conditions do not preclude participation in a group setting in which group members are encouraged to explore their own vulnerabilities. As Hayes and Feldman (2004) note, careful consideration must be given to patients' abilities to face their own negative material without use of their current coping strategies. Guidelines for acceptance into MBSR classes vary among organizations and individual teachers, yet the exclusion parameters set by the CFM programs suggest typical practice. The CFM program specifically excludes from participation patients with active addiction or who have been in recovery less than a year; patients with suicidality, psychosis (refractory to medication), PTSD, depression or other major psychiatric disorders if they interfere with group participation, and social anxiety that makes a group environment difficult. With these exclusion criteria, however, come the significant exceptions that if the patient is highly motivated to participate in the MBSR class, is engaged in appropriate and supportive treatment with other professionals, agrees to the MBSR teacher communicating with the professionals, and the professionals agree to act as primary care givers and first contacts in emergencies, enrollment may be considered, with the teacher making the final decision (CFM, 2004). Other issues that may exclude participation are language comprehension, physical inability to get to class (not physical impairment, but logistical impossibility), and scheduling issues that would result in missing three or more classes.

Integrative psychiatrists may wish to ascertain if MBSR courses are offered in their geographic areas. An extensive, though by no means comprehensive, list of MBSR teachers and programs can be found at http://www.umassmed.edu/cfm/mbsr/. For patients who may be excluded from participation in MBSR groups, it may be that other mindfulness-based group interventions are available in the area. Mindfulness-based approaches and curricula have been developed and evaluated for a range of disorders, including substance abuse (e.g., Witkiewitz, Marlatt, & Walker, 2005), for personality disorders (e.g., Linehan, 1993), for psychosis (e.g., Chadwick, Newman-Taylor, & Abba, 2005), and for PTSD (e.g., Batten, Orsillo, & Walser, 2005). A curriculum of mindfulness-based cognitive therapy (Segal, Williams, & Teasdale, 2002) has been developed and shown to be effective for prevention of relapse in patients with three or more incidences of depression. For some patients who are excluded from group interventions, the individuals or organizations that offer MBSR courses may be willing to provide individual instruction in the basics of the MBSR 8-week curriculum—in effect, titrating the program to the patient's specific needs and capacities.

Cultivating a personal practice. If you have read this far you have no doubt discerned that you might derive significant professional and personal value from the cultivation of mindfulness. In your practice, you may have observed that when you are truly present with patients it affects the encounter in the moment and, perhaps, the clinical outcome over time. Ideally, one is able to maintain attention on both the patient and one's own inner experience (Speeth,

1982). In fact, Martin (1997) has suggested that mindfulness is a "common factor" in all psychotherapeutic encounters, defining it as "[A] state of psychological freedom that occurs when attention remains quiet and limber, without attachment to any particular point of view" (pp. 291–292). This seems congruent with the disposition of "evenly-suspended attention" prescribed for the analyst by Freud (1912/1953, p. 111). Martin (1997) further elaborates two distinct forms of mindful attention and suggests their utility, noting that a *focused* form helps one to see how one is embedded in a habitual pattern and choose to move to another, which is analogous to the processes at the basis of cognitive-behavioral approaches, while an *open* form of mindful attention allows one simultaneously to be aware of alternatives, which is suggestive of exploration from a psychodynamic perspective. A personal, formal practice of mindfulness can help to strengthen and allow more direct and explicit access to these ways of being with patients. This has been shown to effect outcomes: Grepmair et al., (2007) found that patients gave significantly higher ratings to therapists who had meditated before sessions than those who did not, and, further, the patients whose therapists were meditators changed significantly more than the control group on a range of measures of psychological problems and symptoms.

Personal benefits for integrative psychiatrists of participation in mindfulness training and practice are suggested in a review of stress management in medical education (Shapiro, Shapiro, & Schwartz, 2000); participating medical trainees showed more robust immune function, reductions of anxiety and depression, increases in spirituality and empathy, more frequent use of positive coping skills, and capability for resolving role conflicts, among other characteristics. The specific benefits of MBSR are suggested in a controlled study of medical students taking the course (Rosenzweig et al., 2003), which demonstrates reductions in measures of psychological distress in the MBSR group, and concludes that mindfulness is "relevant throughout the lifetime of the physician and is arguably a core characteristic of clinical practice" (p. 90). In another example, results of a qualitative study of graduate counseling students in a 15-week course based on MBSR (Schure, Christopher, & Christopher, 2008) included increases in awareness of the body, awareness and acceptance of emotions and personal issues, mental clarity and organization, tolerance of physical and emotional pain, and sense of relaxation. Impact on work with clients included being more comfortable with silence, more attentive to the process of therapy, and intentions to continue with mindfulness practice personally as well as to bring mindfulness practices to patients.

To begin or refresh a personal practice of mindfulness meditation, participation in an MBSR course may offer a range of benefits. Taking part in an 8-week MBSR course—most of which welcome professionals as well as patients—can provide and reinforce the basic skills of mindfulness for yourself, while allowing you to observe the process and outcome with a variety of other participants. Remember, however, that observation of others is secondary; be sure to make yourself the focus of your experience.

Becoming an MBSR teacher. If you have an established, regular mindfulness practice, and feel attracted to this intervention, we would urge you to test your vocation to teach. There is no better way to do that, at this moment, than to take the 7-day residential training/retreat, "Mindfulness-based stress reduction in mind–body medicine," taught by Jon Kabat-Zinn and Saki Santorelli. This is one of the foundational courses in the training scheme developed by the Center for Mindfulness at University of Massachusetts Medical School (CFM, 2007a). It offers a gateway into further training in MBSR through the CFM. Beyond this, the choice is yours as to when you begin teaching. Santorelli and Kabat-Zinn's (2001) words on this are, perhaps, both a beacon and a boundary for those who would teach: "What we encourage, if and when you yourself decide that you are ready to do this work, is taking the initiative to make this kind of program happen and to do it with as much depth and honesty and integrity as possible."

In the authors' program, as in many of the larger programs around the world, becoming an MBSR teacher is a lengthy process of development, akin to an apprenticeship. By the time a teacher is teaching independently in our program, she will have completed the professional training with Jon Kabat-Zinn and Saki Santorelli, participated in a formal practicum, and passed through an internship custom-designed to address weaknesses and embellish strengths by assuming greater and greater responsibilities while co-facilitating with senior teachers and the program director. The expected skills of a teacher are outlined in this chapter, but these are an overlay on a preexisting and continually developing authenticity of being. Therefore, for self-development, regular intensive practice through retreats, workshops, and trainings is expected of developing teachers and senior staff. MBSR teachers work with and from who they are from moment to moment.

Resources for Teacher Training

Oasis: An international learning center
Comprehensive training in teaching MBSR is available through the Center for Mindfulness in Medicine, Health Care, and Society at the University of Massachusetts. The program includes two foundation courses, two advanced offerings, and a review for certification.

Foundation courses:

- Mindfulness-based stress reduction in mind–body medicine: A 7-day residential training retreat
- Practicum in mindfulness-based stress reduction: Living inside participant–practitioner perspectives.

Advanced offerings:

- Teacher development intensive: An advanced mindfulness-based stress reduction teacher training/retreat
- Supervision in mindfulness-based stress reduction
- MBSR teacher certification review.

For more information: http://www.umassmed.edu/cfm/oasis

Other training opportunities in medical settings

Jefferson-Myrna Brind Center of Integrative Medicine
Offers three programs for which the Oasis MBSR in Mind–Body Medicine Retreat is a prerequisite.

- Practicum in mindfulness-based stress reduction
- Internship in teaching MBSR
- Supervision in teaching MBSR.

For more information: http://www.jeffersonhospital.org/cim

El Camino Hospital Mindfulness Stress Reduction Program
Offers a practicum in mindfulness-based stress reduction that is certified by the Center for Mindfulness at the University of Massachusetts Medical School as partial fulfillment of requirements for MBSR teacher certification.

For more information: http://www.mindfulnessprograms.com/teacher-training.html

Academic Education in Teaching Mindfulness-Based Interventions

Centre for Mindfulness Research and Practice, School of Psychology, Bangor University, UK

Offers a range of degree, diploma, and certificate programs:

- MSc/MA in Mindfulness-Based Approaches
  - Postgraduate Diploma in Mindfulness-Based Approaches
  - Postgraduate Certificate in Mindfulness-Based Approaches
- MSc/MA in Teaching Mindfulness-Based Courses
  - Postgraduate Diploma in Teaching Mindfulness-Based Courses
  - Postgraduate Certificate in Teaching Mindfulness-Based Courses
- Postgraduate Certificate in Advanced Mindfulness-Based Teaching Practice.

For more information: http://www.bangor.ac.uk/imscar/mindfulness

BIBLIOGRAPHY

Agazarian, Y. M. (1997). *Systems centered therapy for groups.* New York: Guilford.

Allen, N. B., Blashki, G., & Gullone, E. (2006). Mindfulness-based psychotherapies: A review of conceptual foundations, empirical evidence and practical considerations. *Australian and New Zealand Journal of Psychiatry, 40*(4), 285–294.

Astin, J. (1997). Stress reduction through mindfulness meditation: Effects on psychological symptomatology, sense of control, and spiritual experience. *Psychotherapy and Psychosomatics, 66,* 97–106.

Andersen, T. (2007). Human participating: Human "being" is the step for human "becoming" in the next step. In H. Anderson & D. Gehart (Eds.), *Collaborative therapy: Relationships and conversations that make a difference.* New York: Routledge.

Baer, R. (2003). Mindfulness training as a clinical intervention: A conceptual and empirical review. *Clinical Psychology: Science and Practice, 10*(2), 125–148.

Batchelor, S. (1997) *Buddhism without beliefs.* New York: Riverhead Books

Batten, S. V., Orsillo, S. M., & Walser, R. D. (2005). Acceptance and mindfulness-based approaches to the treatment of posttraumatic stress disorder. In S. M. Orsillo & L. Roemer (Eds.), *Acceptance and mindfulness-based approaches to anxiety: Conceptualization and treatment.* New York: Springer, pp. 241–269.

Benson, H. (1975). *The relaxation response.* New York: Morrow.

Beutler, L. E., Malik, M. L., Alimohamed, S., Harwood, T. M., Talebbi, H., Noble, S., et al. (2004). Therapist variables. In M. J. Lambert (Ed.), *Bergin and Garfield's handbook of psychotherapy and behavior change.* New York: Wiley, pp. 227–306.

Bevis, W. W. (1988). *Mind of winter: Wallace Stevens, meditation, and literature.* Pittsburgh, PA: University of Pittsburgh Press.

Bion, W. R. (1961/1989). *Experiences in groups and other papers.* New York: Routledge.

Bishop, S. (2002). What do we really know about mindfulness-based stress reduction? *Psychosomatic Medicine, 64,* 71–84.

Bishop, S., Lau, M., Shapiro, S., Carlson, L. Anderson, N., Carmody, J., et al. (2004). Mindfulness: A proposed operational definition. *Clinical Psychology: Science and Practice, 11*(3), 230–241.

Blow, A., Sprenkle, D., & Davis, S. (2007). Is who delivers the treatment more important than the treatment itself? The role of the therapist in common factors. *Journal of Marital and Family Therapy, 33*(3), 298–317.

Boorstein, S. (1996). Clinical aspects of meditation. In B. W. Scotton, A. B. Chinen, & J. R. Battista. (1996). *Textbook of transpersonal psychiatry and psychology.* New York: Basic Books.

Bravewell Collaborative. (2008). Review June 19 of program components listed at http://www.bravewell.org/patient_empowerment/bravewell_clinical_network/

Brody, L. R., & Park, S. H. (2004). Narratives, mindfulness, and the implicit audience. *Clinical Psychology: Science and Practice, 11*(2), 147–154.

Brooks, V. W. (1936). *The flowering of New England, 1815–1865.* New York: E. P. Dutton & Co.

Brooks, V. W. (1962). *Fenollosa and his circle, with other essays in biography.* New York: Dutton.

Brown, K., & Ryan, R. (2004). Perils and promise in defining and measuring mindfulness: Observations from experience. *Clinical Psychology: Science and Practice, 11*(3), 242–248.

Cage, J. (1966). *Silence: Lectures and writings.* Cambridge: The M.I.T. Press.

Carse, J. (1986). *Finite and infinite games.* New York: Ballantine Books.

Carmody, J., & Baer, R. A. (2008). Relationships between mindfulness practice and levels of mindfulness, medical and psychological symptoms and well-being in a mindfulness-based stress reduction program. *Journal of Behavioral Medicine, 31,* 23–33.

Carmody, J., Reed, G., Kristeller, J., & Merriam, P. (2008). Mindfulness, spirituality, and health-related symptoms. *Journal of Psychosomatic Research, 64,* 393–403.

Carrington, P. (1975/1998). *The book of meditation: The complete guide to modern meditation.* Boston, MA: Element. (Rev. ed. of: *Freedom in meditation.* East Millstone, NJ: Pace Educational Systems, 1975).

CFM (Center for Mindfulness in Medicine, Health Care & Society). (2007a). *Oasis: An international learning center. Professional trainings in mindfulness-based stress reduction and other mindfulness-based approaches and interventions.* Worcester, MA: Center for Mindfulness in Medicine, Health Care & Society.

CFM (Center for Mindfulness in Medicine, Health Care & Society). (2007b). http://www.umassmed.edu/Content.aspx?id=43816&linkidentifier=id&itemid=43816 (Downloaded 1/20/08).

CFM (Center for Mindfulness in Medicine, Health Care & Society). (2004). Screening criteria for exclusion from the SRP. Handout provided at Teacher Development Intensive, presented by the Center for Mindfulness in Medicine, Health Care and Society, Worcester, MA, April 6-14, 2005. (Unpaginated).

Chadwick, P., Newman-Taylor, K., & Abba, N. (2005). Mindfulness groups for people with psychosis. *Behavioural and Cognitive Psychotherapy, 33*(3), 351–359.

Claxton, G. (2006). Mindfulness, learning and the brain. *Journal of Rational-Emotive & Cognitive-Behavior Therapy, 23*(4), 301–314.

Clinical Trials. (2008). Downloaded August 10 from http://www.clinicaltrials.gov/ct2/results?term=mindfulness.

Davidson, R. J., Kabat-Zinn, J., Schumaker, J., Rosenkranz, M., Muller, D., Santorelli, S., et al. (2003). Alterations in brain and immune function produced by mindfulness meditation. *Psychosomatic Medicine, 65*, 564–570.

Deikman, A. (1966). De-automatization and the mystic experience. *Psychiatry, 29*, 324–338.

Deikman, A. (1982). *The observing self: Mysticism and psychotherapy.* Boston, MA: Beacon Press.

Drummond, M. S. (2006). Conceptualizing the efficacy of mindfulness of body sensations in the mindfulness-based interventions. *Constructivism in the Human Sciences, 11*(1):2–29.

Dryden, W., & Still, A. (2006). Historical aspects of mindfulness and self-acceptance in psychotherapy. *Journal of Rational-Emotive & Cognitive-Behavior Therapy, 24*(1), 3–28.

Epstein, M. (1995). *Thoughts without a thinker: Psychotherapy from a Buddhist perspective.* New York: Basic Books.

Fields, R. (1981). *How the swans came to the lake: A narrative history of Buddhism in America.* Boulder, CO: Shambhala.

Fowler, J. (1981). *Stages of faith: The psychology of human development and the quest for meaning.* New York: HarperCollins.

Freire, P. (1988). *Pedagogy of freedom: Ethics, democracy, and civic courage.* Lanham, MD: Rowman & Littlefield.

Freud, S. (1912). Recommendations to physicians practicing psycho-analysis. In J. Strachey (Ed.). (1958). *The standard edition of the complete psychological works of Sigmund Freud, Volume XII (1911–1913).* London: Hogarth Press.

Gendlin, E. T. (1962). *Experiencing and the creation of meaning; a philosophical and psychological approach to the subjective.* New York: Free Press of Glencoe.

Gergen, K. (1999). *An invitation to social construction.* Thousand Oaks, CA: Sage Publications.

Goleman, D. (1977/1988). *The meditative mind: The varieties of meditative experience.* Los Angeles: J.P. Tarcher; New York: Distributed by St. Martin's Press. Updated ed. of *The varieties of the meditative experience.*

Grepmair, L., Mitterlehener, F., Loew, Bachler, E., Rother, W., & Nickel, M. (2007). Promoting mindfulness in psychotherapists in training influences the treatment results of their patients: A randomized, double-blind, controlled study. *Psychotherapy and Psychosomatics, 76*, 332–338.

Grossman, P., Niemann, L., Schmidt, S., & Walach, H. (2004). Mindfulness-based stress reduction and health benefits: A meta-analysis. *Journal of Psychosomatic Research, 57*, 35–43.

Hayes, A., & Feldman, G. (2004). Clarifying the construct of mindfulness in the context of emotion regulation and the process of change in therapy. *Clinical Psychology: Science and Practice, 11*(3), 255–262.

Hayes, S., & Shenk, C. (2004). Operationalizing mindfulness without unnecessary attachments. *Clinical Psychology: Science and Practice, 11*(3), 249–254.

Hayes, S. C., & Wilson, K. G. (2003). Mindfulness: Method and process. *Clinical Psychology: Science & Practice, 10*, 161–165.

Hoffman, L. (2007). The art of "withness": A new bright edge. In H. Anderson & D. Gehart (Eds.), *Collaborative therapy: Relationships and conversations that make a difference*. New York: Routledge.

Hovanessian, M. (2003). Zen and the art of corporate productivity. *Business Week,* July 28.

Ivanovski, B. & Malhi, G. S. (2007). The psychological and neurophysiological concomitants of mindfulness forms of meditation. *Acta Neuropsychiatrica, 19,* 76–91.

Jain, S., Shapiro, S., Swanick, S., Roesch, S., Mills, P., Bell, I., et al. (2007). A randomized controlled trial of mindfulness meditation versus relaxation training: Effects on distress, positive states of mind, rumination, and distraction. *Annals of Behavioral Medicine, 3,* 11–21.

Kabat-Zinn, J. (1990). *Full catastrophe living: Using the wisdom of your body and mind to face stress, pain, and illness*. New York: Delta.

Kabat-Zinn, J. (1993). Curriculum outline. In S. F. Santorelli & J. Kabat-Zinn (Eds.) (2003). *Mindfulness-based stress reduction professional training resource manual*. Worcester, MA: Center for Mindfulness in Medicine, Health Care, and Society.

Kabat-Zinn, J. (1994). *Wherever you go, there you are*. New York: Hyperion.

Kabat-Zinn, J. (1996). Mindfulness meditation: What is, what it isn't, and its role in health care and medicine. In Y. Haruki et al. *Comparative and psychological study on meditation*. Netherlands: Eburon.

Kabat-Zinn, J. (1999). Indra's net at work: The mainstreaming of dharma practice in society. In G. Watson, S. Batchelor, & G. Claxton (Eds.), *The psychology of awakening: Buddhism, science and our day-to-day lives*. London: Rider.

Kabat-Zinn, J. (2003). Mindfulness-based interventions in context: Past, present, and future. *Clinical Psychology: Science and Practice, 10*(2), 144–154.

Kabat-Zinn, J. (2004). The uses of language and images in guiding meditation practices in MBSR. Audio Recording from 2nd Annual Conference sponsored by the Center for Mindfulness in Medicine, Health Care and Society at the University of Massachusetts Medical School. March 26.

Kabat-Zinn, J. (2005). *Coming to our senses: Healing ourselves and the world through mindfulness*. New York: Hyperion.

Kalb, C. (2003). Faith & healing. *Newsweek,* November 10.

Kasamatsu, A. and Hirai, T. (1973). An electroencephalographic study of the Zen meditation (Zazen). In D. H. Shapiro & R. N. Walsh (Eds.), (1984). *Meditation, classic and contemporary perspectives*. New York: Aldine.

Ladden, L. (2007). Mindfulness meditation and systems-centered practice. *Systems-Centered News, 15*(1), 8–11.

Langer, E.J. (1989). *Mindfulness*. Reading, MA: Addison-Wesley.

Lebow, J. (2006). *Research for the psychotherapist: From science to practice*. New York: Routledge.

Linden, W. (1973) Practicing of meditation by school children and their levels of field dependence, test anxiety, and reading achievement. *Journal of Consulting and Clinical Psychology, 41*(1), 139–143.

Linehan, M. M. (1993). *Cognitive-behavioral treatment of borderline personality disorder*. New York: Guilford Press.

Mahesh Yogi, M. (1968/1963). *Transcendental meditation.* New York: New American Library.

Martin, J. (1997). Mindfulness: A proposed common factor. *Journal of Psychotherapy Integration, 7*(4), 291–312.

McCown, D. (2004). Cognitive and perceptual benefits of meditation. *Seminars in Integrative Medicine, 2*(4), 148–151.

McCown, D., Reibel, D., & Malcoun, E. (2007). Psychological type and participation in mindfulness-based stress reduction programs. Presentation at *5th Annual Conference: Integrating Mindfulness-Based Interventions into Medicine, Health Care, and Society,* Worcester, MA, March 29–April 1.

Mezirow, J. (2000). Learning to think like an adult: Core concepts of transformation theory. In J. Mezirow & Associates (Eds.), *Learning as transformation.* San Francisco, CA: Jossey-Bass.

Merton, T. (1968). *Zen and the birds of appetite.* New York: New Directions.

Moyers, B. (1993). *Healing and the mind.* New York: Doubleday.

Norum, D. (2000). Mindful solutions: A journey of awareness. *Journal of Systemic Therapies, 19*(1), 16–19.

Palmer, P. (1998). *The courage to teach: Exploring the inner landscape of a teacher's life.* San Francisco, CA: Jossey-Bass Publishers.

Pelletier, K. (1974). Influence of transcendental meditation upon autokinetic perception. In D. H.Shapiro and R. N. Walsh (Eds.), (1984). *Meditation, classic and contemporary perspectives.* New York: Aldine.

Perls, F., Hefferline, R., & Goodman, P. (1969, c1951). *Gestalt therapy: Excitement and growth in the human personality.* New York: Julian Press.

Reibel, D. K., Greeson, J. M., Brainard, G. C., & Rosenzweig, S.(2001). Mindfulness-based stress reduction and health related quality of life in a heterogeneous patient population. *General Hospital Psychiatry, 23,* 183–192.

Rogers, C. (1961). *On becoming a person; a therapist's view of psychotherapy.* Boston, MA: Houghton Mifflin.

Rogers, F. (2004). *The world according to Mr. Rogers: Important things to remember.* New York: Hyperion.

Rosenzweig, S., Reibel, D., Greeson, J., Brainard, G., & Hojat, M. (2003). Mindfulness-based stress reduction lowers psychological distress in medical students. *Teaching and Learning in Medicine, 15*(2), 88–92.

Roth, B. & Calle-Mesa, L. (2006). Mindfulness-based stress reduction with Spanish- and English-speaking inner-city medical patients. In R. A. Baer (Ed.), *Mindfulness-based treatment approaches: Clinician's guide to evidence base and applications.* Boston, MA: Elsevier Academic Press.

Rothwell, N. (2006). The different facets of mindfulness. *Journal of Rational-Emotive & Cognitive-Behavior Therapy, 24,* 79–86.

Safran, J. D. & Segal, Z. (1990). *Interpersonal process in cognitive therapy.* New York: Basic Books.

Santorelli, S. (2004) Three points to consider when teaching mindfulness-based stress reduction. Personal notes provided by Santorelli at Post-Conference Instructional

Institute, *2nd Annual Conference sponsored by the Center for Mindfulness in Medicine, Health Care and Society*, Worcester, MA. March 27, 2004.

Santorelli, S. (1999). *Heal thy self.* New York: Bell Town.

Santorelli, S., & Kabat-Zinn, J. (2001). MBSR curriculum guide and supporting materials: Guidelines for presenting this work. In S. F. Santorelli & J. Kabat-Zinn (Eds.) (2003). *Mindfulness-based stress reduction professional training resource manual.* Worcester, MA: Center for Mindfulness in Medicine, Health Care, and Society. (unpaginated).

Santorelli, S. (2001a). Mindfulness-based stress reduction: Qualifications and recommended guidelines for providers. In S. F. Santorelli & J. Kabat-Zinn (Eds.) (2003). *Mindfulness-based stress reduction professional training resource manual.* Worcester, MA: Center for Mindfulness in Medicine, Health Care, and Society. (unpaginated).

Santorelli, S. (2001b). Mindfulness-based stress reduction (MBSR): Standards of practice. In S. F. Santorelli & J. Kabat-Zinn (Eds.) (2003). *Mindfulness-based stress reduction professional training resource manual.* Worcester, MA: Center for Mindfulness in Medicine, Health Care, and Society. (unpaginated).

Santorelli, S. (2001c). Interview with Saki Santorelli, Stress Reduction Clinic, Massachusetts Memorial Medical Center. In Freedman, L. (Ed.), *Best practices in alternative and complementary medicine.* Frederick, MD: Aspen.

Schure, M. B., Christopher, J., & Christopher, S. (2008). Mind–body medicine and the art of self-care: Teaching mindfulness to counseling students through yoga, meditation, and Qigong. *Journal of Counseling and Development, 86*(1), 47–56.

Seeman, W., Nidich, S., & Banta, T. (1972). Influence of Transcendental Meditation on a measure of self-actualization. *Journal of Counseling Psychology, 19,* 184–187.

Segal, Z. V., Williams, J. M. G., & Teasdale, J. D. (2002). *Mindfulness-based cognitive therapy for depression: A new approach to preventing relapse.* New York: Guilford Press.

Selver, C. & Brooks, C. V. W. (2007). *Reclaiming vitality and presence: Sensory awareness as a practice for life.* Berkeley: North Atlantic Books.

Shapiro, S., Carlson, L., Astin, J., & Freedman, B. (2006). Mechanisms of mindfulness. *Journal of Clinical Psychology, 62*(3), 373–386.

Shapiro, S. L., Shapiro, D. E., & Schwartz, G. E. (2000). Stress management in medical education: A review of the literature. *Academic medicine, 75*(7), 748–759.

Simon, G. M. (2003). *Beyond technique in family therapy: Finding your therapeutic voice.* Boston: Allyn & Bacon.

Simon, G. M. (2006). The heart of the matter: A proposal for placing the self of the therapist at the center of psychotherapy research and training. *Family Process, 45,* 331–344.

Speca, M., Carlson, L. E., Goodey, E., & Angen, M. (2000) A randomized, wait-list controlled clinical trial: The effect of a mindfulness meditation-based stress reduction program on mood and symptoms of stress in cancer outpatients. *Psychosomatic Medicine, 62,* 613– 622.

Speeth, K. R. (1982). On psychotherapeutic attention. *Journal of Transpersonal Psychology, 14*(2), 141–160.

Stein, J. (2003). Just say OM. *Time*, August 4.

Still, A. (2006). Introduction. *Journal of Rational-Emotive & Cognitive-Behavior Therapy, 23*(4), 275–280.

Suzuki, D. T., Fromm, E., & De Martino, R. (1960). *Zen Buddhism & psychoanalysis.* New York: Harper & Row.

Tuckman, B. W. & Jensen, M. C. (1977). Stages of small-group development revisited. *Group & Organization Studies, 2*(4), 419–427.

Tweed, T. A. (1992). *The American encounter with Buddhism, 1844–1912: Victorian culture and the limits of dissent.* Bloomington, IN: Indiana University Press.

Wallace, R. K. (1970). Physiological effects of Transcendental Meditation. *Science, 167,* 1751–1754.

Wampold, B. E. (2001). *The great psychotherapy debate: Models, methods, and findings.* Mahwah, NJ: Erlbaum.

Watts, A. (*c.* 1959). *Beat Zen, square Zen, and Zen.* San Francisco, CA: City Lights Books.

Wátzlawick, P., Weakland, J. H., & Fisch, R. (1974). *Change; principles of problem formation and problem resolution.* New York: Norton.

West, W. (2000). *Psychotherapy and spirituality: crossing the line between therapy and religion.* Thousand Oaks, CA: Sage.

Winnicott, D. W. (1971). *Playing & reality.* New York: Basic Books.

Witkiewitz, K., Marlatt, A., & Walker, D. (2005). Mindfulness-based relapse prevention for alcohol and substance use disorders. *Journal of Cognitive Psychotherapy, 19*(3), 211–228.

Yalom, I. (1985). *The theory and practice of group psychotherapy.* New York: Basic Books.

Zimmerman, J. & Coyle, V. (1996). *The way of council.* Las Vegas, NV: Bramble Books.

14

The Neurobiology of Meditation

ANDREW B. NEWBERG

KEY CONCEPTS

- Meditation is a complex mental process that involves changes in cognition, sensory perception, emotions, hormones, and autonomic activity.
- Many different neurotransmitter systems, including dopamine, serotonin, glutamate, and opiates are likely affected by meditation practices.
- Meditation has also become widely used in psychiatric and medical practices for stress management, as well as for a variety of physical and mental disorders.
- There has been limited understanding of the overall biological mechanism of these practices in terms of the effects in both the brain and body.
- Recent studies using clinical tools and functional neuroimaging have substantially augmented the knowledge of the biology of meditative practices.

■

Introduction

The study of meditation, a complex mental task, is potentially one of the most important areas of research that may be pursued by science in the next decade. Meditation practices offer a fascinating window into human consciousness, psychology, and experience; the relationship between mental states and body physiology; emotional and cognitive processing; and the biological correlates of religious experience. In the past 30 years, scientists have explored the neurobiological effects and mechanism of meditation in great detail. Initial studies measured changes in autonomic activity, such as heart rate and blood pressure as well as electroencephalographic changes. More recent studies have explored changes in hormonal and immunological function associated with meditation practices. While many of these studies have utilized peripheral measurements of different substances, they are consistent with a number of central neurochemical changes. Studies have also explored the clinical effects of meditation in both physical and psychological disorders.

Functional neuroimaging has opened a new window into the investigation of meditative states by exploring the neurological correlates of these experiences. A growing number of imaging studies of meditative practices are currently available in the literature (see Table 14.1). The neuroimaging techniques used in these studies include positron emission tomography (PET: Herzog et al., 1990–1991; Lou et al., 1999), single photon emission computed tomography (SPECT: Newberg et al., 2001; Newberg, Pourdehnad, Alavi, & d'Aquili, 2003), and functional magnetic resonance imaging (fMRI: Beauregard & Paquette, 2006; Brefczynski-Lewis, Lutz, Schaefer, Levinson, & Davidson, 2007; Lazar et al., 2000). Each of these techniques provides different advantages and disadvantages in the study of meditation. Functional MRI has improved resolution over SPECT and the ability of immediate anatomic correlation, but would be very difficult to utilize for the study of meditation because of noise from the machine and the problem of requiring the subject to lie down, an atypical posture for many forms of meditation. In fact, we attempted the use of fMRI with one of our initial meditation subjects in order to determine feasibility, but the subject found it extremely difficult to carry out the meditation practice. While PET imaging also provides better resolution than SPECT, if one strives to make the environment relatively distraction free to maximize the chances of having a strong meditative experience, it is sometimes beneficial to perform these studies during nonclinical times, which may make PET radiopharmaceuticals such as fluorodeoxyglucose difficult to obtain. Functional MRI allows for the ability to measure multiple time points during meditation practices, but PET and SPECT offers an opportunity to evaluate neurotransmitter systems. Thus, functional brain imaging offers important techniques for studying meditation, although the best approach may depend on a number of individual factors.

This chapter reviews the existing data on neurophysiology and physiology with relation to meditation practices and attempts to integrate this data into a comprehensive neurobiological model of such practices. However, there are many possible neurochemical changes that may occur during meditation, even though they may not occur in every type of practice or in each individual. This model is designed to provide a framework of the neurological and

Table 14.1. Imaging Studies of Meditative Practices Currently
Available in the Literature.

Study	Type of Critique Meditation	Imaging Modality	N	Measures	Results
Herzog et al.	Yoga	PET	8	CBF	↑Frontal Lobe, ↓Parietal Lobe Meditation in the scanner, limited regional (1990–1991) analysis, one time point
Lou et al.	Yoga Nidra	PET	9	CBF	↑Parietal during focus on self, subjects listened to tape guiding the meditation (2000) ↑Hippocampus, ↓PFC meditation, different forms of meditation, one time point
Newberg et al.	Tibetan	SPECT	8	CBF	↑PFC, Thalamus, Brainstem, ↓PSPL No cross correlation with other modalities, (2001); SPECT offers lowest resolution, one time point
Lazar et al.	Kundalini	fMRI	5	CBF	↑PFC, Parietal, Hippocampus, Temporal lobe Attempted to factor in MRI noise to prevent (2000) Cingulate Gyrus, Hypothalamus distraction, smallest N, limited ability to detect decreased CBF, multiple time points
Kjaer et al.	Yoga Nidra	PET	5	Dopamine	↑dopamine in the striatum; subjects listened to tape guiding the (2002) meditation
Newberg et al.	Prayer	SPECT	3	CBF	↑PFC, Thalamus, Brainstem, ↓PSPL No cross correlation with other modalities; (2003) Very small number of subjects.
Short et al.	Meditation	fMRI	12	CBF	↑PFC, ↑anterior cingulate, ↑temporal, ↑parietal Short meditation practice, but evaluated (2007) changes over time during meditation

physiological correlates of meditative experiences and create a springboard for future research. Within this model, specific structures, including the prefrontal cortex, parietal lobe, limbic system, autonomic nervous system, appear to interact in an integrated manner. Further, this model suggests that a number of neurotransmitters, including serotonin, dopamine, gamma amino butyric acid, and glutamate, also play an important role.

Types of Meditation

Although there are many specific approaches to meditation, we have typically divided such practices into two basic categories. The first category is one in which the subjects simply attempt to clear all thought from their sphere of attention and includes practices such as Theravada (d'Aquili & Newberg, 1993). This form of meditation is an attempt to reach a subjective state characterized by a sense of no space, no time, and no thought. Further, this state is cognitively experienced as fully integrated and unified, such that there is no sense of a self and other. The second category is one in which the subject focuses his attention on a particular object, image, phrase, or word, and includes practices such as transcendental meditation and various forms of Tibetan Buddhism. This form of meditation is designed to lead to a subjective experience of absorption with the object of focus. Mindfulness meditation (Kabat-Zinn, 2005) is a practice in which attention is focused on whatever thoughts or feelings enter into the mind. The goal is to be more aware of one's inner mental processes. There is another distinction in which some meditation is guided by following along with a leader who is verbally directing the practitioner either in person or on tape. Others merely practice the meditation on their own volition. There are probably important differences between volitional and guided meditation practices that should also be reflected in specific differences in cerebral activation.

Phenomenological analysis suggests that the end result of many practices of meditation is similar, although this result might be described differently depending on the culture and individual. Therefore, it seems reasonable that while the initial neurophysiological activation occurring during any given practice may differ, there may eventually be a convergence of experiences and neurophysiological correlates. This chapter focuses on a description of volitional meditation in which subjects focus on an object that, hopefully, will provide an overall framework from which any given type of meditation can be considered (see Figure 14.1). However, the brain structures and functions described will probably apply to other types of meditation practices, although the specifics will be slightly different.

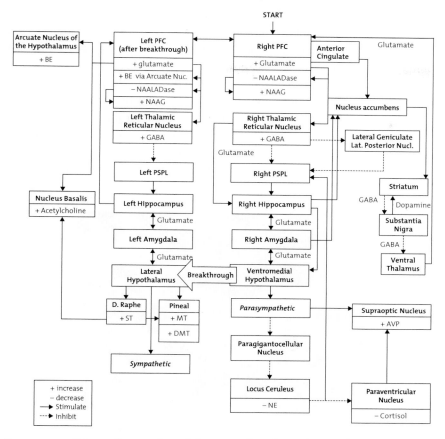

FIGURE 14.1. Schematic overview of the neurophysiological network possibly associated with meditative states. The circuits generally apply to both hemispheres; however, much of the initial activity is on the right.

Activation of the Prefrontal and Cingulate Cortex

Brain imaging studies suggest that willful acts and tasks that require sustained attention are initiated via activity in the prefrontal cortex (PFC), particularly in the right hemisphere (Frith, Friston, Liddle, & Frackowiak, 1991; Ingvar, 1994; Pardo, Fox, & Raichle, 1991; Posner and Petersen, 1990). The cingulate gyrus has also been shown to be involved in focusing attention, probably in conjunction with the PFC (Vogt, Finch, & Olson, 1992). Since meditation requires intense focus of attention, it seems appropriate that a model for meditation begin with activation of the PFC (particularly in the right) as well as the cingulate gyrus.

This notion is supported by the increased activity observed in these regions on several of the brain imaging studies of volitional types of meditation (Herzog et al., 1990–1991; Lazar et al., 2000; Newberg et al., 2001). In a study of Tibetan Buddhist meditators (see Figures 14.2 and 14.3), there was increased activity in the PFC bilaterally (greater on the right) and in the cingulate gyrus during meditation. Therefore, meditation appears to start by activating the prefrontal and cingulate cortex, associated with the will or intent to clear the mind of thoughts or to focus on an object. One PET study of a guided type of meditation did not demonstrate increased prefrontal activity; however, a recent study showed decreased frontal activity during externally guided word generation compared to

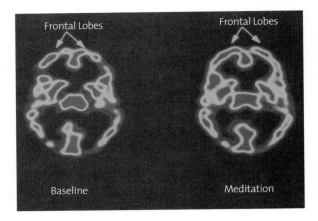

FIGURE 14.2. The SPECT images were obtained during a study of the neurophysiological correlates of Tibetan Buddhist meditation. These axial images show the results from a baseline scan on the left (i.e. at rest) and during a "peak" of meditation shown on the right. The images demonstrate that the frontal lobes, usually involved in focusing attention, are more active during meditation (increased red activity).

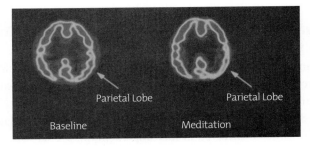

FIGURE 14.3. Axial SPECT images, slightly higher up in the brain demonstrate decreased activity in the superior parietal lobe (lower right shows up as yellow rather than the red on the left image) during meditation compared to the resting state.

internal or volitional word generation (Crosson et al., 2001). Thus, prefrontal and cingulate activation may be associated with the volitional aspects of meditation.

Thalamic Activation

Several animal studies have shown that the PFC, when activated, innervates the reticular nucleus of the thalamus (Cornwall & Phillipson, 1988), particularly as part of a more global attentional network (Portas et al., 1998). Such activation may be accomplished by the PFC's production and distribution of the excitatory neurotransmitter glutamate, which the PFC neurons use to communicate among themselves and to innervate other brain structures (Cheramy, Romo, & Glowinski, 1987). The thalamus itself governs the flow of sensory information to cortical processing areas via its interactions with the lateral geniculate and lateral posterior nuclei, and also probably uses the glutamate system in order to activate neurons in other structures (Armony & LeDoux, 2000). The lateral geniculate nucleus receives raw visual data from the optic tract and routes it to the striate cortex for processing (Andrews, Halpern, & Purves, 1997). The lateral posterior nucleus of the thalamus provides the posterior superior parietal lobule (PSPL) with the sensory information it needs to determine the body's spatial orientation (Bucci, Conley, & Gallagher, 1999).

When excited, the reticular nucleus secretes the inhibitory neurotransmitter gamma aminobutyric acid (GABA) onto the lateral posterior and geniculate nuclei, cutting off input to the PSPL and visual centers in proportion to the reticular activation (Destexhe, Contreras, & Steriade, 1998). During meditation, because of the increased activity in the PFC, particularly on the right, there should be a concomitant increase in the activity in the reticular nucleus of the thalamus. While brain imaging studies of meditation have not had the resolution to distinguish the reticular nuclei, several studies have demonstrated a general increase in thalamic activity that may be proportional to the activity in the PFC. This is consistent with, but does not confirm, the specific interaction between the PFC and reticular nuclei during meditation practices. However, if the activation of the right PFC causes increased activity in the reticular nucleus during meditation, the result may be decreased sensory input entering into the PSPL. Several studies have demonstrated an increase in serum GABA during meditation (see Table 14.2 for an overview of neurochemical changes during meditation), which may reflect increased central GABA activity (Elias, Guich, & Wilson, 2000). This functional deafferentation related to increased GABA would mean that fewer distracting outside stimuli would arrive at the visual cortex and PSPL. This might enhance the sense of focus of the meditator and contribute to the overall experience.

Table 14.2. Summary of Neurochemically Related Changes in Serum Concentration Observed During Meditation Techniques and the Central Nervous System Structures Typically Involved in Their Production.

Neurochemical	Observed Change	CNS Structure
Arginine vasopressin	Increased	Supraoptic nucleus
GABA	Increased	Thalamus, other inhibitory structures
Melatonin	Increased	Pineal gland
Serotonin	Increased	Dorsal raphe
Cortisol	Decreased	Paraventricular nucleus
Norepinephrine	Decreased	Locus ceruleus
β-Endorphin	Rhythm changed; levels unaltered	Arcuate nucleus

It should also be noted that the dopaminergic system, via the basal ganglia, is believed to participate in regulating the glutamatergic system and the interactions between the prefrontal cortex and subcortical structures. A PET study utilizing 11C-Raclopride to measure the dopaminergic tone during Yoga Nidra meditation demonstrated a significant increase in dopamine levels during the meditation practice (Kjaer et al., 2002). They hypothesized that this increase may be associated with the gating of cortical-subcortical interactions that leads to an overall decrease in readiness for action that is associated with this particular type of meditation. Future studies will be necessary to elaborate on the role of dopamine during meditative practices, as well as the interactions between dopamine and other neurotransmitter systems.

PSPL Deafferentation

The PSPL is heavily involved in the analysis and integration of higher-order visual, auditory, and somaesthetic information (Adair et al., 1995). It is also involved in a complex attentional network that includes the PFC and thalamus (Fernandez-Duque & Posner, 2001). Through the reception of auditory and visual input from the thalamus, the PSPL is able to help generate a three-dimensional image of the body in space, provide a sense of spatial coordinates in which the body is oriented, help distinguish between objects, and exert influences in regard to objects that may be directly grasped and manipulated (Lynch,

1980; Mountcastle, Motter, & Anderson, 1980). These functions of the PSPL might be critical for distinguishing between the self and the external world. It should be noted that a recent study has suggested that the superior temporal lobe may play a more important role in body spatial representation, although this has not been confirmed by other reports (Karnath, Ferber, & Himmelbach, 2001). However, it remains to be seen what is the actual relationship between the parietal and temporal lobes in terms of spatial representation.

Regardless, deafferentation of these orienting areas of the brain has been suggested as an important mediator in the physiology of meditation (Newberg & Iversen, 2003). If, for example, deafferentation of the PSPL occurs by the reticular nucleus's GABAergic effects, the person may begin to lose his or her usual ability to define the self spatially and to help orient the self. Such a notion is supported by clinical findings in patients with parietal lobe damage who have difficulty orienting themselves. The effects of meditation are likely to be more selective and do not destroy the sense of self, but alter the perception of it. Deafferentation of the PSPL has also been supported by two imaging studies demonstrating decreased activity in this region during intense meditation (Herzog et al., 1990–1991; Newberg et al., 2001). The lateralization of these decreases has not been fully elucidated, although it is reasonable that depending on the practice and experience, greater decreases might be observed in either the right or left hemisphere. However, more studies will be needed to determine the precise relationship between changes in each of the hemispheres.

Hippocampal and Amygdalar Activation

In addition to the complex cortical-thalamic activity, meditation might also be expected to alter activity in the limbic system, especially since stimulation of limbic structures is associated with experiences similar to those described during meditation (Fish, Gloor, Quesney, & Oliver, 1993; Saver & Rabin, 1997). The hippocampus acts to modulate and moderate cortical arousal and responsiveness, via rich and extensive interconnections with the prefrontal cortex, other neocortical areas, the amygdala, and the hypothalamus (Joseph, 1996). Hippocampal stimulation has been shown to diminish cortical responsiveness and arousal; however, if cortical arousal is initially at a low level, then hippocampal stimulation tends to augment cortical activity (Redding, 1967). The ability of the hippocampus to stimulate or inhibit neuronal activity in other structures probably relies upon the glutamate and GABA systems respectively (Armony & LeDoux, 2000). The partial deafferentation of the right PSPL during meditation may result in stimulation of the right hippocampus because of the inverse modulation of the hippocampus in relation to cortical activity. If, in addition, there is simultaneous direct stimulation of the right hippocampus via the thalamus (as part of the known attentional network) and mediated by glutamate, then a powerful recruitment of stimulation of the right hippocampus occurs. Right hippocampal activity may ultimately enhance the stimulatory function of the PFC on the thalamus via the nucleus accumbens, which gates the neural input from the PFC to the thalamus via the neuromodulatory effects of dopamine (Chow & Cummings, 1999; Newman & Grace, 1999).

The hippocampus greatly influences the amygdala, such that they complement and interact in the generation of attention, emotion, and certain types of imagery (Joseph, 1996). It seems that much of the prefrontal modulation of emotion is via the hippocampus and its connections with the amygdala (Poletti & Sujatanond, 1980). Because of this reciprocal interaction between the amygdala and hippocampus, the activation of the right hippocampus probably stimulates the right lateral amygdala as well. The results of the fMRI study by Lazar et al. support the notion of increased activity in the regions of the amygdala and hippocampus during meditation (Lazar et al., 2000).

Hypothalamic and Autonomic Nervous System Changes

The hypothalamus is interconnected extensively with the limbic system. Stimulation of the right lateral amygdala has been shown to result in stimulation of the ventromedial portion of the hypothalamus, with a subsequent stimulation of the peripheral parasympathetic system (Davis, 1992). Increased parasympathetic activity should be associated with the subjective sensation first of relaxation and, eventually, of a more profound quiescence. Activation of the parasympathetic system would also cause a reduction in heart rate and respiratory rate. All of these physiological responses have been observed during meditation (Jevning, Wallace, & Beidebach, 1992).

Typically, when breathing and heart rate slow down, the paragigantocellular nucleus of the medulla ceases to innervate the locus ceruleus (LC) of the pons. The LC produces and distributes norepinephrine (or NE: Foote, 1987), a neuromodulator that increases the susceptibility of brain regions to sensory input by amplifying strong stimuli, while simultaneously gating out weaker activations and cellular "noise" that fall below the activation threshold (Waterhouse & Moises, 1998). Decreased stimulation of the LC results in a decrease in the level of NE (Van Bockstaele & Aston-Jones, 1995). The breakdown products of catecholamines, such as NE and epinephrine, have generally been found to be reduced in the urine and plasma during meditation (Infante et al., 2001; Walton, Pugh, Gelderloos, & Macrae, 1995), which may simply reflect the systemic change in autonomic balance. However, it is not inconsistent with a cerebral decrease in NE levels as well. During a meditative practice, the reduced firing of the paragigantocellular nucleus probably cuts back its innervation of the locus ceruleus, which densely and specifically supplies the PSPL and the lateral posterior nucleus with NE (Foote, 1987). Thus, a reduction in NE would decrease the impact of sensory input on the PSPL, contributing to its deafferentation.

The locus ceruleus would also deliver less NE to the hypothalamic paraventricular nucleus. The paraventricular nucleus of the hypothalamus typically secretes corticotropin-releasing hormone (CRH) in response to innervation by NE from the locus ceruleus (Ziegler, Cass, & Herman Ziegler, 1999). This CRH stimulates the anterior pituitary to release adrenocorticotropic hormone (ACTH) (Livesey, Evans, Mulligan, & Donald, 2000). ACTH, in turn, stimulates the adrenal cortex to produce cortisol, one of the body's stress hormones (Davies, Kenyon, & Fraser, 1985). Decreasing NE from the locus ceruleus during meditation would probably decrease the production of CRH by the paraventricular nucleus, and ultimately decrease cortisol levels. Most studies have found that urine and plasma cortisol levels are decreased during meditation (Jevning, Wilson, & Davidson, 1978; Sudsuang, Chentanez, & Veluvan, 1991; Walton et al., 1995).

The drop in blood pressure associated with parasympathetic activity during meditation practices would be expected to relax the arterial baroreceptors, leading the caudal ventral medulla to decrease its GABAergic inhibition of the supraoptic nucleus of the hypothalamus. This lack of inhibition can provoke the supraoptic nucleus to release the vasoconstrictor arginine vasopressin (AVP), thereby tightening the arteries and returning blood pressure to normal (Renauld, 1996). AVP has also been shown to contribute to the general maintenance of positive affect (Pietrowsky, 1991), decrease self-perceived fatigue and arousal, and significantly improve the consolidation of new memories and learning (Weingartner et al., 1981). In fact, plasma AVP has been shown to increase dramatically during meditation (O'Halloran et al., 1985). The sharp increase in AVP should result in a decreased subjective feeling of fatigue and increased sense of arousal. It could also help to enhance the meditator's memory of his experience, perhaps explaining the subjective phenomenon that meditative experiences are remembered and described in very vivid terms.

PFC Effects on Other Neurochemical Systems

As a meditation practice continues, there should be continued activity in the PFC associated with the persistent will to focus attention. (PFC activity might also be associated with meditations in which the individual focuses the mind on nothing, but this has not been fully studied.) In general, as PFC activity increases, it produces ever-increasing levels of free synaptic glutamate in the brain. Increased glutamate can stimulate the hypothalamic arcuate nucleus to release beta-endorphin (Kiss, Kocsis, Csaki, Gorcs, & Halasz, 1997). Beta-endorphin (BE) is an opioid produced primarily by the arcuate nucleus of the medial hypothalamus and distributed to the brain's sub-cortical areas (Yadid, Zangen, Herzberg, Nakash, & Sagen, 2000). BE is known to depress respiration, reduce fear, reduce pain, and produce sensations of joy and euphoria (Janal et al., 1984). That such effects have been described during meditation may implicate some degree of BE release related to the increased PFC activity. Meditation has been found to disrupt diurnal rhythms of BE and ACTH, while not affecting diurnal cortisol rhythms (Infante et al., 1998). However, it is probable that BE is not solely responsible for meditative experiences, because simply taking morphine-related substances does not produce equivalent experiences to those in meditation. Furthermore, one very limited study demonstrated that blocking the opiate receptors with naloxone did not affect the experience or EEG associated with meditation (Sim & Tsoi, 1992).

Glutamate activates N-methyl d-Aspartate receptors (NMDAr), but excess glutamate can kill these neurons through excitotoxic processes (Albin & Greenamyre, 1992). We propose that if glutamate levels approach excitotoxic concentrations during intense states of meditation, the brain might limit its production of N-acetylated-alpha-linked-acidic dipeptidase, which converts the endogenous NMDAr antagonist N-acetylaspartylglutamate (NAAG) into glutamate (Thomas, Vornov, Olkowski, Merion, & Slusher, 2000). The resultant increase in NAAG would protect cells from excitotoxic damage. There is an important side effect, however, since the NMDAr inhibitor NAAG is functionally analogous to the disassociative hallucinogens ketamine, phencyclidine, and nitrous oxide (Jevtovic-Todorovic & Wozniak, 2001). These NMDAr antagonists produce a variety of states that may be characterized as either schizophrenomimetic or mystical, such as out-of-body and near-death experiences (Vollenweider et al., 1997).

Autonomic-Cortical Activity

In the early 1970s, Gellhorn and Kiely developed a model of the physiological processes involved in meditation based almost exclusively on autonomic nervous system (ANS) activity. This model is somewhat limited because of the heavy reliance on the ANS, but their work indicated the importance of the ANS during meditative experiences (Gellhorn and Kiely, 1972). These authors suggested that intense stimulation of either the sympathetic or parasympathetic system, if continued, could ultimately result in simultaneous discharge of both systems (what might be considered a "breakthrough" of the other system). Several studies have demonstrated predominant parasympathetic activity during meditation associated with decreased heart rate and blood pressure, decreased respiratory rate, and decreased oxygen metabolism (Sudsuang et al., 1991; Jevning et al., 1992; Travis, 2001). However, a recent study of two separate meditative techniques suggested a mutual activation of parasympathetic and sympathetic systems by demonstrating an increase in the variability of heart rate during meditation (Peng et al., 1999). The increased variation in heart rate was hypothesized to reflect activation of both arms of the autonomic nervous system. This notion also fits the characteristic description of meditative states in which there is a sense of overwhelming calmness as well as significant alertness. Also, the notion of mutual activation of both arms of the ANS is consistent with recent developments in the study of autonomic interactions (Hugdahl, 1996).

Serotonergic Activity

Activation of the autonomic nervous system can result in intense stimulation of structures in the lateral hypothalamus and median forebrain bundle, which are known to produce both ecstatic and blissful feelings when directly stimulated (Olds & Forbes, 1981). Stimulation of the lateral hypothalamus can also result in changes in serotonergic activity. In fact, several studies have shown that, after meditation, the breakdown products of serotonin (ST) in urine are significantly increased suggesting an overall elevation in ST during meditation (Walton et al., 1995). Serotonin is a neuromodulator that densely supplies the visual centers of the temporal lobe, where it strongly influences the flow of visual associations generated by this area (Foote, 1987). The cells of the dorsal raphe produce and distribute ST when innervated by the lateral hypothalamus (Aghajanian, Sprouse, & Rasmussen, 1987) and also when activated by the prefrontal cortex (Juckel, Mendlin, & Jacobs, 1999). Moderately increased levels of ST appear to correlate with positive affect, while low ST often signifies depression (Van Praag & De Haan, 1980). This relationship has clearly been demonstrated with regard to the effects of the selective serotonin reuptake inhibitor medications that are widely used for the treatment of depression. When cortical ST_2 receptors (especially in the temporal lobes) are activated, however, the stimulation can result in a hallucinogenic effect. Tryptamine psychedelics such as psylocybin and LSD seem to take advantage of this mechanism to produce their extraordinary visual associations and mystical or religious experiences (Aghajanian & Marek, 1999; Griffiths, Richards, McCann, & Jesse, 2006). The mechanism by which this appears to occur is that ST inhibits the lateral geniculate nucleus, greatly reducing the amount of visual information that can pass through (Funke & Eysel, 1995; Yoshida, Sasa, & Takaori, 1984). If combined with reticular nucleus inhibition of the lateral geniculate, ST may increase the fluidity of temporal visual associations in the absence of sensory input, possibly resulting in the internally generated imagery that has been described during certain meditative states.

Increased ST levels can affect several other neurochemical systems. An increase in serotonin has a modulatory effect on dopamine suggesting a link between the serotonergic and dopaminergic system, which may enhance feelings of euphoria (Vollenweider, Vontobel, Hell, & Leenders, 1999) frequently described during meditative states. Serotonin, in conjunction with the increased glutamate, has been shown to stimulate the nucleus basalis to release acetylcholine, which has important modulatory influences throughout the cortex (Manfridi, Brambilla, & Mancia, 1999; Zhelyazkova-Savova & Giovannini, 1997). Increased acetylcholine in the frontal lobes has been shown to augment the attentional system, and in the parietal lobes to enhance orienting without altering sensory input (Fernandez-Duque & Posner, 2001). While no studies have evaluated the specific role of acetylcholine in meditation, it appears that this neurotransmitter may enhance the attentional component as well as the orienting response in the face of progressive deafferentation of sensory input into the parietal lobes during meditation. Increased serotonin combined with lateral hypothalamic innervation of the pineal gland may lead the latter to increase production of the neurohormone melatonin (MT) from the conversion of ST (Moller, 1992). Melatonin has been shown to depress the central nervous system and reduce pain sensitivity (Shaji & Kulkarni, 1998). During meditation, blood plasma MT has been found to increase sharply (Tooley, Armstrong, Norman, & Sali, 2000), which may contribute to the feelings of calmness and decreased awareness of pain (Dollins, Lynch, Wurtman, Deng, & Lieberman, 1993). Under circumstances of heightened activation, pineal enzymes can also endogenously synthesize the powerful hallucinogen 5-methoxy-dimethyltryptamine (DMT) (Monti & Christian, 1981). Several studies have linked DMT to a variety of mystical states, including out-of-body experiences, distortion of time and space, and interaction with supernatural entities (Strassman & Clifford, 1994; Strassman, Clifford, Qualls, & Berg, 1996). Hyperstimulation of the pineal at this step, then, could also lead to DMT production, which can be associated with the wide variety of mystical-type experiences associated with that hallucinogen.

Conclusion

Much work still needs to be done to better elucidate the intricate neurobiological mechanisms underlying meditative practices. Most studies of the biological correlates of meditation currently available suffer from a low number of subjects, lack of control conditions, and difficulty in factoring out confounding variables. Furthermore, knowledge of neurotransmitter systems is highly complex and continually being refined. Thus, it may be very difficult to assess if all of the systems would function in the integrated manner described above. However, the neurophysiological effects that have been observed during meditative states seem to outline a consistent pattern of changes involving certain key cerebral structures in conjunction with autonomic and hormonal changes. These changes are also reflected in neurochemical changes involving the endogenous opioid, GABA, norepinephrine, and serotonergic receptor systems. The current research studies have begun to elucidate the mechanism underlying the physical and psychological effects of meditative practices and provide an impetus for future studies of these and other complex mental tasks.

REFERENCES

Adair, K. C., Gilmore, R. L., Fennell, E. B., Gold, M., Heilman, K. M. (1995). Anosognosia during intracarotid barbiturate anaesthesia: unawareness or amnesia for weakness. *Neurology, 45*, 241–243.

Aghajanian, G., Sprouse, J., & Rasmussen, K. (1987). Physiology of the midbrain serotonin system. In H. Meltzer (Ed.), *Psychopharmacology, the third generation of progress.* New York: Raven Press, pp. 141–149.

Aghajanian, G. K., & Marek, G. J. (1999). Serotonin and hallucinogens. *Neuropsychopharmacology, 21*, 16S–23S.

Albin, R., & Greenamyre, J. (1992). Alternative excitotoxic hypotheses. *Neurology, 42*, 733–738.

Andrews, T. J., Halpern, S. D., & Purves, D. (1997). Correlated size variations in human visual cortex, lateral geniculate nucleus, and optic tract. *Journal of Neuroscience, 17*, 2859–2868.

Armony, J. L., & LeDoux, J. E. (2000). How danger is encoded: Toward a systems, cellular, and computational understanding of cognitive-emotional interactions in fear. In M. S. Gazzaniga (Ed.), *The new cognitive neurosciences.* Cambridge, MA: MIT Press, pp. 1067–1079.

Beauregard, M., & Paquette, V. (2006). Neural correlates of a mystical experience in Carmelite nuns. *Neuroscience Letters, 405*(3), 186–190.

Brefczynski-Lewis, J. A., Lutz, A., Schaefer, H. S., Levinson, D. B., & Davidson, R. J. (2007). Neural correlates of attentional expertise in long-term meditation practitioners. *Proceedings of National Academy of Sciences USA, 104*(27), 11483–11488.

Bucci, D. J., Conley, M., & Gallagher, M. (1999). Thalamic and basal forebrain cholinergic connections of the rat posterior parietal cortex. *Neuroreport, 10*, 941–945.

Cheramy, A., Romo, R., & Glowinski, J. (1987). Role of corticostriatal glutamatergic neurons in the presynaptic control of dopamine release. In M. Sandler, C. Feuerstein,

& B. Scatton, et al. (Eds.), *Neurotransmitter interactions in the basal ganglia*. New York: Raven Press.

Chow, T. W., & Cummings, J. L. (1999). *Frontal*-subcortical circuits. In B. L. Miller, & J. L. Cummings (Eds.), *The human frontal lobes*. New York: Guilford Press, pp. 3–26.

Cornwall, J., & Phillipson, O. T. (1988). Mediodorsal and reticular thalamic nuclei receive collateral axons from prefrontal cortex and laterodorsal tegmental nucleus in the rat. *Neuroscience Letters, 88*, 121–126.

Crosson, B., Sadek, J. R., & Maron, L. et al. (2001). Relative shift in activity from medial to lateral frontal cortex during internally versus externally guided word generation. *Journal of Cognitive Neuroscience, 13*, 272–283.

d'Aquili, E. G., & Newberg, A. B. (1993). Religious and mystical states: A neuropsychological model. *Zygon, 28*, 177–200.

Davies, E., Kenyon, C. J., & Fraser, R. (1985). The role of calcium ions in the mechanism of ACTH stimulation of cortisol synthesis. *Steroids, 45*(6), 551–560.

Davis, M. (1992). The role of the amygdala in fear and anxiety. *Annual Review of Neuroscience, 15*, 353–375.

Destexhe, A., Contreras, D., & Steriade, M. (1998). Mechanisms underlying the synchronizing action of corticothalamic feedback through inhibition of thalamic relay cells. *Journal of Neurophysiology, 79*, 999–1016.

Dollins, A. B., Lynch, H. J., Wurtman, R. J., Deng, M. H., & Lieberman, H. R. (1993). Effect of pharmacological daytime doses of melatonin on human mood and performance. *Psychopharmacology, 112*, 490–496.

Elias, A. N., Guich, S., & Wilson, A. F. (2000). Ketosis with enhanced GABAergic tone promotes physiological changes in transcendental meditation. *Medical Hypotheses, 54*, 660–662.

Fernandez-Duque, D., & Posner, M. I. (2001). Brain imaging of attentional networks in normal and pathological states. *Journal of Clinical and Experimental Neuropsychology, 23*, 74–93.

Fish, D. R., Gloor, P., Quesney, F. L., & Oliver, A. (1993). Clinical responses to electrical brain stimulation of the temporal and frontal lobes in patients with epilepsy. *Brain, 116*, 397–414.

Foote, S. (1987). Extrathalamic modulation of cortical function. *Annual Review of Neuroscience, 10*, 67–95.

Frith, C. D., Friston, K., Liddle, P. F., & Frackowiak, R. S. J. (1991). Willed action and the prefrontal cortex in man. A study with PET. *Proceedings of the Royal Society of London, 244*, 241–246.

Funke, K., & Eysel, U. T. (1995). Possible enhancement of GABAergic inputs to cat dorsal lateral geniculate relay cells by serotonin. *Neuroreport, 6*, 474–476.

Gellhorn, E., & Kiely, W. F. (1972). Mystical states of consciousness: Neurophysiological and clinical aspects. *Journal of Nervous and Mental Disease, 154*, 399–405.

Griffiths, R. R., Richards, W. A., McCann, U., & Jesse, R. (2006). Psilocybin can occasion mystical-type experiences having substantial and sustained personal meaning and spiritual significance. *Psychopharmacology (Berl), 187*(3), 268–83.

Herzog, H., Lele, V. R., Kuwert, T., Langen, K., Kops, E. R., & Feinendegenen, L. E. (1990–1991). Changed pattern of regional glucose metabolism during Yoga meditative relaxation. *Neuropsychobiology, 23,* 182–187.

Hugdahl, K. (1996). Cognitive influences on human autonomic nervous system function. *Current Opinion in Neurobiology,* 6: 252–258.

Infante, J. R., Peran, F., Martinez, M., Roldan, A., Poyatos, R., Ruiz, C., et al. (1998). ACTH and beta-endorphin in transcendental meditation. *Physiology & Behavior, 64,* 311–315.

Infante, J. R., Torres-Avisbal, M., Pinel, P., Vallejo, J. A., Peran, E., Gonzalez, E., et al. (2001). Catecholamine levels in practitioners of the transcendental meditation technique. *Physiology & Behavior, 72,* 141–146.

Ingvar, D. H. (1994). The will of the brain: Cerebral correlates of willful acts. *Journal of Theoretical Biology, 171,* 7–12.

Janal, M., Colt, E., & Clark, W., et al. (1984). Pain sensitivity, mood and plasma endocrine levels in man following long-distance running: Effects of naxalone. *Pain, 19,* 13–25.

Jevning, R., Wallace, R. K., & Beidebach, M. (1992). The physiology of meditation: A review. A wakeful hypometabolic integrated response. *Neuroscience Biobehavioral Review, 16,* 415–424.

Jevning, R., Wilson, A. F., & Davidson, J. M. (1978). Adrenocortical activity during meditation. *Hormones and Behavior, 10,* 54–60.

Jevtovic-Todorovic, V., Wozniak, D. F., Benshoff, N. D., & Olney J. W. (2001). A comparative evaluation of the neurotoxic properties of ketamine and nitrous oxide. *Brain Research, 895,* 264–267.

Joseph, R. (1996). *Neuropsychology, neuropsychiatry, and behavioral neurology.* New York: Williams & Wilkins, p. 197.

Juckel, G. J., Mendlin, A., & Jacobs, B. L. (1999). Electrical stimulation of rat medial prefrontal cortex enhances forebrain serotonin output: implications for electroconvulsive therapy and transcranial magnetic stimulation in depression. *Neuropsychopharmacology, 21,* 391–398.

Kabat-Zinn, J. (2005). *Wherever you go, there you are: Mindfulness meditation in everyday life.* New York: Hyperion

Karnath, H. O., Ferber, S., & Himmelbach, M. (2001). Spatial awareness is a function of the temporal not the posterior parietal lobe. *Nature, 411,* 950–953.

Kiss, J., Kocsis, K., Csaki, A., Gorcs, T. J., & Halasz, B. (1997). Metabotropic glutamate receptor in GHRH and beta-endorphin neurons of the hypothalamic arcuate nucleus. *Neuroreport, 8,* 3703–3707.

Kjaer, T. W., Bertelsen, C., Piccini, P., Brooks, D., Alving, J., & Lou, H. C. (2002). Increased dopamine tone during meditation-induced change of consciousness. *Cognitive Brain Research, 13*(2), 255–259.

Lazar, S. W., Bush, G., Gollub, R. L., Fricchione, G. L., Khalsa, **G.,** Benson, H., et al. (2000). Functional brain mapping of the relaxation response and meditation. *Neuroreport, 11,* 1581–1585.

Livesey, J. H., Evans, M. J., Mulligan, R., & Donald, R. A. (2000). Interactions of CRH, AVP and cortisol in the secretion of ACTH from perifused equine anterior pituitary cells: "Permissive" roles for cortisol and CRH. *Endocrine Research*, 26: 445–463.

Lou, H. C., Kjaer, T. W., Friberg, L., Wildschiodtz, G., Holm, S., & Nowak, M. (1999). A 15O-H2O PET study of meditation and the resting state of normal consciousness. *Human Brain Mapping*, 7, 98–105.

Lynch, J.C. (1980). The functional organization of posterior parietal association cortex. *Behavioral and Brain Sciences*, 3: 485–499.

Manfridi, A., Brambilla, D., & Mancia, M. (1999). Stimulation of NMDA and AMPA receptors in the rat nucleus basalis of Meynert affects sleep. *American Journal of Physiology*, 277, R1488–1492.

Moller, M. (1992). Fine structure of pinealopetal innervation of the mammalian pineal gland. *Microscopy Research and Technique*, 21, 188–204.

Monti, J. A., & Christian, S. T. (1981). N-N-Dimethyltryptamine: An Endogenous Hallucinogen. *International Review of Neurobiology*, 22, 83–110.

Mountcastle, V. B., Motter, B. C., & Anderson, R. A. (1980). Some further observations on the functional properties of neurons in the parietal lobe of the waking monkey. *Behavioral and Brain Sciences*, 3, 520–523.

Newberg, A., Pourdehnad, M., Alavi, A., & d'Aquili, E. G. (2003). Cerebral blood flow during meditative prayer: preliminary findings and methodological issues. *Perceptual and Motor Skills*, 97(2), 625–630.

Newberg, A. B., Alavi. A., Baime, M., Pourdehnad, M., Santanna, J., & d'Aquili, E. (2001). The measurement of regional cerebral blood flow during the complex cognitive task of meditation: A preliminary SPECT study. *Psychiatric Research: Neuroimaging*, 106, 113–122.

Newberg, A. B., & Iversen, J. (2003). The neural basis of the complex mental task of meditation: Neurotransmitter and neurochemical considerations. *Medical Hypotheses*, 61(2), 282–291.

Newman, J., & Grace, A. A. (1999). Binding across time: The selective gating of frontal and hippocampal systems modulating working memory and attentional states. *Consciousness and Cognition*, 8, 196–212.

O'Halloran, J. P., Jevning, R., Wilson, A. F., Skowsky, R., Walsh, R. N., & Alexander, C. (1985). Hormonal control in a state of decreased activation: Potentiation of arginine vasopressin secretion. *Physiology & Behavior*, 35, 591–595.

Olds, M. E., & Forbes, J. L. (1981). The central basis of motivation, intracranial self-stimulation studies. *Annual Review of Psychology*, 32, 523–574.

Pardo, J. V., Fox, P. T., & Raichle, M. E. (1991). Localization of a human system for sustained attention by positron emission tomography. *Nature*, 349, 61–64.

Peng, C. K., Mietus, J. E., Liu, Y. et al. (1999). Exaggerates heart rate oscillations during two meditation techniques. *InternationalJournal of Cardiology*, 70: 101–107.

Pietrowsky, R., Braun, D., Fehm, H. L., Pauschinger, P., & Born, J. (1991). Vasopressin and oxytocin do not influence early sensory processing but affect mood and activation in man. *Peptides*, 12, 1385–1391.

Poletti, C. E., & Sujatanond, M. (1980). Evidence for a second hippocampal efferent pathway to hypothalamus and basal forebrain comparable to fornix system: A unit study in the monkey. *Journal of Neurophysiology, 44:* 514–531.

Portas, C. M., Rees, G., Howseman, A. M., Josephs, O., Turner, R. & Frith, C. D. (1998). A specific role for the thalamus in mediating the interaction attention and arousal in humans. *Journal of Neuroscience, 18,* 8979–8989.

Posner, M. I., & Petersen, S. E. (1990). The attention system of the human brain. *Annual Review of Neuroscience, 13,* 25–42.

Redding, F. K. (1967). Modification of sensory cortical evoked potentials by hippocampal stimulation. *Electroencephalography and Clinical Neurophysiology, 22,* 74–83.

Renaud, L. P. (1996). CNS pathways mediating cardiovascular regulation of vasopressin. *Clinical and Experimental Pharmacology & Physiology, 23,* 157–160.

Saver, J. L., & Rabin J. (1997). The neural substrates of religious experience. *Journal of Neuropsychiatry and Clinical Neurosciences, 9,* 498–510.

Shaji, A. V., & Kulkarni, S. K. (1998). Central nervous system depressant activities of melatonin in rats and mice. *Indian Journal of Experimental Biology, 36,* 257–263.

Short, E. B., Kose, S., Mu, Q., Borckardt, J., Newberg, A. B., George, M. S., et al. (2007). Regional brain activation during meditation shows time and practice effects: An exploratory fMRI study. *Evidence-Based Complementary and Alternative Medicine, 10,* 1–7.

Sim, M. K., & Tsoi, W. F. (1992). The effects of centrally acting drugs on the EEG correlates of meditation. *Biofeedback Self Regulation, 17,* 215–220.

Strassman, R. J., & Clifford, R. (1994). Dose–response study of N, N-Dimethyltrypamine in humans. I: Neuroendocrine, autonomic, and cardiovascular effects. *Archives of General Psychiatry, 51,* 85–97.

Strassman, R. J., Clifford, R., Qualls, R., & Berg, L. (1996). Differential tolerance to biological and subjective effects of four closely spaced doses of N, N-Dimethyltrypamine in humans. *Biological Psychiatry, 39,* 784–795.

Sudsuang, R., Chentanez, V., & Veluvan, K. (1991). Effects of Buddhist meditation on serum cortisol and total protein levels, blood pressure, pulse rate, lung volume and reaction time. *Physiology & Behavior, 50,* 543–548.

Thomas, A. G., Vornov, J. J., Olkowski, J. L., Merion, A. T., & Slusher, B. S. (2000). N-Acetylated alpha-linked acidic dipeptidase converts N-acetylaspartylglutamate from a neuroprotectant to a neurotoxin. *Journal of Pharmacology and Experimental Therapeutics, 295,* 16–22.

Tooley, G. A., Armstrong, S. M., Norman, T. R., & Sali, A. (2000). Acute increases in night-time plasma melatonin levels following a period of meditation. *Biological Psychology, 53,* 69–78.

Travis, F. (2001). Autonomic and EEG patterns distinguish transcending from other experiences during Transcendental Meditation practice. *International Journal of Psychophysiology, 42,* 1–9.

Van Bockstaele, E. J., & Aston-Jones, G. (1995). Integration in the ventral medulla and coordination of sympathetic, pain and arousal functions. *Clinical and Experimental Hypertension, 17,* 153–165.

Van Praag, H., & De Haan, S. (1980). Depression vulnerability and 5-Hydroxytryptophan prophylaxis. *Psychiatric Research, 3,* 75–83.

Vogt, B. A., Finch, D. M., & Olson, C. R. (1992). Functional heterogeneity in cingulate cortex: The anterior executive and posterior evaluative regions. *Cerebral Cortex, 2,* 435–443.

Vollenweider, F. X., Leenders, K. L., Scharfetter, C., Antonini, A., Maguire, P., Missimer, J., et al. (1997). Metabolic hyperfrontality and psychopathology in the ketamine model of psychosis using positron emission tomography (PET) and [18F]fluorodeoxyglucose (FDG). *European Neuropsychopharmacology, 7,* 9–24.

Vollenweider, F.X., Vontobel, P., Hell, D., & Leenders, K.L. (1999). 5-HT modulation of dopamine release in basal ganglia in psilocybin-induced psychosis in man—a PET study with [11C]raclopride. *Neuropsychopharmacology, 20,* 424–433.

Walton, K. G., Pugh, N. D., Gelderloos, P., & Macrae, P. (1995). Stress reduction and preventing hypertension: Preliminary support for a psychoneuroendocrine mechanism. *Journal of Alternative and Complementary Medicine, 1,* 263–283.

Waterhouse, B. D., Moises, H. C., & Woodward, D. J. (1998). Phasic activation of the locus coeruleus enhances responses of primary sensory cortical neurons to peripheral receptive field stimulation. *Brain Research, 790,* 33–44.

Weingartner, H., Gold, P., Ballenger, J. C., Smallberg, S., Post, R. M. & Goodwin, F. D. (1981). Effects of vasopressin on human memory functions. *Science, 211,* 601–603.

Yadid, G., Zangen, A., Herzberg, U., Nakash, R., & Sagen, J. (2000). Alterations in endogenous brain beta-endorphin release by adrenal medullary transplants in the spinal cord. *Neuropsychopharmacology, 23,* 709–716.

Yoshida, M., Sasa, M., & Takaori, S. (1984). Serotonin-mediated inhibition from dorsal raphe neurons nucleus of neurons in dorsal lateral geniculate and thalamic reticular nuclei. *Brain Research, 290,* 95–105.

Zhelyazkova-Savova, M., Giovannini, M. G., & Pepeu, G. (1997). Increase of cortical acetylcholine release after systemic administration of chlorophenylpiperazine in the rat: An in vivo microdialysis study. *Neuroscience Letters, 236,* 151–154.

Ziegler, D. R., Cass, W. A., & Herman, J. P. (1999). Excitatory influence of the locus coeruleus in hypothalamic-pituitary-adrenocortical axis responses to stress. *Journal of Neuroendocrinology,* 11: 361–36.

15

Hypnosis and Biofeedback as Prototypes of Mind–Body Medicine

MARIE STONER AND LINDA SHRIER

KEY CONCEPTS

- In recent years, 17% of the adult population used mind–body techniques and in 2006, $16 million was committed to research in this area.
- Hypnotizability is a strong moderator for treatment outcome.
- Biofeedback has strong support for use with migraine headaches.
- Hypnosis is able to reduce distress and pain in short procedures and has been particularly studied in cancer procedures.
- Biofeedback for hypertension is successful when clinical practice guidelines identifying patient characteristics are followed.
- Hypnosis and biofeedback are both useful in establishing a relaxation response.
- Feedback for normalization of pCO_2 levels in Panic Disorder shows promise for significant symptom reduction.
- PTSD, OCD, and Eating Disorders patients may be selectively responsive to hypnotic suggestion.
- Heart rate variability biofeedback shows promise as a technique to directly target self-regulatory mechanisms.

■

Background: Mind–Body Medicine

Mind–body medicine is one of four major domains of complementary and alternative medicine (CAM) designated by the National Center for Complementary and Alternative Medicine (NCCAM) (What is CAM? 2007). Within this category are those interventions that emphasize the interactions among the brain, mind, body, and spirit. The interest in techniques such as relaxation, hypnosis, visual imagery, meditation, yoga, biofeedback, tai chi, qi gong, cognitive-behavioral therapies, group support, autogenic training, and spirituality share the common goals of actively training the mind to positively affect physiology, modulate behavior, and enhance wellness.

Mind–body interventions constitute a major portion of overall CAM patient visits and expenditures. In 2002, mind–body techniques were used by approximately 17% of the adult U.S. population (Barnes, Powell-Griner, McFann, & Nahin, 2004). As these techniques become more mainstream, research interest has followed. In 2006, NCCAM's budget was $122.7 million, with about $16 million committed to research of mind–body medicine (Brower, 2006).

Hypnosis and biofeedback are two well-established mind–body medicine techniques that can be integrated with biomedicine to further the biopsychosocial model of health and illness. Around the same time that this paradigm was introduced by Engel (1977) to broaden the biological disease model to include psychological and social determinants of illness, hypnosis and biofeedback were being increasingly studied and integrated into clinical practice.

Research Challenges

This chapter will emphasize those conditions for which research-based evidence supports efficacy in clinical practice. Tables 15.1 and 15.2 highlight diagnoses and references that are discussed and represent best practices for hypnosis and biofeedback.

However, there are methodological research limitations to much of the mind–body literature. The gold standard of traditional medical research has been that neither the subject nor the researcher knows whether an active standardized treatment or a placebo is being assigned to a subject. This concept is difficult to apply to the mind–body techniques of biofeedback and hypnosis because their success is dependent upon the patient's interactive participation in the treatment. For example, the most potent hypnotic suggestions are elicited from the subject's internal experience, not from a standard protocol.

Table 15.1. Indications for Biofeedback with Representative Research.

Disorder	Symptoms	Reference
Elimination disorders	Incontinence	Glazer & Laine, 2006
	Functional anorectal	Burgio et al., 1998
		Palsson et al., 2004
Repetitive stress	Pain, muscle weakness	Peper et al., 2003
ADHD	Hyperactivity, inattention	Monastra et al., 2005
Depression	Mood	Waldkoetter & Sanders, 1997
		Katsamanis et al., 2007
Migraine	Throbbing	Nestouriuc & Martin, 2007
	Head pain	
Tension headache	Muscle tightness	McCory et al., 1996
		Holroyd et al., 2001
Chronic pain	Back pain	Flor & Birbaumer, 1993
	TMD	Appelbaum, 1988
	Rheumatoid	
	Arthritis	Flor et al., 1983
	Pain threshold	deCharms et al., 2005
Hypertension	BLP>140/90	Nakao, 2003
		Linden, 2006
Anxiety	Worry	Hiebert, 1981
	Sleep difficulties	Rice et al., 1993
	Panic	Mauret, 2007

In biofeedback training, accurate information about physiology precludes double- or even single-blind procedures. The use of sham feedback or placebo (inactive) conditions dependent on the subject's lack of awareness of the intervention is an inappropriate and contradictory concept for these techniques (Yucha & Gilbert, 2004).

Another problem confronting research in this area is the question of which patients are most likely to respond to a specific mind/body intervention. Failure to understand and consider moderators of response can lead to poor research

Table 15.2. Indications for Hypnosis with Representative References.

Disorder	Symptoms	Reference
Headaches	Prevention of recurrence	Spinhoven et al., 1992
Invasive procedures	Anxiety, pain, length of time, distress and complications, pain, procedure time	Clinton, 1992; Lang et al., 2002; Schupp, 2005
Stress	Negative emotion Autonomic arousal	Sebastiani et al., 2007
PTSD	Flashbacks anxiety	Bryant et al., 2005
	Affective arousal Helplessness	Spiegel et al., 1988; Gordon et al., 2004

design and meaningless results (Nisholson, Hursey, & Nash, 2005). In fact, individual response sets in behavioral treatments will create more variability than in pharmaceutical research because these treatments require patients to make complex behavioral changes over time (Nielson, Weir, & Robin, 2001).

Introduction to Hypnosis

Hypnosis is a state of consciousness that is characterized by intense absorption with internal experience and a voluntary suspension of normal awareness of outside stimuli. In this dissociated state of focused awareness, it is possible to influence voluntary and involuntary behavior through suggestion (Hilgard, 1986). The clinician typically uses an induction technique that may incorporate focus on the breath, relaxation, directing attention, confusion, and/or imagery that evokes memories of previous dissociative experience. Some researchers have achieved comparable responsiveness using an induction in which relaxation was prevented (Banyai & Hilgard, 1976), suggesting that patients in awkward circumstances can be hypnotized.

The first use of hypnosis in medicine was by Franz Mesmer (1734–1815), a French physician, who is considered to be the father of hypnosis (Gauld, 1992). Interest in hypnosis increased in the United States after World War II, when Weitzenhofer and Hilgarde founded a laboratory to study hypnosis at Stanford University where they developed the Stanford Hypnotic Susceptibility Scale (Weitzenhofer & Hilgard, 1959). Hypnotizability is measured by this scale, which is made up of a series of hypnotic behaviors. Table 15.3 lists some common hypnotic phenomena that are associated with hypnotizability. With this research tool, hypnosis could be studied scientifically, and began to be integrated into conventional medical and psychological treatment.

Table 15.3. Common Hypnotic Phenomena from Edgette and Edgette (1995).

Amnesia	Catalepsy
Hypermnesia	Ideomotor movement
Posthypnotic suggestion	Analgesia and anaesthesia
Time distortion	Dissociation
Age regression	Positive hallucination
Future progression	Negative hallucination

Table 15.4. Characteristics of Highly Hypnotizable People.

Factor	Example	Reference
Age	Between ages 8 and 10 maximum susceptibility	Hilgard, 1967
	Children show higher amounts of amnesia and hallucination	
IQ	Slight positive correlation	Udolf, 1987
Absorptive capacity	Positive-constructive daydreaming	Brown, 1991
	Use of vivid imagery; greater intensity of affect	
EEG findings	Longer alpha durations	London, 1967

Hypnotizability is a stable trait (Piccione, Hilgard, & Zimbardo, 1989). Within a random population there is evidence that 15%–20% will demonstrate a high level of hypnotic propensity (sometimes referred to as hypnotic "talent"), 70%–75% score in the intermediate range, and the remaining have low hypnotizability (Sacerdote, 1982). Hypnotizability seems to be affected by childhood experiences of normal dissociation, and the trait seems relatively stable through adulthood (Hilgard, 1970). Table 15.4 provides some characteristics of the highly hypnotizable population.

As a stable characteristic, hypnotizability is an example of the class of research and treatment variables known as moderators, which are variables that can predict the level of impact a treatment will have. Barabasz and Perez (2007) review evidence for hypnotizabiity as a moderating core construct. Three recent well-controlled studies with large samples established that hypnotizability is an outcome predictor that is significantly stronger than expectations and context (Benham, Woody, Wilson, & Nash, 2006; Liossi, White, & Hatira, 2006; Milling, Reardon, & Carosella, 2006). One of these studies demonstrated the importance of hypnotizability as a trait for response to hypnotic suggestion for pain treatments, even when participants were not told that they were being hypnotized (Milling, Reardon, & Carosella, 2006). Finally, in a study of pediatric cancer patients undergoing lumbar puncture, Liossi et al. (2006) concluded that baseline hypnotizability was significantly and strongly associated with the magnitude of the therapeutic benefit for the hypnosis intervention group only.

Mechanisms of Hypnosis

Genetic and neuroimaging data have contributed to our understanding of hypnotizabilty. Genetic determinants were explored by Morgan (1973) in a comparison of monozyotic and dizygotic twins. She computed a heritability index of .64, strongly suggestive of a genetic contribution. Horton (2004) in an fMRI comparison of high and low hypnotizable normal subjects found that high hypnotizables show a significantly ($p < 0.003$) larger (31.8%) rostrum area. This is the area of the brain involved in allocation of attention and transfer of information between the two prefrontal cortices, suggesting that high hypnotizables possibly have more efficient frontal attention systems that allow them to inhibit stimuli in a trance state. Lichtenberg (2000) traced individual differences in DNA (polymorphism of the catechol O-methyltransferase gene) to hypnotizability, more significantly in males than females.

Recent investigations using neuroimaging techniques have focused on changes in the brain during hypnosis in an effort to understand the process of hypnosis. In a comprehensive discussion of the literature to date, Raz (2005) concludes that results from neuroimaging studies support a potential common mechanism of dopaminergic modulation affecting both attentional and hypnotic performance, and that these mechanisms operate differently in high and low hypnotizables.

Although some describe hypnosis in terms of behavior that is elicited by cues and context, it is clearly a phenomenon of body and mind that at least involves a complex interplay of genetics, brain structure, imagination, and neurochemical processes. Further research is needed to understand the dynamic interaction of all these variables.

Introduction to Biofeedback

Biofeedback training (bfb) is a technique in which an individual learns to consciously control involuntary responses, such as heart rate, brain waves, and muscle contractions. Information about a normally unconscious physiologic process is electronically monitored and relayed back to the patient as part of a program to enact change, initially with the support of the reinforcing properties of the computerized signal and the biofeedback therapist, then generalized to self-regulation in everyday life.

Miniaturization of electronics after World War II, combined with research documenting the ability to train normal subjects to isolate separate motor units within a muscle and to activate them consciously, helped to launch the field of biofeedback (Basmajian, 1963). Early bfb applications in the 1960s were neuromuscular (EMG), and included protocols for stroke patients (Andrews, 1964; Marinacci & Horande, 1960) and those with tension headaches (Budzynski, Stoyva, Adler, & Mullaney, 1973).

Subsequently, biofeedback procedures were applied to clinical problems associated with the autonomic nervous system, building on the work of researchers such as Miller (1969) with animals and Kimmel (1974) with humans that demonstrated that the ANS could be modified through operant conditioning. Researchers at the Menninger Foundation developed a clinical protocol for migraines with a 74% improvement in subjects treated with thermal (bloodflow) biofeedback (Sargent, Green, & Walters, 1972). This work led to the establishment of the Menninger Voluntary Controls Program for research and clinical applications in biofeedback and the first NIH grant for the study of biofeedback in 1967 (Green, Ferguson, Green, & Walters, 1970).

Mechanisms of Biofeedback

The psychophysiological pathways of biofeedback are complex, and at least involve several levels of the central nervous system that interact with the autonomic nervous system. A simple example of a pathway is neuromuscular feedback. A sensor is placed on a muscle area of interest and the patient, through trial and error, learns to either recruit or inhibit the electrical activity under the sensor. Work with elimination disorders over the past 30 years has validated this model for these conditions. In reviews of well-designed randomized studies, biofeedback was deemed efficacious for most functional anorectal disorders (Palsson, Heymen, & Whitehead, 2004) and efficacious and specific in females for training of pelvic floor musculature in incontinence (Glazer & Laine, 2006). In a randomized trial by Burgio, Locher, and Jaquet (1998) biofeedback was more effective than drug treatment for reducing incontinence episodes in elderly women. Biofeedback is also used successfully to increase awareness of muscle tension in the prevention of repetitive strain injury (Peper et al., 2003).

As the technique of biofeedback moved into disorders of the autonomic nervous system, the main system of interest was the sympathetic branch of the

ANS and the "fight-flight response" first discussed by Cannon (1929). Prolonged and repeated activation of the hypothalamic-pituitary-adrenal axis (HPAC) triggered by this response is posited to underlie stress-related disorders. More recently, some physiologists have shown interest in the influence of the vagal withdrawal of the parasympathetic branch of the ANS in response to stress (Porges, 1995). Self-regulation of the ANS with biofeedback is accomplished via monitoring and training of the parameters of vasoconstriction (hand-cooling), heart rate, electrodermal activity, muscle tension, and breathing, all potential indicators of stress reactivity. Repeated conditioning of lower arousal states leads to less reactivity and lowered baselines within the sympathetic system. With the help of the biofeedback therapist, patients learn to recognize stress cues and practice their conditioned response.

New technology has supported the clinical use of neurofeedback (eeg biofeedback), which is the conditioning of changes in specific brainwave patterns leading to changes in behavior. This pathway for biofeedback is being studied for disorders as diverse as clinical depression and ADHD. Preliminary case studies (Kumano et al., 1996; Rosenfeld, 2000) and a pilot study (Waldkoetter & Sanders, 1997) show that neurofeedback may decrease depressive symptoms. Three decades of case studies and controlled group studies using neurofeedback to treat ADHD have been reviewed by Monastra et al. (2005) with a report of significant clinical improvement in approximately 75% of patients in each of the studies.

Best Evidence for Common Disorders Treated by Hypnosis and Biofeedback

BIOFEEDBACK FOR HEADACHES

Four decades after work at the Menninger Clinic demonstrated that thermal bfb was an effective treatment for migraine headaches; bfb continues to hold a prominent place in headache management. The treatment of migraine and tension-type headaches utilizes a range of physiological feedback: temperature, blood volume pulse (bvp), electromyography and any of these modalities in combination. The most recent meta-analysis found that all of these forms of biofeedback produced significant medium-to-large effect sizes for migraine treatment (Nestouriuc & Martin, 2007). Compared to other treatment and control groups, there was a medium significance for bfb versus no-treatment control, a small-to-medium significance for bfb versus placebo control or pharmacotherapy, and a lack of significance for bfb versus relaxation.

Table 15.5. Evidence-Based Guidelines for Migraine Headaches, US Headache Consortium (Campbell, 2000).

Grade A: For prevention of migraine	1. Relaxation training 2. Thermal biofeedback combined with relaxation training 3. EMG biofeedback 4. Cognitive-behavioral therapy
Grade B: Behavior therapy combined with drug tx for prevention of migraine	1. Thermal biofeedback plus relaxation plus cognitive-behavioral therapy 2. Thermal biofeedback plus relaxation 3. EMG biofeedback

Grade A. Multiple well-designed randomized clinical trials.
Grade B. Some evidence from randomized clinical trials.

Similarly positive, but less robust studies for tension-type headaches have been reported. McCory, Penszien, and Rains (1996) performed a meta-analysis in which EMG biofeedback was modestly effective for tension-type headaches compared to wait-list, but not significantly different from cognitive or relaxation therapies or hypnosis. For chronic tension headache, a comparison between amitriptyline and a brief stress management therapy (combining three 1-hour office visits with home practice in relaxation and cognitive coping skills) found no difference in rate of improvement (35% versus 38%), but 64% of patients were helped by a combination of the two treatments (Holroyd et al., 2001).

Within hypnosis research on headaches, Spinhoven, Linssen, BanDyck, and Zitman (1992) found a significant and specific symptom reduction for hypnotic subjects who received a future-oriented suggestion to imagine themselves 6 months later pain free. This was in contrast to a group trained in autogenic relaxation and a hypnosis group that did not get the future-oriented suggestion. At 6-month follow-up, the future-oriented hypnosis group maintained the statistically significant symptom improvement.

This body of evidence has brought mind–body practices to the attention of a number of expert panels, including the multidisciplinary U.S. Headache Consortium (Campbell, 2000). Table 15.5 presents guidelines for migraine prevention and treatment based on review of evidence.

Acute and Chronic Pain (Hypnosis and Biofeedback)

The variable experience of pain prompted Melzack and Wall's gate control theory (1965), which recognized many factors, including psychological, that can modulate pain. This theory, even with subsequent modifications and exceptions, makes the treatment of pain conditions very amenable to the biopsychosocial model and multi-modal treatment approaches involving mind–body techniques. A 1996 NIH Technology Assessment Panel found strong evidence for the use of relaxation in reducing chronic pain, and hypnosis for pain associated with cancer. Moderate evidence was cited for the effectiveness of biofeedback in relieving chronic pain (NIH Technology Panel, 1996).

A hypnotic trance state, with its potential to alter sensory experience, has shown promise in alleviating the experience of pain and distress during invasive procedures and surgery. Even before the development of modern anesthesiology, Esdaile pioneered the use of hypnosis in surgery in 1845. He was surprised to notice that the mortality rate in surgery patients went from 50% before the use of hypnosis to 5% among the patients who had hypnosis (Mutter, 1998).

More recently, the increase in short procedures, and procedures for which the patient is awake, has highlighted the effects of anxiety and distress as variables in outcome. In 1992, the U.S. Department of Health and Human Services released a position paper on anxiety and pain management in short procedures and discussed relaxation strategies to supplement or substitute for conscious sedation (Clinton, 1992). Schupp, Berbaum, Berbaum, and Lang (2005) found a significant correlation between patients' baseline anxiety prior to the procedures and the amount of anxiety and pain during the procedure. Further, the amount of medication needed, and the duration of the procedure, were also predicted by baseline anxiety (Lang & Rosen, 2002).

Lang et al. conducted two large prospective randomized trials of 241 patients undergoing radiological intervention in the kidneys and vascular system (1999) and 236 women undergoing large-core breast biopsies in out-patient surgery (2006). All received local anesthesia. In both studies the self-hypnosis relaxation condition reported significantly less distress than the control conditions. In Lang's radiological group, the self-hypnosis group had a procedure time averaging 17 minutes shorter and fewer complications; resulting in a savings of $330.00 per procedure.

Hypnosis has been studied specifically for its use with cancer populations. In pediatric populations, there is evidence that hypnosis has a beneficial effect on anxiety and pain associated with bone marrow aspiration (Liossi & Hatira, 1999) and lumbar puncture (Liossi & Hatira, 2003). Montgomery et al. (2002) reached similar conclusions with a randomized group of breast biopsy patients assigned to a brief presurgery hypnosis intervention. Hypnosis treatment has also been associated with less nausea and vomiting for chemotherapy patients (Jacknow, Tschann, Link, & Boyce, 1994), and there is some evidence for use with pain in terminally ill patients (Iglexias, 2004).

Biofeedback has demonstrated efficacy for specific chronic pain disorders and for patients with certain characteristics, often as part of a multi-modal package. Flor and Birbaumer (1993) compared the efficacy of EMG biofeedback, cognitive-behavioral therapy, and conservative medical treatment in two patient populations: chronic back pain and chronic temporomandibular pain. The biofeedback group (trained in muscle relaxation at the site of pain) obtained the most substantial improvement and was the only group to maintain improvement at the 6- and 24-month follow-up. Pain chronicity was negatively correlated with patient improvement.

Thermal and EMG bfb have been studied for rheumatoid populations as part of a relaxation and cognitive-behavioral treatment, and have shown positive changes in pain activity (Appelbaum, Blanchard, Hickling, & Alfonso, 1988; Bradley et al., 1987). In a rheumatoid back pain population, EMG biofeedback treatment was compared to a pseudotherapy condition in which subjects were told that a machine would relax their muscles. The treatment group reported positive effects post-intervention and at 4- to 5-month follow-up in both pain and cognitions about pain (Flor, Haag, Turk, & Koehler, 1983).

In one study, the use of a real-time functional MRI to provide feedback about brain areas involved in pain perception and regulation generated media attention in 2005. Working with an image of a flame reflecting activation of the rostral anterior cingulate cortex, normal subjects were able to increase and decrease perception of pain caused by a noxious stimulus. This research was extended to chronic pain patients who were able to significantly decrease pain perception in comparison to traditional autonomic feedback methods (deCharms et al., 2005).

Biofeedback and Hypertension

The most extensively researched mind–body cardiac disorder is hypertension. After positive findings by Blanchard (1986) and McGrady (1981) for EMG and thermal biofeedback interventions on systolic and diastolic blood pressure, subsequent research did not replicate these findings (Blanchard et al., 1993). A 2003 meta-analysis (Nakao, 2003) of 22 randomized, controlled studies with 905 essential hypertensive subjects found biofeedback to be superior to no treatment, but only better than a sham treatment or nonspecific behavioral treatment when the biofeedback was combined with relaxation, leaving doubt as to the antihypertensive effect of biofeedback as separate from effects of the general relaxation response.

A review of more than 100 randomized controlled trials testing efficacy of all behavioral treatments for hypertension (Linden, 2006) found a modest

Tables 15.6. Prediction Models for Response to Biofeedback and Behavioral Treatment for Essential Hypertension.

(a) Based on McGrady (1996)

Who Responds?	*How Much Will BP Decrease?*
Patients with:	Factors are:
High heart rate	High heart rate
Cool hands	Cool hands
High EMG	High anxiety
High PRA	High-normal cortisol

(b) Based on Yuccha et al. (2005)

Factors predicting outcome of 5 mmHg or more decrease in SPB

- Not taking hypertensive medicine
- Lowest starting finger temperature
- Smallest standard deviation in daytime mean arterial pressure
- Lowest score on Multidimensional Health Locus of Control-internal scale

decrease in blood pressure in those treated with bfb over wait-list or other inactive controls. Noted in this review are the variable effect sizes and difficulty reaching conclusions based on many different selection criteria, trial designs and measurement choices. The recommendation for clinical practice guidelines that match behavioral treatments for hypertension with patient characteristics has been addressed by two researchers (McGrady, 1996; Yucha, 2005) and is outlined in Tables 15.6a and b. Matching patient characteristics with disease management is an important challenge for mind–body research and treatment.

Mind–Body and Stress Management

The use of hypnosis and biofeedback for relaxation is rooted in concepts of stress reactivity and research supporting the benefits of a general relaxation response proposed by Benson (1975). In this view, relaxation is a system-wide, nonspecific response that can be helpful for anxiety and stress reduction.

In support of this view, Hiebert (1981) studied 10 different bfb and cognitive multi-modal treatment groups with an anxiety population and found that all treatment groups showed significant anxiety reductions. In a 1988 long-term follow-up to a biofeedback treatment group that included chronic psychiatric patients as two subgroups (anxiety $n = 115$, phobia $n = 16$), there was a 75.6% and 87.6% reduction in symptoms reported. However, in a follow-up assessment, almost twice as many subjects rated relaxation training (in office and home practice) more helpful than the biofeedback experience (Olson, 1988). Rice, Blanchard, and Purcell (1993) studied three different bfb conditions and a pseudomeditation condition compared to a waiting list control of Generalized Anxiety patients and found that all treated subjects showed significant reductions in STAI-trait anxiety and psychophysiological symptoms.

Hypnosis has also proven effective in helping individuals develop a relaxation response through direct suggestion and refocusing, and can do so even under adverse conditions. Sebastiani, D'Alessandro, Menicucci, Ghelarducci, and Santarcangelo (2007) observed changes in physiology, including cardiovascular, EEG patterns, and tonic skin conductance, in response to suggestion. Specifically, subjects produced autonomic relaxation in response to suggestions for relaxation and numbing. They maintained low arousal even during a fearful guided imagery associated with threat suggestions. This lower arousal continued even when subjects reported experiencing high negative emotion.

Hypnosis, as used by most contemporary clinicians, evokes a generalized relaxation response. While dissociation is the defining characteristic of the hypnotic state (Hilgard, 1986), when the induction is based on relaxing imagery, the subject's involvement evokes relaxation, allowing for distress, worrisome thoughts, and physical discomfort to be out of awareness.

Biofeedback for Panic Disorder

Within the context of a global relaxation response, there has emerged research supporting specific treatment effects. Mauret, Wilhelm, Ritz, and Walton (2007) have targeted a breathing feedback treatment for panic disorder that uses pCO_2 as an outcome measure. Patients were given immediate feedback via a capnometer and were instructed on breath pacing and normalization of pCO_2 levels during a period of 5-weekly treatment sessions and home training. In comparison to a wait-list control group, the treatment group showed a moderate-to-large effect size improvement in anxiety symptoms, disability, and respiratory measures, maintained at 2- and 12-month follow-up. Replication of this treatment effect holds the promise of a simple and effective treatment for panic disorder with or without agoraphobia.

Hypnosis-Assisted CBT for Mental Health Populations

Although there are mixed findings for hypnosis and psychiatric disorders, an indication for use with populations that may be more susceptible to its effect is clearer. In a meta-analysis of 18 studies in which a CBT therapy was compared with the same therapy plus hypnosis, treatment outcome was substantially enhanced by the addition (Kirsch, Montgomery, & Sapirstein, 1995). Combining this finding with evidence of higher hypnotizability for certain disorders provides a promising avenue for the use of hypnosis. Representative diagnoses in these studies included Obsessive Compulsive Disorder (OCD), Eating Disorders, and Post-Traumatic Stress Disorder (PTSD).

Hypnosis-Facilitated CBT for OCD

Behavioral and cognitive therapies combined with psychopharmacology are the treatment of choice for Axis I OCD. Unfortunately, up to 25% of patients do not respond to this treatment combination (Bjorgvinsson, Hart, & Heffelinger, 2007). Frederick (2007) presents an argument that the strong link between dissociation and OCD reported in three studies by Watson, Wu, and Cutshall (2004) strengthens Shusta's 1999 recommendation that all OCD refractory patients be screened for dissociation. She further presents case material in which hypnotically facilitated treatment of refractory OCD had good results.

Hypnosis-Facilitated CBT for Eating Disorders

Bulimic patients have been shown to be significantly more hypnotizable than a control group and scored higher on a self-report of dissociative experiences (Covino, Jimerson, Wolfe, Franko, & Frankel, 1994). Barabasz (2007) reviews several studies of treatments combining CBT and hypnosis using a standardized manual detailing both behavior modification and hypnotic suggestions provided from a script (Griffiths, 1995; Griffiths, Hadzi-Pavlovic, & Channon-Little, 1996). To address methodological issues, Barabasz reports on a more recent study by Barga and Barabasz (in press) that compared CBT to CBT plus hypnosis, also in a highly scripted protocol. Results included significantly lower binge frequency for the CBT+Hypnosis group at post-treatment; and within-treatment measures for this group indicated statistically significant improvement on all measures from pre-treatment to post-treatment to 3-month follow-up.

Even though anorexic patients show similar levels of hypnotizability, the control issues central to this disorder necessitate a more permissive and individualized approach. Baker and Nash (1987) treated 36 women within this paradigm of hypnosis for self-control with 76% showing remission of symptoms at 5 and 12 months, compared to 53% of a group who did not receive hypnosis as part of their psychotherapy treatment. The contrast of the methods used for these two highly hypnotizable populations (bulimia and anorexia) highlights the necessity of choosing an approach that will allow the patient to activate hypnotic potential.

Hypnosis for Post-Traumatic Stress Disorder

The incidence of post-traumatic stress disorder in the United States is estimated to be as high as 5% in men and 10% in women (Kessler, Sonnega, Bromet, Hughes, & Nelson, 1995). According to the DSM-IV (Frances, Pincus, & First, 1994) PTSD results when a person experiences or witnesses an event that is perceived as life threatening, experiences horror and/or helplessness, and dissociates for some part of the event, with these symptoms persisting for more than a month. Because of the persistent arousal, it is considered to be primarily an anxiety disorder.

It may be that PTSD patients are selectively more responsive to hypnotic suggestion than other populations (Spiegel, Hunt, & Dondershine, 1988), and hypnotizability among this population has been associated with successful outcome (Cardena, 2000). A randomized controlled study comparing hypnosis to systematic desensitization of distressing cues showed both to be effective with a trend toward fewer sessions for the hypnosis condition (Brom, Kleber, & Defare, 1989).

In a 3-year follow-up to a study treating trauma survivors diagnosed with acute stress disorder (Bryant et al., 2005), a combined intervention of hypnosis plus CBT appeared initially to have greater benefit than CBT alone. However, this additional benefit did not hold at 6-month and 3-year follow-up as predicted. The authors of this study hypothesized that the treatment effect didn't hold because hypnosis was only used for imaginal exposure and not explicitly tied to anxiety management or in vivo exposure strategies. They conclude that a broader use of hypnosis should be the focus of future research.

Adolescents in Kosovo diagnosed with PTSD 4 months after the NATO bombing were trained in a variety of techniques including guided imagery, biofeedback, movement, and breathing. This pilot study did target the individual's capacity to alter psychological and physiological states and linked techniques learned with life situations, which may explain the significantly reduced PTSD symptoms (pre versus post $p < .001$). This mind–body treatment group did report continued improvement at 9- and 15-month follow-up (Gordon, Staples, Blyta, & Bytyqi, 2004). This study and others suggest a common mechanistic thread among biofeedback, hypnosis, and other mind–body techniques. Monti, Sufian, and Peterson (2008) characterize this thread in terms of affecting self-regulation pathways that govern the stress response.

Heart Rate Variability Biofeedback for ANS Disorders

The expanding knowledge base regarding mechanisms of mind/body interaction and increasingly sophisticated technology to measure and monitor those interactions are leading to biofeedback treatments that target complex homeostatic mechanisms in the body, rather than end-organ symptoms. A new biofeedback approach that uses breathing as a pacemaker for oscillatory variability in heart rate is an example of this approach.

Heart rate variability (HRV) refers to the beat-to-beat alterations in heart rate and has historically been associated with cardiovascular health. Low HRV is the best predictor for nonsurvival in severe cardiovascular disease (La Rovere et al., 1998) and is also associated with hypertension (Mancia, 1978), presence and severity of ischemic heart disease (Huikuri & Makikallio, 2001), and rejection risk after heart transplant (Izrailtyan et al., 2000). Disorders of autonomic dysregulation such as asthma (Kazuma, Otsuka, Matsuoka, & Murata, 1997) and depression (Agelink, Boz, Ulrich, & Andrich, 2002) also show decreased amplitude and complexity of HRV.

The broad range of disorders that can be tracked by this physiological marker has led some to suggest that HRV is a measure of general adaptability, and diminished HRV a sign of vulnerability to stress of any type. Biofeedback training to increase HRV is conceptualized as directly targeting the complex self-regulatory reflexes of the body (Lehrer, 2007). Pilot studies with fibromyalgia (Hassett et al., 2007) and major depression (Katsamanis et al., 2007) report positive outcomes correlated with practicing breathing to increase amplitude of HRV. A more controlled study taught this paced breathing to a group of patients with coronary artery disease, a population with diminished HRV known to be a risk factor. In comparison to a control group, the subjects were able to increase HRV over a 6-week period, and these changes were maintained at 3-month follow-up (Del Pozo, 2004).

Conclusions

Consumers of health services are increasingly utilizing mind–body medicine techniques, and there is a substantive evidence-base for some modalities, particularly hypnosis and biofeedback. There are research challenges to find more sophisticated models to assess mediators and moderators of treatment effect, overcome limitations of blinded controls, and better determine which populations are most responsive to given techniques.

With long histories of clinical applications and research, hypnosis and biofeedback are good representatives of the transition from the biomedicine to biopsychosocial model. Hypnosis appears to be best for alterations of thought and sensation. This can be an especially powerful treatment for the subgroup of the population that is highly hypnotizable. More research is needed to elucidate this important moderating variable.

Biofeedback engages mental activities to create objective physiological changes and has an impact in the way in which it can lead to healthier and more balanced self-regulatory patterns. Like hypnosis, there is much to understand about mechanisms of action, and also like hypnosis, there are problems and illnesses that can be positively affected by treatment. Research in this area can explore the fluid boundaries of mind/body distinctions.

REFERENCES

Agelink, M. W., Boz, C., Ulrich, H., & Andrich, J. (2002). Relationship between major depression and heart rate variability. Clinical consequences and implications for antidepressive treatment. *Psychiatry Research, 113*, 139–149.

Andrews, J. M. (1964). Neuromuscular re-education of hemiplegic with aid of electromyography. *Archives of Physical Medicine and Rehabilitation, 45*, 530–532.

Appelbaum, K. A., Blanchard, E. B., Hickling, E. J., & Alfonso, M. (1988). Cognitive behavioral treatment of a veteran population with moderate to severe rheumatoid arthritis. *Behavioral Therapy, 19*, 489–502.

Baker, E. L., & Nash, M. R. (1987). Applications of hypnosis in the treatment of anorexia nervosa. *American Journal of Clinical Hypnosis, 29*, 185–193.

Banyai, E. I., & Hilgard, E. R. (1976). A comparison of active-alert hypnotic induction with traditional relaxation induction. *Journal of Abnormal Psychology*, APR, 85(2), 218–224.

Barabasz, A., & Perez, N. (2007) Salient findings: Hypnotizability as core construct and the utility of hypnosis. *International Journal of Clinical and Experimental Hypnosis, 55*, 372–379.

Barabasz, M. (2007). Efficacy of hypnotherapy in treatment of eating disorders. *International Journal of Clinical and Experimental Hypnosis, 55*, 318–335.

Barga, J., & Barabasz, M. (in press). Effects of hypnosis as an adjunct to cognitive-behavioral therapy in the treatment of bulimia. *International Journal of Clinical and Experimental Hypnosis.*

Barnes, P. M., Powell-Griner, E., McFann, K., & Nahin, R. L. (2004). Complementary and alternative medicine use among adults: United States, 2002. *CDC Advance Data Report #343.*

Basmajian, J. V. (1963). Control and training of individual motor units. *Science, 141,* 440–441.

Benham, G., Woody, E. Z., Wilson, K. S., & Nash, M. R. (2006). Expect the unexpected: Ability, attitude, and responsiveness to hypnosis. *Journal of Personality and Social Psychology, 91,* 342–350.

Benson, H. (1975). *The relaxation response.* New York: Morrow.

Bjorgvinsson, T., Hart, J., & Heffelinger, S. (2007). Obsessive-compulsive disorder: Update on assessment and treatment. *Journal of Psychiatric Practice, 13,* 362–372.

Blanchard, E. B., McCoy, C. C., Musso, A., Gerardi, M. A., Pallmeyer, T. P., Gerardi, R. J., et al. (1986). A controlled comparison of thermal biofeedback and relaxation training in the treatment of essential hypertension: I short-term and long-term outcome. *Behavior Therapy, 17,* 563–579.

Blanchard, E. B., Eisele, G., Gordon, M. A., Cornish, P. J., Wittrock, D. A., Gillmore, L., et al. (1993). Thermal biofeedback as an effective substitute for sympatholytic medication in moderate hypertension: A failure to replicate. *Biofeedback and Self Regulation, 18,* 237–253.

Bradley, L. A., Young, L. D., Anderson, K. O., Turner, R. A., Agudelo, C. A., McDaniel, L. K., et al. (1987). Effects of psychological therapy on pain behavior of rheumatoid arthritis patients: Treatment outcome and six-month followup. *Arthritis and Rheumatism, 30,* 1105–1114.

Brom, D., Kleber, R. J., & Defare, P. B. (1989). Brief psychotherapy for posttraumatic stress disorder. *Journal of Consulting and Clinical Psychology, 57,* 607–612.

Brower, V. (2006). Mind–body research moves towards the mainstream. *EMBO Reports, 7*(4), 358–361.

Brown, P. (1991). *The hypnotic brain.* New Haven, CT: Yale University Press.

Bryant, R. A., Moulds, M. L., Nixon, R. D., Mastrodomenico, J., Felmingham, K. & Hopwood, S. (2005). Hypnotherapy and cognitive behavior therapy of acute stress disorder: A 3-year follow-up. *Behavioral and Research Therapy, 44,* 1331–1335.

Budzynski, T. H., Stoyva, J. M., Adler, C. S., & Mullaney, D. J. (1973). EMG biofeedback and tension headache: A controlled outcome study. *Psychosomatic Medicine, 35,* 484–496.

Burgio, K. L., Locher, B., & Jaquet, A. (1998). Behavioral vs drug treatment for urge urinary incontinence in older women: A randomized controlled trial. *Journal of American Medical Association, 280,* 1995–2000.

Campbell, J. K., Penzien, D. B., & Wall, E. M. (2000). Evidence-based guidelines for migraine headaches: Behavioral and physical treatments. Available at http://www.aan.com/

Cannon, W. B. (1929). Organization for physiological homeostasis. *Physiological Reviews, 9*, 399–431.

Cardena, E. (2000). Hypnosis in the treatment of trauma:A promising, but not fully supported, efficacious intervention. *International Journal of Clinical and Experimental Hypnosis, 48*, 225–238.

Clinton (1999). (Clinical Practice Guideline). Publication No. AHCPR 92–0032. Rockville, MD: Self.

Covino, N. A., Jimerson, D. C., Wolfe, B. E., Franko, D. C., & Frankel, F. H. (1994). Hypnotizability, dissociation, and bulimia nervosa. *Journal of Abnormal Psychology, 103*, 455–459.

deCharms, R. C., Maeda, F., Glover, G. H., Ludlow, D., Pauly, J. M., Soneji, D., et al. (2005). Control over brain activation and pain learned by using real-time functional MRI. *PNAS, 102*, 18626–18631.

Del Pozo, J. M., Gevirtz, R. N., Scher, B., & Guarneri, E. (2004). Biofeedback treatment increases heart rate variability in patients with known coronary artery disease. *American Heart Journal, 147*, G1–G1.

Edgette, J., & Edgette, E. (1995). *The handbook of hypnotic phenomena in psychotherapy*, New York, NY: Bruner/Mazel, Inc.

Engel, G. L. (1977). The need for a new medical model: a challenge for biomedical science. *Science, 196*, 129–136.

Flor, H., Haag, G., Turk, D. C., & Koehler, H. (1983). Efficacy of EMG biofeedback, pseudotherapy, and conventional medical treatment for chronic rheumatic back pain. *Pain, 17*, 21–31.

Flor, H., & Birbaumer, N. (1993). Comparison of the efficacy of electromyographic biofeedback, cognitve-behavioral therapy and conservative medical interventions in the treatment of chronic musculoskeletal pain. *Journal of Consulting and Clinical Psychology, 61*, 653–658.

Frederick, C. (2007). Hypnotically facilitated treatment of obsessive-compulsive disorder: Can it be evidence-based? *International Journal of Clinical and Experimental Hypnosis, 55*, 189–206.

Gauld, A. (1992). *A history of hypnotism*. New York: Cambridge University Press.

Glazer, H. I., & Laine, C. D. (2006). Pelvic floor muscle biofeedback in the treatment of urinary incontinence: A literature review. *Applied Psychophysiology and Biofeedback, 31*, 187–201.

Gordon, J., Staples, J. K., Blyta, A., & Bytyqi, M. (2004). Treatment of posttraumatic stress disorder in postwar Kosovo high school students using mind–body skills groups: A pilot study. *Journal of Traumatic Stress, 17*, 143–147.

Green, E. E., Ferguson, D. W., Green, A. M., & Walters, E. D. (1970). Preliminary report on the voluntary controls project: Swami Rama. Voluntary Controls Project: The Menninger Foundation. Topeka, KS (Mimeograph).

Griffiths, R. (1995). Hypnobehavioural treatment for bulimia nervosa: A treatment manual. *Australian Journal of Clinical and Experimental Hypnosis, 21*(1), 25–46.

Griffiths, R. A., Hadzi-Pavlovic, D., & Channon-Little, L. (1996). The short-tem follow-up effects of hypnobehavioural and cognitive behavioural treatment for bulimia nervosa. *European Eating Disorders Review, 4,* 12–31.

Hassett, A. L., Radvanski, D. C., Vaschillo, E. G., Vaschillo, B., Sigal, L. H., Karavidas, M. K., et al. (2007). A pilot study of the efficacy of heart rate variability (hrv) biofeedback in patients with fibromyalgia. *Applied Psychophysiology and Biofeedback, 32,* 1–10.

Hiebert, B. A., & Fitzsimmons, G. (1981). A comparison of emg feedback and alternative anxiety treatment programs. *Biofeedback and Self-Regulation, 6,* 501–516.

Hilgard, E. R. (1986). *Divided consciousness: Multiple controls in human thought and action* (expanded edn). New York: Wiley.

Hilgard, E. R. (1967). Individual differences in hypnotizability. In J. E. Gordon (Ed.), *Handbook of clinical and experimental hypnosis.* New York: The Macmillan Company, pp. 391–443.

Hilgard, J. R. (1970). *Personality and hypnosis: A study of imaginative involvement.* Chicago, IL: U. of Chicago Press.

Holroyd, K. A., O'Donnell, F. J., Stensland, M., Lipchik, G. L, Cordingley, G. E., & Carlson, B. W. (2001). Management of chronic tension-type headache with tricyclic antidepressant medication, stress management therapy and their combination: a randomized controlled trial. *JAMA, 285,* 2208–2215.

Horton, J. E., Crawford, H. J., Harrington, G., & Downs, J. H. (2004). Increased corpus callosum size associated with hypnotizability and the ability to control pain. *Brain, 127,* 1741–1747.

Huikuri, H. V., & Makikallio, T. H. (2001). Heart rate variability in ischemic heart disease. *Autonomic Neuroscience: Basic and Clinical, 90,* 95–101.

Iglexias, A. (2004). Hypnosis and existential psychotherapy with end-stage terminally ill patients. *American Journal of Clinical Hypnosis, 46,* 201–213.

Izrailtyan, I., Kresh, J. Y., Morris, R. J., Brozena, S. C., Kutalik, S. P., & Wechsler, A. S. (2000). Early detection of acute allograft rejection by linear and nonlinear analysis of heart rate variability. *Journal of Thoracic and Cardiovascular Surgery, 120,* 737–745.

Jacknow, D. S., Tschann, J. M., Link, M. P., & Boyce, W. T. (1994). Hypnosis in the prevention of chemotherapy-related nausea and vomiting in children: a prospective study. *Journal of Developmental and Behavior Pediatrics, 15,* 258–264.

Katsamanis Karavidas, M, Lehrer, P. M., Vaschillo, E., Vaschillo, B., Marin, H., Buyske, S., et al. (2007). Preliminary results of an open label study of heart rate variability biofeedback for the treatment of major depression. *Applied Psychophysiology and Biofeedback, 32,* 19–30.

Kazuma, N., Otsuka, K., Matsuoka, I., & Murata, M. (1997). Heart rate variability during 24 hours in asthmatic children. *Chronobiology International, 14,* 597–606.

Kessler, R., Sonnega, A., Bromet, E., Hughes, M., & Nelson, C. (1995). Post-traumatic stress disorder in the National Comorbididity Survey. *Archives of General Psychiatry, 52,* 1048–1060.

Kimmel, H. (1974). Instrumental conditioning of autonomically mediated responses in human beings. *American Journal of Psychology, 29*, 325.

Kirsch, I., Montgomery, G., & Sapirstein, G. L. (1995). Hypnosis as an adjunct to cognitive-behavioral psychotherapy: a meta-analysis. *Journal of Consulting and Clinical Psychology, 63*, 214–220.

Kumano, H., Horie, H., Shidara, T., Kuboki, T., Suematsu, H., & Yasushi, M. (1996). Treatment of a depressive disorder patient with eeg-driven photic stimulation. *Biofeedback and Self Regulation, 21*, 323–334.

Lang, E. V., Lutgendorf, S., Logan, H., Benotsc, E., Laser, E., & Spiegel, D. (1999). Nonpharmacologic analgesia and anxiolysis for interventional radiological procedures. *Seminars in Interventional Radiology, 16*, 113–123.

Lang, E. V., & Rosen, M. (2002). Cost analysis of adjunct hypnosis for sedation during outpatient interventional procedures. *Radiology, 222*, 375–382.

Lang, E. V., Berbaum, K. S., Faintuch, S., Hatsiopoulou, O., Halsey, N., Li, X., et al. (2006). Adjunctive self-hypnotic relaxation for outpatient medical procedures: A prospective reandomized trial with women undergoing large core breast biopsy. *Pain, 126*(1–3): 3–4.

La Rovere, M. T., Bigger, J. T. J., Marcus, F. I., Mortara, A., & Schwartz, P. J. (1998). Baroreflex sensitivity and heart-rate variability in predictions of total cardiac mortality after myocardial infarction. *Lancet, 351*, 478–484.

Lehrer, P. M. (2007). Biofeedback training to increase heart rate variability. In P. M. Lehrer, R. L. Woolfolk, & W. E. Sime (Eds.), *Principles and practice of stress management* (3rd edn). New York: Guilford Press, pp. 227–248.

Lichtenberg, P., Bachner-Melman, R., Gritsenko, I., & Ebstein, R.P. (2000). Exploratory association between catechol-O-methyltransferase (COMT) high/low enzyme activity polymorphism and hypnotizability. *American Journal of Medical Genetics, 96*, 771–774.

Linden, W., & Moseley, J. V. (2006). The efficacy of behavioral treatment for hypertension. *Applied Psychophysiology and Biofeedback, 31*, 51–63.

Liossi, C., & Hatira, P. (1999). Clinical hypnosis versus cognitive behavioral training for pain management with pediatric cancer patients undergoing bone marrow aspirations. *International Journal of Clinical and Experimental Hypnosis, 47*, 104–116.

Liossi, C., & Hatira, P. (2003). Clinical hypnosis in the alleviation of procedure-related pain in pediatric oncology patients. *International Journal of Clinical and Experimental Hypnosis, 51*, 4–28.

Liossi, C., White, P., & Hatira, P. (2006). Randomized clinical trial of local anesthetic versus a combination of local anesthetic with self-hypnosis in the management of pediatric procedure-related pain. *Health Psychology, 25*, 307–315.

London, P., Hart, J. T., Leibovitz, M. P., & McDevitt, P. A. (1967). The psychophysiology of hypnotic susceptibility. In L. Chertok (Ed.), *Psychophysiological mechanisms of hypnosis*. Berlin, Germany: Springer-Verlag, pp. 151–172.

Mancia, G., Ludbrook, J., Ferrari, A., Gregorini, L., & Zanchetti, A. (1978). Baroreceptor reflexes in human hypertension. *Circulation Research, 43*, 170–177.

Marinacci, A. A., & Horande, M. (1960). Electromyogram in neuromuscular re-education. *Bulletin Los Angeles Neurological Society, 25*, 57–71.

Mauret, A. E., Wilhelm, F. H., Ritz, T., & Walton, T. R. (2004). Respiratory feedback for treating panic disorder. *Journal of Clinical Psychology, 60*, 197–207.

McCrory, D. C., Penszien, D. B., & Rains, J.C. (1996). Efficacy of behavioral treatments for migraine and tension-type headache: Meta-analysis of controlled trials. *Headache, 36*, 272.

McGrady, A. V., Yonker, R., Tan, S. Y., Fine, T. H., & Woerner, M. (1981). The effect of biofeedback-assisted relaxation training on blood pressure and selected biochemical parameters in patients with essential hypertension. *Biofeedback and Self Regulation, 6*, 343–353.

McGrady, A. (1996). Good news-bad press: Applied psychophysiology in cardiovascular disorders. *Biofeedback and Self-Regulation, 21*, 335–346.

Melzack, R., & Wall, P. D. (1965). Pain mechanisms: A new theory. *Science, 150*, 171–179.

Miller, N. (1969). Learning of visceral and glandular responses. *Science, 163*, 434–445.

Milling, L. S., Reardon, J. M., & Carosella, G. M. (2006). Mediation and moderation of psychological pain treatments: response expectancies and hypnotic suggestibility. *Journal of Consulting & Clinical Psychology, 74*, 253–262.

Monastra, V. J., Lynn, S., Linden, M., Lubar, J. E., Gruzelier, J., & LaVaque, T. J. (2005). Electroencephalographic biofeedback in the treatment of attention-deficit/hyperactivity disorder. *Applied Psychophysiology and Biofeedback, 30*, 95–114.

Montgomery, G. H., Welta, C. R., Selta, M. & Bovberg, D. H. (2002). Brief presurgery hypnosis reduces distress and pain in excisional breast biopsy patients. *International Journal of Clinical and Experimental Hypnosis, 50*, 17–32.

Monti, D., Sufian, M., & Peterson, C. (2008). Potential role of mind–body therapies in cancer survivorship. *Cancer, 112*(11 suppl), 2607–2616.

Morgan, A. H. (1973). The heritability of hypnotic susceptibility in twins. *Journal of Abnormal Psychology, 82*, 55–61.

Mutter, C.B. (1998). History of hypnosis. In C. D. Hammond (Ed.), *Hypnotic induction & suggestion*. Chicago, IL: American Society of Clinical Hypnosis, pp. 10–12.

Nakao, M., Yano, E., Nomura, S., & Kuboki, T. (2003). Blood pressure-lowering effects of biofeedback treatment in hypertension: A meta-analysis of randomized controlled trials. *Hypertension Research, 26*, 37–46.

Nestoriuc, Y., & Martin, A. (2007). Efficacy of biofeedback for migraine: A meta-analysis. *Pain, 128*, 111–127.

Nicholson, R. A., Hursey, K., & Nash, J. M. (2005). Moderators and mediators of behavioral treatment for headache. *Headache, 45*, 513–519.

Nielson, W. R., & Weir, R. (2001). Biopsychosocial approaches to the treatment of chronic pain. *Clinical Journal of Pain, 17*, S114–127.

NIH Technology Assessment Panel on Integration of Behavioral and Relaxation Approaches into the Treatment of Chronic Pain and Insomnia (1996) *JAMA, 276*: 313–318.

Olson, R. P. (1988). A long-term, single group follow-up study of biofeedback therapy with chronic medical and psychiatric patients. *Biofeedback and Self-Regulation, 13*, 331–346.

Palsson, O. S., Heymen, S., & Whitehead, W. E. (2004). Biofeedback treatment for functional anorectal disorders: a comprehensive efficacy review. *Applied Psychophysiology and Biofeedback, 29,* 153–174.

Peper, E., Wilson, V. S., Gibney, K. H., Huber, K., Harvey, R., & Shumay, D. M. (2003). The integration of electromyography (semg) at the workstation: Assessment, treatment, and prevention of repetitive strain injury (rsi). *Applied Psychophysiology and Biofeedback, 28,* 167–182.

Piccione, C., Hilgard, E. R., & Zimbardo, P. G. (1989). On the degree of stability of measured hypnotizability over a 25-year period. *Journal of Personality and Social Psychology, 56,* 289–295.

Pincus, H. A., & First, M. B. (1994). *Task force on DSM-IV. Diagnostic and statistical manual of mental disorders* (4th edn). Washington, DC: American Psychiatric Association.

Porges, S. W. (1995). Cardiac vagal tone: A physiological index of stress. *Neuroscience and Biobehavioral Reviews, 19,* 225–233.

Raz, A. (2005). Attention and hypnosis: neural substrates and genetic associations of two converging processes. *International Journal of Clinical and Experimental Hypnosis, 53,* 237–258.

Rice, K. M., Blanchard, E. B., & Purcell, M. (1993). Biofeedback treatments of generalized anxiety disorder: Preliminary results. *Biofeedback and Self-Regulation, 18,* 93–105.

Rosenfeld, J. P. (2000). An EEG biofeedback for affective disorders. *Clinical Electroencephalography, 31,* 7–12.

Sacerdote, P. (1982). Why is hypnosis effective in pain control? In D. Waxman, P. Misra, M. Gibson, M. A. Basker (Eds.), *Modern trends in hypnosis.* New York: Plenum Press, pp. 249–258.

Sargent, J. D., Green, E. E., & Walters, E. D. (1972). The use of autogenic feedback in a pilot study of migraine and tension headaches. *Headache, 12,* 120–125.

Schupp, C., Berbaum, D., Berbaum, M., & Lang, E. V. (2005). Pain and anxiety during interventional radiological procedures. Effect of patients'state anxiety at baseline and modulation by nonpharmacologic analgesia adjuncts. *Journal of Vascular & Interventional Radiology, 16,* 1585–1592.

Sebastiani, L., D'Alessandro, L., Menicucci, D., Ghelarducci, B., & Santarcangelo, E. L. (2007). Role of relaxation and specific suggestions in hypnotic emotional numbing. *International Journal of Psychophysiology, 63,* 125–132.

Shusta, S. R. (1999). Successful treatment of refractory obsessive-compulsive disorder. *American Journal of Psychotherapy, 53,* 377–391.

Spiegel, D., Hunt, T., & Dondershine, H. E. (1988). Dissociation and hypnotizability in posttraumatic stress disorder. *American Journal of Psychiatry, 145,* 301–305.

Spinhoven, P., Linssen, A. C., BanDyck, R., & Zitman, F. G. (1992). Autogenic training and self-hypnosis in the control of tension headaches. *General Hospital Psychiatry, 14,* 408–415.

Udolf, R. (1987). *Handbook of hypnosis for professionals* (2nd edn.). New York: Van Nostrand Reinhold Company.

Waldkoetter, R. O., & Sanders, G. O. (1997). Auditory brainwave stimulation in treating alcoholic depression. *Perceptual and Motor Skills, 84,* 226.

Watson, D., Wu, K., & Cutshall, C. (2004). Symptom subtypes of obsessive-compulsive disorder and their relation to dissociation. *Journal of Anxiety Disorders, 18,* 435–458.

Weitzenhofer, A. M., & Hilgard, E. R. (1959). *Stanford hypnotic susceptibility scale, form A.* Palo Alto, CA: Consulting Psychologist Press.

What is CAM? (2007). Available from http://nccam.nih.gov/health/backgrounds/mindbody.htm

Yucha, C., & Gilbert, C. (2004). *Evidence-based practice in biofeedback and neurofeedback.* Wheat Ridge: AAPB.

Yucha, C. B., Tsai, P. S., Calderon, K. S., & Tian, L. (2005). Biofeedback-assisted relaxation training for essential hypertension: who is most likely to benefit? *Cardiovascular Nursing, 20,* 198–205.

16

Facilitating Emotional Health and Well-Being

PATRICIA A. COUGHLIN

> Happiness is the whole aim and end of human existence.
>
> —*Aristotle*

Introduction

The shift from a focus on pathology to potential, from illness to wellness, and from treatment to prevention lies at the foundation of integrative medicine. In the field of psychiatry, this requires practitioners to study resilience and emotional health, in addition to disorders and disease. The mere absence of emotional distress does not constitute happiness, vitality, or emotional well-being. In 1946, the World Health Organization defined health as "a state of complete physical, mental, and social well-being and not merely the absence of disease or infirmity." Currently, those studying wellness (Owen, 1999) include spiritual well-being and occupational satisfaction in the definition of vibrant good health.

Our grandmothers seemed to know intuitively what science has now validated—"If you want to be healthier, you should eat a balanced diet, exercise regularly, and not smoke. You should have good relationships with other people and pursue activities that are fulfilling" (Peterson, 2006, p. 235). Who follows this advice and who doesn't? Research suggests that optimists are healthier than pessimists because, in large part, they take better care of themselves and behave in ways that enhance well-being. Most evidence now suggests that emotional factors, like optimism, are primary predictors of physical, as well as emotional, health. Other factors include: acceptance of self and other; playing to your strengths and using your talents; creating strong and lasting relationships with others, especially a happy marriage; low levels of defensiveness and openness to emotional experience; autonomy, mastery, and competence; clear values and a strong character; creating meaning and purpose in life; passionate engagement; and the ability to learn and grow from trauma and adversity. Each of these factors will be considered in some detail in this chapter.

Given the centrality of emotional health and well-being for physical health, quality of relationships, and longevity, it is surprising and disheartening to find that, in the field of psychiatry, the study of emotional well-being has been sorely neglected. George Vaillant (2003) wrote, "Psychiatry is always talking about mental health, but no one ever does anything about it." This volume is an attempt to address that neglect. Even the field of psychology, which began, at least in part, as the study of normal development and human potential, got caught up in the medical model—studying illness and dysfunction to the exclusion of healthy and extraordinary adaptation to life. It was not until 1998, when Martin Seligman became the new president of the American Psychological Association, that he reclaimed the heritage of the field and declared his intention to study genuine happiness. Since then, there has been an explosion in the study of mental health and resilience. Advances in interdisciplinary studies of mental health, including a "focus on the mind, the brain, and human relationships" (Siegel, 2003, p. 2), are increasing our knowledge base. We are now in a position to learn a great deal about what does and does not reliably contribute to a state of mental health. Further, as clinicians, we can learn how to intervene in order to bolster strengths and capacities within our patients, rather than focus exclusively on their difficulties.

In this chapter, the author will review the literature on emotional health, in order to discover the necessary elements of genuine and lasting happiness. There is a significant pool of data providing clear evidence regarding the factors that support mental health, as well as those that do not. For example, some factors frequently assumed to have a positive impact on longevity actually have no predictive value. The longevity of one's ancestors, cholesterol level at the age of 50, and the occurrence of traumatic life events prior to the age of 65 have no identifiable impact on longevity, while emotional and social factors, like optimism and positive relationships, have a very strong impact on longevity (Peterson, 2006; Reis & Gable, 2003; Snowdon, 2001; Vaillant, 2004).

Empirically validated methods for facilitating potentials, enhancing strengths, and promoting neural and behavioral growth will also be included in this chapter. Neuroscientific findings can inform and enhance our clinical effectiveness by providing guidelines for facilitating "the occurrence of specific learning experiences that are likely to exert a positive influence" (Grawe, 2007, p. 7) on growth and development. In fact, the combination of neuroscientific evidence and psychotherapy outcome research (Smith & Grawe, 2001, 2005) suggests that a focus on problems alone is limited in therapeutic value and may even be counterproductive. Rather, it is essential to "facilitate changes in a positive direction, to establish the emergence of new neural activation patterns" (Grawe, 2007, p. 41). In order to achieve these ends, focused and directed intervention on the part of the therapist is absolutely essential. Examples of such interventions will be included here.

Recent Research

EMOTIONAL FACTORS

Since emotional factors have such a profound impact on health and longevity, as well as happiness and emotional well-being, we will begin the chapter with an examination of this cornerstone of "the life well lived." Our founding fathers included "the pursuit of happiness" as an inherent human right—yet there remains considerable confusion about what constitutes happiness. Often we mistake *pleasure* for genuine happiness, something which is frequently encouraged by Madison Avenue. While we all seem to know, somewhere deep inside, that "money can't buy me love," our culture promotes the idea that snagging an attractive mate, obtaining wealth and fame, or creating physical beauty will pave the road to happiness. All one needs to do is catch the headlines in the tabloids to discover that these external factors do not reliably create happy and fulfilled human beings.

Since transient pleasures and external factors are not reliably associated with genuine happiness, what is? We are talking about the factors that make life worth living. It turns out that human beings are not very good predictors of what will actually sustain or disrupt their experience of happiness and well-being (Gilbert et al., 1998; Wilson et al., 2000). Research findings suggest that we consistently overestimate how long we will be emotionally affected by both desirable and undesirable life events. One of the most dramatic examples of this was a study on the lasting effects of extreme events, like winning the lottery or being permanently paralyzed (Brickman, Coates, & Janoff-Bulman, 1978). Most people anticipate that winning millions will enhance their sense of happiness, but the research does not support that prediction. Even more surprising was the finding that those who had become permanently paralyzed assessed their happiness and pleasure in everyday life as higher than the lottery winners—a finding few would have predicted. They were also more optimistic about the future! Humans tend to adapt to their given circumstances, whether positive or negative, fairly rapidly, returning to their "set point" within a relatively brief amount of time. However, this is not cast in stone, and the "set point" can be changed with certain kinds of emotional "exercises."

Learning to "savor" positive experiences can reliably extend their lasting effects (Bryant, 2003). Those who tend to savor sweetness and victories in life are happier and more satisfied than those for whom such experiences are fleeting. By consciously and intentionally sharing positive experiences, building strong memories of the peak moments in life, as well as celebrating the best of one's self, we can enhance well-being considerably (Bryant, 2003). This practice has an impact on couples, families, and business organizations, as well as on the individual. In fact, couples who make a practice of sharing positive memories with their partner have more satisfying marriages than those who don't (Gottman, 2002).

"Emotional intelligence" (Goleman, 1995), defined as the ability to accurately label, directly experience, and appropriately express feelings, while being aware of and sensitive to the feelings of others, is highly related to happiness and satisfaction in life. Human beings vary widely in their awareness of emotions and ability to intentionally regulate their feelings. Studies indicate that those who are emotionally facile have a clear advantage when it comes to adjustment and well-being, as well as physical health and longevity (Goleman, 1995; Pennebaker, 1997). Antonio Damasio (1994, 1999), one of the leading neuroscientists of our time, has suggested that our ability to be aware of and reflect on our feelings is one of the factors that make us uniquely human. Emotions have been selected for in evolution because they help us navigate, survive, and thrive in an interpersonal world. These emotions serve as a kind of internal guidance system, offering important information, as well as energy to fuel effective action. "The more we can laugh when happy, cry when sad, use anger to set firm limits, make love passionately, and give and receive tenderness fully and openly, the further one is from suffering" (McCullough-Vaillant, 1997). Conversely, those who habitually avoid and repress their emotions suffer physically, socially, and occupationally (Pennebaker, 1997).

Emotions are physiological events and, when mismanaged or avoided, can lead to adverse health and behavioral consequences (Abbass, 2005; Damasio, 1999; Pennebaker, 1997). Those who rely heavily on defensive avoidance of their feelings simultaneously suppress their immune system and fall ill far more often than their expressive counterparts (Pennebaker, 1997). When encouraged to express painful emotions—especially feelings of grief and anger—patients suffering from rheumatoid arthritis reported a significant decrease in physical pain (Kelly et al., 1997). In fact, the more deeply and authentically patients experienced and shared their anger, the greater the pain relief they reported. This is a very important finding, since anger has gotten a bad rap as some sort of toxic emotion (Tavris, 1989). Anger has been built in as a way to alert us to danger and the threat of trespass. When detected and channeled properly, the experience of anger aids us in self- protection and limit setting. A recent study also found that moderate levels of anger aided cognitive functioning and powers of discrimination (Moons & Mackie, 2007). Anger is a clarifying and energizing emotion. Anger seems to help people pay attention to what really matters, while screening out irrelevant and distracting information (Moons & Mackie, 2007). Those who characteristically suppress their anger tend to be passive and susceptible to depression, and are often used and abused by others (Coughlin Della Selva, 1996; Tavris, 1989).

We are literally (Damasio, 1999) wired for emotion. Our spontaneous feelings emerge from the cingulated region of the brain, over which we have no conscious control. "We are about as effective at stopping an emotion as we are at preventing a sneeze" (Damasio, 1999, p. 49). While we can not stop ourselves from registering an emotion, we can ignore it or suppress its expression, often at our own peril. We need access to our feelings of desire to motivate action and prime learning; we need to experience love to establish and maintain attachments; we need to feel fear to make us pause and assess our situation; and we need to register anger to get clear about what is important and how to protect what is precious. Without access to these feelings, one is driving blind through life.

In addition to the negative consequences of chronic avoidance of emotion, the habitual suppression of feelings increases the likelihood of physical illness and even early death (Pennebarker, 1997). It looks like the chronic repression of emotions leads to suppression of the immune response, rendering one more susceptible to illnesses of all kinds. The lesson from these studies is clear: we can help our patients be healthier, happier, more connected to others, and more effective at work if we help them gain direct access to their emotions and express them constructively.

POSITIVE EMOTIONS

The study of positive emotions is relatively new. From Darwin (1873) to Tompkins (1962, 1973, 1991, 1992) and Ekman (1993), those who have studied emotional expression in humans have tended to focus on "negative" emotions, such as fear, disgust, grief, and anger. Typically, only one (joy) or two (love) "positive" emotions are even mentioned in the study of affective experience. As we shift our focus from mere survival to the life well-lived, an examination of positive emotions becomes essential (Baker, 2003; Fredrickson, 2004).

Barbara Fredrickson (1998, 2001) is a pioneer in this area of research, and has developed the "broaden and build" theory of positive emotion. Negative emotions alert us to danger and enhance survival. Positive emotions seem to signal safety, and enable us to broaden our attention, enhance memory, and verbal fluency, facilitate new learning, and increase the integration of new information (Fredrickson & Branigan, 2005). Joy and delight provide the fuel for learning. We also need a certain degree of challenge to be primed for new learning. There seems to be an optimal level at which peak performance is most likely to occur. Too little challenge, and we get bored—too much and we get overly anxious and give up. When one's skill and capacity is adequate for the challenge, motivation is heightened, moderate levels of cortisol are produced, attention is focused and new learning is facilitated (Abercrombie et al., 2003).

In addition to facilitating learning, research has discovered that the experience of positive emotion can undo the damaging physiological effects of negative emotions, like anger and fear (Fredrickson & Levenson, 1998; Tugade & Fredrickson, 2004). The activation of positive feelings has been shown to aid cardiovascular recovery and reduce anxiety. These findings suggest that using humor in the face of hardship can boost well-being and bolster physical health. This has clear implications for clinicians, who would be well advised to facilitate the direct experience of positive feelings, as well as working to simply reduce anxiety and depression in their patients.

Those who have ready access to positive emotions tend to have better relationships and more success in life than their grumpy peers. Our emotions color everything, from our perceptions to our behavior. In the 1970s, Paul Meehl began studying what he called "positive affectivity"—an innate capacity to experience joy and interest. He found that this quality was independent of "negative affectivity," suggesting they are not inversely related. In other words, some people are able to experience the full range of human emotion in an intense fashion, whether those emotions are positive or negative in tone. Affective tone proved quite stable over time and circumstance (Costa & Mc Crae, 1992). Those who score on the upper end of positive affectivity tend to be outgoing and gregarious, having lots of friends and being socially active—another factor highly associated with genuine happiness. While one's level of positive and negative affectivity tends to remain fairly stable over time, evidence of heritability is only moderate. New studies suggest that therapy can readily change affectivity, as can recently devised practices formulated by Seligman to enhance happiness (www.reflectivehappiness.com).

EMOTIONS AND EMPATHY

Emotions are contagious (Goleman, 2006; Numann & Strack, 2000), for good or for ill. The process of contagion is typically subtle and unconscious. Just seeing a picture of a happy face tends to induce a smile on the face of the observer (Dimberg & Thunberg, 2000). The closer we feel to another, the more power they have to affect us emotionally. Empathic connection seems to foster physiological synchrony. For example, marital partners tend to mimic one another's biological responses during an argument, often resulting in escalation of conflict (Levinson & Ruef, 1992). Empathy and rapport increase with "mutual attention, shared positive feelings and a well-co-ordinated nonverbal duet"

(Goleman, 2006, p. 28). The more "in synch" a couple is on a nonverbal level, each mirroring the other, the more positive feelings they experience. This kind of empathic resonance is the result of multiple mirror neuron systems that have been designed to enhance our feelings of connection with others (Stern, 1999). This type of compassion propels us into empathic action, while self-absorption seems to kill empathy.

Virtually from birth, babies cry when they hear another baby cry (though not when they hear a recording of their own wails). By 14 months, toddlers attempt to console or help others in distress (Goleman, 2006). These fndings suggest that we are wired for kindness, empathy, and altruism. Yet, the experience of isolation and disconnection many Americans experience on a daily basis can undermine the very empathy that fuels connection. A comprehensive study on narcissism among college students has documented a 30% increase in the prevalence of this disorder from 1982 to 2006. Jean Twenge (2006) has written a book about these findings called *Generation Me: Why Today's Young Americans are more Confident, Assertive, Entitled—and Miserable—Than Ever Before.* The title pretty much says it all. Those who focus on themselves and what they are entitled to receive, rather than focusing on what they have to give, end up feeling miserable. Parents who have overindulged their children and asked for nothing in return—an all too common phenomenon among American baby-boom parents—have inadvertently set their children up for this kind of narcissistic existence (McGrath, 2007).

APPRECIATION AND GRATITUDE

Appreciation is considered by some the purest and strongest form of love, as it is freely given and requires nothing in return (Baker, 2003). Being in a state of loving appreciation is the antidote to fear, both emotionally and neurologically. While in a state of appreciation, messages from the amygdala, the brain's fear center, don't register (Baker, 2003). This is an amazing finding and one with direct implications for our work. Rather than simply try to reduce anxiety and depression, we can help patients plagued with anxiety by helping them develop "an attitude of gratitude." "During active appreciation, your brain, heart, and endocrine system work in synchrony and heal in harmony" (Baker, 2003, p. 81). The simple practice of writing down three things that went well each day has proven remarkably effective in reducing anxiety and depression, as well as increasing well-being, in subjects studied by Seligman and his colleagues at the University of Pennsylvania. The "Appreciation Audit," a focused meditation on the people, places, and things you are most grateful for, done three times a day for 3–5 minutes, has been shown in numerous studies "to have a powerful impact upon the autonomic nervous system, the brain's neurotransmitter profile, the cardiovascular profile, muscular tension and the psyche" (Baker, 2003, p. 101). Put very simply, "To be happy, you must overcome fear, and the best way to overcome fear is with love" (Baker, 2003, p. 106).

EMOTIONAL SUPPORT AND CONNECTION

Bowlby (1969, 1979, 1980) and Harlow (1971) have probably contributed more to our understanding of the basic need for attachment over the life span than anyone else in the field. Other collaborators (Ainsworth et al., 1978; Main, 1995; Siegel, 1999) have confirmed that the nature of early attachments has a profound impact on our sense of well-being throughout life. Neuroscientific studies have substantiated the view that we are wired for emotional connection with others (Goleman, 2006). Mirror neurons and spindle cells, more plentiful in the human brain than in any other primate, attune us to others and facilitate close interactions. The more closely connected we are to another, the more profoundly our brains affect one another. It is becoming clear that our relationships affect our biology as well as our biography. Nurturing and satisfying relationships are an enormous boon to our health and well-being, while stressful and contentious relationships are toxic to our system. Emotionally charged interactions stimulate hormones that regulate all kinds of biological systems, from our hearts to our immune systems (Cocioppo & Berntson, 1992; Lieberman & Ochsner, 2001; Siegel, 1999).

We now know that the capacity to love and be loved is absolutely crucial to health and well-being from birth until death. In fact, loving relationships may be the single most important factor in determining happiness and well-being, a finding that is robust across age and culture (Reis & Gable, 2003). When in love, the brain is bathed in oxytocin and dopamine, increasing happiness and buffering the effects of negative emotions (Bartels & Zeki, 2000; Porges, 1998). Isolation and lack of love create a "pain in the brain." Panskepp's research (2003), using MRI technology to study blood flow in the brain has documented that psychological pain, grief, and loneliness share some of the same neural pathways that elaborate physical pain. Only love seems to alleviate the pain of social isolation.

Social connection and support enhance physical health, as well as happiness, by buffering stress and its negative effects (Cassel, 1976). Yet, not just any social support will do. Mutually supportive relationships seem to be most beneficial (Berkman et al., 2000). Rapport is another way to define the quality of connection that mutual relationships contain. Rapport requires full attention, positive feelings, and nonverbal synchrony (Goleman, 2006). All the right words, without the nonverbal affective tone of warmth, will not be registered as supportive. Having true friends, rather than a group of acquaintances, is most important for health and well-being.

Beyond feelings of love, human beings have a basic need to be seen and acknowledged. Getting this need met in a reliable way seems to bolster happiness and contribute to longevity. A study of Academy Award-winning actors makes this point. Over a 70-year period, winners lived 4 years longer than those who were nominated but did not win the award. Multiple winners, like Katherine Hephurn, lived longest of all. This finding suggests that it is not success in financial terms (most of the big moneymakers don't win Academy Awards), but recognition for excellence among one's peers, that has such a potent effect.

Doing what you love and receiving recognition for your contribution enhances well-being and longevity. Unfortunately for those working in large corporations, the likelihood of achieving this end is in doubt. Studies suggest that the majority (65%) of employees in the United States feel disconnected at work, and did not receive a single appreciation in the past year (Rath & Clifton, 2004). This lack of connection, along with a feeling of being unappreciated, contributes to poor productivity, high absenteeism, and cynicism. What a waste for all of us! Conversely, giving and receiving genuine acknowledgement greatly increases well-being, productivity, and morale (Gottman, 2002). Of interest, affective tone has a greater impact on employees receiving feedback from their managers than the content of that feedback. Newcombe and Ashkanasy (2002) systematically altered tone and content of feedback in order to study this phenomenon. Employees responded much more positively to negative feedback delivered in a warm and encouraging tone than they did when given positive feedback in a cold and perfunctory manner.

In our society of narcissism and isolation, many of us suffer from a lack of connection with others. Sadly, as of 2003, single-person households became the most common living situation for adults in the United States. Our brains are wired for connection, yet most Americans are chronically deprived of this basic human need (Goleman, 2006). Both our emotional and physical health depend upon the state of our closest relationships. When people, even children as young as 2 years of age, are spending 3–4 hours a day in front of a television or computer, and less and less time in close interaction with other human beings (Goleman, 2006), we all suffer. In contrast, when we attend to the needs of those around us and behave in an altruistic fashion, we gain even more than those whom we choose to help (Baker, 2003; Dulin & Hill, 2003). We can also have a profound impact on those around us in a vicarious manner. Studies suggest that witnessing, or even hearing, a stirring story about the actions of a Good Samaritan, causes "elevation"—a kind of emotional glow that inspires further altruistic impulses in one who views such an act (Darley & Bateson, 1973).

Just as we have begun to establish the vital necessity of emotional support for mental health and emotional well being, the deprivation of such support has been shown to adversely affect physical, as well as emotional, health—even leading to death (Mayer, 1967). During the Korean War, more prisoners of war died while in captivity (an astounding 38%) than in any other conflict in U.S. military history, despite the fact that they were given plenty of food and water and received very little in the way of physical torture. Instead, the Korean captors focused almost exclusively on social isolation and deprivation of our innate need for the support of others. They used four primary tactics: informing on others, self-criticism, breaking loyalty to leadership and country, and withholding all positive emotional support. Prisoners were amply rewarded for informing on others, insuring the breakdown of support between the men held hostage. In order to promote self-criticisms, the captors created groups in which soldiers were forced to stand up and confess all the bad things they had ever done, along with a recitation of all the times they failed to do something positive. It was essential that this self-flagellation take place in the company of their peers, eroding the soldiers' respect and affection for themselves and each other. All good news was systematically withheld from the prisoners, while bad news (such as a letter from home revealing a death in the family or unpaid bills that were threatening their family's stability) was delivered promptly. The result was a state that doctors labeled "Mirasmus"—a profound kind of learned helplessness and meaninglessness that robbed these men of motivation, hope, and the desire to live. As a result, half of all the men who died in captivity died of hopelessness, rather than an identifiable organic cause.

THE BENEFITS OF A GOOD MARRIAGE

A good marriage dramatically enhances health, happiness, financial stability, and longevity (Keicolt-Glaser, 2005; Keicolt-Glaser & Newton, 2001; Peterson, 2006), though dramatically more so for men than for women. When exploring the effects of a bad marriage on health and happiness, the gender difference is even more striking. While a bad marriage is much worse for women than men, even a bad marriage is better for a man than living alone. Some suggest that women tend to have more friends and emotional connections that sustain them, while many men rely almost exclusively on their wives for a sense of emotional connection. Since marriage can so dramatically effect happiness, it is an important topic to explore in some depth. It is often assumed that those who have an unhappy marriage will be happier if they divorce. With the exception of those in a violent marriage, a longitudinal study of over 5,000 adults clearly disputes this assumption (Waite et al., 2002). Six hundred and forty-five of 5,232 adults interviewed reported being "very unhappy" in their marriages. When interviewed again 5 years later, many interesting and unexpected results were discovered. Most surprising was the finding that two-thirds of this group reported being happy in their marriage 5 years later. Those who divorced, however, experienced no reduction in depression or increase in self-esteem following their divorce, especially if they remained single. Twenty-four percent of the divorced group had remarried and 81% of them were happy in this second marriage. This suggests that being married, rather than single or divorced, is the decisive factor when it comes to happiness.

This investigation (Waite et al., 2002) discovered that external stressors like unemployment, financial hardship, and difficult children, often appeared to be the culprit in the unhappy marriages (Waite et al., 2002). Couples who persevered and worked through difficulties together, rather than divorcing, found that their marriages improved significantly over time. These couples reported that their efforts to comfort each other, make time for themselves by going out on dates, and getting help from a trusted family member, therapist, or minister enhanced their ability to develop resilience as a couple. Even threats of divorce were noted as a vital factor in making the shift from unhappiness to a happy, productive union.

It is certainly possible that the couples who stayed together were different from the start than those who divorced, but the results of this study should still inform our work with patients. Gottman (1993, 2001, 2002), who has probably done more and better research on success and failure in marriage than anyone on the planet, has found that a couple's ability to make and accept attempts at repair when things go awry is of crucial importance. Women tend to be much better at this than men. In fact, women in distressed marriages made just as many repair attempts as those in happy marriages. The difference was in how their husbands responded. Husbands in happy marriages accepted their wives' attempts to repair a rupture far more often (80% of the time), than men in distressed marriages (18%). Helping men reduce their defensiveness and allow for forgiveness will go a long way to improving their capacity to accept repair attempts and preserve their marriages.

Hanging in there with those we love, and working to resolve difficulties together, clearly confers tremendous benefits to the adult partners in marriage, as well as to their children. Since developing and maintaining close emotional ties appears to be the most important factor in overall happiness, we are well-advised to focus a good deal of therapeutic attention on enhancing our patients' ability to stay connected, instead of withdrawing and breaking off contact with others.

CHARACTER, STRENGTHS, AND VIRTUE

Other things being equal, human beings enjoy the exercise of their realized
capacities.

—*Aristotle*

Sometimes, it requires courage to choose love and appreciation over fear
and scarcity. Courage is most often defined, not as an absence of fear, but the
willingness to take decisive action in the face of fear. When desire and value predominate over fear, we behave in a courageous manner. What is most important
to you in life? Is your life focused on your most deeply held values and principles, or are you motivated by greed? Perhaps you are living on automatic pilot,
simply responding to external circumstances.

Research shows that leading a purpose-driven life greatly enhances life
satisfaction (Collins, 2007; Csikszentmihalyi, 2006). Obtaining rewards without effort does not confer happiness. Remember those studies on the lottery
winners? Human beings like to feel powerful, effective, and masterful. In order
to achieve that, we must be able to see a direct connection between our efforts
and the outcomes we create. Exercising our talents and playing to our strengths
contributes enormously to our level of happiness and satisfaction in life.

Having choice in the matter also has a huge impact on life satisfaction
(Sheldon, 2004). Our power to make choices gives us a sense of self-determi-
nation and efficacy (Bandura, 1989). Feeling as if we are in charge of our lives
and our destiny increases autonomy and self-esteem, and bolsters well-being
(Sheldon, 2004). Goals are only motivating insofar as they are our own personal
goals. When we try to achieve goals that others have set for us, even if we reach
them, we don't end up with the same feelings of competence and well-being as
when these goals are our own.

Jerry Porras and his associates (2006) decided to conduct a study on what
it takes to build a life that matters by doing in-depth interviews with over 200
people who have made a profound difference in the world. They eliminated
people like Tiger Woods and Yo Yo Ma, who, were born with an exceptional gift.
What they found was a group of ordinary people doing extraordinary things.
In fact, many of these people, like Sir Richard Branson and Chuck Schwab,
had significant obstacles to overcome in life, like poverty and serious learning disabilities. Jimmy Carter was another example in their study. The son of a
poor peanut farmer, and the first in his family to attend college, Jimmy Carter
became President of the United States and won the Nobel Peace Prize. How did
they do it? Every single one of these people experienced significant failures,

defeats, losses, and disappointments in life, but they all bounced back, learning from adversity and staying focused on desired outcomes. Their reliance on self-validation, rather than relying on validation from others, along with an unwillingness to play victim or blame others, made them determined, resilient, and successful in overcoming obstacles to reach their desired goals. Most importantly of all, they define success as the ability to make a difference and have a lasting impact on the lives of others.

These highly successful people embody the character traits long associated with the best of humanity: determination, persistence, humility, generosity, and integrity. Truly successful people are passionate about what they believe in and are more likely to be geeks than charismatic celebrities. Contrary to popular belief, the CEOs who transformed good solid companies into truly great organizations that out-performed all their competition, were humble and self-effacing individuals who displayed no ego and were devoted to something much bigger than themselves (Collins, 2001). They proved to be internally motivated and held themselves accountable, blaming no one else for their mistakes and generously acknowledging the contribution of others when successful. Put very simply, these folks "are more emotionally committed to doing what they love, than being loved by others" (Collins, 2001).

By combining their strengths, abilities, passions, and beliefs with the needs of others, truly successful people construct lives that make a difference and have a lasting impact on others (Porras et al., 2006). Three central qualities differentiated them from the rest: 1) a focus on meaning—what matters deeply, what they lose track of time doing, and would do for free; 2) accountability, audacity, passion and optimism; and 3) willingness to take decisive and effective action. Buffet said, "it is dangerous not to do what you love, as someone who does have passion will always outperform you." For folks who work just to make a living, expecting rewards to come later in life, he said, "It is like saving sex for old age." Steven Jobs, in his commencement speech at Stanford, encouraged graduates to "find something you love, then get good at it. Your time is limited, so don't waste it living someone else's life." Again and again, this focus on self- determined goals and an unwillingness to sell out for approval, emerge as defining qualities of the life well lived.

PLAYING TO YOUR STRENGTHS

Knowing what your strengths are, and playing to those strengths, is crucial in constructing a life of meaning and purpose. In fact, Seligman found that, while gratitude exercises have the largest overall effect on happiness and well-being, the most *lasting* effects were achieved by combining this practice with that of using your signature strengths in novel ways (Peterson, 2006; Seligman et al., 2005). The most successful people in life have an accurate sense of their own strengths and play to them everyday. Some people have a skewed perception of self and don't appreciate their own gifts. The Values in Action Classification of Character Strengths (Peterson & Seligman, 2004) can help to identify strengths in those who don't seem to know themselves very well. Some of these strengths include a love of learning, an appreciation of beauty and excellence, creativity, and fairness. Knowing what your "signature" strengths are and making use of them everyday goes a long way toward creating a meaningful and satisfying life. Conversely, constructing a life that is at odds with these strengths predicts frustration and dissatisfaction. Sadly, a Gallop poll revealed that 80% of American employees reported having no opportunity to play to their strengths on a daily basis at work. This is a prescription for low morale and high levels of dissatisfaction for all involved. Companies like Google, who encourage employees to do what they love and have fun in the process, develop loyal and productive employees who are creative, happy, and healthy.

FLOW

Discovering your passion and finding a way to have that passion serve others is a key to creating a life that matters. When we are deeply involved in a passionate pursuit, we are often "in the flow." "Flow" has been defined as a psychological state that accompanies highly engaging voluntary activities (Csikszentmihalyi, 1990). This state involves a sense of timelessness and complete presence and involvement, as if one is working to full capacity. Learning to balance one's interest, skill, and challenge is an essential component of the experience of flow. Csikszentmihalyi (1990) has conducted studies using the "Experience Sampling Method," in which participants wear electronic pagers for a week and fill out a questionnaire about their current experience whenever it goes off. While many assume they will feel most relaxed and happy when resting, quite the opposite turned out to be the case. Almost all respondents reported feeling "happier, more cheerful, stronger, more active, more creative, more concentrated and more motivated" when involved in a demanding and challenging activity. Participants felt better when dealing with adversity, than during leisure time when they reported feeling sad, dull, and dissatisfied. As mental health professionals, we are in a position to pass on this information, which is not common knowledge.

It is important to recognize, that leisure activites are, in fact, a vital part of the equation when we study happy and successful lives. However, this type of leisure does not mean doing nothing. The kind of leisurely activity that promotes well-being is that which is highly engaging—whether it is a sport like tennis or golf, a pastime like gardening, or an artistic mode of expression like playing a musical instrument or painting. In fact, having voluntary activities one is passionate about increases levels of positive emotion, vitality, and aliveness. In many cases, these activities provide a sense of identity and social connection with other, like- minded individuals, adding further to their positive impact.

RESILIENCE

While there has been a lot of focus in the past couple of decades on the phenom-enon of Post-Traumatic Stress Disorder, only 8% of those exposed to traumatic circumstances develop this disorder (Bonnano, 2004). Most of us are resilient and bounce back after traumatic experiences, while a significant number of people experience what is now referred to as "Post-traumatic Growth" (Park & Helgeson, 2006). Going through traumatic circumstances frequently moti-vates us to reassess our lives and to focus on what is most important. Traumatic events can be a "wake up call" that serves a very useful purpose in realigning our actions with deeply held values and beliefs. While the notion that we grow through trials and tribulations in not new, the systematic study of this phe-nomenon is quite recent (Ickovics et al., 2006). A meta-analysis of 77 research studies on the subject revealed that growth through distress was related to the experience of positive consequences. The longer the follow-up from the time of the trauma, the clearer the relationship between that trauma and its positive effects became. So, it looks like it takes time for people to realize the positive benefits of these jarring events, creating wisdom from their wounds.

Studies of the process through which traumatic events create positive out-comes suggests that growth is a consequence of reflection, self-inquiry, and re-evaluation of the basic assumptions about life that were challenged by the trauma. Once again, the implications for psychotherapy seem quite clear. The data suggest that it is possible to benefit and grow considerably through very difficult experiences. By helping our patients consider the positive benefits of the worst experiences in their life, we can facilitate growth, something rarely advocated previously (Root & Cohen, 2006).

A study of neural correlates of post-traumatic growth (Rabe, Sollner, Maercher, & Karl, 2006) following severe auto accidents demonstrated a clear relationship between increased left frontal brain activation (associated with the approach system and positive emotion) and post-traumatic growth. In partic-ular, "left pre-frontal activity was associated with . . . new possibilities, changed relationships, appreciation of life, and personal strength, but not with spiri-tual changes" (p. 882). These results suggest that therapists should focus on activating the approach system, an orientation to psychotherapeutic intervention advocated by Grawe (2005). In other words, encouraging patients to approach what they want in life, rather than avoiding what they fear, greatly enhances well-being. Focusing on what has been learned, rather than on what has been lost, facilitates recovery from trauma.

So what exactly is resilience, and how can it be fostered? Definitions of resilience vary widely, depending upon the context. In psychological terms, resilience generally refers to the ability to recover, or even grow from, traumatic experiences. In physics and engineering, resilience refers to the amount of energy that can be absorbed by a given material "elastically" (without shattering). This definition could be applied to humans as well. The ability to absorb shock and respond flexibly, without breaking down, is another way to define resilience.

It is important to remember than resilience is an on-going process of development, requiring time and effort. Being resilient *does not* refer to an absence of distress. In fact, it is the ability to tolerate the distressing affects, pain, grief, rage, and anxiety, that seems to result in new learning, greater compassion for self and other, and what is often referred to as "wisdom."

Hebb (1949) discovered that "neurons that fire together, wire together." Many of our patients are stuck in automatic ways of responding that maintain their symptoms and contribute to their suffering. In order to be effective, we must these ingrained, pathological connections (say, between self-assertion and anxiety), while stimulating the activation of new and healthier connections. In patients who are clinically depressed, for example, "it is not sensible to work directly on the problem behavior. First we must build the impoverished brain regions, because their easy activation will be necessary to enable the patient to pursue positive goals and to experience joy and happiness" (Grawe, 2005). In fact, both neuroscientific findings and the results of psychotherapy outcomes studies suggest that a focus on problems will only be effective if conducted within the context of pursuing an important, and currently activated, goal. In other words, we can only help someone complaining of social anxiety and inhibition once their desire for contact, connection, and affinity is palpably activated. So, the delineation of positive approach goals is an essential task for all therapists. Despite this information, most therapists remain focused on problems and deficits when intervening with their patients.

OPTIMISM

It is important to point out that some people are more likely to respond to challenging and traumatic life circumstances in a positive, growth-oriented manner than are others. A study by Rimi and colleagues (2004) found that only mothers who were optimistic displayed a positive adjustment 6 months after their child had undergone stem cell transplantation. So, once again, optimism turns out to be a central factor in positive adjustment. Optimism is often defined as an ability to maintain realistic hope and a sense of personal efficacy in relation to one's life goals. Optimists are not Pollyannas. They are realistic in their assessment of their own abilities, and tend to focus on their efforts rather than on variables outside of their control. Those who strive to control outcomes beyond their sphere of influence tend to create stress and depression (Peterson, 2006; Seligman, 1991).

While some seem to be optimistic by nature, or as a result of being raised in a home that focused on personal mastery, studies suggest that this capacity can also be learned later in adulthood (Seligman, 1991). Pessimists view difficult circumstances as permanent, while optimists see them as temporary. Consequently, optimists try harder the next time. It is almost never what happens that affects us over time, but the story we tell ourselves about what happens. If we tell ourselves we are victims—losers in life who have gotten a raw deal—we will be depressed, bitter, and hopeless. In the very same circumstances, if we adopt an optimistic mind set and focus on what we can learn, choosing to make the best of it, we will build resilience and well-being. Mental health professionals can actively help patients cultivate an optimistic mindset that supports emotional and physical health, buffers stress, and aids resilience by encouraging this kind of reframing.

Conclusions and Recommendations

While the systematic study of interventions specifically designed to boost well-being, happiness, and self-efficacy is relatively new, the data are strong and unequivocal. These practices work to increase life satisfaction and decrease depression. In fact, Seligman's data (www.reflectivehappiness.com) suggest that simple practices such as counting your blessings on a daily basis can increase happiness and decrease depression dramatically (90% or more on average). While all studies have some limitations, different levels of evidence are required for different kinds of interventions being studied. Just as there are different levels of evidence admissible in court—from DNA samples to eye-witness testimony—there are different levels of scientific evidence—from double-blind studies to observational studies. When the risks and possible side effects of a given procedure are high (as with surgery and medication), the level of evidence required to support its use is quite high. When the possible benefits are high and risks are low or nonexistent, as in the case with all the interventions and practices designed to enhance well-being described in this chapter, we can accept all levels of evidence to support their use. There is simply no reason not to add these interventions to those specifically designed to treat symptoms in order to speed recovery and aid in the development of happiness and resilience.

How can clinicians bolster health, well-being, and resilience, as well as treating symptoms and disorders? The research reviewed here provides clear guidelines for interventions that build strength and capacity. If we remember that we never cure anyone, and that it is the patient's innate capacity for growth and optimal functioning that is responsible for healing, our focus will remain on what we can do to (1) encourage the patient's ability to tolerate anxiety for growth; (2) encourage patients to relinquish defenses; and (3) facilitate the direct experience and expression of their feelings, needs, and desires.

First and foremost, the studies reviewed in this chapter suggest that it is essential to assess a patient's strengths, as well as their areas of weakness (Coughlin Della Selva, 1996/2004). We need to create an alliance with the healthy part of patients so that, together, we can tackle their difficulties head on (Davanloo, 1990). In order to build on strength and capacity, as well as facilitate new learning, we need to establish a strong therapeutic alliance with the patient. Once this bond is established, we need to induce moderate levels of stress by creating a challenging atmosphere in order to help the patient face what he has been avoiding. Therapists often intervene to lower anxiety to the point where no new learning takes place. This inadvertently keeps the patient functioning at a low level of capacity. By taking over the anxiety regulating function of the ego for the patient, the therapist promotes dependence, rather than mastery. So, learning to work at an optimal level of anxiety is a crucial skill for every therapist to learn.

Second, we need to work actively to mobilize the approach system. By activating the desire for valued goals, and working to increase the patient's capacity to tolerate anxiety for gain, we will facilitate rapid growth and build capacity in our patients. Many patients get stuck in life because they allow fear and anxiety to dominate them. By activating the approach system and getting patients in touch with their deepest convictions and strongest desires, we can help them overcome this log jam.

Research also clearly indicates that unencumbered access to affect promotes health and well-being, while reliance on defenses undermines health and interferes with attachment. Focusing on the breakdown of defenses and activation/exposure to core emotions facilitates health by helping the patient get to know himself or herself in an intimate and unguarded way (Coughlin Della Selva, 1996/2004; Davanloo, 1990). Intimate knowledge of self, and the ability to accept rather than avoid one's own feelings, puts the patient in a position of choice when it comes to opening up to others. This ability also promotes empathy and compassion with others. Since having and maintaining close, nurturing bonds is such an essential element in health and well-being, anything we can do to remove barriers to closeness and facilitate secure attachments will greatly enhance therapeutic effectiveness. Additionally, facing the feelings one has long avoided creates a sense of mastery and competence, which builds confidence and fuels resilience (Weinberger, 1995).

In summary, adding strength-enhancing interventions to our therapeutic arsenal should reliably increase our effectiveness. The practice of integrative medicine involves boosting the healthy immune system, as well as treating acute illness. In a similar fashion, the practice of Integrative Psychiatry should focus on interventions designed to boost our patients' levels of happiness and satisfaction in life, in order to enhance therapeutic outcomes and prevent relapse.

BIBLIOGRAPHY

Abercrombie, H.C., Kalin, N.H., Thurow, M.E., Rosenkranz, M.A., Davidson, R.J. (2003). Cortisol variation in humans affects memory for emotionally laden and neurtral information. *Behavioral Neuroscience, 117,* 505–516.

Ainsworth, M.D.S., Blehar, M.C., Waters, E., Wall, S. (1978). *Patterns of Attachment: A psychological study of the Strange Situation.* Hillsdale, NJ: Erlbaum.

Argyle, M. (1996). *The social psychology of leisure.* London: Routledge.

Argyle, M. (2001). *The psychology of happiness* (2nd ed.). East Sussex, England: Routledge.

Baker, D. (2003). *What happy people know.* U.S.: Rodale, Inc.

Bandura, A. (1989). Human agency in social cognitive theory. *American Psychologist, 44,* 175–184.

Bartels, A., Zeki, S. (2000). The neural basis of romantic love. *NeuroReport, 11,* 3829–3834.

Bergin, A.E., Jensen, J.P. (1990). Religiosity and psychotherapists: A national study. *Psychotherapy, 27,* 3–7.

Berkman, L.F., Glass, T., Brisette, I., Seeman, T.E. (2000). From social integration to health: Durkheim in the new millennium. *Social Science and Medicine, 51,* 843–857.

Bonnano, G.A. (2004). Loss, trauma, and human resilience: Have we underestimated the human capacity to thrive after extremely aversive events? *American Psychologist, 55,* 20–28.

Bowlby, J. (1969). *Attachment and loss: Vol. 1: Attachment.* New York: Basic.

Bowlby, J. (1973). *Attachment and loss, Vol. 2: Separation, anxiety and anger.* New York: Basic.

Bowlby, J. (1979). *The making and breaking of affectional bonds.* London: Tavistock.

Bowlby, J. (1980). *Attachment and loss, Vol. 3: Loss, sadness, and depression.* New York: Basic.

Brickman, P., Coates, D., Janoff-Bulman, R. (1978). Lottery winners and accident victims: Is happiness relative? *Journal of Personality and Social Psychology, 36,* 917–927.

Brown, S.L., Nesse, R.M., Vinokur, A.D., Smith, D.M. (2003). Providing social support may be more beneficial than receiving it: Results from a prospective study of morality. *Psychological Science, 14,* 320–327.

Bryant, F.B. (2003). Savoring Beliefs Inventory (SBI): A scale for measuring beliefs about savoring. *Journal of Mental Health, 12,* 175–196.

Byrd, R.C. (1988). Positive therapeutic effects of intercessory prayer in a coronary care unity population. *Southern Medical Journal, 81,* 826–829.

Capra, F. (1995). The emerging new culture. www.intuition.org/text/capra.html.

Cassel, J. (1976). The contribution of the social environment to host resistance. *American Journal of Epidemiology, 104,* 107–123.

Clark, D., Watson, D. (1999). Temperament: A new Paradigm for Trait Psychology. In L.A. Pervin, O.P. John (Eds), *Handbook of Personality* (2nd ed., pp. 399–423). New York: Guilford.

Cocioppo, J., Berntson, G. (1992). Social psychological contributions to the Decade of the Brain: Doctrine of Multiple Analysis. *American Psychologist, 47,* 1019–1028.

Cohen, S., Tyrell, D.J., Smith, A.P. (1991). Psychological stress and susceptibility to the common cold. *New England Journal of Medicine, 325,* 606–612.

Collins, J. (2001). *Good to great.* New York: Harper Collins.

Coughlin Della Selva, P. (1996/2004). *Intensive short-term dynamic psychotherapy: Theory and technique.* New York: Wiley/London: Karnac.

Csikszentmihalyi, M. (1990). *Flow: The psychology of optimal experience.* New York: Harper and Row.

Dahlsgaard, K., Peterson, C., Seligman, M.E.P. (2005). Shared virtue: The convergence of valued human strengths across cultures and histories. *Review of General Psychology, 9,* 203–213.

Damasio, A. (1994). *Decartes error: Emotion, reason, and the human brain.* New York: Avon Books.

Damasio, A. (1999). *The feeling of What Happens.* NY: Harcourt, Brace & Company.

Damon, W. (2004). What is positive youth development? *Annals of American Academy of Political and Social Science, 591,* 13–24.

Darley, J.M., Bateson, C.D. (1973). On the Good Samaritan experiment, a classic in social psychology. *Journal of Personality and Social Psychology, 27,* 100–108.

Davanloo, H. (1990). *Unlocking the unconscious.* New York: Wiley.

Dimberg, U., Thunberg, M. (2000). Rapid facial reactions to emotional facial expression. *Scandinavian Journal of Psychology, 39,* 39–46.

Dulin, P., Hill, R. (2003). Relationship between altruistic activity and positive and negative affect among lower income older adult service providers. *Aging and Mental Health, 7,* 294–299.

Fredrickson, B.L. (1998). What good are positive emotions? *Review of General Psychology, 2,* 300–319.

Fredrickson, B.L. (2000). Cultivating positive emotions to optimize health and well-being. *Prevention and Treatment, 3.* Document available at http://journals.apa.org/prevention.

Fredrickson, B.L. (2001). The role of positive emotions in positive psychology: The broaden-and-build theory of positive emotions. *American Psychologist, 56,* 218–226.

Fredrickson, B.L., Branigan, C. (2005). Positive emotions broaden the scope of attention and thought-action repertoires. *Cognition and Emotion, 19,* 313–332.

Fredrickson, B.L., Mancuso, R.A., Branigan, C., Tugade, M.M. (2000). The undoing effects of positive emotions. *Motivation and Emotion, 24,* 237–258.

Fried, R.L. (2001). *The passionate learner.* Boston: Beacon.

Fromm, E. (1956). *The art of loving.* New York: Harper & Row.

Gilbert, D.T., Pinel, E.C., Wilson, T.D., Blumberg, S.J., Wheatley, T. (1998). Immune neglect: A source of durability bias in affective forecasting. *Journal of Personality and Social Psychology, 75,* 617–638.

Goleman, D. (1995). *Emotional intelligence.* New York: Bantam.

Goleman, D. (2005) *Social intelligence.* New York: Bantam.

Gottman, J. (1993). *What predicts divorce: The relationship between marital processes and marital outcomes.* Hillsdale, N.J.: Erlbaum.

Gottman, J. (2000). *The seven principles for making marriage work.*

Gottman, J. (2002). *The relationship Cure.* New York: Three Rivers Press.

Grawe, K. (2007). *Neuropsychotherapy: How the neurosciences inform effective psychotherapy.* Mahwah, New Jersey: Lawrence Erlbaum Associates, Publishers.

Guarneri, M. (2006). *The heart speaks.* New York: Touchstone.

Gupta, V., Korte, C. (1994). The effects of a confidant and a peer group on the well being of single elders. *International Journal of Aging and Human Development, 39,* 293–302.

Harlow, H.F. (1974). *Learning to love.* New York: Aronson.

Harris, W.S., Gowda, M., Kolb, J.W., Strychacz, C.P., Vacek, J.L., Jones, P.G., et al. (1999). A randomized controlled trial of the effects of remote intercessory prayer on outcomes in patients admitted to coronary care unit. *Archives of General Medicine, 159,* 2273–2278.

Hebb, D. (1949). The organization of behavior. New York: Wiley.

Hendricks, G. (1999). *The ten second miracle: creating relationship breakthroughs.* New York: Harper Collins.

Ickovics, J.R., Meade, C.S., Kershaw, T.S., Milan, S., Lewis, J.B., Ethier, A (2006). Urban teens: Trauma, posttraumatic growth, and emotional distress among adolescent girls. *Journal of Consulting and Clinical Psychology, 74,* 841–850.

Jahoda, M. (1958). *Current concepts of positive mental health.* New York: Basic.

Kandel, E. (2005). Psychiatry, Psychoanalysis and

Kaplan, G.A. (1988). Social connection and mortaility from all causes and cardiovascular disease: Prospective evidence from Eastern Finland. *American Journal of Epidemeology, 128,* 370–380.

Keicolt-Glaser, J. (2005). Marriage, stress, immunity and wound healing: How relationships influence health. *Archives of General Psychiatry, 62,* 1377–1384.

Keicolt-Glaser, J., Newton, T. (2001). Marriage and Health: His and Hers. *Psychological Bulletin, 127,* 472–503.

King, M.B., Dein, S. (1998). The spiritual variable in psychiatric research. *Psychological Medicine, 28,* 1259–1262.

Levinson, R., Ruef, A. (1992). Empathy: A physiological substrate. *Journal of Personality and Social Psychology, 63,* 234–246.

Lieberman, M., Ochsner, K (2001). The emergence of social cognitive neuroscience. *American Psychologist, 56,* 717–734.

Lyubomersky, S., King, L.A., Diener, E. (2005). The benefits of frequent positive affect: Does happiness lead to success? *Psycological Bulletin, 131,* 803–855.

Main, M. (1995). Attachment: Overview, with Implications for Clinical Work. In S. R. Goldberg, R. Muir, J. Kerr (Eds), *Attachment Theory: Social, Developmental and Clinical Perspectives.* Hillsdale, NJ: Analytic Press.

McCullough, M.E., Kilpatrick, S.D., Emmons, R.A., Larson, D.B. (1999). Gratitude as moral affect. *Psychological Bulletin, 127,* 249–266.

McCullough, M.E., Root, L.M., Cohen, A.D. (2006). Writing about the benefits of an interpersonal transgression facilitates forgiveness. *Journal of Consulting and Clinical Psychology, 74,* 887–897.

McCullough Valliant, L. (1997). *Changing character.* New York: Basic Books.

McGrath, T. (2007). Bad parents. *Philadelphia Magazine.* September, 100–107.

Mickley, J.R., Carson, V., Soecken, K.L. (1995). Religion and adult mental health: The state of science in nursing. *Issues in Mental Health Nursing, 16,* 345–360.

Moons, W.G., Mackie, D.M. (2007). Thinking straight while seeing red: The influence of anger on information processing. *Personality and Social Psychology Bulletin, 33,* 706–720.

Neugarten, B.L. (1970). Adaptation and the life cycle. *Journal of Geriatric Psychiatry, 4,* 71–87.

Neumann, R., Strack, F. (2000). Mood contagion: The automatic transfer of mood between persons. *Journal of Personality and Social Psychology, 78,* 3022–3514.

Newcombe, M.J., Ashkanasy, N.M. (2002). The code of affect and affective congruence in perceptions of leaders: An experimental study. *Leadership Quarterly, 13,* 601–604.

Owen, T.R. (1999). The reliability and validity of a wellness inventory. *American Journal of Health Promotion, 13,* 180–182.

Panskepp, J. (2003). Feeling the pain of social loss. *Science, 302,* 237–239.

Park, N. (2004). Character strengths and positive youth development. *Annals of the American Academy of Political and Social Science, 591,* 40–54.

Park, C.L., Helgeson, V.S. (2006). Introduction to special section: Growth following highly stressful life events—current status and future directions. *Journal of Consulting and Clinical Psychology, 74,* 791–796.

Park, N., Peterson, C. (2005). The Values in Action Inventory of Character Strengths for Youth. In K.A. Moore, L.H. Lippman (Eds), *What Do Children Need to Flourish? Conceptualizing and Measuring Indicators of Positive Development.* (pp. 13–23). New York: Springer.

Park, N., Peterson, C., Seligman, M.E.P. (2004). Strengths of character and well being. *Journal of Social and Clinical Psychology, 23,* 603–619.

Pennebaker, J. (1997). *Opening up: The healing power of expressing emotions.* New York: Morrow.

Peterson, C. (2006). *A primer in positive psychology.* New York: Oxford University Press.

Peterson, C., Seligman, M.E.P. (2004). *Character strengths and virtues: A handbook and classification.* New York: Oxford University Press.

Pilch, J.J. (2000). *Healing in the New Testament: Insights from medical and Mediterranean anthropology.* Minneapolis: Fortress Press.

Porges, S.W. (1998). Love: An emergent property of the mammalian autonomic nervous system. *Psychoneuroendocrinology, 23,* 837–861.

Porras, J., Emery, S., Thompson, M. (2006). *Success built to last: Creating a life that matters.* Upper Saddle River, New Jersey: Wharton School Publishing.

Rabe, S., Zollner, T., Maercker, A., Karl, Al (2006). Neural correlates of posttraumatic growth after severe motor vehicle accidents. *Journal of Consulting and Clinical Psychology, 74,* 880–886.

Rath, T., Clifton, D.O. (2004). *How full is your bucket: Positive strategies for work and for life.* New York: Gallup Press.

Redelmeier, D., Singh, S. (2001). Survival in Academy Award-winning actors and actresses. *Annals of Internal Medicine, 134,* 955–962.

Reis, H.T., Gable, S.L. (2003). Toward a Positive Psychology of Relationships. In C.L.M. Keyes, J. Haidt (Eds), *Flourishing: Positive Psychology and the Life Well-lived* (pp. 129–159). Washington, DC: American Psychological Association.

Rimi, C., Manne, S., Duttanel, K.N., Austin, J., Ostroff, J., Boulad, F., et al. (2004). Mother's perceptions of benefit following pediatric stem cell transplantation: A longitudinal investigation of the roles of optimism, medical risk and sociodemographic resources. *Annals of Behavioral Medicine, 28,* 132–141.

Root, L.M., Cohen, A.D. (2006). Writing about the benefits of an interpersonal transgression facilitates forgiveness. *Journal of Consulting and Clinical Psychology, 74,* 887–897.

Ruff, G.F., Korchin, S.J. (1964). Personality Characteristics of the Mercury Astronauts. In G. G.H. Grosser, H., Wechsler, & Greenblatt (Eds.), *The Threat of Impending Disaster* (pp. 197–207). Boston: MIT Press.

Rutter, M. (1981). Stress, coping and development: Some issues and some questions. *Journal of Child Psychology and Psychiatry, 22,* 323–356.

Rutter, M. (1986). Myerian Psychobiology, Personality development and the role of life experiences. *American Journal of Psychiatry, 143,* 1077–1087.

Ryff, C.D. (1995). Psychologyical well being in adult life. *Current Directions in Psychological Science, 4,* 99–104.

Ryff, C.D., Singer, B.H. (2001). *Emotions, social relationships, and health.* New York: Oxford University Press.

Scheier, M.F., Carver, C.S. (1987). Dispositional optimism and physical well being: The influence of generalized outcome expectancies on health. *Journal of Personality, 55,* 169–210.

Schwartz, C., Meisenhelder, J.B., Ma, Y., Ried, G. (2003). Altruistic social interest behaviors are associated with better mental health. *Psychosomatic Medicine, 75,* 778–785.

Segerstrom, S.C., Miller, G.E. (2004). Psychological stress and the human immune system: A meta analytic study of 30 years of inquiry. *Psychological Bulletin, 130,* 601–630.

Seligman, M.E.P. (1991). *Learned optimism.* New York: Knopf.

Seligman, M.E.P. (2002). *Authentic happiness.* New York: Free Press.

Selgiman, M.E.P. (2004). Can happiness be taught? *Daedalus, 133,* 80–87.

Seligman, M.E.P., Steen, T.A., Park, N., Peterson, C. (2005). Positive psychology progress: Empirical validation of interventions. *American Psychologist, 60,* 410–421.

Sheldon, K.M. (2004). *Optimal human being: An Integrated multi-level perspective.* NJ: Erlbaum.

Siegel, D.J. (1999). *The developing mind: How relationships and the brain interact to shape who we are.* New York: Guilford.

Siegel, D.J. (2003). An Interpersonal Neurobiology of Psychotherapy: The Developing Mind and the Resolution and of Trauma. In M.F. Solomon, D.J. Siegel (Eds), *Healing Traums: Attachment, Mind, Body and Brain.* New York: W.W. Norton.

Smith, E., Graw, K. (2005). Which therapeutic mechanism works when? A step towards the formulation of empirically validated guidelines for therapists' session-to-session decisions. *Clinical Psychology and Psychotherapy, 12,* 112–123.

Smith, E., Grawe, K. (2003). What makes psychotherapy sessions productive? A new approach to bridging the gap between process research and practice. *Clinical Psychology and Psychotherapy, 10,* 275–285.

Snowdon, D. (2001). *Age with grace: What the nun study tells us about leading longer, healthier, and more meaningful lives.* New York: Bantum.

Swinton, J. (2001). *Spirituality and mental health care: Rediscovering a "Forgotten" dimension.* London: Jessica Kingsley Publishers.

Swinton, J., Kettel, S. (1997). Resurrecting the person: Redefining mental illness—a spiritual perspective. *Psychiatric Care, 4,* 1–4.

Tavris, C. (1989). *Anger: The misunderstood emotion.* Cambridge, Massachusetts: Harvard University Press.

Taylor, S.E., Klein, L.C., Lewis, B.P., Gruenewald, T.L, Gurung, R.A., Updegroff, J. (2000). Biobehavioral responses to stress in females: Tend-and-befriend, not fight or flight. *Psychological Review, 107,* 422–429.

Tiger, L. (1979). *Optimism: The biology of hope.* New York: Simon & Schuster.

Trevarthen, C. (1993). The Self Born in Intersubjectivity: The Psychology of Infant Communicating. In U. Neisser (Ed.), *The Perceived Self: Ecological and Interpersonal Sources of Self-knowledge* (pp. 121–173). New York: Cambridge University Press.

Twenge, J.M. (2006). *Generation me: Why today's young Americans are more confident, assertive, entitled—and miserable than ever before.* New York: Free Press.

Vaillant, G.E. (1993). *The wisdom of the ego.* Cambridge, Massachusetts: Harvard University Press.

Vaillant, G.E. (2000). Adaptive mental mechanisms: Their role in a positive psychology. *American Psychologist, 55,* 89–98.

Vaillant, G.E. (2003). Mental health. *American Journal of Psychiatry, 160,* 1373–1384.

Vaillant, G.E. (2004). Positive Aging. In P.A. Linley, S. Joseph (Eds), *Positive Psychology in Practice* (pp. 561–578). New York: Wiley.

Waite, L., Browning, D., Doherty, W.J., Gallagher, M., Lou, Y., Stanley, S.M. (2002). *Does divorce make people happy? Findings from a study of unhappy marriages.* New York: Institute for American Values.

Watson, D. (2000). *Mood and temperament.* New York: Guildord.

Watson, D., Hubbard, B., Wiese, D. (2000). General traits of personality and affectivity as predictors of satisfaction in intimate relationships: Evidence from self- and partner-ratings. *Journal of Personality, 68,* 413–449.

Weaver, A.J., Flannelly, L.T., Flannelly, K.J., Koenig, H.G., Larson, D.B. (1998). An analysis of research on religious and spiritual values in three major mental health journals. *Issues in Mental Health Nursing, 15,* 2632–2676.

Werner, E.E., Smith, R.S. (1982). *Vulnerable but Invincible.* New York: McGraw-Hill.

Wilson, T.D., Wheatley, T.P., Meyers, J.M., Gilbert, D.T., Assom, D. (2000). Focalism: A source of durability bias in affective forecasting. *Journal of Personality and Social Psychology, 78,* 821–836.

Wolf, S., Bruhn, J. (1979). *The Rosetta story: An anatomy of health.* Norman: University of Oklahoma Press.

Wright, R. (1994). *The moral animal: The new science of evolutionary Psychology.* New York: Random House.

Yankelovich, D. (1981). *New rules.* New York: Random House.

17

The Interaction of Religion and Health

BRUCE Y. LEE AND ANDREW B. NEWBERG

Introduction

Throughout history, religion and health care have oscillated between cooperation and antagonism. In ancient times, many of the world's most advanced civilizations (such as the Assyrians, Chinese, Egyptians, Mesopotamians, and Persians) equated physical illnesses with evil spirits and demonic possessions and devised treatments to exorcize these spirits. Since then, religious groups have labeled physicians and other health care providers as everything from evil sorcerers to charlatans to conduits of God's healing powers. Similarly, views on religion of physicians, scientists, and health care providers have ranged from interest to disinterest to disdain.

In recent years, the medical and scientific communities have grown increasingly interested in the effects of religion on health (Levin, 1996). Coverage of the interplay of religion and health has become much more frequent in popular magazines, such as *Time* and *Newsweek*, and on television shows (Begley, 2001a, 2001b; Greenwald, 2001; Woodward, 2001). There has been a surge in the popularity of spiritual activities, such as yoga, that aim to improve or maintain health (Corliss, 2001; van Montfrans, Karemaker, Wieling, & Dunning, 1990b). Moreover, many patients consider religion to be very important and have indicated that they would like their physicians to discuss religious issues with them. We will review what is currently known about clinical effects of religious and spiritual practices, and the challenges that researchers and health care practitioners may face in designing appropriate studies and translating results to clinical practice. We also will discuss future directions in the roles of religion and spirituality in health care.

The Importance of Religion and Spirituality to Patients and Physicians

Religion and spirituality play significant roles in many people's lives. Over 90% of Americans believe in God or a higher power, 90% pray, 67%–75% pray on a daily basis, 69% are members of a church or synagogue, 40% attend a church or synagogue regularly, 60% consider religion to be very important in their lives, and 82% acknowledge a personal need for spiritual growth (Bezilla, 1992–1993; Miller, & Thoresen, 2003; Poloma & Pendleton, 1991; Shuler, Gelberg, & Brown, 1994; The Gallup Report, 1994). Additionally, many patients seem interested in integrating religion with their health care. Over 75% of surveyed patients want physicians to include spiritual issues in their medical care, approximately 40% want physicians to discuss their religious faith with them, and nearly 50% would like physicians to pray with them (Daaleman & Nease, 1994; King & Bushwick, 1994; King, Hueston, & Rudy, 1994; Matthews et al., 1998). Although many physicians seem to agree that spiritual well-being is an important component of health that should be addressed with patients, only a minority (less than 20%) do so with any regularity (MacLean et al., 2003; Monroe et al., 2003). According to surveyed physicians, lack of time, inadequate training, discomfort in addressing the topics, and difficulty in identifying patients who want to discuss spiritual issues are responsible for this discrepancy (Armbruster, Chibnall, & Legett, 2003; Chibnall & Brooks, 2001; Ellis, Vinson, & Ewigman, 1999).

Educators have responded by offering courses, conferences, and curricula in medical schools, post-graduate training, and continuing medical education (Pettus, 2002). However, some question the relevance and appropriateness of discussing religion and spirituality in the health care setting, fearing that health care workers may impose personal religious beliefs on others and replace necessary medical interventions with religious interventions. Sloan and colleagues cautioned that patients may be forced to believe that their illnesses are due solely to poor faith (Sloan & Bagiella, 2002; Sloan, Bagiella, & Powell, 1999). Moreover, there is considerable debate over how religion should be integrated with health care and who should be responsible, especially when health care providers are agnostic or atheist (Levin, Larson, & Puchalski, 1997).

The Role of Religion in Health Care

Despite this controversy, the role of religion in health care seems to be growing. For instance, the *Diagnostic and Statistical Manual of Mental Disorders* (Fourth Edition) recognizes religion and spirituality as relevant sources of either emotional distress or support (Kutz, 2002; Lukoff, Lu, & Turner, 1992; Turner, Lukoff, Barnhouse, & Lu, 1995). Also, the guidelines of the Joint Commission on Accreditation of Health care Organizations (JCAHO) require hospitals to meet the spiritual needs of patients (La Pierre, 2003). The medical literature reflects this trend as well. The frequency of studies on religion and spirituality and health has increased over the past decade (Levin et al., 1997). Stefanek and colleagues tallied a 600% increase in spirituality and health publications and a 27% increase in religion and health publications from 1993 to 2002 (Stefanek, McDonald, & Hess, 2004).

Some have recommended that physicians and other health care providers routinely take religious and spiritual histories of their patients to better understand the patients' religious background, determine how he or she may be using religion to cope with illness, open the door for future discussions about any spiritual or religious issues, and help detect potentially deleterious side effects from religious and spiritual activities (Kuhn, 1988; Lo et al., 2002; Lo, Quill, & Tulsky, 1999; Matthews & Clark, 1998). It may also be a way of detecting spiritual distress (Abrahm, 2001): There also has been greater emphasis in integrating various religious resources and professionals into patient care, especially when the patient is near the end-of-life (Lo et al., 2002). Some effort has been made to train health care providers to listen appropriately to patients' religious concerns, perform clergy-like duties when religious professionals are not available, and better understand spiritual practices (Morse, & Proctor, 1998; Proctor, Morse, & Khonsari, 1996).

Methodological Issues with Clinical Studies

Like most nascent research areas, the study of religion and health has had to contend with lack of adequate funding, institutional support, and training for investigators. These challenges have helped limit the number of well-designed studies in the medical literature. Rather than true scientific studies, many "studies" actually have been anecdotes and editorials, which can galvanize discussions, germinate ideas, and fuel future studies, but cannot establish causality or scientifically justify the use of specific interventions. In fact, many of the "scientific" studies have only been correlational, and while they have demonstrated interesting associations, they have not always adjusted for all possible confounding variables, such as socioeconomic status, ethnicity, and different lifestyles or diets, and as a result have not clearly established causality. In some cases, religious variables were included in a larger study that did not focus on the effects of religion. Since these studies were not necessarily designed and powered primarily to study the religious variables, results must be considered cautiously. There have been a limited number of randomized controlled trials (RCTs). For example, in a systematic review of studies from 1966 to 1999, Townsend and colleagues counted nine RCTs. But as the study of religion and health progresses, the number and sophistication of scientific studies should continue to grow.

In addition to external challenges, the clinical study of religion has some inherent challenges as well. Understanding these inherent challenges is crucial when either designing or interpreting studies. Otherwise, you may conduct significantly flawed studies, draw inappropriate conclusions, administer unnecessary or even dangerous interventions, pursue the wrong research questions, or neglect to pursue further necessary research. These challenges include the following:

1. How do you do you define religion and spirituality?

"Religion" and "spirituality" are two distinct yet difficult to define terms that many often mistakenly use synonymously (Powell, Shahabi, & Thoresen, 2003; Tanyi, 2002). Even if universal definitions were established, which specific practices would be classified as either or neither? For example, where does one draw the line between religions and cults? In fact, the Merriam Webster Dictionary defines cult as "a religion regarded as unorthodox or spurious." What then is the criterion for being "unorthodox and spurious"? In fact, as history has often demonstrated, what formerly was considered a cult and spurious can eventually become a major religion, and vice-versa.

2. Can you recruit and retain enough study subjects?

Finding appropriate and compliant subjects is not easy. The beliefs and practices relevant to your study may be rare in your vicinity. The further a subject has to travel, the less likely that subject is to participate in your study. Some beliefs and practices may be incompatible with your study design or environment (e.g., some religions do not allow subjects to travel or use electronic devices on certain days). Subjects may be unwilling or unable to alter their religious beliefs and practices for your study.

3. How do you monitor and maintain subject compliance?

Many religious and spiritual activities such as prayer and meditation are private, silent, subtle, integrated with, or indistinguishable from, social interactions. How do you verify if and how often a subject prays or meditates? How do you ensure that a subject performs a religious or spiritual activity in a "proper" or certain manner? A subject may inadvertently be noncompliant. The environment and other people may influence whether and how a subject behaves. For example, a subject may be more likely to pray when she is in a church or surrounded by others who frequently pray.

4. Which measures of religiousness or spirituality should you use?

Many possible measures of religiousness and spirituality exist. Someone who scores high in one dimension of religiousness may not necessarily score high in others. For example, individuals who describe themselves as "very religious" (high *subjective religiosity*) may not necessarily score high on more objective measures (low *religious commitment/motivation*). An individual may not participate significantly in formal church, synagogue, or temple activities (low *organizational religiosity*), but may regularly perform private religious activities, such as praying, reading religious scriptures, and watching religious television (high *nonorganizational religiosity*). A number of other potential measures exist, including how closely an individual's beliefs conform to the established doctrines of a religious body (*religious belief*), how knowledgeable or informed an individual is about the doctrines of his or her religion (*religious knowledge*) and how well his or her actions, such as working for the church and acts of altruism, support his or her religion (*religious consequences*). Finally, spirituality and religiousness are not always commensurate with some individuals considering themselves spiritual and not religious, or religious and not spiritual. Thus, studies should always clearly state the exact measures used and avoid making claims about measures not used.

5. Is your measure of religiousness accurate and valid?

Directly observing a subject's behavior frequently is the most accurate and valid way of measuring religiousness. For example, you may determine organizational religiosity by measuring how often a person attends church, reads religious scriptures, and prays over a period of time. However, direct observation may not be practical or easy. Shadowing each of your subjects throughout the duration of the study would be incredibly time consuming and expensive. Even if you were able to follow and observe a subject's every move, counting and interpreting such activities can be challenging. You may miss subtle religious displays (e.g., a momentary pause or gesture can represent prayer, meditation, or a religious thought). Moreover, what are the correct units of measure? Is the duration or intensity of an activity more important than the frequency? Is reading scriptures everyday for 1 hour equivalent to reading scriptures 5 days a week for four hours? What if someone reads the scriptures as a rote ritual instead of truly feeling connected with what is being read? To establish a true cause and effect relationship, it would be helpful to elicit a dose-response curve, that is, determine if increased religiosity corresponds to better health. Many studies simply divided patients into dichotomous groups (e.g., did they belong to a church?), which do not account for significant variation within each of the two groups. Should certain religious activities be considered more important than others? Someone who does not belong to a church but regularly prays and follows religious doctrine may in fact have greater religious commitment than a person who belongs to a church but does not believe in, or care to comprehend, religious doctrine.

Since direct observation is difficult, many investigators have relied on questionnaires or interviews of subjects. As you can imagine, depending on subjects' views and descriptions of themselves is problematic. People may consciously or unconsciously misrepresent their actual behavior. Subjects may be forgetful or distracted. Dutifully keeping track of one's activities and thoughts requires significant organization, focus, and compulsiveness. Some patients may be unwilling to admit lapses in religiousness. Moreover, the quality of data depends on the quality of the instrument collecting the data. Poorly worded questions and vague instructions can mislead or confuse subjects. Some questions may not elicit the information they are supposed to elicit. Unfortunately, many studies do not indicate whether and how their questionnaires or interviews were tested and validated.

6. The positive externalities of religion may confound results.
Participating in religious activities can alter a person's life in many ways. Church groups often provide a social support network. Many church activities also function as social and recreational activities. They may offer opportunities for people to exercise and to stay away from unhealthy environments. Through church activities people may meet future spouses, physicians, other health care workers, exercise partners, nutritionists, potential employers, or any other individuals that may help their professional and personal lives. Participating in religious activities may be reprieves from daily stress and time for reflection. Religion can provide structure and discipline to a person's life. These favorable secondary effects of religious activities (i.e., "positive externalities" of religion) may be responsible for some health benefits. So when a study shows a positive effect of religion, differentiating what is truly responsible for the effect can be difficult.

7. Is a patient's religious activity causing the observed effects on his or her health, or is the patient's health status affecting his or her religious activity?

Establishing the direction of causality can be challenging. A person's health status may influence whether he or she participates in a religious activity. Physical disabilities or problems may prevent a person from traveling to or engaging in certain activities. A person with a contagious disease may not want to expose others. Someone depressed or anxious may feel unmotivated or embarrassed to see others. Conversely, serious health problems may motivate patients to attend religious activities to seek solace or healing.

8. Practices and doctrines vary significantly among and within different religious affiliations and denominations.

People practice religion in many different ways. For example, prayers may be silent or vocal, restrained or demonstrative, short or long in duration, and performed alone or in groups. Some groups may require specific words to be said or garments to be worn. What constitutes devoted religious behavior in one sect or denomination may be inadequate or irreverent in other sects or denominations. For example, proper dress in one denomination may be sacrilegious in more orthodox denominations.

9. A person's sense of well-being may depend on the degree of hierarchy in a religion, and his or her place in that hierarchy.

Some religions are more hierarchical than others. A person's status within a religious group may affect his or her psychological and physical well-being. Those near the top of the organization may feel more powerful and have many benefits, while those near the bottom may feel more stress or be forced to do unpleasant work. Religious groups vary in how their leaders treat and take care of their members. Different members do not receive equal treatment. A person's degree of acceptance by a given religious group may depend on his or her socioeconomic status, gender, ethnicity, or appearance.

10. Religions are affected by the local environment.

Different religions hold different social statuses in different countries during different times. Practically all religions have faced persecution, discrimination, and isolation at some time and place during history. Belonging to the dominant religion in a society can confer greater social acceptance, a stronger and more extensive social network, and more access to resources, all of which can have subtle psychological and physical consequences. Minority religious sects may endure psychological or physical stress, or in some severe cases, physical punishment. Moreover, minority or fringe religious sects who are unable to convince mainstream individuals to join their cause may have to recruit among societal outcasts, many of whom could have psychological or physical illness. Therefore, any study of a specific religious sect should account for the location of the study group, and the sect's relationship with the ambient society.

11. What is a proper time frame for the study?

How long should you follow and observe individuals or populations before seeing any effects? Some spiritual activities, such as prayer, yoga, and meditation, may have immediate effects on physical parameters, such as heart rate and blood pressure. But the potential effects of other religious and spiritual activities may take longer to manifest. Therefore, observing subjects over only a short period of time may miss findings. However, the longer the follow-up, the more difficult the study is to perform, and the greater chance that more confounders will enter the picture.

12. Multidisciplinary research is challenging.

The study of religion and health involves individuals from different disciplines and professions. Ultimately, interdisciplinary research can be more productive than research confined to a single discipline. People from different fields and professions bring different interests, experiences, perspectives, and abilities to the table. However, multidisciplinary research must confront and overcome communicative, administrative, and cultural hurdles. Every discipline and profession has its own language, culture, structure, and motivations. Health researchers and religion researchers often are not familiar with important publications in each others' specialty journals. Separate meetings, separate departments, different methodologies, and different lexicons have hindered collaboration. However, the emergence of interdisciplinary journals and conferences has alleviated this problem.

The Positive Effects of Religion on Health

DISEASE INCIDENCE AND PREVALENCE

Various systematic reviews and meta-analyses have demonstrated that religious involvement correlates with decreased morbidity and mortality (Ball, Armistead, & Austin, 2003; Braam, Beekman, Deeg, Smit, & Van Tilburg, 1999; Brown, 2000; Kark et al., 1996; Kune, Kune, & Watson, 1993; McCullough, Hoyt, Larson, Koenig, & Thoresen, 2000; McCullough & Larson, 1999; Oman, Kurata, Strawbridge, & Cohen, 2002), and high levels of religious involvement may be associated with up to 7 years of longer life expectancy (Helm, Hays, Flint, Koenig, & Blazer, 2000; Hummer, Rogers, Nam, & Ellison, 1999; Koenig et al., 1999; Oman & Reed, 1998; Strawbridge, Cohen, Shema, & Kaplan, 1997). A study by Kark and colleagues over a 16-year period revealed that belonging to a religious collective in Israel was associated with lower mortality (Kark et al., 1996). In Comstock and Partridge's analysis of 91,000 people in a Maryland county, those who regularly attended church had a lower prevalence of cirrhosis, emphysema, suicide, and death from ischemic heart disease (Comstock & Partridge, 1972). Several studies have implied that religious participation and higher religiosity may have a beneficial effect on blood pressure (Armstrong, van Merwyk, & Coates, 1977; Hixson, Gruchow, & Morgan, 1998; Koenig et al., 1998; Walsh, 1998).

Some studies have suggested that members of different religions may have different mortality and morbidity, even when adjusting for major biological, behavioral, and socioeconomic differences (Rasanen, Kauhanen, Lakka, Kaplan, & Salonen, 1996; Van Poppel, Schellekens, & Liefbroer, 2002). However, as mentioned previously, the experience of individuals within a given religion can depend significantly on the local environment, the person's status within the religious group, and the religious group's status within the surroundings. Therefore, one should interpret the results of such comparisons with caution. For instance, a study of contemplative monks in the Netherlands showed that mortality compared with the general population varied with time during the 1900s (de Gouw, Westendorp, Kunst, Mackenbach, & Vandenbroucke, 1995). Greater morbidity and mortality have been reported among Irish Catholics in Britain, which may reflect their disadvantaged socioeconomic status in that country (Abbotts, Williams, & Ford, 2001; Abbotts, Williams, Ford, Hunt, & West, 1997). A study in Holland suggested that smaller religious groups may be less susceptible to infectious disease because of social isolation (Van Poppel et al., 2002). In general, there have not been enough studies looking at how mortality and morbidity for different religions vary over time and place. Moreover, many religions and religious sects have received little attention from investigators. Consequently, the body of literature comparing morbidity and mortality rates among religions is not large enough to draw any definitive conclusions.

As a whole, broad epidemiological studies that use crude outcome measures such as morbidity and mortality cannot establish causality, but suggest that something about religion may protect health. Many study populations may have been too large to account for all possible confounders. Religious participation may be associated with a number of socioeconomic, lifestyle, ethnic, and geographic factors that may affect health. Further, epidemiological studies looking at different subgroups may help refine and define associations.

DISEASE AND SURGICAL OUTCOMES

Studies also have suggested that people with high religiousness may have better outcomes after major illnesses and medical procedures. In Oxman and colleagues' analysis of 232 patients following elective open heart surgery, lack of participation in social or community groups, and absence of strength and comfort from religion, were consistent predictors of mortality (Oxman, Freeman, & Manheimer, 1995). In Pressman and colleagues' look at 30 elderly women after hip repair, religious belief was associated with lower levels of depressive symptoms and better ambulation status (Pressman, Lyons, Larson, & Strain, 1990). Contrada and colleagues found that in patients who underwent heart surgery, stronger religious beliefs were associated with shorter hospital stays and fewer complications, but attendance at religious services predicted longer hospitalizations (Contrada et al., 2004). On the other hand, Hodges and colleagues did not find spiritual beliefs to significantly affect recovery from spinal surgery (Hodges, Humphreys, & Eck, 2002).

Studies have examined whether religiosity improves the survival of patients with different illnesses as well. In a study of African American women with breast cancer, patients who did not belong to a religion tended not to survive as long (Van Ness, Kasl, & Jones, 2003). In a study by Zollinger and colleagues, Seventh-day Adventists had better breast cancer survival than non-Seventh-day Adventists, but this was probably due to earlier diagnosis and treatment (Zollinger, Phillips, & Kuzma, 1984). Several other studies of various cancers, including colorectal, lung, and breast cancer, showed no statistically significant effect of religious involvement on cancer survival (Kune, Kune, & Watson, 1992; Loprinzi et al., 1994; Ringdal, Gotestam, Kaasa, Kvinnsland, & Ringdal, 1996; Yates, Chalmer, St. James, Follansbee, & McKegney, 1981). A study by Blumenthal and colleagues showed no correlation between post-myocardial infarction outcomes and self-reported spirituality, frequency of church attendance, or frequency of prayer (Blumenthal et al., 2007).

GENERAL BEHAVIOR AND LIFESTYLES

Studies have looked at whether people with high religiosity live generally healthier and less risky lifestyles than those with lower religiosity, which may account for some of the observed health benefits of religion. One hypothesis is that religion may provide structure, teaching, role models, and support to individuals, so that they do not have the desire or time to engage in risky behavior.

Some studies have supported this hypothesis. The study of Texas adults by Hill and colleagues showed that regular religious activity attendance correlated with use of preventive care, vitamins, and seatbelts, decreased bar attendance, and decreased smoking and drinking, walking, strenuous exercise, and sound sleep quality (Hill, Burdette, Ellison, & Musick, 2006). Oleckno and Blacconiere's study of college students revealed an inverse correlation between religiosity and behaviors that adversely affect health (Oleckno & Blacconiere, 1991). Religious involvement has been shown to be associated with greater use of seat belts (Oleckno & Blacconiere, 1991) and preventative services (Comstock & Partridge, 1972). Compared to the general population, Mormons and Seventh-day Adventists have been found to have lower incidence of and mortality rates from cancers that have been linked to tobacco and alcohol (Grundmann, 1992; Fraser, 1999). However, other studies have shown no relationship, or even an inverse relationship, between religiosity and certain risky behaviors (Hasnain, Sinacore, Mensah, & Levy, 2005; Poulson, Eppler, Satterwhite, Wuensch, & Bass, 1998).

DIET AND NUTRITION

Could dietary differences explain some of the observed health benefits of religion? A 2005 study found that African American women with high religiosity consumed more fruits and vegetables than those with low religiosity (Holt, Haire-Joshu, Lukwago, Lewellyn, & Kreuter, 2005). Studies in Israel showed that compared to religious residents, secular residents had diets higher in total fat and saturated fatty acids (Friedlander, Kark, Kaufmann, & Stein, 1985), and higher plasma levels of cholesterol, triglyceride, and low-density lipoprotein (Friedlander, Kark, & Stein, 1987). Some religions enforce certain specific diets, such as periodic fasting or vegetarianism (Roky, Houti, Moussamih, Qotbi, & Aadil, 2004; Sarri, Linardakis, Codrington, & Kafatos, 2007). For example, a large, prospective epidemiologic study of Seventh-day Adventists revealed that a diet rich in nuts, as advocated by Adventists, was associated with a lower risk of cardiovascular disease (Sabate, 1999). However, the benefits and harms of specific religious diets have not been clearly established.

ALCOHOL, TOBACCO, AND DRUG ABUSE

Religion can affect alcohol and substance use at several stages. It may affect whether a person initiates use, how significant the use becomes, how the use affects the person's life, and whether the person is able to quit and recover

(Miller, 1998). The attitudes of religions towards alcohol and substance use vary considerably. Some religious sects strictly prohibit alcohol and substance use (Enstrom & Breslow, 2007). Others are less stringent, but discourage excessive use. Some allow the use of alcohol and have incorporated drinking wine into their rituals, and others use psychoactive substances, such as peyote, khat, and hashish to achieve spiritual goals (Lyttle, 1988).

Indeed, some evidence suggests that individuals involved in religion are less likely to use alcohol and other substances (Heath et al., 1999; Luczak, Shea, Carr, Li, & Wall, 2002; Stewart, 2001). Even among alcohol and drug users, religiously involved individuals are more likely to use them moderately and not heavily (Gorsuch & Butler, 1976; Miller, 1998). Leigh and colleagues' study of college students revealed that students with higher spirituality scores smoked and binge-drank less frequently (Leigh, Bowen, & Marlatt, 2005). In a nationally representative sample of adolescents, Miller and colleagues determined that personal devotion—which they defined as a personal relationship with the Divine—and affiliation with more fundamentalist denominations were inversely associated with alcohol and illicit drug use (Miller, Davies, & Greenwald, 2000). This effect was seen outside the United States as well, in Latin America (Chen, Dormitzer, Bejarano, & Anthony, 2004). There are a number of possible reasons for these findings. Fear of violating religious principles and doctrines can have a powerful effect. Religions can play a role in educating people about the dangers of alcohol and drugs (Stylianou, 2004). Religious involvement and the accompanying positive externalities may keep people occupied and prevent idleness and boredom that can lead to substance abuse. There may be peer pressure from other members of the church to remain abstinent, and an absence of peer pressure to try alcohol and other substances. Moreover, religious involvement could be the effect rather than the cause. Substance abuse may prevent religious involvement. Larson and Wilson noted that alcoholics compared to non-alcoholic subjects had less involvement in religious practices, less exposure to religious teachings, and fewer religious experiences (Larson & Wilson, 1980).

Many, including patients, believe that incorporating religion and spirituality into alcohol, tobacco, and drug cessation programs may enhance their efficacy (Arnold, Avants, Margolin, & Marcotte, 2002; Dermatis, Guschwan, Galanter, & Bunt, 2004). Indeed, spirituality already permeates many established programs, such as Alcoholics Anonymous (AA) (Brush & McGee, 2000; Forcehimes, 2004; Li, Feifer, & Strohm, 2000; Moriarity, 2001). Studies have suggested that religious and spiritual practices may aid recovery (Aron & Aron, 1980; Avants, Warburton, & Margolin, 2001; Carter, 1998). A significant number of recovering intravenous drug abusers seem to use religious healing, relaxation techniques, and meditation (Manheimer, Anderson, & Stein, 2003). Data suggests that patients often experience spiritual awakenings or religious conversion during recovery (Green, Fullilove, & Fullilove, 1998). However, not all studies showed that religiously involved patients have better outcomes. The first randomized controlled trials failed to demonstrate sufficient clinical benefit from meditation (Murphy, Pagano, & Marlatt, 1986) or intercessory prayer (Walker, Tonigan, Miller, Corner, & Kahlich, 1997). In a study by Tonigan and colleagues, while subjects self-labeled as religious were more likely than agnostics and atheists to initiate and continue attending AA meetings, their outcomes were not clearly better (Tonigan, Miller, & Schermer, 2002).

SEXUAL BEHAVIOR

Some religions may play a role in preventing risky sexual behavior. In a study of African American adolescent females, religiosity correlated with more frank discussions about the risks of sex and avoidance of unsafe sexual situations (McCree, Wingood, DiClemente, Davies, & Harrington, 2003). Miller and Gur's study of over 3,000 adolescent girls found positive associations between personal devotion and fewer sexual partners outside a romantic relationship, religious event attendance and proper birth control use, and religious event attendance and a better understanding of human immunodeficiency virus or pregnancy risks from unprotected intercourse (Miller & Gur, 2002). But these findings are not universal. Some have found no relationship between religiosity and sexual practices (Dunne, Edwards, Lucke, Donald, Raphael, 1994; McCormick, Izzo, & Folcik, 1985). Based on data from the 1995 National Survey of Family Growth, Jones and colleagues concluded that young women with more frequent religious service attendance tended to have delayed first intercourse but did not exhibit significantly different sexual behavior from others once they began having sex (Jones, Darroch, & Singh, 2005). In fact, religious traditions or environments may actually suppress open discussion of sex and contraception. Lefkowitz and colleagues found that adolescents who discussed safe sex with their mothers tended to be less religious (Lefkowitz, Boone, Au, & Sigman, 2003).

EXERCISE

Some religious or spiritual practices promote or even involve exercise. Religious activities can motivate people to leave their homes, walk to different locations, and participate in physical activities. Some church-related activities, such as softball leagues or dances, involve even more strenuous exercise. Among Utah residents, Merill and Thygerson found that people who attended church weekly were more likely to exercise regularly. However, differences in smoking and general health status seemed to account for this effect (Merrill & Thygerson, 2001). A study by McLane and colleagues suggested incorporating faith-based practices in exercise programs may be attractive to certain people and improve participation in physical activity (McLane, Lox, Butki, & Stern, 2003). To date, church-based initiatives to promote exercise have yielded mixed results (Wilcox et al., 2007; Young & Stewart, 2006).

ACCESS TO HEALTH CARE RESOURCES

Along with encouraging healthy lifestyles, religious groups may promote or provide access to better health care, and sponsor health improvement programs (e.g., blood pressure screening, blood drives, soup kitchens, and food drives) (Heath et al., 1999; Koenig et al., 1998; Stewart, 2001; Zaleski & Schiaffino, 2000). Groups, such as the Catholic Church, have substantial resources and positions that allow them to influence people positively in ways that many secular organizations cannot. Additionally, many hospitals and health care clinics are supported by, affiliated with, or even owned by religious groups.

GENERAL MENTAL HEALTH

The impact of religion on mental health has been studied more extensively than the impact of religion on physical health. Studies have demonstrated religiosity to be positively associated with feelings of well-being in White American, Mexican American (Markides, Levin, & Ray, 1987), and African American populations (Coke, 1992), as well as in different age groups (Yoon & Lee, 2007). Krause observed that older African American individuals were more likely than similarly aged White Americans to derive life satisfaction from religion (Krause, 2003). Religious service attendance was predictive of higher life satisfaction among elderly Chinese Hong Kong residents (Ho et al., 1995) and elderly Mexican American women (Levin & Markides, 1988). Members of religious kibutzes in Israel reported a higher sense of coherence and less hostility and were more likely to engage in volunteer work than nonmembers (Kark, Carmel, Sinnreich, Goldberger, & Friedlander, 1996). Similar findings occurred in a population of nursing home residents (House, Robbins, & Metzner, 1982). Hope and optimism seemed to run higher among religious individuals than nonreligious individuals in some study populations (Idler & Kasl, 1997a, 1997b; Raleigh, 1992). Using religious attendance as one of the markers of social engagement, Bassuk and colleagues determined that social disengagement was linked with cognitive decline in the noninstitutionalized elderly (Bassuk, Glass, & Berkman, 1999).

A few studies compared different religions. For example, one study showed that among elderly women in Hong Kong, Catholics and Buddhists enjoyed better mental health status than Protestants (Boey, 2003). However, not enough data exist to generate meaningful conclusions.

DEPRESSION

A number of investigators have looked at the effects of religion on depression. Prospective cohort studies have shown religious activity to be associated with remission of depression in Protestant and Catholic Netherlanders (Braam, Beekman, Deeg, Smit, van Tilburg, 1997) and in ill older adults (Koenig, George, & Peterson, 1998). Prospective studies have also found religious activity to be strongly protective against depression in Protestant and Catholic offspring who share the same religion as their mother (Miller, Warner, Wickramaratne, & Weissman, 1997), and weakly protective in female twins (Kennedy, Kelman, Thomas, & Chen, 1996). Cross-sectional studies have yielded significant (Koenig et al., 1997) and nonsignificant (Bienenfeld, Koenig, Larson, & Sherrill, 1997; Koenig, 1998; Musick, Koenig, Hays, & Cohen, 1998) associations between different indicators of religiosity and a lower prevalence of depression in various populations. Chen and colleagues found that in patients already diagnosed with depression, religious participation may lead to better outcomes (Chen, Cheal, McDonel Herr, Zubritsky, & Levkoff, 2007).

Studies also have suggested an inverse correlation between religiosity and suicide. This was found to be the case in Nisbet's analysis of 1993 National Mortality Followback Survey data (Nisbet, Duberstein, Conwell, & Seidlitz, 2000) and Neeleman and colleagues' analysis of cross-sectional data of Judaeo-Christian older adults from 26 countries (Neeleman & Lewis, 1999). Suicide may be less acceptable to people with high religious devotion and orthodox religious beliefs (Neeleman, Halpern, Leon, & Lewis, 1997; Neeleman, Wessely, & Lewis, 1998). But again, it is unclear whether suicidal individuals are less likely to hold strong religious beliefs, or individuals with strong religious beliefs are less likely to be suicidal.

Several RCTs have been performed. One RCT demonstrated that directed and nondirected intercessory prayer correlated favorably with multiple measures of self-esteem, anxiety, and depression, but did not clearly state the randomization technique and did not account for multiple confounders (O'Laoire, 1997). Another RCT suggested that using religion-based cognitive therapy had a favorable impact on Christian patients with clinical depression, but may have contained too many comparison groups for strong cause-and-effect relationships to be established (Propst, Ostrom, Watkins, Dean, & Mashburn, 1992). Three RCTs suggested that religious (Islamic-based) psychotherapy appeared to speed recovery from anxiety and depression in Muslim Malays, but did not control for the use of antidepressants and benzodiazepines (Azhar & Varma, 1995; Azhar, Varma, & Dharap, 1994; Razali, Hasanah, Aminah, & Subramaniam, 1998).

COPING WITH MEDICAL PROBLEMS

Religious belief may provide meaning to and, in turn, help patients better cope with their diseases (Autiero, 1987; Foley, 1988; Patel, Shah, Peterson, & Kimmel, 2002). Although many major religions have deemed illness and suffering the result of sin, many believe that pain and suffering can be strengthening, enlightening, and purifying. According to various religious teachings, pain and suffering are inevitable and can be cleansing, test virtue, educate, readjust priorities, stimulate personal growth, and define human life (Amundsen, 1982).

Different religions may differ in how they confront suffering. While generalizations are difficult to draw since considerable variability exists within each religion, many Buddhists believe in enduring pain matter-of-factly (Tu, 1980), many Hindus stress understanding and detachment from pain (Shaffer, 1978), many Muslims and Jews favor resisting or fighting pain (Bowker, 1978), and many Christians stress seeking atonement and redemption (Amundsen, 1982).

Evidence suggests that religion provides more than just a distraction from suffering. The "diverting attention" and "praying" factors on the Coping Strategies Questionnaire (CSQ) have correlated with pain levels (Geisser, 1994; Swartzman, Gwadry, Shapiro, & Teasell, 1994; Swimmer, Robinson, & Geisser, 1992). The social network and support provided by religions may be associated with lower pain levels, and religious belief may improve self-esteem and sense of purpose (Hays et al., 1998; Musick et al., 1998; Swimmer et al., 1992). After following 720 adults, Williams concluded that religious attendance buffered the effects of stress on mental health (Williams, Larson, Buckler, Heckmann, & Pyle, 1991). In Coward's study of 107 women with advanced breast cancer, spirituality appeared to improve emotional well-being (Coward, 1991).

The Negative Effects of Religion on Health

Although most studies have shown positive effects, religion and spirituality also may negatively impact health. For example, religious groups may directly oppose certain health care interventions, such as transfusions or contraception, and convince patients that their ailments are due to noncompliance with religious doctrines rather than to organic disease (Donahue, 1985). Asser and colleagues demonstrated that a large number of child fatalities could have been prevented had medical care not been withheld for religious reasons (Asser & Swan, 1998). After interviewing 682 North Carolina women, Mitchell and colleagues concluded that belief in religious intervention may delay African American women from seeing their physicians for breast lumps (Mitchell, Lannin, Mathews, & Swanson, 2002). In addition, religions can stigmatize those with certain diseases to the point that they do not seek proper medical care (Lichtenstein, 2003; Madru, 2003).

Moreover, as history has shown, religion can be the source of military conflicts, prejudice, violent behaviors, and other social problems. Religions may ignore, sterotype, ostracize, or abuse those who do not belong to their church. Those not belonging to a dominant religion may face obstacles to obtaining resources hardships, and stress that deleteriously affect their health (Bywaters, Ali, Fazil, Wallace, & Singh, 2003; Walls & Williams, 2004). Religious leaders may abuse their own members physically, emotionally, or sexually (Rossetti, 1995; Tieman, 2002). Religious laws or dictums may be invoked to justify harmful, oppressive, and injurious behavior (Kernberg, 2003).

Additionally, perceived religious transgressions can cause emotional and psychological anguish, manifesting as physical discomfort. This "religious" and "spiritual pain" can be difficult to distinguish from pure physical pain (Satterly, 2001). In extreme cases, spiritual abuse—convincing people that they are going to suffer eternal purgatory—and spiritual terrorism—an extreme form of spiritual abuse—can occur either overtly or insidiously, that is, it can be implied, though not actually stated, that a patient will be doomed (Purcell, 1998a, 1998b). When a mix of religious, spiritual, and organic sources is causing physical illness, treatment can become complicated. Health care workers must properly balance treating each source.

The Effects of Specific Religious and Spiritual Activities

Religious and spiritual activities have become highly prevalent and may be practiced in either a religious or a secular manner. Although many of these activities have been correctly or incorrectly linked to specific religions, practicing them does not necessarily connote certain beliefs. In fact, hundreds of variations of each spiritual activity exist, since many have been altered and combined with other activities, such as aerobics, to develop hybrid techniques. As a result, some forms barely resemble the original versions. Thus, investigators must be very specific in describing the technique or activity that they are examining. Results from one form of meditation or yoga may not apply to other forms. A review of literature shows that many studies do not clearly describe the form of spiritual activity under investigation.

PRAYER

In Eisenberg and colleagues' survey of alternative medicine usage among Americans, one-fourth of respondents used prayer to cope with physical illness (Eisenberg et al., 1998). There is evidence that prayer may be associated with less muscle tension, improved cardiovascular and neuroimmunologic parameters, psychologic and spiritual peace, a greater sense of purpose, enhanced coping skills, less disability and better physical function in patients with knee pain (Rapp, Rejeski, & Miller, 2000), and a lower incidence of coronary heart disease (Gupta, 1996; Gupta, Prakash, Gupta, & Gupta, 1997).

Poloma and Pendleton found that *petitionary* and *ritualistic prayers* were associated with lower levels of well-being and life satisfaction, while *colloquial prayers* were associated with higher levels (Poloma, & Pendleton, 1991). Leibovici reported on a double-blinded RCT that showed that remote, retroactive intercessory prayer was associated with shorter length of fever and hospital stay in patients with bloodstream infection (Leibovici, 2001). A very small, limited double-blind study showed that intercessory prayer used as adjunct therapy appeared to decrease mortality among children with leukemia (Collipp, 1969). In Byrd and colleagues' double-blind study of patients admitted to a coronary care unit, *intercessory prayer* was linked to significantly more "good" outcomes (163 versus 147) than "bad" outcomes (27 versus 44) (Byrd, 1988). Harris and colleagues found similar outcomes with remote *intercessory prayer* (Harris et al., 1999). However, similar subsequent studies were not able to replicate these findings (Aviles et al., 2001; Matthews, Conti, & Sireci, 2001; Matthews, Marlowe, & MacNutt, 2000; Townsend, Kladder, Ayele, Mulligan, 2002). Interestingly, the Study of the Therapeutic Effects of Intercessory Prayer (STEP), a multicenter randomized clinical trial, showed that patients who knew that they were receiving intercessory prayer had worse post-coronary artery bypass graft surgery outcomes than patients who did not receive intercessory prayer. The same study showed no difference between patients who unknowingly received intercessory prayer and patients who did not receive intercessory prayer (Benson et al., 2006). In fact, a Cochrane systematic review of all major studies on intercessory prayer yielded equivocal results, precluding any definitive conclusions (Roberts, Ahmed, & Hall, 2007).

MEDITATION

Meditation and meditation-related practices are widely used as alternative therapy for physical ailments (Eisenberg et al., 1998). Many physicians routinely recommend meditation techniques to their patients and include them as part of integrated health programs, such as Dean Ornish's popular heart disease programs and a Stanford arthritis self-care course. Meditative and relaxation techniques are often part of childbirth preparation classes.

While evidence is not yet definitive, preliminary studies suggest that meditation may have a number of health benefits, helping people achieve a state of restful alertness with improved reaction time, creativity, and comprehension (Domino, 1977; Solberg, Berglund, Engen, Ekeberg, & Loeb, 1996); decreasing anxiety, depression, irritability, and moodiness, and improving learning ability, memory, self-actualization, feelings of vitality and rejuvenation, and emotional stability (Astin, 1977; Astin et al., 2003; Bitner, Hillman, Victor, & Walsh, 2003; Jain et al., 2007; Solberg et al., 1996; Walton, Pugh, Gelderloos, & Macrae, 1995). Preliminary studies suggest that meditative practices may benefit and provide acute and chronic support for patients with hypertension, psoriasis, irritable bowel disease, anxiety, epilepsy, premenstrual symptoms, menopausal symptoms, and depression (Arias, Steinberg, Banga, & Trestman, 2006; Barrows & Jacobs, 2002; Jacobs, Carlson, Ursuliak, Goodey, Angen, & Speca, 2001; Castillo-Richmond et al., 2000; Kabat-Zinn et al., 1992, 1998; Kaplan, Goldenberg, & Galvin-Nadeau, 1993; Keefer & Blanchard, 2002; King, Carr, & D'Cruz, 2002; Manocha, Marks, Kenchington, Peters, & Salome, 2002; Reibel, Greeson, Brainard, & Rosenzweig, 2001; Williams, Kolar, Reger, & Pearson, 2001). There is also evidence that meditation can improve chronic pain (Kabat-Zinn, 1982; Kabat-Zinn, Lipworth, & Burney, 1985). In a study by Kaplan and colleagues, all 77 men and women with fibromyalgia who completed a 10-week stress-reduction program using meditation had symptom improvement (Kaplan et al., 1993). Moreover, in several studies, meditators had better respiratory function (vital capacity, tidal volume, expiratory pressure, and breath holding), cardiovascular parameters (diastolic blood pressure and heart rate), and lipid profiles than nonmeditators (Cooper & Aygen, 1979; Wallace, Silver, Mills, Dillbeck, & Wagoner, 1983; Wenneberg et al., 1997).

Unfortunately, many studies did not specify or describe the type of meditation used. A wide variety of methods may be used, including some in which the body is immobile (e.g., Zazen, Vipassana), others in which the body is let free (e.g., Siddha Yoga, the Latihan, the chaotic meditation of Rajneesh), and still others in which the person participates in daily activities while meditating (e.g., Mahamudra, Shikan Taza, Gurdjieff's "self-remembering"). So it is not clear which forms may be beneficial and what aspects of meditation are providing the benefits.

Although physically noninvasive, meditation can be harmful in patients with psychiatric illness, potentially aggravating and precipitating psychotic episodes in delusional or strongly paranoid patients and heightening anxiety in patients with overwhelming anxiety. Moreover, it can trigger the release of repressed memories. Therefore, all patients using meditative techniques should be monitored, especially when a patient first starts using meditation.

YOGA

Yoga is also widely used, often for regular exercise. Contrary to popular misconception, yoga predated Hinduism by several centuries, and as The American Yoga Association emphasizes, since yoga practice does not specify particular higher powers or religious doctrines, it can be compatible with all major religions. In fact, many religions, including many Christian denominations, have adopted yoga techniques.

Yoga is based on a set of theories that have not yet been scientifically proven. Yoga practitioners believe that blockages or shortages of life force can cause disease or decreased resistance to disease and that yoga can restore the flow of life force to different parts of the body. They use a series of stretching, breathing, and relaxation techniques to prepare for meditation and use stretching movements or postures (*asanas*) that aim to increase blood supply and *prana* (vital force) as well as increase the flexibility of the spine, which is thought to improve the nerve supply. They also use breathing techniques (*pranayamas*) to try to improve brain function, eliminate toxins, and store reserve energy in the solar plexus region.

The relatively few, limited clinical studies on yoga have been encouraging, showing reduced serum total cholesterol, LDL cholesterol, and triglyceride levels, decreased basal metabolic rates, and improved pulmonary function tests in yoga practitioners (Arambula, Peper, Kawakami, & Gibney, 2001; Birkel, & Edgren, 2000; Chaya, Kurpad, Nagendra, & Nagarathna, 2006; Sarang & Telles, 2006; Schell, Allolio, & Schonecke, 1994; Selvamurthy et al., 1998; Stancak, Kuna, Srinivasan, Dostalek, & Vishnudevananda, 1991; Stanescu, Nemery, Veriter, & Marechal, 1981; Udupa, Singh, & Yadav, 1973). They also suggest that yoga may be associated with acute- and long-term decreases in blood pressure (Murugesan, Govindarajulu, & Bera, 2000; Sundar et al., 1984) and acute increases in brain gamma-aminobutyric (GABA) levels (Streeter et al., 2007). Preliminary evidence indicates that yoga may benefit patients with asthma, hypertension, heart failure, mood disorders, insomnia, migraine headaches, irritable bowel syndrome, end-stage renal disease, and diabetes (Jain, Uppal, Bhatnagar, & Talukdar, 1993; John, Sharma, Sharma, & Kankane, 2007; Khalsa, 2004; Kuttner et al., 2006; Malhotra, Singh, Singh, et al., 2002; Malhotra, Singh, Tandon, et al., 2002; Manocha et al., 2002; van Montfrans, Karemaker, Wieling, & Dunning, 1990a; Yurtkuran, Alp, & Dilek, 2007) and improve pregnancy outcomes (Narendran, Nagarathna, Narendran, Gunasheela, & Nagendra, 2005). Two small controlled, but nondouble-blinded studies showed Hatha Yoga to significantly alleviate pain in osteoarthritis of the fingers and in carpal tunnel syndrome (Garfinkel et al., 1998; Garfinkel, Schumacher, Husain, Levy, & Reshetar, 1994). However, yoga is not completely benign, as certain asanas may be strenuous and cause injury. In fact, yoga practitioners believe some asanas cause disease.

More studies are needed to determine the benefits (and potential dangers) of yoga. Like meditation, many forms of yoga have emerged. Some involve significant aerobic exercise. Others involve significant strength and conditioning work. Many yoga practices include changes in diet and lifestyles. It may be difficult to draw the line between yoga and other practices that have established health benefits, such as exercise. Therefore, future studies should focus on specific yoga forms and movements, and avoid making general conclusions about all yoga practices.

FAITH HEALING

Faith healers use prayer or other religious practices to combat disease. Surveys have found that a fair number of patients in rural (21%) and inner city (10%) populations have used faith healers, and many physicians (23%) believe that faith healers can heal patients (McKee & Chappel, 1992). Despite numerous anecdotes of healing miracles, there has been no consistent and convincing scientific proof that faith healers are effective (King & Bushwick, 1994). Additionally, it has not been determined whether faith healers affect patients psychologically or physiologically, and what factors may make them effective. Conclusions cannot be drawn until further research is performed.

Conclusions and Future Directions

Existing evidence suggests that religious and spiritual practices may have beneficial effects on health. But the reasons behind these findings are not clearly understood. We know that religious and spiritual practices can bring social and emotional support, motivation, healthy lifestyles, and health care resources to their practitioners. However, are there other mechanisms involved? The medical world is just starting to answer this question.

In general, performing clinical studies that can establish cause-and-effect relationships is difficult. This is especially true in the study of religion and health. Confounding factors abound. Religious and spiritual doctrines and practices vary significantly among and within different sects and denominations. Measuring religious and spiritual activity, and monitoring and ensuring compliance among study subjects, are challenging. Moreover, available resources, properly-trained investigators, and institutional support for clinical studies have been scarce. As a result, the current body of medical literature is short on well-designed clinical studies.

Future studies should address a number of different issues. What are the roles of different potential confounding factors? What physiologic mechanisms may be involved? What are the clinical implications of existing physiologic studies? How much does a person's health affect his or her ability to engage in religious and spiritual activities? Do findings hold across different practices, sects, and denominations? Existing studies have only looked at a limited population of religious groups and sects. What are the effects of varying demographic parameters, such as age, gender, and location? How do different practices affect different diseases? Many practices and diseases have not been studied. How should religious and spiritual issues be incorporated into the health care system?

The findings to date already have clinical implications. Religion is clearly important to many patients. Health care providers may need to better address patients' religious concerns, and be aware of how religious involvement can affect patients' symptoms, quality of life, and willingness to receive treatment. Moreover, religious and spiritual activities may serve as adjunct therapy in various disease and addiction treatment programs. The future may see the development of more specific spiritual interventions for particular medical problems.

In the coming years, the study of religion and health, as well as the integration of religion into health care, should continue to grow. New research methods, designs, techniques, and instruments may emerge. As long as the worlds of religion, science, and health care cooperate, many exciting new findings may appear in coming decades, hopefully for the betterment of all.

REFERENCES

Abbotts, J., Williams, R., & Ford, G. (2001). Morbidity and Irish Catholic descent in Britain. Relating health disadvantage to socio-economic position. *Social Science & Medicine, 52*, 999–1005.

Abbotts, J., Williams, R., Ford, G., Hunt, K., & West, P. (1997). Morbidity and Irish Catholic descent in Britain, an ethnic and religious minority 150 years on. *Social Science & Medicine, 45*, 3–14.

Abrahm, J. (2001). Pain management for dying patients. How to assess needs and provide pharmacologic relief. *Postgraduate Medicine, 110*, 99–100, 8–9, 13–4.

Amundsen, D. W. (1982). Medicine and faith in early Christianity. *Bulletin of the History of Medicine, 56*, 326–350.

Arambula, P., Peper, E., Kawakami, M., & Gibney, K. H. (2001). The physiological correlates of Kundalini Yoga meditation: a study of a yoga master. *Applied Psychophysiology and Biofeedback. 26*, 147–153.

Arias, A. J., Steinberg, K., Banga, A., & Trestman, R. L. (2006). Systematic review of the efficacy of meditation techniques as treatments for medical illness. *Journal of Alternative and Complementary Medicine, 12*, 817–832.

Armbruster, C. A., Chibnall, J. T., & Legett, S. (2003). Pediatrician beliefs about spirituality and religion in medicine: associations with clinical practice. *Pediatrics, 111*, e227–e235.

Armstrong, B., van Merwyk, A. J., & Coates, H. (1977). Blood pressure in Seventh-day Adventist vegetarians. *American Journal of Epidemiology, 105*, 444–449.

Arnold, R., Avants, S. K., Margolin, A., & Marcotte, D. (2002). Patient attitudes concerning the inclusion of spirituality into addiction treatment. *Journal of Substance Abuse Treatment, 23*, 319–326.

Aron, A., & Aron, E. N. (1980). The transcendental meditation program's effect on addictive behavior. *Addictive Behaviors, 5*, 3–12.

Asser, S. M., & Swan, R. (1998). Child fatalities from religion-motivated medical neglect. *Pediatrics, 101*, 625–629.

Astin, J. A. (1997). Stress reduction through mindfulness meditation. Effects on psychological symptomatology, sense of control, and spiritual experiences. *Psychotherapy and Psychosomatics, 66*, 97–106.

Astin, J. A., Berman, B. M., Bausell, B., Lee, W. L., Hochberg, M., & Forys, K. L. (2003). The efficacy of mindfulness meditation plus Qigong movement therapy in the treatment of fibromyalgia: a randomized controlled trial. *Journal of Rheumatology, 30*, 2257–2262.

Autiero, A. (1987). The interpretation of pain: the point of view of Catholic theology. *Acta Neurochirurgica Supplement* (Wien), *38*, 123–126.

Avants, S. K., Warburton, L. A., & Margolin, A. (2001). Spiritual and religious support in recovery from addiction among HIV-positive injection drug users. *Journal of Psychoactive Drugs, 33*, 39–45.

Aviles, J. M., Whelan, S. E., Hernke, D. A., Williams, B. A., Kenny, K. E., O'Fallon, W. M., et al. (2001). Intercessory prayer and cardiovascular disease progression in a coronary care unit population: a randomized controlled trial. *Mayo Clinic Proceedings, 76*, 1192–1198.

Azhar, M. Z., & Varma, S. L. (1995). Religious psychotherapy in depressive patients. *Psychotherapy and Psychosomatics, 63*, 165–168.

Azhar, M. Z., Varma, S. L., & Dharap, A. S. (1994). Religious psychotherapy in anxiety disorder patients. *Acta Psychiatrica Scandinavica, 90,* 1–3.

Ball, J., Armistead, L., & Austin, B. J. (2003). The relationship between religiosity and adjustment among African-American, female, urban adolescents. *Journal of Adolescence, 26,* 431–446.

Barrows, K. A., & Jacobs, B. P. (2002). Mind-body medicine. An introduction and review of the literature. *Medical Clinics of North America, 86,* 11–31.

Bassuk, S. S., Glass, T. A., & Berkman, L. F. (1999). Social disengagement and incident cognitive decline in community-dwelling elderly persons. *Annals of Internal Medicine, 131,* 165–173.

Begley, S. (2001). Religion and the brain. *Newsweek, 137,* 50–57.

Begley, S. (2001). Searching for the God within. *Newsweek, 137,* 59.

Benson, H., Dusek, J. A., Sherwood, J. B., Lam, P., Bethea, C. F., Carpenter, W., et al. (2006). Study of the Therapeutic Effects of Intercessory Prayer (STEP) in cardiac bypass patients: a multicenter randomized trial of uncertainty and certainty of receiving intercessory prayer. *American Heart Journal, 151,* 934–942.

Bezilla, R. (Ed.). (1992–1993). *Religion in America.* Princeton, NJ: Princeton Religious Center (Gallup Organization).

Bienenfeld, D., Koenig, H. G., Larson, D. B., & Sherrill, K. A. (1997). Psychosocial predictors of mental health in a population of elderly women. Test of an explanatory model. *American Journal of Geriatric Psychiatry, 5,* 43–53.

Birkel, D. A., & Edgren, L. (2000). Hatha yoga: improved vital capacity of college students. *Alternative Therapies in Health and Medicine, 6,* 55–63.

Bitner, R., Hillman, L., Victor, B., & Walsh, R. (2003). Subjective effects of antidepressants: a pilot study of the varieties of antidepressant-induced experiences in meditators. *Journal of Nervous and Mental Disease, 191,* 660–667.

Blumenthal, J. A., Babyak, M. A., Ironson, G., Thoresen, C., Powell, L., Czajkowski, S., et al. (2007). Spirituality, religion, and clinical outcomes in patients recovering from an acute myocardial infarction. *Psychosomatic Medicine, 69,* 501–508.

Boey, K. W. (2003). Religiosity and psychological well-being of older women in Hong Kong. *International Journal of Psychiatric Nursing Research, 8,* 921–935.

Bowker, D. (1978). Pain and suffering-Religious perspective. In: Reich, W. T., (Ed.), *Encyclopedia of Bioethics.* New York, NY, Free Press, pp. 1185–1189.

Braam, A. W., Beekman, A. T., Deeg, D. J., Smit, J. H., & van Tilburg, W. (1997). Religiosity as a protective or prognostic factor of depression in later life; results from a community survey in The Netherlands. *Acta Psychiatrica Scandinavica, 96,* 199–205.

Braam, A., Beekman, A. T., Deeg, D. J., Smit, J. H., & Van Tilburg, W. (1999). Religiosity as a protective factor in depressive disorder. *American Journal of Psychiatry, 156,* 809; author reply 10.

Brown, C. M. (2000). Exploring the role of religiosity in hypertension management among African Americans. *Journal of Health Care for the Poor and Underserved, 11,* 19–32.

Brush, B. L., & McGee, E. M. (2000). Evaluating the spiritual perspectives of homeless men in recovery. *Applied Nursing Research, 13,* 181–186.

Byrd, R. C. (1988). Positive therapeutic effects of intercessory prayer in a coronary care unit population. *Southern Medical Journal, 81*, 826–829.

Bywaters, P., Ali, Z., Fazil, Q., Wallace, L. M., & Singh, G. (2003). Attitudes towards disability amongst Pakistani and Bangladeshi parents of disabled children in the UK: considerations for service providers and the disability movement. *Journal of Health Care for the Poor and Underserved, 11*, 502–509.

Carlson, L. E., Ursuliak, Z., Goodey, E., Angen, M., & Speca, M. (2001). The effects of a mindfulness meditation-based stress reduction program on mood and symptoms of stress in cancer outpatients: 6-month follow-up. *Support Care Cancer, 9*, 112–123.

Carter, T. M. (1998). The effects of spiritual practices on recovery from substance abuse. *Journal of Psychiatric and Mental Health Nursing, 5*, 409–413.

Castillo-Richmond, A., Schneider, R. H., Alexander, C. N., Cook, R., Myers, H., Nidich, S., et al. (2000). Effects of stress reduction on carotid atherosclerosis in hypertensive African Americans. *Stroke, 31*, 568–573.

Chaya, M. S., Kurpad, A. V., Nagendra, H. R., & Nagarathna, R. (2006). The effect of long term combined yoga practice on the basal metabolic rate of healthy adults. *BMC Complementary and Alternative Medicine, 6*, 28.

Chen, C. Y., Dormitzer, C. M., Bejarano, J., & Anthony, J. C. (2004). Religiosity and the earliest stages of adolescent drug involvement in seven countries of Latin America. *American Journal of Epidemiology, 159*, 1180–1188.

Chen, H., Cheal, K., McDonel Herr, E. C., Zubritsky, C., & Levkoff, S. E. (2007). Religious participation as a predictor of mental health status and treatment outcomes in older persons. *International Journal of Geriatric Psychiatry, 22*, 144–153.

Chibnall, J. T., & Brooks, C. A. (2001). Religion in the clinic: the role of physician beliefs. *Southern Medical Journal, 94*, 374–379.

Coke, M. M. (1992). Correlates of life satisfaction among elderly African Americans. *Journal of Gerontology, 47*, P316–P320.

Collipp, P. J. (1969). The efficacy of prayer: a triple-blind study. *Medical Times, 97*, 201–204.

Comstock, G. W., & Partridge, K. B. (1972). Church attendance and health. *Journal of Chronic Diseases, 25*, 665–672.

Contrada, R. J., Goyal, T. M., Cather, C., Rafalson, L., Idler, E. L., & Krause, T. J. (2004). Psychosocial factors in outcomes of heart surgery: the impact of religious involvement and depressive symptoms. *Health Psychology, 23*, 227–238.

Cooper, M. J., & Aygen, M. M. (1979). A relaxation technique in the management of hypercholesterolemia. *Journal of Human Stress, 5*, 24–27.

Corliss, R. (2001). The power of yoga. *Time, 157*, 54–63.

Coward, D. D. (1991). Self-transcendence and emotional well-being in women with advanced breast cancer. *Oncology Nursing Forum, 18*, 857–863.

Daaleman, T. P., & Nease, D. E., Jr. (1994). Patient attitudes regarding physician inquiry into spiritual and religious issues. *Journal of Family Practice, 39*, 564–568.

de Gouw, H. W., Westendorp, R. G., Kunst, A. E., Mackenbach, J. P., & Vandenbroucke, J. P. (1995). Decreased mortality among contemplative monks in The Netherlands. *American Journal of Epidemiology, 141*, 771–775.

Dermatis, H., Guschwan, M. T., Galanter, M., & Bunt, G. (2004). Orientation toward spirituality and self-help approaches in the therapeutic community. *Journal of Addictive Diseases, 23,* 39–54.

Domino, G. (1977). Transcendental meditation and creativity: an empirical investigation. *Journal of Applied Psychology, 62,* 358–362.

Donahue, M. J. (1985). Intrinsic and extrinsic religiousness: review and meta-analysis. *Journal of Personality and Social Psychology, 48,* 400–419.

Dunne, M. P., Edwards, R., Lucke, J., Donald, M., & Raphael, B. (1994). Religiosity, sexual intercourse and condom use among university students. *Australian Journal of Public Health, 18,* 339–341.

Eisenberg, D. M., Davis, R. B., Ettner, S. L., Appel, S., Wilkey, S., Van Rompay, M., et al. (1998). Trends in alternative medicine use in the United States, 1990-1997: results of a follow-up national survey. *Journal of American Medical Association, 280,* 1569–1575.

Ellis, M. R., Vinson, D. C., & Ewigman, B. (1999). Addressing spiritual concerns of patients: family physicians' attitudes and practices. *Journal of Family Practice, 48,* 105–109.

Enstrom, J. E., & Breslow, L. (2007). Lifestyle and reduced mortality among active California Mormons, 1980–2004. *Preventive Medicine.*

Foley, D. P. (1988). Eleven interpretations of personal suffering. *Journal of Religion and Health, 27,* 321–328.

Forcehimes, A. A. (2004). De profundis: spiritual transformations in Alcoholics Anonymous. *Journal of Clinical Psychology, 60,* 503–517.

Fraser, G. E. (1999). Associations between diet and cancer, ischemic heart disease, and all-cause mortality in non-Hispanic white California Seventh-day Adventists. *American Journal of Clinical Nutrition, 70,* 532S–538S.

Friedlander, Y., Kark, J. D., Kaufmann, N. A., & Stein, Y. (1985). Coronary heart disease risk factors among religious groupings in a Jewish population sample in Jerusalem. *American Journal of Clinical Nutrition, 42,* 511–521.

Friedlander, Y., Kark, J. D., & Stein, Y. (1987). Religious observance and plasma lipids and lipoproteins among 17-year-old Jewish residents of Jerusalem. *Preventive Medicine, 16,* 70–79.

Garfinkel, M. S., Schumacher, H. R., Jr., Husain, A., Levy, M., & Reshetar, R. A. (1994). Evaluation of a yoga based regimen for treatment of osteoarthritis of the hands. *Journal of Rheumatology, 21,* 2341–2343.

Garfinkel, M. S., Singhal, A., Katz, W. A., Allan, D. A., Reshetar, R., & Schumacher, H. R., Jr. (1998;). Yoga-based intervention for carpal tunnel syndrome: a randomized trial. *Journal of American Medical Association, 280,* 1601–1603.

Geisser, M. E., Robinson, M. E., & Henson, C. D. (1994). The Coping Strategies Questionnaire and chronic pain adjustment: a conceptual and empirical reanalysis. *Clinical Journal of Pain, 10,* 98–106.

Gorsuch, R. L., & Butler, M. C. (1976). Initial drug abuse: a review of predisposing social psychological factors. *Psychological Bulletin, 83,* 120–137.

Green, L. L., Fullilove, M. T., & Fullilove, R. E. (1998). Stories of spiritual awakening. The nature of spirituality in recovery. *Journal of Substance Abuse Treatment, 15,* 325–331.

Greenwald, J. (2001). Alternative medicine. A new breed of healers. *Time, 157,* 62–5, 8–9.

Grundmann, E. (1992). Cancer morbidity and mortality in USA Mormons and Seventh-day Adventists. *Archives d'Anatomie Et De Cytologie Pathologiques, 40,* 73–78.

Gupta, R. (1996). Lifestyle risk factors and coronary heart disease prevalence in Indian men. *Journal of the Association of Physicians of India, 44,* 689–693.

Gupta, R., Prakash, H., Gupta, V. P., & Gupta, K. D. (1997). Prevalence and determinants of coronary heart disease in a rural population of India. *Journal of Clinical Epidemiology, 50,* 203–209.

Harris, W. S., Gowda, M., Kolb, J. W., Strychacz, C. P., Vacek, J. L., Jones, P. G., et al. (1999). A randomized, controlled trial of the effects of remote, intercessory prayer on outcomes in patients admitted to the coronary care unit. *Archives of Internal Medicine, 159,* 2273–2278.

Hasnain, M., Sinacore, J. M., Mensah, E. K., & Levy, J. A. (2005). Influence of religiosity on HIV risk behaviors in active injection drug users. *AIDS Care, 17,* 892–901.

Heath, A. C., Madden, P. A., Grant, J. D., McLaughlin, T. L, Todorov, A. A., & Bucholz, K. K. (1999). Resiliency factors protecting against teenage alcohol use and smoking: influences of religion, religious involvement and values, and ethnicity in the Missouri Adolescent Female Twin Study. *Twin Research, 2,* 145–155.

Helm, H. M., Hays, J. C., Flint, E. P., Koenig, H. G., & Blazer, D. G. (2000). Does private religious activity prolong survival? A six-year follow-up study of 3,851 older adults. *Journals of Gerontology. Series A Biological Sciences and Medical Sciences, 55,* M400–M405.

Hill, T. D., Burdette, A. M., Ellison, C. G., & Musick, M. A. (2006). Religious attendance and the health behaviors of Texas adults. *Preventive Medicine, 42,* 309–312.

Hixson, K. A., Gruchow, H. W., & Morgan, D. W. (1998). The relation between religiosity, selected health behaviors, and blood pressure among adult females. *Preventive Medicine, 27,* 545–552.

Ho, S. C., Woo, J., Lau, J., Chan, S. G., Yuen, Y. K., & Chan, Y. K., et al. (1995). Life satisfaction and associated factors in older Hong Kong Chinese. *Journal of the American Geriatrics Society, 43,* 252–255.

Hodges, S. D., Humphreys, S. C., & Eck, J. C. (2002). Effect of spirituality on successful recovery from spinal surgery. *Southern Medical Journal, 95,* 1381–1384.

Holt, C. L., Haire-Joshu, D. L., Lukwago, S. N., Lewellyn, L. A., & Kreuter, M. W. (2005). The role of religiosity in dietary beliefs and behaviors among urban African American women. *Cancer Control, 12*(Suppl 2), 84–90.

House, J. S., Robbins, C., & Metzner, H. L. (1982). The association of social relationships and activities with mortality: prospective evidence from the Tecumseh Community Health Study. *American Journal of Epidemiology, 116,* 123–140.

Hummer, R. A., Rogers, R. G., Nam, C. B., & Ellison, C. G. (1999). Religious involvement and U.S. adult mortality. *Demography, 36,* 273–285.

Idler, E. L., & Kasl, S. V. (1997). Religion among disabled and nondisabled persons II: attendance at religious services as a predictor of the course of disability. *Journals of Gerontology. Series B Psychological Sciences and Social Sciences, 52,* S306–S316.

Idler, E. L., & Kasl, S. V. (1997). Religion among disabled and nondisabled persons I: cross-sectional patterns in health practices, social activities, and well-being. *Journals of Gerontology. Series B Psychological Sciences and Social Sciences, 52*, S294–S305.

Jain, S., Shapiro, S. L., & Swanick, S., Roesch, S. C., Mills, P. J., Bell, I. et al. (2007). A randomized controlled trial of mindfulness meditation versus relaxation training: effects on distress, positive states of mind, rumination, and distraction. *Annals of Behavioral Medicine, 33*, 11–21.

Jain, S. C., Uppal, A., Bhatnagar, S. O., & Talukdar, B. (1993). A study of response pattern of non-insulin dependent diabetics to yoga therapy. *Diabetes Research and Clinical Practice , 19*, 69–74.

John, P. J., Sharma, N., Sharma, C. M., & Kankane, A. (2007). Effectiveness of yoga therapy in the treatment of migraine without aura: a randomized controlled trial. *Headache, 47*, 654–661.

Jones, R. K., Darroch, J. E., & Singh, S. (2005). Religious differentials in the sexual and reproductive behaviors of young women in the United States. *Journal of Adolescent Health, 36*, 279–288.

Kabat-Zinn, J. (1982). An outpatient program in behavioral medicine for chronic pain patients based on the practice of mindfulness meditation: theoretical considerations and preliminary results. *General Hospital Psychiatry, 4*, 33–47.

Kabat-Zinn, J., Lipworth, L., & Burney, R. (1985). The clinical use of mindfulness meditation for the self-regulation of chronic pain. *Journal of Behavioral Medicine, 8*, 163–190.

Kabat-Zinn, J., Massion, A. O., Kristeller, J., Peterson, L. G., Fletcher, K., Pbert, L., et al. (1992). Effectiveness of a meditation-based stress reduction program in the treatment of anxiety disorders. *American Journal of Psychiatry, 149*, 936–943.

Kabat-Zinn, J., Wheeler, E., Light, T., Skillings, A., Scharf, M.S., Cropley, T. G., et al. (1998). Influence of a mindfulness meditation-based stress reduction intervention on rates of skin clearing in patients with moderate to severe psoriasis undergoing phototherapy (UVB) and photochemotherapy (PUVA). *Psychosomatic Medicine, 60*, 625–632.

Kaplan, K. H., Goldenberg, D. L., & Galvin-Nadeau, M. (1993). The impact of a meditation-based stress reduction program on fibromyalgia. *General Hospital Psychiatry, 15*, 284–289.

Kark, J. D., Carmel, S., Sinnreich, R., Goldberger, N., & Friedlander, Y. (1996). Psychosocial factors among members of religious and secular kibbutzim. *Israel Journal of Medical Sciences, 32*, 185–194.

Kark, J. D., Shemi, G., Friedlander, Y., Martin, O., Manor, O., & Blondheim, S. H. (1996). Does religious observance promote health? Mortality in secular vs religious kibbutzim in Israel. *American Journal of Public Health, 86*, 341–346.

Keefer, L., & Blanchard, E. B. (20020. A one year follow-up of relaxation response meditation as a treatment for irritable bowel syndrome. *Behaviour Research and Therapy, 40*, 541–546.

Kennedy, G. J., Kelman, H. R., Thomas, C., & Chen, J. (1996). The relation of religious preference and practice to depressive symptoms among 1,855 older adults. *Journals of Gerontology. Series B Psychological Sciences and Social Sciences, 51*, P301–P308.

Kernberg, O. F. (2003). Sanctioned social violence: a psychoanalytic view. Part II. *International Journal of Psycho-analysis, 84*, 953–968.

Khalsa, S. B. (2004). Treatment of chronic insomnia with yoga: a preliminary study with sleep-wake diaries. *Applied Psychophysiology and Biofeedback, 29*, 269–278.

King, D. E., & Bushwick, B. (1994). Beliefs and attitudes of hospital inpatients about faith healing and prayer. *Journal of Family Practice, 39*, 349–352.

King, D. E., Hueston, W., & Rudy, M. (1994). Religious affiliation and obstetric outcome. *Southern Medical Journal, 87*, 1125–1128.

King, M. S., Carr, T., & D'Cruz, C. (2002). Transcendental meditation, hypertension and heart disease. *Australian Family Physician, 31*, 164–168.

Koenig, H. G. (1998). Religious attitudes and practices of hospitalized medically ill older adults. *International Journal of Geriatric Psychiatry, 13*, 213–224.

Koenig, H. G., George, L. K., Cohen, H. J., Hays, J. C., Larson, D. B., & Blazer, D. G. (1998). The relationship between religious activities and cigarette smoking in older adults. *Journals of Gerontology. Series A Biological Sciences and Medical Sciences, 53*, M426–M434.

Koenig, H. G., George, L. K., Hays, J. C., Larson, D. B., Cohen, H. J., & Blazer, D. G. (1998). The relationship between religious activities and blood pressure in older adults. *International Journal of Psychiatry in Medicineicine, 28*, 189–213.

Koenig, H. G., George, L. K., & Peterson, B. L. (1998). Religiosity and remission of depression in medically ill older patients. *American Journal of Psychiatry, 155*, 536–542.

Koenig, H. G., Hays, J. C., George, L. K., Blazer, D. G., Larson, D. B., & Landerman, L. R. (1997). Modeling the cross-sectional relationships between religion, physical health, social support, and depressive symptoms. *American Journal of Geriatric Psychiatry, 5*, 131–144.

Koenig, H. G., Hays, J. C., Larson, D. B., George, L. K., Cohen, H. J., McCullough, M. E., et al. (1999). Does religious attendance prolong survival? A six-year follow-up study of 3,968 older adults. *Journals of Gerontology. Series A Biological Sciences and Medical Sciences, 54*, M370–M376.

Krause, N. (2003). Religious meaning and subjective well-being in late life. *Journals of Gerontology. Series B Psychological Sciences and Social Sciences, 58*, S160–S170.

Kuhn, C. C. (1988). A spiritual inventory of the medically ill patient. *Psychiatric Medicine, 6*, 87–100.

Kune, G. A., Kune, S., & Watson, L. F. (1992). The effect of family history of cancer, religion, parity and migrant status on survival in colorectal cancer. The Melbourne Colorectal Cancer Study. *European Journal of Cancer, 28A*, 1484–1487.

Kune, G. A., Kune, S., & Watson, L. F. (1993). Perceived religiousness is protective for colorectal cancer: data from the Melbourne Colorectal Cancer Study. *Journal of the Royal Society of Medicine, 86*, 645–647.

Kuttner, L., Chambers, C. T., Hardial, J., Israel, D. M., Jacobson, K., & Evans, K. (2006). A randomized trial of yoga for adolescents with irritable bowel syndrome. *Pain Research and Management, 11*, 217–223.

Kutz, I. Samson, the Bible, and the DSM. (2002). *Archives of General Psychiatry, 59*, 565; author reply, 6.

La Pierre, L. L. (2003). JCAHO safeguards spiritual care. *Holistic Nursing Practice, 17,* 219.

Larson, D. B., & Wilson, W. P. (1980). Religious life of alcoholics. *Southern Medical Journal, 73,* 723–727.

Lefkowitz, E. S., Boone, T. L., Au, T. K., & Sigman, M. (2003). No sex or safe sex? Mothers' and adolescents' discussions about sexuality and AIDS/HIV. *Health Education and Research, 18,* 341–351.

Leibovici, L. (2001). Effects of remote, retroactive intercessory prayer on outcomes in patients with bloodstream infection: randomised controlled trial. *British Medical Journal, 323,* 1450–1451.

Leigh, J., Bowen, S., & Marlatt, G. A. (2005). Spirituality, mindfulness and substance abuse. *Addictive Behaviors, 30,* 1335–1341

Levin, J., & Markides, K. (1988). Religious attendance and psychological well-being in middle-aged and older Mexican Americans. *Sociological Analysis, 49,* 66–72.

Levin, J. S. (1996). How religion influences morbidity and health: reflections on natural history, salutogenesis and host resistance. *Social Science & Medicine, 43,* 849–864.

Levin, J. S., Larson, D. B., & Puchalski, C. M. (1997). Religion and spirituality in medicine: research and education. *Journal of American Medical Association, 278,* 792–793.

Li, E. C., Feifer, C., & Strohm, M. (2000). A pilot study: locus of control and spiritual beliefs in alcoholics anonymous and smart recovery members. *Addictive Behaviors, 25,* 633–640.

Lichtenstein, B. (2003). Stigma as a barrier to treatment of sexually transmitted infection in the American deep south: issues of race, gender and poverty. *Social Science & Medicine, 57,* 2435–2445.

Lo, B., Quill, T., & Tulsky, J. (1999). Discussing palliative care with patients. ACP-ASIM End-of-Life Care Consensus Panel. American College of Physicians-American Society of Internal Medicine. *Annals of Internal Medicine, 130,* 744–749.

Lo, B., Ruston, D., & Kates, L.W., et al. (2002). Discussing religious and spiritual issues at the end of life: a practical guide for physicians. *Journal of American Medical Association, 287,* 749–754.

Loprinzi, C. L., Laurie, J. A., Wieand, H. S., Krook, J. E., Novotny, P. J., Kugler, J. W., et al. (1994). Prospective evaluation of prognostic variables from patient-completed questionnaires. North Central Cancer Treatment Group. *Journal of Clinical Oncology, 12,* 601–607.

Luczak, S. E., Shea, S. H., Carr, L. G., Li, T. K., & Wall, T. L. (2002). Binge drinking in Jewish and non-Jewish white college students. *Alcoholism, Clinical and Experimental Research, 26,* 1773–1778.

Lukoff, D., Lu, F., & Turner, R. (1992). Toward a more culturally sensitive DSM-IV. Psychoreligious and psychospiritual problems. *Journal of Nervous and Mental Disease, 180,* 673–682.

Lyttle, T. (1988). Drug based religions and contemporary drug taking. *Journal of Drug Issues, 18,* 271–284.

MacLean, C. D., Susi, B., Phifer, N., Schultz, L., Bynum, D., Franco, M., et al. (2003). Patient preference for physician discussion and practice of spirituality. *Journal of General Internal Medicine, 18,* 38–43.

Madru, N. (2003). Stigma and HIV: does the social response affect the natural course of the epidemic? *Journal of the Association of Nurses in AIDS Care* , *14*, 39–48.

Malhotra, V., Singh, S., Singh, K. P., Gupta, P., Sharma, S. B., Madhu, S. V., et al. (2002). Study of yoga asanas in assessment of pulmonary function in NIDDM patients. *Indian Journal of Physiology and Pharmacology, 46*, 313–320.

Malhotra, V., Singh, S., Tandon, O. P., Madhu, S. V., Prasad, A., & Sharma, S. B. (2002). Effect of yoga asanas on nerve conduction in type 2 diabetes. *Indian Journal of Physiology and Pharmacology, 46*, 298–306.

Manheimer, E., Anderson, B. J., & Stein, M. D. (2003). Use and assessment of complementary and alternative therapies by intravenous drug users. *American Journal of Drug Alcohol Abuse, 29*, 401–413.

Manocha, R., Marks, G. B., Kenchington, P., Peters, D., & Salome, C. M. (2002). Sahaja yoga in the management of moderate to severe asthma: a randomised controlled trial. *Thorax, 57*, 110–115.

Markides, K. S., Levin, J. S., & Ray, L. A. (1987). Religion, aging, and life satisfaction: an eight-year, three-wave longitudinal study. *Gerontologist, 27*, 660–665.

Matthews, D. A., & Clark, C. (1998). *The faith factor: proof of the healing power of prayer.* New York, NY: Viking (Penguin-Putnam).

Matthews, D. A., Marlowe, S. M., & MacNutt, F. S. (2000). Effects of intercessory prayer on patients with rheumatoid arthritis. *Southern Medical Journal, 93*, 1177–1186.

Matthews, D. A., McCullough, M. E., Larson, D. B., Koenig, H. G., Swyers, J. P., & Milano, M. G. (1998). Religious commitment and health status: a review of the research and implications for family medicine. *Archives of Family Medicine, 7*, 118–124.

Matthews, W. J., Conti, J. M., & Sireci, S. G. (2001). The effects of intercessory prayer, positive visualization, and expectancy on the well-being of kidney dialysis patients. *Alternative Therapies in Health and Medicine, 7*, 42–52.

McCormick, N., Izzo, A., & Folcik, J. (1985). Adolescents' values, sexuality, and contraception in a rural New York county. *Adolescence, 20*, 385–395.

McCree, D. H., Wingood, G. M., DiClemente, R., Davies, S., & Harrington, K. F. (2003). Religiosity and risky sexual behavior in African-American adolescent females. *Journal of Adolescent Health, 33*, 2–8.

McCullough, M. E., & Larson, D. B. (1999). Religion and depression: a review of the literature. *Twin Research, 2*, 126–136.

McCullough, M. E., Hoyt, W. T., Larson, D. B., Koenig, H. G., & Thoresen, C. (2000). Religious involvement and mortality: a meta-analytic review. *Health Psychology, 19*, 211–222.

McKee, D. D., & Chappel, J. N. (1992). Spirituality and medical practice. *Journal of Family Practice, 35*, 201, 5–8.

McLane, S., Lox, C. L., Butki, B., & Stern, L. (2003). An investigation of the relation between religion and exercise motivation. *Perceptual and Motor Skills, 97*, 1043–1048.

Merrill, R. M., & Thygerson, A. L. (2001). Religious preference, church activity, and physical exercise. *Preventive Medicine, 33*, 38–45.

Miller, L., Davies, M., & Greenwald, S. (2000). Religiosity and substance use and abuse among adolescents in the National Comorbidity Survey. *Journal of the American Academy of Child and Adolescent Psychiatry, 39*, 1190–1197.

Miller, L., & Gur, M. (2002). Religiousness and sexual responsibility in adolescent girls. *Journal of Adolescent Health, 31*, 401–406.

Miller, L., Warner, V., Wickramaratne, P., & Weissman, M. (1997). Religiosity and depression: ten-year follow-up of depressed mothers and offspring. *Journal of the American Academy of Child and Adolescent Psychiatry, 36*, 1416–1425.

Miller, W. R. (1998). Researching the spiritual dimensions of alcohol and other drug problems. *Addiction, 93*, 979–990.

Miller, W. R., & Thoresen, C.E. (2003). Spirituality, religion, and health. An emerging research field. *American Psychologist , 58*, 24–35.

Mitchell, J., Lannin, D. R., Mathews, H. F., & Swanson, M. S. (2002). Religious beliefs and breast cancer screening. *Journal of Womens Health* (Larchmt), *11*, 907–915.

Monroe, M. H., Bynum, D., Susi, B., Phifer, N., Schultz, L., Franco, M., et al. (2003). Primary care physician preferences regarding spiritual behavior in medical practice. *Archives of Internal Medicine, 163*, 2751–2756.

Moriarity, J. (2001). The spiritual roots of AA. *Minnesota Medicine, 84*, 10.

Morse, J. M., & Proctor, A. (1998). Maintaining patient endurance. The comfort work of trauma nurses. *Clinical Nursing Research, 7*, 250–274.

Murphy, T. J., Pagano, R. R., & Marlatt, G. A. (1986). Lifestyle modification with heavy alcohol drinkers: effects of aerobic exercise and meditation. *Addictive Behaviors, 11*, 175–186.

Murugesan, R., Govindarajulu, N., & Bera, T. K. (2000). Effect of selected yogic practices on the management of hypertension. *Indian Journal of Physiology and Pharmacology, 44*, 207–210.

Musick, M. A., Koenig, H. G., Hays, J. C., & Cohen, H. J. (1998). Religious activity and depression among community-dwelling elderly persons with cancer: the moderating effect of race. *Journals of Gerontology. Series B Psychological Sciences and Social Sciences, 53*, S218–S227.

Narendran, S., Nagarathna, R., Narendran, V., Gunasheela, S., & Nagendra, H. R. (2005). Efficacy of yoga on pregnancy outcome. *Journal of Alternative and Complementary Medicine, 11*, 237–244.

Neeleman, J., Halpern, D., Leon, D., & Lewis, G. (1997). Tolerance of suicide, religion and suicide rates: an ecological and individual study in 19 Western countries. *Psychological Medicine , 27*, 1165–1171.

Neeleman, J., & Lewis, G. (1999). Suicide, religion, and socioeconomic conditions. An ecological study in 26 countries, 1990. *Journal of Epidemiology and Community Health, 53*, 204–210.

Neeleman, J., Wessely, S., & Lewis, G. (1998). Suicide acceptability in African- and white Americans: the role of religion. *Journal of Nervous and Mental Disease, 186*, 12–16.

Nisbet, P. A., Duberstein, P. R., Conwell, Y., & Seidlitz, L. (2000). The effect of participation in religious activities on suicide versus natural death in adults 50 and older. *Journal of Nervous and Mental Disease, 188*, 543–546.

O'Laoire, S. (1997). An experimental study of the effects of distant, intercessory prayer on self-esteem, anxiety, and depression. *Alternative Therapies in Health and Medicine, 3*, 38–53.

Oleckno, W. A., & Blacconiere, M. J. (1991). Relationship of religiosity to wellness and other health-related behaviors and outcomes. *Psychological Reports, 68*, 819–826.

Oman, D., Kurata, J. H., Strawbridge, W. J., & Cohen, R. D. (2002). Religious attendance and cause of death over 31 years. *International Journal of Psychiatry in Medicine, 32,* 69–89.

Oman, D., & Reed, D. (1998). Religion and mortality among the community-dwelling elderly. *American Journal of Public Health, 88,* 1469–1475.

Oxman, T. E., Freeman, D. H., Jr., & Manheimer, E. D. (1995). Lack of social participation or religious strength and comfort as risk factors for death after cardiac surgery in the elderly. *Psychosomatic Medicine, 57,* 5–15.

Patel, S. S., Shah, V. S., Peterson, R. A., & Kimmel, P. L. (2002). Psychosocial variables, quality of life, and religious beliefs in ESRD patients treated with hemodialysis. *American Journal of Kidney Disease, 40,* 1013–1022.

Pettus, M. C. (2002). Implementing a medicine-spirituality curriculum in a community-based internal medicine residency program. *Academic Medicine, 77,* 745.

Poloma, M., & Pendleton, B. (1991). The effects of prayer and prayer experience on measures of general well being. *Journal of Psychology and Theology, 10,* 71–83.

Poulson, R. L., Eppler, M. A., Satterwhite, T. N., Wuensch, K. L., & Bass, L. A. (1998). Alcohol consumption, strength of religious beliefs, and risky sexual behavior in college students. *Journal of American College Health, 46,* 227–232.

Powell, L. H., Shahabi, L., & Thoresen, C. E. (2003). Religion and spirituality. Linkages to physical health. *American Psychologist, 58,* 36–52.

Pressman, P., Lyons, J. S., Larson, D. B., & Strain, J. J. (1990). Religious belief, depression, and ambulation status in elderly women with broken hips. *American Journal of Psychiatry, 147,* 758–760.

Proctor, A., Morse, J. M., & Khonsari, E. S. (1996). Sounds of comfort in the trauma center: how nurses talk to patients in pain. *Social Science & Medicine, 42,* 1669–1680.

Propst, L. R., Ostrom, R., Watkins, P., Dean, T., & Mashburn, D. (1992). Comparative efficacy of religious and nonreligious cognitive-behavioral therapy for the treatment of clinical depression in religious individuals. *Journal of Consulting and Clinical Psychology, 60,* 94–103.

Purcell, B. C. (1998). Spiritual abuse. *American Journal of Hospice & Palliative Care, 15,* 227–231.

Purcell, B. C. (1998). Spiritual terrorism. *American Journal of Hospice & Palliative Care, 15,* 167–173.

Raleigh, E. D. (1992). Sources of hope in chronic illness. *Oncology Nursing Forum, 19,* 443–448.

Rapp, S. R., Rejeski, W. J., & Miller, M. E. (2000). Physical function among older adults with knee pain: the role of pain coping skills. *Arthritis Care and Research, 13,* 270–279.

Rasanen, J., Kauhanen, J., Lakka, T. A., Kaplan, G. A., & Salonen, J. T. (1996). Religious affiliation and all-cause mortality: a prospective population study in middle-aged men in eastern Finland. *International Journal of Epidemiology, 25,* 1244–1249.

Razali, S. M., Hasanah, C. I., Aminah, K., & Subramaniam, M. (1998). Religious-sociocultural psychotherapy in patients with anxiety and depression. *Australian and New Zealand Journal of Psychiatry, 32,* 867–872.

Reibel, D. K., Greeson, J. M., Brainard, G. C., & Rosenzweig, S. (2001). Mindfulness-based stress reduction and health-related quality of life in a heterogeneous patient population. *General Hospital Psychiatry, 23,* 183–192.

Ringdal, G. I., Gotestam, K. G., Kaasa, S., Kvinnsland, S., & Ringdal, K. (1996). Prognostic factors and survival in a heterogeneous sample of cancer patients. *British Journal of Cancer, 73,* 1594–1599.

Roberts, L., Ahmed, I., & Hall, S. (2007). Intercessory prayer for the alleviation of ill health. *Cochrane Database of Systematic Reviews,* CD000368.

Roky, R., Houti, I., Moussamih, S., Qotbi, S., & Aadil, N. (2004). Physiological and chronobiological changes during Ramadan intermittent fasting. *Annals of Nutrition & Metabolism, 48,* 296–303.

Rossetti, S. J. (1995). The impact of child sexual abuse on attitudes toward God and the Catholic Church. *Child Abuse & Neglect, 19,* 1469–1481.

Sarang, P. S., & Telles, S. (2006). Oxygen consumption and respiration during and after two yoga relaxation techniques. *Applied Psychophysiology and Biofeedback, 31,* 143–153.

Sarri, K., Linardakis, M., Codrington, C., & Kafatos, A. (2007). Does the periodic vegetarianism of Greek Orthodox Christians benefit blood pressure? *Preventive Medicine, 44,* 341–348.

Satterly, L. (2001). Guilt, shame, and religious and spiritual pain. *Holistic Nursing Practice, 15,* 30–39.

Schell, F. J., Allolio, B., & Schonecke, O. W. (1994). Physiological and psychological effects of Hatha-Yoga exercise in healthy women. *International Journal of Psychosomatics, 41,* 46–52.

Selvamurthy, W., Sridharan, K., Ray, U. S., Tiwary, R. S., Hegde, K. S.,. Radhakrishan, U., et al. (1998). A new physiological approach to control essential hypertension. *Indian Journal of Physiology and Pharmacology, 42,* 205–213.

Shaffer, J. A. (1978). Pain and suffering: philosophical perspectives. In: Reich, W. T. (Ed.), *Encyclopedia of bioethics.* New York, NY: Free Press, pp. 1181–1185.

Shuler, P. A., Gelberg, L., & Brown, M. (1994). The effects of spiritual/religious practices on psychological well-being among inner city homeless women. *Nurse Practitioner Forum, 5,* 106–113.

Sloan, R. P., & Bagiella, E. (2002). Claims about religious involvement and health outcomes. *Annals of Behavioral Medicine, 24,* 14–21.

Sloan, R. P., Bagiella, E., & Powell, T. (1999). Religion, spirituality, and medicine. *Lancet, 353,* 664–667.

Solberg, E. E., Berglund, K. A., Engen, O., Ekeberg, O., & Loeb, M. (1996). The effect of meditation on shooting performance. *British Journal of Sports Medicine, 30,* 342–346.

Stancak, A., Jr., Kuna, M., Srinivasan, Dostalek , C., & Vishnudevananda, S. (1991). Kapalabhati—yogic cleansing exercise. II. EEG topography analysis. *Homeostasis in Health and Disease, 33,* 182–189.

Stanescu, D. C., Nemery, B., Veriter, C., & Marechal, C. (1981). Pattern of breathing and ventilatory response to CO_2 in subjects practicing hatha-yoga. *Journal of Applied Physiology, 51*, 1625–1629.

Stefanek, M., McDonald, P. G., & Hess, S. A. (2004). Religion, spirituality and cancer: Current status and methodological challenges. *Psychooncology, 14, 450–463.*

Stewart, C. (2001). The influence of spirituality on substance use of college students. *Journal of Drug Education, 31, 343–351.*

Strawbridge, W. J., Cohen, R. D., Shema, S. J., & Kaplan, G. A. (1997). Frequent attendance at religious services and mortality over 28 years. *American Journal of Public Health, 87, 957–961.*

Streeter, C. C., Jensen, J. E., Perlmutter, R. M., Cabral, H. J., Tian, H., Terhune, D. B., et al. (2007). Yoga Asana sessions increase brain GABA levels: a pilot study. *Journal of Alternative and Complementary Medicine, 13, 419–426.*

Stylianou, S. (2004). The role of religiosity in the opposition to drug use. *International Journal of Offender Therapy and Comparative Criminology, 48, 429–448.*

Sundar, S., Agrawal, S. K., Singh, V. P., Bhattacharya, S. K., Udupa, K. N., & Vaish, S. K. (1984). Role of yoga in management of essential hypertension. *Acta Cardiologica, 39,* 203–208.

Swartzman, L. C., Gwadry, F. G., Shapiro, A. P., & Teasell, R. W. (1994). The factor structure of the Coping Strategies Questionnaire. *Pain, 57,* 311–316.

Swimmer, G. I., Robinson, M. E., & Geisser, M. E. (1992). Relationship of MMPI cluster type, pain coping strategy, and treatment outcome. *Clinical Journal of Pain, 8,* 131–137.

Tanyi, R. A. (2002). Towards clarification of the meaning of spirituality. *Journal of Advanced Nursing, 39,* 500–509.

The Gallup Report: Religion in America:1993–1994. (1994). Princeton, NJ: Gallup Poll.

Tieman, J. (2002). Priest scandal hits hospitals. As pedophilia reports grow, church officials suspend at least six hospital chaplains in an effort to address alleged sexual abuse. *Modern Healthcare, 32,* 6–7, 14, 1.

Tonigan, J. S., Miller, W. R., & Schermer, C. (2002). Atheists, agnostics and Alcoholics Anonymous. *Journal of Studies on Alcohol, 63,* 534–541.

Townsend, M., Kladder, V., Ayele, H., & Mulligan, T. (2002). Systematic review of clinical trials examining the effects of religion on health. *Southern Medical Journal, 95,* 1429–1434.

Tu, W. (1980). A religiophilosophical perspective on pain. In: Koster, H. W., Kosterlitz, D., Terenius, L. Y. (Eds.), *Pain and society.* Verlag Chemie, Weinheim-Deerfield Beach, Florida, pp. 63–78.

Turner, R. P., Lukoff, D., Barnhouse, R. T., & Lu, F. G. (1995). Religious or spiritual problem. A culturally sensitive diagnostic category in the DSM-IV. *Journal of Nervous and Mental Disease, 183,* 435–444.

Udupa, K. N., Singh, R. H., & Yadav, R. A. (1973). Certain studies on psychological and biochemical responses to the practice in Hatha Yoga in young normal volunteers. *Indian Journal of Medical Research, 61,* 237–244.

van Montfrans, G. A., Karemaker, J. M., Wieling, W., & Dunning, A. J. (1990a). Relaxation therapy and continuous ambulatory blood pressure in mild hypertension: a controlled study. *British Medical Journal, 300,* 1368–1372.

van Montfrans, G. A., Karemaker, J. M., Wieling, W., & Dunning, A. J. (1990b). Yoga and massage: If it's physical, it's therapy. *Newsweek, 140,* 74–75.

Van Ness, P. H., Kasl, S. V., & Jones, B. A. (2003). Religion, race, and breast cancer survival. *International Journal of Psychiatry in Medicineicine, 33,* 357–375.

Van Poppel, F., Schellekens, J., & Liefbroer, A. C. (2002). Religious differentials in infant and child mortality in Holland, 1855–1912. *Population Studies* (Camb), *56,* 277–289.

Walker, S. R., Tonigan, J. S., Miller, W. R., Corner, S., & Kahlich, L. (1997). Intercessory prayer in the treatment of alcohol abuse and dependence: a pilot investigation. *Alternative Therapies in Health and Medicine, 3,* 79–86.

Wallace, R. K., Silver, J., Mills, P. J., Dillbeck, M. C., & Wagoner, D. E. (1983). Systolic blood pressure and long-term practice of the Transcendental Meditation and TM-Sidhi program: effects of TM on systolic blood pressure. *Psychosomatic Medicine, 45,* 41–46.

Walls, P., & Williams, R. (2004). Accounting for Irish Catholic ill health in Scotland: a qualitative exploration of some links between "religion," class and health. *Sociology of Health & Illness, 26,* 527–556.

Walsh, A. (1998). Religion and hypertension: testing alternative explanations among immigrants. *Behavioral Medicine, 24,* 122–130.

Walton, K. G., Pugh, N. D., Gelderloos, P., & Macrae, P. (1995). Stress reduction and preventing hypertension: preliminary support for a psychoneuroendocrine mechanism. *Journal of Alternative and Complementary Medicine, 1,* 263–283.

Weaver, A. J., Koenig, H. K., Flannelly, K. J., et al. (2003). Spiritual assessment required in all settings. *Hospital Peer Review, 28,* 55–56.

Wenneberg, S. R., Schneider, R. H., MacLean, C., Levitsky, D. K., Walton, K. G., Mandarino, J. V., et al. (1997). A controlled study of the effects of the Transcendental Meditation program on cardiovascular reactivity and ambulatory blood pressure. *International Journal of Neuroscience, 89,* 15–28.

Wilcox, S., Laken, M., & Bopp, M., Gethers, O., Huang, P., McClorin, L., et al. (2007). Increasing physical activity among church members: community-based participatory research. *American Journal of Preventive Medicine, 32,* 131–138.

Williams, D. R., Larson, D. B., Buckler, R. E., Heckmann, R. C., & Pyle, C. M. (1991). Religion and psychological distress in a community sample. *Social Science & Medicine, 32,* 1257–1262.

Williams, K. A., Kolar, M. M., Reger, B. E., & Pearson, J. C. (2001). Evaluation of a wellness-based mindfulness stress reduction intervention: a controlled trial. *American Journal of Health Promotion, 15,* 422–432.

Woodward, K. L. (2001). Faith is more than a feeling. *Newsweek, 137,* 58.

Yates, J. W., Chalmer, B. J., St. James, P., Follansbee, M., & McKegney, F. P. (1981). Religion in patients with advanced cancer. *Medical and Pediatric Oncology, 9,* 121–128.

Yoon, D. P., & Lee, E. K. (2007). The impact of religiousness, spirituality, and social support on psychological well-being among older adults in rural areas. *Journal of Gerontology and Social Work, 48,* 281–298.

Young, D. R., & Stewart, K. J. (2006). A church-based physical activity intervention for African American women. *Family Community Health, 29,* 103–117.

Yurtkuran, M., Alp, A., & Dilek, K. (2007). A modified yoga-based exercise program in hemodialysis patients: a randomized controlled study. *Complementary Therapies in Medicine, 15,* 164–171.

Zaleski, E. H., & Schiaffino, K. M. (2000). Religiosity and sexual risk-taking behavior during the transition to college. *Journal of Adolescence, 23,* 223–227.

Zollinger, T. W., Phillips, R. L., & Kuzma, J. W. (1984). Breast cancer survival rates among Seventh-day Adventists and non-Seventh-day Adventists. *American Journal of Epidemiology, 119,* 503–509.

18

Synchronicity and Healing

BERNARD D. BEITMAN, ELIF CELEBI,
AND STEPHANIE L. COLEMAN

KEY CONCEPTS

- Jung defined synchronicity as coincidence in time of two or more causally unrelated events which have the same or similar meaning.
- The term "synchron" refers to a single coincidence event that is characterized by (1) low probability, (2) mind–environment connection, (3) similarity or parallel, (4) increased emotional intensity, and (5) ambiguity of meaning.
- Aside from probability and statistics, theories of synchronicity are derived from ideas beyond current scientific causality principles including archetypes, nonlocality, and econmens as well as theological explanations.
- Higher frequency synchron detectors tend to be more spiritual and religious.
- During psychotherapy the discussion of synchrons can (1) reassure patients that these are common experiences, (2) help strengthen the working alliance, (3) engender feelings of spirituality and gratitude, and (4) increase awareness of subjective–contextual connections.
- Patient problems sometimes closely parallel therapist problems offering the possibility of furthering psychological development for each participant.

As a psychiatrist organizes the history of her similarly aged patient, it becomes apparent that she and one of her patients share almost identical problems with their fathers-in-law. Both psychiatrist and patient are currently confronting an overbearing, critical, intrusive man who is interfering with their respective spousal relationships. The psychiatrist had also recently heard a colleague mention that "my problems walk into my office," which meant that perhaps this is not an isolated incident for clinical psychiatrists and other mental health professionals. In addition, she had read that reports by the general public of meaningful coincidences were increasing. As an English literature major, she had touched upon the use of coincidence in nineteenth century English literature, including the novels of Charles Dickens and Jane Austen (e.g., Dannenberg, 2004).

Typically these occurrences are called just coincidence, fate, chance, happenstance, serendipity, or cited as examples of God influencing the world or the interconnectedness of human minds. They can also represent symptoms associated with ideas of reference and psychosis. The event was very meaningful to the psychiatrist and fit into a broad, commonly experienced set of meaningful coincidences called "synchronicity," a term coined by Carl Jung (1973). By working with this patient with a similar problem, the psychiatrist had the opportunity to observe parallel emotional responses, and the consequences of those responses before she, herself, attempted to address her own similar situation.

In the past 20 years, the number of books and papers on meaningful coincidences has expanded exponentially (Figure 18.1). This chapter summarizes some key philosophical concepts and research findings related to these types of events,

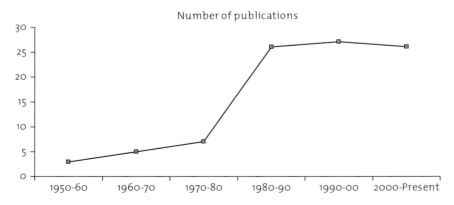

FIGURE 18.1. Number of journal articles and books on synchronicity as a function of the date of publication between 1950 and 2006.

which often are referred to as "synchronicities," or as being "synchronistic." We explore the ramifications of personal meanings ascribed to such events, and consider the potential utility of discussing them with patients in the clinical setting.

Why this on-going interest? We can look to the development of Integrative Medicine for a clue. In regard to meeting the multidimensional needs of patients, allopathic medicine has clear limitations in the many specialties covered in this Oxford Integrative Medicine Series. The introduction of old and new paradigms into Western medicine concepts is invigorating our practices. Similarly, the psychotherapy paradigms, while quite useful, are generally limited cause–effect models of Freudian psychoanalysis and Cognitive-Behavior therapy, and might benefit from an expansion of current paradigm limits. Integrative medicine often incorporates principles, concepts, and philosophies of ancient times and healing approaches from non-Western lands, many of which embrace the idea that a single human mind is not distinctly separate from other minds or from its surroundings. Furthermore, integrative medicine recognizes the importance of spirituality as a component of health and wellness. In this chapter we consider the possibility that the everyday occurrence of meaningful coincidences provides a useful means of helping us to navigate the often troublesome waters of daily life and can add a vital transpersonal dimension to the practice of psychotherapy.

We begin with the concept of synchronicity and a proposed definition. Next, we present brief descriptions of several of its many theoretical explanations and end with the recognition that, while we have no satisfactory explanation for it, synchronicity may offer several benefits, including encouragement, psychological insight, guidance, confirmation of decisions, and increased spirituality. We then provide a brief overview of synchronicity- related research, with major emphasis on our *Weird Coincidence Survey*. Finally, we address the problem of interpreting synchronicities, followed by their potential use in psychotherapy and implications for future research.

Concept of Synchronicity

Each human life is intersected by chance events. Each chance event appears, by definition, as unlikely and unpredictable. Yet the likelihood of chance events occurring in one's daily life remains quite high. When two or more chance events are interrelated in a way that has personal meaning, most people disregard the association as coincidence.

Our lives are marked by the intersections of events—meeting a friend, arriving on time, reading a book, finding a job, falling in love, appreciating a sunset, discovering useful information.

The simultaneous occurrence of two events would not generally be called a coincidence. For example, seeing lightning and then hearing thunder would be considered a causal relationship. Hearing an air conditioner turn on at the same time someone starts speaking would appear to be unrelated events happening at the same time and not called a coincidence. We recognize that the lightening caused the thunder and that there was no causal connection between the speaker and the air conditioner. The speaker and air conditioner would not usually be considered to be related to each other.

There also are times when two co-occurring events may not be "just a coincidence." They may at first seem unrelated, yet, depending upon the perceived similarity as well as the emotion the connection generates, the events could possibly be related. Such thinking might form the subtext of paranoid thinking, or it could present a sharper view of what may be really going on. For example, a woman learns that her husband decides to make a quick trip to Chicago just when her best friend is leaving for Chicago. Just a coincidence?

The term "coincidence" is reserved for two or more events occurring in close physical or temporal proximity that seem to be surprisingly related. One of your patients arriving at the time of his appointment does not qualify as a coincidence. There must be some mystery, something unexplained to make it surprising. The quality of surprise may initiate a search for meaning. If you run into a patient at a Farmer's Market at which you rarely shop, the coincidence is likely to be surprising but not particularly meaningful to you. If the patient has paranoid tendencies, he might read a great deal of significance into the chance encounter. Optimal use of coincidences requires the ability to consider how they might have personal meaning while at the same time not over-interpreting or over-valuing them. The meaningfulness of a coincidence is to be found in the eyes of the beholder (Hopke, 1997, pp. 19–21). The same scene in a television show or movie can elicit varying responses from different viewers. Similarly, some coincidences elicit strong emotional responses, while others generate "so what?" responses. The degree of meaningfulness can be reflected by the intensity of the experiencer's emotional response. This emotional response may then be "unpacked" for its particular significance.

Jung defined synchronicity in many different ways. (For a thorough review of Jung's various definitions, see Clark, 1996.) His classical definition of synchronicity was "a coincidence in time of two or more causally unrelated events which have the same or similar meaning" (Jung, 1973). One event is in the mind, the other in the environment. There is a conjunction between inner and outer states: between thoughts, feelings, and images in one's mind and features of and events in one's environment. His most often-quoted example involves the appearance of a scarab-like beetle at the window of his consulting room at the same time that a resistant patient was describing a dream involving a scarab.

The startling simultaneity, according to Jung, broke the therapeutic impasse, thereby freeing the patient to explore her unconscious more fully than she had before the event (Jung, 1973). While many meaningful coincidences involve parallels between inner and outer worlds, many others, outside the classical Jungian definition, occur *between* minds or involve meaningfully related external events (Main, 2007, pp. 18–19). Some people report having the same dream—an example of mind-to-mind synchronicities (Ryback & Sweitzer, 1988). The same number or idea repeatedly appearing in external reality provides an example of outer–outer synchronicities (Kammerer, 1919).

Jung also insisted that simultaneity be a distinguishing feature of synchronicity, as illustrated by the scarab dream story in which the beetle appeared at the window just as the dreamer was describing the scarab in the dream. While simultaneity often startles an experiencer to pay attention, many coincidences take place in sequence—hours or days later, or perhaps even months or years— that could still qualify. For example, Main described a man who, while immersing himself in Zechariah's vision of the four horsemen, whose horses were red, black, dapple, and white, went out on the balcony of his hotel to be greeted with four horses (red, black, dapple, and white) grazing below. Eleven months later, while exploring a natural area, he turned to see grazing nearby another 4 horses of the same colors. The coincidences astounded him.

In his discussion of parallelisms that can occur between inner and outer events, Jung also included the following phenomena: (1) clairvoyance—"seeing" or becoming aware of something that is out of range of the five senses and is later verified; (2) precognition—gaining knowledge about something that is going to happen in the future that eventually comes to pass; and (3) telepathy— communicating with another mind or minds without use of visual, tactile, or auditory sensory inputs. The debate continues about the overlap between these psi phenomena and synchronicity (see Mansfield, 1997; Storm, 1999). Psi phenomena may be providing information in an anomalous way outside of the other usual methods that extend the reach of our senses, such as telephone calls, email, text messaging, books, and other media (Mayer, 2007). Because psi and the more narrow definition of synchronicity share some common features, we include psi events in this discussion.

To simplify the words used here, we propose that a synchronistic event be called a "synchron," and that the person experiencing a synchron be called a "synchroner."

We offer the following criteria for defining a synchron:

1. *Low probability/simultaneous.* Low probability occurrence of two or more events usually (but not always) within a narrow time frame that cannot be explained by commonly accepted causes. The narrow

"window of time" often makes the occurrence of the two events seem improbable and therefore significance-generating. The lower the probability of the co-occurrence of the events, the more significant the coincidence will seem.

2. *Thought-environment connection.* The co-occurrence of events usually involves thought or image and an environmental event. The co-occurrence may also involve mental events between two or more people or between two or more environmental events.

3. *Similarity.* The co-occurring events are, in some way, similar; their underlying patterns seem parallel.

4. *Emotional intensity.* The low probability stirs an emotional response in the synchroner. The stronger the emotion, the greater the motivation to find meaning.

5. *Acausal meaning.* The meaning is not explained by known principals of cause and effect, thereby requiring subjective analysis to understand as opposed to causally related coincidences, like thunder accompanying lightening, which are readily explained.

Synchronicity Theories

As reflected in our criteria above, Jung characterized synchronicity as *acausal*: the coincidences were not explainable by conventional scientific and philosophical principles of cause and effect (Jung, 1973). This characterization was not intended to suggest that there were no possible causes, but rather that to understand them we must extend currently accepted scientific views. Attempts to explain synchronicity have utilized several theories, including Jung's concept of archetypes, as well as observations from quantum physics— especially "non-locality." We add the concept of "eco-mens" (mind embedded in environment). Many insist that synchrons can be best explained by the laws of probability as chance occurrences. None of these theories is yet to be a proven explanation. We are, at this point, left with accepting this limitation and to consider whether there is practical reality to meaningful coincidences, even though we may not understand why they occur. Like dreams, synchrons appear to our consciousness. Like dreams, synchrons may be considered useless byproducts of our active brains or images with varying potentials for useful commentary on our personal existence.

Cause. Causal thinking holds that an effect is preceded in time by another event: the first event causes the second. Humans learn: "If I do X, then Y will happen." Since "Y" does not always happen, we associate a high probability for the connection between X and Y. Cause then may be defined by statistical probability (Storm, 1999). The events comprising a synchron have no apparent statistical association, cannot be understood by causal associations, and therefore seem to lie outside the current conventional laws of our current ideas of reality. The speculations that are being developed to explain meaningful coincidences use complex theories to explain difficult to understand events. Where the balance lies between meaninglessness and meaningfulness is determined by the beliefs of each observer: we are either embedded in a world of symbols awaiting our recognition and use of them, or in a world that is cold, uninvolved, and empty of relationship to us. To touch upon the paradox of these polarities, consider the meanings of the word "chance" as direct reflections of this conflict. In probability contexts, *chance* implies "unlikely" as in *chance* events. In other contexts, *chance* means "opportunity" as in "give peace a chance." *Chance* can be construed as drily statistical or ripe with possibilities.

Archetypes. Within each human mind, at various levels of awareness, are patterns of psychic function that order and condition human knowledge and experience. As elements of brain function, they operate in the primarily unconscious modes that filter and organize both external and internal inputs (Viamontes & Beitman, 2007). In Greek philosophy, they were known as Platonic Ideas and Forms that give the world its shape and meaning, and, for Aristotle, they lent purpose to the processes of life. For Kant, they were the a priori categories; for Blake, mythic gods and goddesses (The Immortals); and for Freud, the primordial instincts. These universal principles impel, structure, and permeate the world of human experience (Tarnas, 2006, pp. 81–84). Summarizing Jung, Tarnas suggested that

> They seem to move from both within and without, manifesting as impulses, emotions, images, ideas and interpretive structures in the interior psyche yet also as concrete forms, events, and contexts in the world, including synchronistic phenomena. (Tarnas, p. 84)

Examples of archetypal situations include death and dying, birth, marriage, romance, war, financial ruin, sudden wealth, betrayal, losing a job, heroism, wonder, beauty, despair, isolation, sex, aggression, feminine and masculine, sickness, joy. The archetypes vary and merge with each other; they are interdependent. They are like chords in music, each standing alone yet together creating the opera of our lives.

Jung believed in a correlation between archetypes and synchronicity—that synchrons were related to the activation of archetypes. He suggested that archetypes become "constellated" or activated during powerful synchronistic events but hesitated to ascribe a causal relationship between an activated archetype and a synchron (Jung, 1973). Evidence from stories and surveys strongly indicates that the frequency of meaningful coincidences increases during birth, death, marriage, and other major life transitions. Each of these transitions is associated with an archetype (birth and rebirth; death and transfiguration), offering support to Jung's belief. How an activated archetype leads to a synchron is not clear. A practical conceptual approach for understanding the relationship between archetype and meaningful coincidence is to consider that there is a correspondence between them, rather than that they are connected through a causal chain of events. Identifying the category of activated archetype may help to clarify the meaning of the coincidence.

For example, if an emotionally powerful synchron takes place during a dramatic life event, its meaning can be understood within the context of the activated archetype. A woman on an airplane, returning to San Francisco from her widowed father's wedding to his second wife is seated next to a man returning to San Francisco after his father's funeral. They are attracted to each other. This is a remarkable coincidence of two lives. Should the major life events within which familial loss and change are so emphasized be interpreted to suggest that they proceed into exploring a relationship with each other? That exploration must, of course, take into consideration objective traits of potential compatibility. The archetypal power of death and transfiguration accelerates the movement toward exploration, and perhaps an openness to both possibilities—a coincidence with future significance, or an emotion-packed chance event to be remembered only as an interesting encounter.

Quantum Physics. The findings of quantum physics are changing philosophical and psychological views of reality. Quantum experiments demonstrate that, at least in the microworld of subatomic particles, electrons change their motion while they are under observation. Known as the Heisenberg Uncertainty Principle, physicists are teaching us that we may know only one of the two complementary characteristics of a particle. For example, when measuring the speed (or momentum) of an electron, its location becomes uncertain; when measuring its location, its speed becomes uncertain. This uncertainty results from the "interaction" of the measuring device with what is being measured. The photons of light used to determine the position of an electron "push" the electron from its course, obscuring its location or changing its speed.

In quantum physics, space and time are more elastic, and more interdependent. The concept of "now" is becoming more ambiguous, more difficult to define (Mansfield, 1995). Cause and effect are also becoming more mysterious. For example, no one can predict or control which of the many radioactive particles in a set of such particles are going to decay at a given moment. As a group they decay at a fixed rate, but no one can know when a specific particle is going to decay. Similarly, actuarial tables tell us that a certain number of people at a certain age with a certain history will die at particular time, but the data cannot tell us who will specifically die.

Uncertainty-complementarities, time-space elasticities, and the problem of causality or "acausality" all underscore that, the more we explore non-Newtonian physics, the clearer it is that we cannot rely purely on the tidy principles of cause and effect in the study of synchronicity. In quantum physics, it is *nonlocality* that seems most parallel to telepathy. If two paired electrons of opposite spin are separated, and the spin of one of them is changed, then the spin of the other is *instantaneously* changed, no matter what the distance. No energy or information can be exchanged between them because the effect takes place immediately, faster than the speed of light. The two particles seem connected—entangled, not separate. By analogy, deeply involved ("entangled") people, like twins, sometimes know at a distance when the co-twin is experiencing pain (Mann & Jaye, 2007). Perhaps telepathy works through paired bonds in a similar way. The quantum connection, however, lacks the meaningful quality that defines synchronicity. Theorizing by analogy can be a first step toward better understanding. As with archetypal reasoning, we can state with confidence that two events *correspond* with each other—particle with particle, loved one with loved one. We cannot, however, attribute causation to telepathy and synchronicity in any of the ways currently accepted by scientific convention.

Eco-mens. Meaningful coincidences are not only hot-house orchids, but also like weeds, wildflowers, and daisies. They run the full range of intensity from minor and insignificant to interesting, funny, and curious types to highly dramatic life-changing ones. More "down to earth" explanations for synchrons are required. The eco-mens idea can do just that. The word suggests that mind (mens) is embedded in environment (eco).

Our bodies are embedded in our environments. Without interaction, human babies fail to thrive, in part because stimulation helps the cortex to expand. Persons placed in sensory isolation chambers may experience strange, sometimes terrifying, journeys (Lilly, 1967). The Central Intelligence Agency (CIA) has added sensory isolation to its list of torture methods. By putting headphones over the ears, blindfolds over the eyes, and cardboard over the hands and arms of prisoners, agents can starve prisoners of stimulation, and easily make them susceptible to outside influence (CIA, 1983). To remain coherent, our sense of self requires continuing input from "outside" of us.

Scientific epistemology would have us believe that we are separate from our surroundings; and that we draw principled conclusions about external events from those observations. Quantum physics has clearly shown that, at least at the micro-atomic level, observation changes what we observe. This, along with other observations, supports the notion that ours appears to be a participatory universe, rather than simply an object-observer universe (Mansfield, 1995). For example, the Hawthorne effect shows that when humans are observed by others, their behavior changes (Mayo, 1933). Human motivation and decision making are strongly determined by the "demand characteristics of the situations." We, then, often try to fulfill these expectations. Synchronicity may indicate that we are connected to our surroundings more than we realize. A simple everyday example is when we "sense" someone is staring at us. We turn around, and there are those eyes on us. We seem to be able to perceive the connection. Sheldrake (2003) has shown that we are, indeed, sensitive to people staring at us.

Recent technological advances have further connected our minds to our surroundings. The Internet, cell phones (with text messaging), television, radio, and print media link human minds as never before. Advertisers, politicians, business leaders seek to use the variety of means available to control what each person thinks. Similarly, when one person communicates with another person, the speaker is trying to influence the response of the listener. Interpersonal behavior is characterized by unconscious attempts to induce desired roles in the other person (Beitman & Viamontes, 2007). Our minds resemble fish swimming in a sea of information sources continuously influencing what we feel and think.

Before the explosion of media inputs into each brain, prehistoric human beings lived in small groups, each of whom had a clear role in the group. Each person was important to the whole (Wilson, 1975). It is possible then to theorize that individuals took on specialized functions for the group. A few registered the group's emotional tone, being able to sense if someone was in trouble. While conventional sensory inputs could be relied upon to know when someone was missing, the "sensitives" could know if the missing person was in danger, or had died or was about to return. This reasoning is based upon frequent reports of such extraordinary knowing (Feather & Schmicker, 2005), suggesting the possibility that these abilities (such as knowing when someone important to the person is in danger, is returning, or has died) are evolutionary capabilities still within us.

Our Cartesian legacy induces us to believe that each of us is separate not only from our social environment but also from the Earth itself. Yet almost everything we see, hear, and touch comes out of the Earth: trees, cars, buildings, dogs, and human beings. Our bodies are created and maintained from ingredients like water and calcium that can only have come from the ground of our being. Our brains are Earth dependent; our minds, then, so deeply enmeshed in brain function, have at least part of their origin in the Earth. Their Earth-mind interface suggests that mind and matter, *psyche* and *terra firma*, may be more connected than we think.

Our connection with the environment sets the stage for meaning-seeking human beings to find purpose, guidance, and encouragement in the coincidences between mind and environment. Is the meaning out there somehow, implicit in the mind–environment interaction, or is it, as suggested by probability theorists, a false attribution of significance to the caprice of chance?

Probability theory. Conventional science advances through controlled experiments that test for the statistical likelihood of perceived effects happening by chance. If the probability of the difference between the experimental process and a standard process falls well below chance occurrence, then the experiment supports the hypothesis that the differences between the experimental process and the control process are "real." Statistics, then, provides a major method by which we know what is true and what is false. Since highly meaningful coincidences are often also highly personal, finding an experimental design with a standard control process appears practically impossible. (How does an experimenter control for the subjective meaning-making variable?)

Synchronicity also creates a statistical paradox: these low probability events have a high probability of occurring. The reason, well articulated by skeptical statisticians, lies with the huge number of potential coincidences available between an active human mind in ordinary environments.

> How likely is it that someone will recall a person he knew (or knew of) in the last 30 years and, within exactly five minutes, learn of that person's death? One such calculation suggests that the chance occurrence is about 0.00003. But in a population of 100,000, this means that about 10 of these experiences should occur everyday. (Schick & Vaughn, 1995, p. 55)

Statistical perspectives on synchronicity assume that ordinary people underestimate the probability of "unlikely" events. The Birthday Surprise is used to demonstrate this human "weakness." Also known as the Birthday Problem and the Birthday Paradox, it asks the following question: "In a room of 23 people, what is the probability that 2 of them will have the same birthday?" Common answers usually are quite low—1%, 5%, maybe 10%. After all there are 365 days in the year so how could two people out of 23 have the same birthday? The surprising answer is 50%.

The birthday problem asks whether any of the 23 people have a matching birthday with any of the others—not one person in particular. The probability for one person to match with any other person is much lower. If on a list of 23 persons you compare the birthday of the first person on the list to the others, you have 22 chances of success, but if you compare each and everyone to the others, you have 253 chances. This is because in a group of 23 people there are $23 \times 22/2 = 253$ pairs, which is more than half of the number of days in the year. So the chance that one of these pairs has a matching birthday is not small.

Statisticians use this example to suggest that highly meaningful coincidences are far more likely to happen than most of us think, since we seem to underestimate the probabilities of certain events.

The surprising frequency of reported synchrons may be due to the following: (1) everyday life provides numerous opportunities to find connections between events; (2) people allow themselves excessive flexibility in identifying meaningful relationships between events that have a relatively high chance of co-occurring; (3) similarly, people are willing to include near misses (Diaconis & Mosteller, 1989); and (4) people desire to consider personal experiences as somehow extraordinary (Falk & MacGregor, 1983).

When a person finds meaning in an unlikely experience, statistics cannot explain why the person finds meaning. Statistics can only suggest that the perception of "unlikely" is overestimated. Research suggests that a coincidence may be judged meaningful when perceivers sense that it violates their notions of randomness (Griffiths & Tennenbaum, 2001). This subjective sense of the violation of randomness triggers high emotion and the search for meaningfulness. Research also suggests that the meaningfulness of a seemingly low probability event is much stronger for the person experiencing the event than for those hearing the story about someone else's synchron (Falk, 1989).

Pragmatics. The scientific method usually requires the formulation of a testable theory for an observation to be considered possibly "real." When a testable theory is not easily developed, detailed description of the phenomenon may help in its development. Pragmatists argue that we use many ideas and perform many behaviors without a strongly held theory and without statistical support. We give antidepressants for depression without much knowledge of how they work and with even less knowledge about the pathophysiology of depression. Similarly, much hypertension is idiopathic, yet many different and effective medication treatments have been developed. Even less clear are the mechanisms of action of psychotherapy, yet there is good evidence that psychotherapy is helpful.

Whether or not synchrons are random chance occurrences or something more, they can be useful. As described later, synchrons may offer a sense of comforting support, interpersonal and intrapsychic insights, assistance, and guidance. Experiences of synchronicity may be able to increase the sense of being connected to others and our surroundings, as well as inspire appreciation, gratitude, and spirituality, and clarify purpose in life. As described by Coughlin (in this volume), these life-affirming forces promote health and well-being. We may not know the mechanism by which synchrons are formed, but utilizing synchronicity may help people live better lives.

Evidence for Synchronicity

Reports of stories fitting the broad definition of synchronicity number in the thousands (Adrienne, 1998; Begg, 2003; Belitz & Lundstrom, 1998; Cousineau, 1997; Eyre, 1997; Gaulden, 2003; Halberstam & Leventhal, 1997; Hay, 2006; Spangler, 1996; Watkins, 2005). Casual conversations about meaningful coincidences generate many more unreported stories (personal communication from G. Nachman, August, 2007). Does the onslaught of stories, particularly the recent surge of books and websites devoted to synchronicity, provide convincing evidence? Not for scientists. Clinicians use the anecdotes of clinical experience to collect case reports into a series that then can lead to controlled, randomized trials. Currently, we have failed to develop a satisfactory and testable theory. But first, as with any new science, we must start with description. Does the phenomenon exist? What are its many forms? What are the varieties of synchronistic experiences?

RESEARCH OVERVIEW

We review research into these anomalous events by first explicating the differences and overlaps between psi and synchronicity.

They may be differentiated by qualities of *verifiability* and *meaningfulness*. The information received through telepathy, clairvoyance, and precognition can be *verified* by external validation. The event seen or predicted through psi either happened or did not happen. Synchronicity, on the other hand, gains its relevance by rendering an ambiguous experience personally *meaningful*.

Psi and synchronicity can overlap because psi information, like information gained through our usual sensory organs, can form the basis of a synchron. For instance, knowing who is calling before picking up the phone can be considered a telepathic experience. The context within which this telepathic event is experienced can make it synchronistic. If an individual is in need of comfort, begins thinking about a long-estranged relative, and that relative calls offering comfort, then the psi information will more likely help to create meaning in this coincidence, and therefore a synchron has occurred.

A continuum of research approaches can be constructed for various degrees of meaningfulness. On the lowest end would be the study of anomalous events that have no meaning attached—the context is depersonalized. This approach characterizes pure psi research. In one paradigm for studying telepathy, a subject's task is to acknowledge receiving telepathic information from a sender in another room. The sender is staring at one of four diagrams. For each trial, the receiver picks one of the four diagrams while being open to the sender's message. There is no personal meaning for the receiver for any of the diagrams.

The difference between a "random," highly informative phone call and telepathically received clip art is the meaningfulness of the stimulus. For example, a distressed woman received a phone call from a woman she did not know. The caller had dialed the wrong number. The receiver was about to go to the airport to reunite with her abusive husband, who had recently kidnapped their children. He wanted to reconcile, again. The caller began talking about her own abusive husband and how difficult, but liberating, divorcing him had been. The receiver decided not to pick up her husband. The phone call was highly meaningful; it helped to change her mind. The information was personally relevant in a direct way. She was in a highly charged emotional state and received information that helped to redirect her. The class to which coincidence belongs could be studied through a survey by asking respondents how often "an unexpected phone call has kept me out of trouble." The degree of "trouble" will vary and could be rated on a continuum. The bigger challenge would be to design an experiment contrasting a control and experimental group for these highly personal experiences.

Where research is positioned along the continuum of meaning is reflected in a tradeoff between *experimental control* and *ecological validity*. Experimental control refers to a scientist's ability to specify a cause-and-effect relationship by eliminating extraneous variables that could potentially explain an event. Ecological validity refers to the extent to which an experiment resembles the natural context in which it is observed. Studying phenomena in both contexts is important in order to attain a comprehensive understanding of them that is, at the same time, realistic and objective. This tradeoff is especially salient in psi and synchronicity research, where natural observations of these phenomena are powerful and striking, but experimental replications can seem weak and irrelevant.

Current research falls within two methodologies: 1) surveys to assess frequencies and beliefs in synchronicity and psi; and 2) experiments attempting to replicate and validate these anomalous experiences under controlled conditions.

SURVEYS

A particular type of type of telepathic experience, anticipation of telephone calls, was assessed by survey several times by Sheldrake and colleagues (Brown

& Sheldrake, 2001; Sheldrake, 2000). This collection of surveys included informal means (e.g., by raised hand at conferences), and with randomized large-scale samples (in London and Bury, England, and Santa Cruz, California). Several questions were asked of respondents, for instance, *Have you ever had a thought about a person you haven't seen for a while, who has then telephoned you the same day?* and *Have you ever felt that someone was going to telephone you just before they did, and you had no reason to expect that person to call?* These researchers found that within large samples (200, 387, and 200, respectively), individuals experienced telephone "telepathy" in high frequencies. For instance, 80%–95% of individuals assessed informally at conferences had experienced telephone synchrons. In the formal survey (from the three locations), the researchers found between 47% and 78% individuals in the samples had experienced telephone telepathies, with the variable results found in questions tapping specific aspects (e.g., knowing who is calling before picking up the phone, having someone say they were just thinking about you when you call), as well as from the different locations. There was no assessment of the "meaning" for these coincidences. There was also no assessment of what percentage of calls received over a person's lifetime had this associated synchronicity; hence, there was no way of knowing how likely it was that the occasional correct guessing/sensing was due to chance.

Many people experience bodily sensations that coincide with the bodily sensations of significant others who are in a different location. These experiences may be called "telesomatic," from *tele* (at a distance) and *soma* (body), and are likely to generate greater emotion and meaning than telephone telepathy. Mann and Jaye (2007) interviewed twenty adult twins in depth about their illness experiences. The researchers built their research on the clinical findings of Schwartz (1967; 1973), suggesting that many people experience the pain of a loved one, both simultaneously and at a distance from each other. The twins reported that the illness or injury of one twin was commonly experienced by the other (Mann & Jaye, 2007). The 20 participants reported over 50 telesomatic experiences: four were in relationship to accidents, five to surgeries, nine to various aspects of pregnancy, and nine to intense emotional states—anxiety, dread, or depressed mood. The twins took these coincidences to mean that they were more connected and less separate than other pairs of people.

Henry (1993) surveyed the coincidence experiences among readers of *The Observer* (London). Nine hundred and ninety people responded to a survey appearing alongside a newspaper article on coincidence. From the sample, the vast majority (84%) reported experiencing meaningful coincidences. Large numbers (above 60%) of respondents reported coincidences such as *spontaneous association*, through which an internal thought (such as a name) is manifested externally (such as on the radio) and *small-world encounters*, which refer to meeting someone connected to one's past in improbable circumstances. Participants reported that these experiences were personally meaningful, significant, and useful, and offered "intuition," "psi," and "chance" as explanations for their occurrence. This data must be considered within the context of a self-selected population, which adds considerable bias to the results. Moreover, the survey appeared with an article on coincidence, which meant most respondents probably came from a subset of the population who were already interested in the topic. Thus, the Henry results, although interesting, cannot be taken to reflect the general population.

The frequency of meaningful chance encounters has been explored within the career counseling literature. Several studies have incorporated questions regarding the frequencies of these chance experiences and their relative impact on career choices. For instance, Meyer's (1989) synchronicity survey noted that significant life-changing events tended to cluster around employment situations. A survey conducted by Betsworth and Hansen (1996) revealed a clear majority (60%) of the sample reporting a serendipitous event in their career development. Furthermore, Bright, Pryor, and Harpham (2005) found that 74% of their respondents had been influenced by a chance event in their career development. Participants reported an average of 7.7 chance events influencing their career paths.

An unpublished dissertation conducted by Meyer (1989) investigated relationships between personality variables and synchronistic experiences. A total of 88 undergraduate students took part in the study, which included several personality instruments as well as a nine-item synchronicity index. Commonly reported specific experiences were: saying what someone else is thinking (or vice versa), thinking of a song and hearing it on the radio, and thinking of a friend who then contacts you. Furthermore, approximately one-quarter of the sample reported that they experienced a life-changing coincidence. These experiences clustered around life challenges (e.g., life-threatening situations), death of others, employment problems, and relationship difficulties.

The tendency to find meaning in ambiguity is likely to be normally distributed, but has not been studied systematically. Some people seem to live their lives through following perceived meaningful coincidences, while others pay them little attention. Of those who pay the most attention, some are likely to use them successfully, while others may create meanings that distort their decision making (Brugger, 2001).

Psi abilities have been studied more systematically. Some people score much higher than others in psi testing (see Parker & Brusewitz, 2003, for specific psi studies with such individuals). Neither age nor gender seems to correlate with special abilities, although extraversion (the tendency to be gregarious and outgoing) appears to increase the probability of psi reports. Believing in the possibility of telepathy, clairvoyance, and precognition also appears to increase the likelihood of reporting them (Rhine-Feather & Schmicker, 2005, pp. 20–21).

High emotionality and/or familiarity between sender and receiver seem to increase the probability of telepathic communication, as suggested by Sheldrake's telephone telepathy study of sisters (Sheldrake & Smart, 2003a, b), and the telesomatic studies of twins reported above (Mann & Jaye, 2007). As discussed in the following section, participants who scored highest in the *Weird Coincidence Survey* described themselves as more religious and more spiritual than those who scored lowest.

CONTROLLED RESEARCH

A preponderance of statistical evidence lends some credibility to the notion that psi abilities exist and can be replicated under controlled conditions. Radin (2006) reported on many of these studies. One of the most popular methods for studying the psi phenomenon (and telepathy specifically) is the "ganzfeld" procedure. This procedure is said to mimic the natural occurrence of psi (reportedly found in a meditation-like state) and to reduce the interference of external sensory "noise" from information transfer (Bem, 1994). In these studies, a receiver is isolated in a room, wears halved ping-pong balls over the eyes, and is stimulated by red light. He or she also wears headphones carrying white noise. The participant may also undergo progressive muscle relaxation to reduce internal somatic noise. A sender, separated from the receiver, concentrates on a visual stimulus that is randomly selected from a large pool of images. At the same time, the receiver continuously describes his or her mental imagery. The receiver is given several visual stimuli and asked to rate the degree to which each image matches his or her mental image. If the receiver's highest-ranked image is the image being "sent," it is called a "hit." The random chance for the receiver to pick the "sent" image is one of four or 25%.

This particular method of studying telepathy has gained favor with both researchers and skeptics over the years. Based on a meta-analysis which combines results across studies, researchers have found statistically significant effects. Across 88 studies with 3,145 trials, Radin (2006) describes a combined hit rate of 32% (compared to the chance rate of 25 or $p < .000000000001$).

As noted in the survey section, a common synchronistic experience is knowing who is calling before picking up the phone. Sheldrake and his colleagues (2003a) attempted to replicate the survey findings under controlled conditions, but in more ecologically valid contexts than traditional telepathic research. A target individual was asked to generate a list of four friends. At a given time, the experimenters would contact one of the four callers (chosen randomly) and ask that person to call the target subject. The subject would predict who was calling by the first ring and an accuracy rate was calculated. By chance alone, the subject should be able to correctly predict 25% of the phone calls. Using this procedure, Sheldrake found success rates significantly higher than chance (usually around 40%). Furthermore, these studies have revealed much higher accuracy rates for familiar rather than unfamiliar callers, and found that distance had little impact on the accuracy rates of the target individual. These elevated success rates could be partially explained by the high degree of emotional closeness between callers, presumably facilitating a telepathic connection. Similar results were found with the more rigorous stipulations (Sheldrake & Smart, 2003b). The researcher found similar results using emails rather than telephone calls (Sheldrake & Smart, 2005).

Braud (1983) examined *sequential synchronicity* in several case examples using himself as the subject. By identifying words with "special feeling" or "anomalous attention" attached to them, he recorded these instances, as well as instances of a control word for 24 hours. Ten instances of synchronicity were found, and the synchronistic instances were found sooner than the control. Another study had Braud searching for key and control words in a newspaper. The meaningful coincidence hypothesis was again confirmed. Braud suggests that these very preliminary methods for investigating serial meaningful coincidences may be further developed. The crudeness of these studies illustrates the need for far better experimental designs.

Another study examined the synchronistic experience of obtaining unexpected money. Landon (2001) attempted to test how "paying attention" to the possibility of receiving unexpected money during the discrete time period of the study influenced the actual incidence of such experiences. In an effort to integrate the spirit of psi experimentation as it relates to archetypes and the synchronicity principle, this ecologically based study chose money (a universally meaningful "substance") as the dependent variable and sought to determine: (1) if the participants would experience more events related to money within the "field" of the experiment than they had in the month previously; and (2) if different methods for paying attention had any effect on the quantity or number of times money was received.

Her 60 participants were split into three groups during an experimental period of 4 weeks. The control group was asked just to pay attention to unexpected money; the two experimental groups were asked to alter their behavior (by lighting a candle and focusing attention, or focusing attention in their own way). Results were compared to pre-test incidences of receiving unexpected money (money that came surprisingly and suddenly).

Several findings are noteworthy: (1) by simply enrolling in the study, participants generally reported receiving unexpected money nearly twice the number of times during the entire study period than they had the month before; (2) those who initially reported high expectations for such results also reported a significantly higher incidence of receiving unexpected money; (3) highly focused concentration generally produced a lower frequency of receiving money than the control group.

Additional studies that systematically manipulate the experiences of individuals to create synchronicities would be useful, especially in regard to clarifying the role of attention and expectation in reported experiences (see Falk, 1989).

MISSOURI WEIRD COINCIDENCE SURVEY

A survey was conducted in 2007 by Beitman and colleagues to identify the frequency of synchronistic experiences in a university population of students, faculty, and staff. An initial item pool of 53 items was constructed from expert ratings, prototypes from other scales (e.g., Belitz & Lundstrom, 1997*; Meyer, 1989), and exemplars of common synchronistic experiences found in stories of synchronicity. These frequency-related items (47 total) were combined with items asking about how respondents analyzed and interpreted the items (6 total), as well as items selected from The Brief Multidimensional Measure of Religiousness/Spirituality(BMMRS) designed for use in health research (Fetzer Group/National Institute on Aging Working Group, 1999). Also included was a simple continuum scale asking for self-rankings of "religious" and "spiritual." These two scales and the BMMRS were included with the hypothesis that those who scored higher on the synchronicity scales would score higher on measures of spirituality and religion. Participants were also asked to provide personal examples of synchronistic experiences. After refinement of the synchronicity experience items through factor analysis, participants in Sample 2 were presented with 36 core synchronicity items, 6 analysis/interpretation items, as well as the other scales measuring strength of religious and spiritual beliefs.

Participants were affiliated with the University of Missouri and were recruited through a mass email announcement sent in a weekly newsletter to members of the university community. Participants were informed that there would be a random drawing from the participant pool for a total of 20 prizes of $20 each. The survey was introduced with the following story:

Kelly is a 28-year-old female member of Alcoholics Anonymous. She was struggling with a great deal of anger and resentment focused on

* We thank Meg Lundstrom for permission to use some of the items in their scale.

her father, an active alcoholic whom she has been with from the age of 10. She described their relationship as one of emotional turmoil and "dysfunctional."

One day, as she was reading the text, *Alcoholics Anonymous,* she came across a passage that described alcoholics as sick people and how we would not treat a cancer patient or someone suffering from another serious medical illness with disdain and resentment. She suddenly had this "revelation" about her father and felt the anger and resentment melt into empathy and concern. She realized how he was suffering and ill from his alcoholism just as she had been suffering from the same illness: "I felt like all those feelings that I carried around my dad were gone. I guess I see this now as God removing my resentments." She suddenly "felt a sense of peace."

As she pondered these new feelings and perceptions her cell phone rang; it was her father calling. The two had been so alienated that she didn't even think he knew her phone number. Surprisingly, he confessed to her how important she had been in his life, how sorry he was, how he cared about her and would do anything to help her. He wept as he spoke

Table 18.1. Weird Coincidence Survey.

Demographic Information	Sample 1*	Sample 2*
Males	19.5%	17%
Females	80.5%	83%
White	90.8%	88.9%
African American	1.9%	1.5%
Asian	2.5%	3.1%
Hispanic/Latino	1.6%	1.2%
Biracial/Multiracial	2.5%	3.7%
Native American	<1%	1.5%
Protestant Christian	33.2%	38.5%
Agnostic/Atheist	19.3%	19.4%
Roman Catholic	16.9%	19.7%
Some college	50.8%	46.8%
Bachelor's/4-year degree	23%	28%
Grad/Professional degree	22%	20.6%

*Of those who reported demographic information

openly about their troubled relationship. Kelly later told the interviewer that the coincidence of her father calling just at the moment when her heart was opening up struck her as "amazing." (Cameron, 2004)

Two data collections were conducted. A total of 760 people from both studies with a mean age of about 28.5 participated in them. Other demographic information from the samples is presented in Table 18.1.

Table 18.2 contains the highest scoring items including (1) thinking of someone and having that person call you; (2) analyzing the meaning of synchronicity; (3) knowing who is calling before picking up the phone; and (4) thinking of a song and then hearing it on the radio. These rankings make sense, given the high base rate of these events: receiving phone calls and hearing songs on the

Table 18.2. Weird Coincidence Survey: Highest Scored Items.

Item	Never	Seldom	Occasionally	Often	Very Frequently
I think of calling someone, only to have that person unexpectedly call me. ($n = 681, M = 3.16$)	5.3%	21.0%	37.4%	25.1%	11.2%
After experiencing meaningful coincidence, I analyze the meaning of that experience. ($n = 680, M = 3.07$)	14.5%	20.7%	26.1%	20.4%	18.1%
When my phone rings, I know who is calling (without checking the cell phone screen or using personalized ring tones). ($n = 681, M = 3.03$)	10.3%	22.0%	31.9%	26.1%	9.7%
I think about a song and then hear it on the radio. ($n = 680, M = 2.96$)	10.9%	24.1%	34.7%	18.8%	11.5%
I run into a friend in an out-of-the-way place. ($n = 681, M = 2.85$)	7.0%	28.3%	41.3%	18.8%	4.6%
I am introduced to people who unexpectedly further my work/career/education. ($n = 679, M = 2.82$)	10.7%	31.9%	28.8%	21.4%	6.9%

(continued)

Table 18.2. (Continued)

Item	Never	Seldom	Occasionally	Often	Very Frequently
I think about someone and then that person unexpectedly drops by my house or office or passes me in the hall or street. ($n = 678$, $M = 2.78$)	10.4%	30.0%	37.0%	15.9%	6.3%
In attempting to reach a goal, obstacle after obstacle prevented me from continuing on a path, which I discovered later was better for me not to have taken. ($n = 681$, $M = 2.77$)	18.9%	23.9%	28.3%	18.9%	9.8%
I am late to get somewhere and find the way surprisingly open, so that I arrive just in time. ($n = 679$, $M = 2.76$)	7.8%	32.0%	40.5%	14.7%	4.7%
I advance in my work/career/education through being at the "right place at the right time." ($n = 681$, $M = 2.71$)	15.1%	32.6%	26.0%	18.8%	7.5%
I need something, and the need is met without my having to do anything. ($n = 679$, $M = 2.69$)	11.9%	32.3%	35.1%	15.9%	4.6%
When I am in a hurry, I find a parking spot right where I need it. ($n = 681$, $M = 2.65$)	13.7%	30.5%	38.0%	12.3%	5.4%
In a desperate search for information, the information amazingly shows up. ($n = 680$, $M = 2.62$)	14.0%	30.8%	36.4%	16.2%	2.5%
The same name or word has appeared several times in close proximity in different contexts. ($n = 681$, $M = 2.61$)	21.0%	28.6%	24.8%	19.4%	6.2%
I think of an idea and hear or see it on the radio, television, or Internet. ($n = 681$, $M = 2.61$)	17.3%	30.0%	32.6%	14.7%	5.4%

Notes: The highest scoring items (by means) of core synchronicity items across both surveys displayed as percentages in each ranking. $N=750$ (some items were not answered by some participants).

Table 18.3. Weird Coincidence Survey.

*Analysis/Interpretation Items**

Survey 1

Item	Strongly Disagree	2	3	Strongly Agree	N/A
I believe God speaks to us through meaningful coincidences. ($n = 335$)	18.2%	14.6%	24.8%	33.1%	9.3%
Meaningful coincidences help me grow spiritually. ($n = 334$)	15.5%	18.6%	28.4%	26.9%	10.5%
I believe fate works through meaningful coincidences. ($n = 333$)	17.1%	19.5%	29.4%	27.0%	6.9%
I feel that meaningful coincidences point to a connection between my internal and external worlds. ($n = 336$)	14.8%	21.4%	31.0%	22.3%	10.4%
I believe that human minds are interconnected. ($n = 337$)	16.3%	26.7%	31.2%	20.2%	5.6%
I believe coincidences can be explained by the laws of probability or chance. ($n = 335$)	18.2%	30.1%	23.3%	18.5%	9.9%

Survey 2 (All items: $n = 344$)

Item	Strongly Disagree	2	3	4	Strongly Agree
I believe God speaks to us through meaningful coincidences.	20.3%	12.2%	17.4%	20.6%	29.4%
I believe fate works through meaningful coincidences.	14.5%	14.8%	26.7%	25.6%	18.3%
Meaningful coincidences help me grow spiritually.	17.4%	16.3%	26.5%	19.8%	20.1%
I believe that human minds are interconnected.	12.8%	20.6%	28.2%	23.3%	15.1%
I feel that meaningful coincidences point to a connection between my internal and external worlds.	17.2%	14.8%	30.8%	23.8%	13.4%
I believe coincidences can be explained by the laws of probability or chance.	15.1%	23.3%	32.0%	18.0%	11.6%

*These results are split because the questions differed slightly between the two surveys.

radio regularly take place in daily life; their high base rate increases the probability that some of these events will coincide with an individual's thoughts. On the other hand, because they are higher frequency events *in general*, the co-occurrences are likely to trigger less emotion and a weaker drive for meaning. More surprising is the high frequency by which people analyze their synchrons.

Respondents often experienced synchronicity through unexpected meetings with others. Several of the highest frequency items included: (1) running into a friend in an out-of-the-way place; (2) experiencing an unexpected introduction that leads to the development of an opportunity; and (3) thinking of someone who unexpectedly appears.

Respondents reported that various needs were met by synchronistic experiences. These included (1) being prevented by obstacles from continuing on a less optimal path; (2) being at the right place at the right time to receive a career opportunity; (3) having a need met without having to do anything. These results suggest that synchrons can aid people in a practical way.

Table 18.3 contains ratings of various explanations for the occurrence of synchrons. Many respondents view synchrons as a means by which God communicates with them and these experiences as helping them to grow spiritually. Conversely, relatively few endorsed the statement that synchronicity is a result of probability or chance.

Based on the mean of all items of synchronistic experiences, individuals were classified into highest and lowest groups. These two groups were compared on self-ratings as being religious and spiritual. High scorers ranked themselves as more religious and more spiritual than low scorers. This difference was statistically significant.[1]

In summary, the *Weird Coincidence Survey* suggests that meaningful coincidences occur commonly in many people's lives, that they are often analyzed, can be useful, and are likely to be associated with spirituality. Interpretations vary. In the next section we discuss principles to consider when analyzing synchrons.

Interpreting Synchrons

The available data suggest that people commonly analyze their synchrons for personal meaning. Jung and others have felt that doing so can be clinically useful by facilitating introspection, insight, and behavior change (Hopke, 1997). In this context, the usefulness of a synchron may emerge from the emotional drive ignited by observation of an external cue. On the other hand, coincidences can

---

[1] For self ranking for religiosity: $t(60) = -3.76, p < .001$; for self-ranking for spirituality: $t(60) = -6.45, p < .001$

be used to empower paranoid ideation, ideas of reference, and magical thinking. Hence, if there is potential value in analyzing synchrons, it would be for
those who have the capacity to objectively observe life events and consider carefully the relationship between external and internal events. Some people mis-
use synchrons in problematic ways: for example, "the fire began when I started
to become angry," and "the boss's new secretary has the same birthday as my
mother so that means I'm going to get promoted." They are misinterpreting the
relationship between their thoughts and external observations. The following
example illustrates the difficulty in interpreting emotionally powerful coincidences during romance:

> I really loved him, like no one else I have ever loved. We seemed to be able
> to communicate telepathically without being in the same room. When he
> was in the same building, I could feel his presence. I melted into his arms.
> His mother's name was the same as my sister's. His father's name was the
> same as my brother's. I could tell how he was feeling when we were apart.
> I told him these things because they seemed like evidence that our love
> was meant to be, that WE should last for all time. After about two years,
> our relationship was over. The coincidences were meaningful only for the
> time we were together. They did not mean forever.

Being in love seems to breed synchrons, but their meaning can be overly interpreted by a lover. The timeless quality of these synchrons encouraged this
woman to believe that the love she was feeling stretched into eternity. Her lover
acted differently. The interpretation of high impact synchrons must include
the forces of ordinary reality. Do they both care about each other? Can they
actually live together?

Consider the following synchron and its interpretation:

> A 32-year-old man living in Boston had driven his car around that con-
> fusing city without incident for 4 years. No accidents, no break-ins. He
> considered himself lucky when he thought about it. He also had a few
> dates, but finally he was going to a restaurant in a busy part of the city with
> a woman he had met at the gym. He was excited. As he walked out of the
> restaurant back to his car (she had come in her own car), he noticed that
> his car door was wide open. He looked inside and found that his prized
> CD player had been stolen. Shaken by the break-in, he interpreted this
> coincidence as indicating he should stay away from this woman.

Did the meaning he ascribed to the event fit his need to disengage from the
relationship? Did the break-in allow him to "break into" subtle information

about this woman, information which told him to avoid her at all costs, information he kept out of his awareness because he was excited about the prospect of having a girlfriend? Or was he primarily displacing his ambivalent feelings about getting involved onto this ambiguous set of symbols? In other words, was his interpretation of this external event triggering the eruption of some ideas and feelings he was denying, or was he using the emotional charge to support his fear of being involved with any woman? Hence, the interpretation of the synchron is not about its "correctness," but rather provides an opportunity to consider, appraise, and challenge the emotional content of the event elicited by the event.

MEANING

As with other potentially significant events, some meanings feel quite clear, and some do not. A person about whom you care touches your hand when you are feeling miserable. This touch is meaningful—"I am cared about." However, a touch on the knee by an acquaintance of the opposite sex under neutral circumstances may have more ambiguous meaning—"Are there sexual implications here?" Being called abruptly into your boss's office may trigger thoughts of anxious implications, even though there is little reason to believe so. In ambiguous circumstances, where the meaning is unclear, we tend to look for a pattern, an organized explanation, to reduce our anxiety. Human beings seem driven to find patterns in the apparent chaos around us (Brugger, 2001).

The specific meaning of a synchron is usually to be found in the mind of the synchroner, just as the potential meanings of dream symbols arise from the subjective experiences of the dreamer. Meaning and emotion are closely connected. Complex synchrons may be characterized by feelings of awe, wonder, amazement, and gratitude. These events contain more than information: they can touch the heart and nourish the spirit. They may provide the synchroner with a sense of contact with something greater, a sense of being guided by a vast intelligence or higher power. Synchrons are sometimes interpreted as a way that God speaks nonverbally to human beings (e.g., Gaulden, 2003). Strong emotions, however, can be associated with distorted meanings, like the sense of being extraordinarily special; that is, "the Universe speaks directly to me because I am very different from other people." However, many others react in quite opposite manner: they believe that seeing meaning in coincidences suggests that they are psychotic, and try to hide their embarrassment by telling no one about these experiences.

PATTERN RECOGNITION AND CREATION

The brain seeks patterns in the vast rush of stimuli reaching it. Furthermore, human brains seem to reward themselves when they find coherence in chaos. (Notice the small sense of reward when you recognize something.) Pattern recognition precedes logic (Edelman, 2006, p. 64) both in evolution and in individual development, because we may need to react before we have had a chance to rationally assess a situation. This pattern-seeking tendency can cause the brain to find patterns that do not exist. The finding of patterns in random data accompanied by a "specific experience of an abnormal meaningfulness" has been called *apophenia* (Konrad, 1958) and characterizes some psychotic people (Brugger, 2001), as well as relatively normal ones.

Meaning is strongly influenced by personal beliefs. People tend to seek evidence to support their strongly held beliefs. They also tend to reject information that contradicts their cherished ones (Nickerson, 1998). For example, those who believe that synchrons may be useful will be more likely to find them useful than those who do not believe they may be useful. Believers will see more synchrons than those who do not believe in their usefulness. Skeptics will cry "apophenia," while spiritual people will claim proof for interconnectedness.

Some psychotic people believe that they can predict the future and read other people's minds, and may see many connections between their external and internal worlds (e.g., people on television are talking to me). Helping psychiatric patients make the distinction between helpful considerations of synchrons and distorted thinking can be quite useful, since they may believe that their synchronicity experiences are part of their psychiatric illness.

A 33-year-old photographer enjoyed finding similarities in apparently dissimilar or unrelated forms and events. His mind sometimes caught significance in coincidences and used the coincidences to inform the way he organized his photo shoots. Sometimes they helped him to title the shoots. He hesitatingly told his psychiatrist about them. His psychiatrist labeled them "synchrons," letting the patient know that these were the subject of study by many people. The patient felt relieved to know that he was not the only one to have such experiences.

Social context influences the frequency with which people recognize and use synchronicity. Religious groups that believe their deity speaks to them through synchrons will encourage their members to watch for and report them to help solidify their religious beliefs. On the other hand, members of agnostic-skeptical groups will carefully avoid observing and discussing synchrons except as potential objects of derision.

Base rates

Base rates refer to the probability that a particular event or class of events will take place. For example, telephone calls from familiar people have high base rates. Each of us receives phone calls, primarily from people we know. Thinking of a person and having that person call is not so surprising since that person calls sometimes. But thinking of someone about whom you have not thought about for many months or years is a lower probability event. Probabilities correlate with emotion—the lower the probability the stronger the emotion is likely to be. Low base rate events rarely occur. They are more improbable. When they do occur, they are more likely to generate higher intensity emotion. For instance, the experience of feeling inexplicable physical pain while a loved one in a far-away place is suffering starts with a low base rate/ low probability event—the suffering of a loved one. To feel any intense pain is also usually associated with a low base rate. There is then even a lower probability that the two experiences will occur simultaneously; consequently, the discovery of such a co-occurrence is often experienced as a powerful emotion-provoking event. There appears to be a principle here: *the lower the base rate of one or both events as well as the likelihood of their co-occurence, the higher the improbability and the greater the emotional response.*

Factors Influencing Interpretations of Synchrons

Using synchrons effectively begins with recognizing the primacy of subjective experience. For example, a 25-year-old man walks down the street in front of four people. Each person has a different reaction to him: (1) curiosity: he looks like my son; (2) attraction: I'd like to go out with him; (3) criticism: his clothes don't fit him; (4) suspicion: he looks like he is up to no good. Like this ambiguous event, synchrons vary in their potential interpretations. An outside viewer cannot know, until told, the subject's emotional/ psychological reaction. The final judge of meaning lies with the synchroner, because the conjunction of events involve that person's concurrent inner experiences.

Using Synchronicity during Psychotherapy

Jung and his followers have employed synchronicity in their therapeutic work for much of the twentieth century. As described above, Jung's paradigmatic scarab appeared on the window of the consulting room just as his psychotherapeutically blocked patient was describing her dream of the scarab. The event startled the woman into considering Jung's ideas about her difficulties (Jung, 1973). This "provocation by the unexpected" provides one of many means by which to use synchronicity during psychotherapy. Following is another resistance-melting psychotherapy synchron:

> Money was an important but unspoken issue. One month, the patient wrote 15 or 20 checks including one to her psychiatrist. Only the psychiatrist's check bounced! The patient began the next session with: "I didn't want to talk about money, but I guess I'm going to have to." Psychotherapy infuriated her because she had trouble spending money on herself, especially for psychotherapy. The chance occurrence of the bounced check made this subject unavoidable. (Bolen, 1979, p. 28)

Potential Value of Synchrons in Psychotherapy

Including discussions of synchronicity in psychotherapy can have several benefits. They may

- Reassure patients that it is okay to contemplate the personal meanings of coincidences.
- Strengthen the working alliance, because the therapist is receptive to something that is personally meaningful to the patient.
- Help some patients feel more connected to other people and their surroundings, which can engender feelings of gratitude and spirituality (Marlo and Kline, 1998, p. 22).
- Encourage patients to continue to examine subjective experiences.
- Help to negotiate life choices.
- Provide opportunities for introspection and reflection for the psychiatrist (Bolen, 1979).

Strengthen the Working Alliance

The therapist's knowledge of synchronicity can be helpful to patients in several ways. An unknown subset of patients report frequent synchrons. They come to treatment for the usual reasons, but hidden within their personal stories is the fear that synchron awareness further indicates that they are "crazy." The Weird Coincidence Survey and the many anecdotes describing similar variations on major themes can assist therapists in reassuring patients that they are indeed not crazy, and that these types of coincidental events are commonly reported. Of course, this applies for patients who have intact reality testing.

The following example shows how recognition by a psychiatrist of seeking synchrons as within normal limits can provide support and relief to some patients.

> A 37 year-old-woman with bipolar disorder reported several synchronicity experiences while not manic, including hearing a song on the radio after she began thinking about it many years after last hearing or thinking about it or the singer. The reassurance that these were experiences reported by "normals" helped to reduce her anxiety about being crazy. Like the many reassurances psychiatrists can offer to people who are afraid of being psychotic, the normalizing of synchrons increases patients' self-confidence as well as trust in the expertise of the psychiatrist.

Synchronicity experiences cut across all human social classes, professional classes, and cultures (Peat, 1987). A paralleling between patient and therapist makes the basic humanity of both patient and therapist even more evident:

> The patient is a married man who presents for treatment of depression related to his daughter's serious medical illness. In initial consultation with the patient, it becomes clear that the patient and therapist share similar histories.
>
> 1. The therapist and the patient are of the same age.
> 2. They have been married for the same length of time.
> 3. They have daughters born within 1 month of one another.
> 4. Both the therapist's and the patient's daughters were born with severe congenital defects that were life-threatening.

The patient is very worried about his daughter's long-term prognosis, and is struggling with making complicated medical decisions. The therapist is faced with similar decisions. As the therapist hears the story, she starts to cry. She reveals to the patient the remarkable coincidences in their children. The patient is moved by the therapist's disclosure. He holds the therapist in very high esteem, as he understands that the therapist is not only an expert in this area, but also knows a considerable amount of his experience from her own.

Symbols to Be Understood

Some synchrons seem like poetry or dreams—symbols to be interpreted and used. The "bird-man" case described next provides an illustration:

The patient wanted to be a bird. The therapist elaborated on the wish by commenting on the patient's desire for a strong mother bird to nourish him. The following session, the patient walked to the office window, and, for the first time in therapy, noticed a baby bird in a nest that had been perched in an adjacent window for several weeks. At that moment, the mother bird flew to the nest to give the baby bird a worm. This synchron had a poignancy which permitted the patient to more freely discuss his needs for nurturance. (Marlo and Kline, pp. 16–17)

Patients may report odd events in their lives, including synchrons that puzzle them. As with dreams and striking interpersonal encounters, patients call upon therapists to help them to decipher the meaning of these symbols.

The 22-year-old patient reported that she had begun dating a man the same age as her father, who was born on the same day in the same year as her father. They were talking about living together. What did the therapist think of this strange coincidence of birthdates? The patient believed that this coincidence meant the relationship was destined to be. One possible response by the therapist is to suggest that this coincidence might be a warning to the patient about not creating a father–daughter relationship with her new boyfriend. (Hopke, 1997)

The following case illustrates how events outside the office could be used to reflect what is going on in the office.

Her therapist was about to go on vacation, and the patient did not want to see him go. For the first time in many years, as she attempted to keep her appointment, her car engine started and then sputtered and died, sputtered, then died, several times. Finally, she got the car going—only to arrive 10 minutes late. As she apologized and began describing why she was late, she and her therapist began laughing. The "stop-start" car mirrored her feelings about the therapist's leaving (Keutzer, 1989)

The patient in the following case often recognized meaningful coincidences. When the following event took place, he quickly reported it to his therapist. The synchron for this patient was used to finally confront the grief of losing his wife.

I went to the grocery store last week. I get melancholy when I go there because I remember my deceased wife: that was one of our favorite things to do. I was standing in the shampoo aisle remembering being with her there. I have not let her go. I have not mourned my loss of her. I suddenly hear the sound of the Rolling Stones coming from somewhere. Not from the store speakers but from my pocket! My phone has to go through three steps before music plays. The key lock was on, which meant the phone could not be activated without me opening the phone which I had not done. It was the song "Mona," which I have many times told friends that this song told the way I feel about her.

I recognized it as synchronicity. It was the Stones song about her. The coincidence meant that I was truly in touch with my feelings, because I could feel again the wonderful times I had with her in the store, and I could also feel my sad feelings in a pure form. The synchronicity helped give my life more meaning—the external environment validated what I was feeling. I feel more confident now to mourn the loss of my wife.

The freedom to tell his psychiatrist about this major synchron facilitated his embarking on his long-avoided grieving of the death of his wife.

Career and Personal Guidance

The planned happenstance notions of career counseling have a distinct place within psychotherapy. By expecting the unexpected, patients may learn to seize opportunities for which they had not planned. Only 15% of the outcome variance in psychotherapy can be ascribed to techniques themselves, with a full 40% being due to variables outside the therapist's office. (The other percentages are 15% for common factors and 30% for the working alliance—Lambert, 2003.) Synchronicities can be one of many extra-therapeutic variables that influence a patient's life choices. Therapist support for examining the thoughts and feelings that the weird coincidences elicit can be useful to patients.

> For months, I've been "searching" for a job, though I never felt motivated to do actual searching. I had a strong irrational pull to go to my ex-girlfriend's wedding. Through various complications, we left town late and missed the ceremony, to arrive in time for the reception. When we entered the room, everyone was already seated, and I saw an open seat next to my advisor, the only person I knew there. During dinner, I mentioned my problems with employment, and he mentioned a research position that had just opened up and who I could contact to get the job. This opening then lead to me being able to get into grad school against the odds, and to further my education from a position where it would otherwise have been impossible.

Patient's Problems Parallel the Therapist's Problems

Jungian therapists have observed that the therapist's problems often walk into their office. Some eagerly anticipate the next new patient to see what message to the therapist might be delivered (Bolen, 1979). Skeptics can argue probabilities based upon the limited number of problems human beings experience. Those therapists who overly interpret patient–therapist synchrons may find too many matches and lose objectivity. Nevertheless, the stories abound of connections between the psyches of the therapist and the patient.

> The 53-year-old psychiatrist had come through a very rocky time with his wife. They had almost separated and divorced. The patient, whom he had seen for many years, was about the same age as his wife. Their names resembled each other: Maria and Mary. Their problems with their husbands seemed somewhat similar over the years. The patient's husband, like the therapist, appeared too caught up in work—"I gave at the office and have nothing to give at home," the therapist would often say. But his wife persisted. And there was something else going on. The patient tearfully told the therapist about the death of her mother—how her husband had not come to support her in the hospital, how he had left the next day on a skiing trip with his buddies. She had spent the day after her mother's death alone. The therapist heard the patient say, "He just does not get it," the very same phrase his own wife had been using to get his attention. He had done almost the same thing to his own wife—abandoned her the day after major surgery to go on a business trip. How glad he was to have made the transition to "getting it"! He could now better help the patient in her

struggle with her husband. From his patient, he also understood more deeply how he had neglected—and harmed—his wife.

The parallels do not even have to be as profoundly emotional. Sometimes they can take a simple, pragmatic turn:

> A psychiatrist had twisted her ankle. Her orthopedic surgeon put a light cast on her ankle and said it would be OK. Several months later, it was not OK. A tennis friend suggested that the psychiatrist go to a physical therapist named Bart for rehabilitation. The therapist thought to herself that, because her tennis friend was 10 years older, her solution would not apply to herself. Shortly afterward, a patient of hers walked into her office, who had recovered from a sprained ankle. The patient was wearing the same tennis shoes that the therapist had worn when she twisted her ankle. "Well, hello" said the therapist to herself. She then asked the patient to whom she had gone for physical therapy. "To Bart," was the reply! The therapist got the message, went to Bart and soon her ankle was healing.

Some patients are avid observers of synchronistic events. Can therapy be tuned to utilize this personal characteristic? Writers about synchronicity in the popular press have reported that many people seem to live their lives through synchronicity guidance. These reports suggest high degrees of emotional and spiritual satisfaction (Anderson, 1999). Should some of our patients who are highly tuned synchroners be encouraged to rely on this form of guidance increasingly in their lives? More research is required.

If the observations of this chapter can be more fully supported by other researchers, then we can place more confidence in "expecting the unexpected," in believing in the promise of chance. Like psychotherapy, synchronicity relies upon establishing basic trust in the helper, which, in this case is completely unknown. Like psychotherapy, synchronicity can offer support, confirmation, useful information, insight, guidance, as well as some not so good or clear guidance. Attention to synchrons both within and outside of psychotherapy can, like many other subjects in therapy, provide a fulcrum around which change can be created. Developing an awareness of synchrons can increase one's sense of connectedness and spirituality. Increased levels of spirituality are associated with better health outcomes.

Limitations and Potential Problems of Using Synchrons in Psychotherapy

Like other psychotherapeutic interventions, synchronicity analysis must be applied to serve the patient's best interests. Patients with weak ego boundaries may be most likely to experience and report synchrons; they are also most likely to find some inner-outer connections that either support their grandiosity or provide evidence for plots against them. Some patients may become overly fascinated with synchrons and limit their focus on pressing interpersonal and work challenges (Keutzer, 1989). They may seek them in coincidences that deserve no analysis and elaborate excessively upon the meaning of others. An over-emphasis on leading a life guided by synchronicity may devalue personal responsibility by requiring that decisions should be inspired primarily by synchron guidance. Ideally, synchronistic events and quotidian cause-effect reality should interact with each other in the minds of patients to illuminate and expand an understanding of each. Clearly, more research and clinical experience is required to know how best to use synchronicity in psychotherapy.

Future Implications

The surveys reported here, as well as the numerous stories illustrating the basic concepts, provide a foundation for future research into frequency, categories, and contexts. Some suggested research topics and areas are contained in Table 18.4.

This future science requires the development of firm, consensually agreed, validated definitions.

Table 18.4. Possible Synchronicity Research Projects.

- *Hospice*: Anecdotal reports from Hospice nurses suggest more synchrons. Define their frequency and character in this context and begin to analyze potential meanings.

- *Psychotherapy:* Make predictions based on current issues the therapist is facing, and correlate with problems seen—a good situation for testing. Synchrons are likely to be increased because of greater access to internal states for both patient and therapist.

- *Career counseling*: Collect synchrons and prospectively analyze the value of their interpretation and effect in career trajectories.

- *High vs low synchronicity experiencers* based on various criteria: locus of control orientation, spirituality, social web (and other measures of interaction with their environments for both content and frequency)

- *Subpopulations*: professional groups (business, religious, help-professionals, physicians by specialty); demographic groups by age, gender, location, population density; religious groups along fundamentalist to liberal continuum; countries and cultures

- *Self-report instrument*: valid, reliable survey adaptable to various contexts and populations

The Weird Coincidence Survey conflates two subcategories of events that may be called synchronicity. At this writing, we see two categories of events falling within this general idea. These categories are defined by the originating source of the coincidence and the means by which to validate the information. Is the source of validation primarily the subjective evaluation of the experiencer, or is the truth of the conclusion verifiable by external observation?

By these criteria, psi (telepathy, clairvoyance, precognition) form one category: these events begin *outside* the mind of the observer, are picked up by the observer's mind, and can be externally validated.

Synchrons begin outside the mind of the observer and then trigger a memory of something similar within the mind of the observer. The connections between the events are usually ambiguous and have varying emotional charges. The ambiguity requires subjective interpretation. Validation then comes primarily from the subjective evaluation, and includes the synchron's practical application.

Also necessary for a future synchronicity science are reliable guidelines for interpreting synchrons. These guidelines need to address the difficult balance between personal, idiosyncratic, emotional, and attribution biases on the one hand, and the question whether the likelihood that certain remarkable, improbable intersections of similar events will present as objectively meaningful to third party observers.

Outside of medicine, what is the place of synchronicity in career development, management and administration, politics, religion, philosophy, anthropology, sociology, and physics? Meaningful coincidences may challenge us to re-examine the nature of reality.

REFERENCES

Adrienne, C. (1998). *The purpose of your life*. New York: Eagle Brook.

Anderson, K. (1999). *The coincidence file*. Blanford: London

Begg, D. (2003). *Synchronicity: The promise of coincidence*. Wilmette, IL: Chiron Publishers.

Beitman, B., & Yue D. (2004). *Learning psychotherapy*. New York: WW Norton.

Beitman, B. D., & Viamontes G. L. (2007). Unconscious role induction: Implications for psychotherapy. *Psychiatric Annals, 37*, 259–268.

Belitz, C., & Lundstrom, M. (1997). *The power of flow: Practical ways to transform your life with meaningful coincidence*. New York: Harmony Books.

Belitz, C., & Lundstrom, M. (1998). *The power of flow: A practical way to transform your life with meaningful coincidence*. New York: Three Rivers Press.

Bem D. J., & Honorton, C. (1994). Does psi exist? Replicable evidence for an anomalous process of information transfer. *Psychological Bulletin, 115*, 4–18.

Betsworth, D. G., & Hansen, J.-I. C. (1996). The categorization of serendipitous career development events. *Journal of Career Assessment, 4*(1), 91–98.

Bolen, J. S. (1979). The Tao of psychology: Synchronicity and the self. San Francisco, CA: Harper & Row

Braud, W. (1983). Toward the quantitative assessment of "meaningful coincidence." *Parapsychology Review, 14*, 5–10.

Brown, D. J., & Sheldrake, R. (2001). The anticipation of telephone calls: A survey in California. *Journal of Parapsychology, 65*(2), 145–156.

Bright, J. E., Pryor, R. G., & Harpham, L. (2005). The role of chance events in career decision making. *Journal of Vocational Behavior, 66*(3), 561–576.

Brugger, P. (2001). From haunted brain to haunted science. In J. Houran and R. Lange (Eds), *Hauntings and Poltergeists: Multidisciplinary Perspectives.* Jefferson, NC: McFarland, pp. 175–213.

Clark, M.W. (1996). *Synchronicity and post-structuralism.* Doctoral Dissertation. Quebec University. http://web.ncf.ca/dy656/earthpages3/cv.htm.

Cameron, M. A. (2004). *Synchronicity and spiritual development in alcoholics anonymous: A phenomenological study.* St. Louis, MO: Saint Louis University.

CIA. (1983). "Human Resource Exploitation Training Manual." Retrieved July 30, 2007, from http://www.gwu.edu/~. From http://www.neverinournames.com/showDiary.do?diaryId=1905

Coughlin, P. (2008). Facilitating emotional health and well-being. In D. Monti & B. D. Beitman (Eds.), *Integrative psychiatry.* New York: Oxford University Press.

Cousineau, P. (1997). *Soul moments.* Berkeley, CA: Conari Press.

Dannenberg, H. (2004). A poetics of coincidence in narrative fiction. *Poetics Today, 25*, 299–436.

Diaconis, P., & Mosteller, F. (1989). Methods for studying coincidences. *Journal of the American Statistical Association, 84*, 853–861.

Edelman, G. M. (2006). *Second nature: Brain science and human knowledge.* New Haven, CT: Yale University Press.

Eyre, R. (1997). *Spiritual serendipity.* New York: Simon & Schuster.

Falk, R. (1989). Judgment of coincidences: Mine versus yours. *American Journal of Psychology, 102*, 477–493.

Falk, R., & MacGregor, D. (1983). The surprisingness of coincidences. In P. Humphreys, O. Stevenson, & A. Vari, (Eds.), *Analyzing and aiding decision processes.* New York: North Hollywood, pp. 489–502.

Feather, S., & Schmicker, M. (2005). *The gift: ESP, the extraordinary experiences of ordinary people.* New York: St. Martin's Press.

Fetzer (1999). Group/National Institute on Aging Working Group.

Gaulden, A. C. (2003). *Signs and wonders.* New York: Atria Books.

Griffiths, T. L., & Tenenbaum, J. B. (2001). Randomness and coincidences: Reconciling intuition and probability theory. *Proceedings of the 23rd Annual Conference of the Cognitive Science Society*, pp. 370–375.

Halberstam, Y., & Leventhal, J. (1997). *Small miracles.* Holbrook, MA: Adams Media Corporation.

Hay, L. L. & friends, compiled and edited by Kramer, J. (2006). *The times of our lives: Extraordinary true stories of synchronicity, destiny, meaning, and purpose.* Carlsbad, CA: Hay House.

Henry, J. (1993). Coincidence experience survey. *Journal of the Society for Psychical Research, 59,* 97–108.

Hopcke, R. H. (1997). *There are no accidents.* New York: Penguin Putnam.

Jung, C. G.(1973). *Synchronicity: An acausal connecting principle.* Princeton, NJ: Princeton University Press

Kammerer, P. (1919). *Das gesetz der serie.* Stuttgart: Deutches Verlags-Anstalt.

Keutzer, C. S. (1989). Synchronicity awareness in psychotherapy. In F. S. Flach (Ed.), *Psychotherapy.* New York: WW Norton, pp. 159–169.

Konrad, C. (1958). Die beginnende Schizophrenie. Versuch einer Gestaltanalyse des Wahns. Stuttgart: Thieme.

Lambert, M. J., & Ogles, B. M. (2003). The efficacy and effectiveness of psychotherapy. In M. J. Lambert (Ed.), *Bergin and Garfield's handbook of psychotherapy and behavior change* (5th edn.). New York: Wiley, pp. 139–193.

Landon, M. K. (2001). On receiving unexpected money: A theoretical and empirical investigation of anomalous mind–matter interactions within archetypal fields. Unpublished doctoral dissertation. San Francisco: California Institute of Integral Studies.

Lilly, J. (1967). *Programming and metaprogramming the human biocomputer.* New York: Julian Press.

Main, R. (2007). *Revelations of chance.* Albany, NY: State University of New York.

Mann, B. S., & Jaye, C. (2007). "Are we one body?" Body boundaries in telesomatic experiences. *Anthropology & Medicine, 14*(2), 183–195.

Mansfield, V. (1995). *Synchronicity, science and soulmaking.* Chicago, IL: Open Court Pub.

Marlo, H., & Kline, J. S. (1998). Synchronicity and psychotherapy: Unconscious communication in the psychotherapeutic relationship. *Psychotherapy: Theory, Research, Practice, and Training, 35,* 13–22.

Mayer, L. M. (2007). *Extraordinary knowing.* New York: Bantam Books

Meyer, M. B. (1989). Role of personality and cognitive variables in the reporting of experienced meaningful coincidences or "synchronicity." Unpublished doctoral dissertation, Saybrook Institute, California.

Mayo, E. (1933). *The human problems of an industrial civilization.* New York: MacMillan.

Nickerson, R. S. (1998). Confirmation bias: A ubiquitous phenomenon in many guises. *Review of General Psychology, 2,* 175–220.

Parker, A., & Brusewitz, G. (2003). A compendium of evidence for psi. *European Journal of Parapsychology, 18,* 33–51.

Peat, D. (1987). *The bridge between matter and mind.* New York: Random House

Radin, D. (2006). *Entangled minds: Extrasensory experiences in a quantum reality.* New York: Simon and Schuster

Redfield, J., & Adrienne, C. (1995). *The celestine prophecy: An experiential guide.* New York: Warne.

Rhine-Feather, S., & Schmicker, M.(2005). *The gift.* New York: Random House

Ryback, D., & Sweitzer, L. (1988). *Dreams that come true.* New York: Ivy Books.

Schick, T. S., & Vaughn, L. (1995). *How to think about weird things.* Mountain View, CA: Mayfield.

Schwartz, B. E. (1967). Possible telesosomatic reactions. *Journal of Med Soc N J., 64*(11), 600–603.

Schwartz, B. E. (1973). Clinical studies of telesomatic reactions. *Medical Times, 10,* 171–184.

Sheldrake, R. (2000). Telepathic telephone calls: Two surveys. *Journal of the Society for Psychical Research, 64*(861), 224–232.

Sheldrake, R. (2003). *The sense of being stared at.* New York: Crown.

Sheldrake, R., & Smart, P. (2003a). Experimental tests for telephone telepathy. *Journal of the Society for Psychical Research, 67*(872), 184–199.

Sheldrake, R., & Smart, P. (2003b). Videotaped experiments on telephone telepathy. *Journal of Parapsychology, 67*(1), 147–166.

Sheldrake, R., & Smart, P. (2005). Testing for telepathy in connection with e-mails. *Perceptual and Motor Skills, 101*(3), 771–786.

Spangler, D. (1996). *Everyday miracles: The inner art of manifestation.* New York: Bantam Books.

Storm, L. (1999). Synchronicity, causality, and acausality. *Journal of Parapsychology, 63*(3), 247–269.

Tarnas, R. (2006). *Cosmos and psyche.* New York: Viking.

Viamontes, G. I.& Beitman, B.D.(2007). Mapping the unconscious in the brain. *Psychiatric Annals, 37,* 259–268.

Wampold, B. (2001) *The great psychotherapy debate.* Mahwah, N.J.: Erlbaum.

Watkins, S. M. (2005). *What a coincidence! The wow factor in synchronicity and what it means in everyday life.* Needham, MA: Moment Point Press.

Weil, A. T. (1972). *The natural mind.* Boston, MA: Houghton-Mifflin.

Wilson, E. O. (1975) *Sociobiology, the new synthesis.* Cambridge, MS: Belknap.

Appendix 1

The key to understanding this problem is to think about the chances of *no two people* sharing a birthday: what are the chances that Person 1 has a different birthday from Person 2, *and* that Person 3 has a different birthday again, *and* Person 4, etc. Each time another person is added to the room, it becomes less and less likely that their birthday is not already taken by someone else. If one has a sample space of *n* people, the first person has 365 possible birthdays to choose from. The second person would have only 364, the third would have 363, and so on. This would be compared with any person being able to have any birthday with no restrictions (in short, all people have 365 possible birthdates.)

INDEX

Note: Page numbers in *Italics* are refer to figures and tables respectively.